THIRD EDITION

Health Fitness Instructor's Handbook

Edward T. Howley, PhD
University of Tennessee at Knoxville

B. Don Franks, PhD
Louisiana State University at Baton Rouge

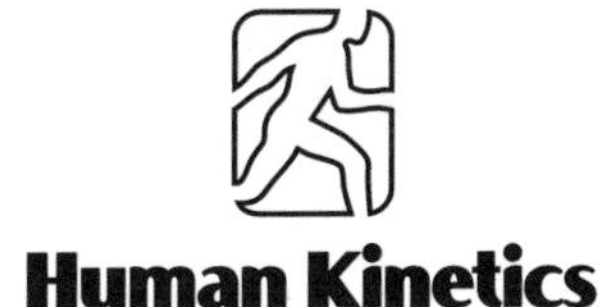

Human Kinetics

Library of Congress Cataloging-in-Publication Data

Howley, Edward T., 1943-
Health fitness instructor's handbook / Edward T. Howley, B. Don Franks. -- 3rd ed.
p. cm.
Includes bibliographical references (p.) and index.
ISBN 0-87322-958-4 (alk. paper)
1. Physical fitness--Handbooks, manuals, etc. 2. Physical fitness--Testing--Handbooks, manuals, etc. 3. Exercise--Physiological aspects--Handbooks, manuals, etc. 4. Health. I. Franks, B. Don. II. Title.
GV481.H734 1997 96-53061
CIP

ISBN: 0-87322-958-4

Acquisitions Editors: Rick Frey, PhD and Scott Wikgren; **Developmental Editor**: Holly Gilly; **Assistant Editors**: Chad Johnson and Rebecca Crist; **Editorial Assistant**: Amy Carnes; **Copyeditor**: Amie Bell; **Proofreader**: Erin Cler; **Indexer**: Joan Griffitts; **Graphic Designer**: Judy Henderson; **Graphic Artists**: Sandra Meier and Julie Overholt; **Photo Manager**: Boyd LaFoon; **Cover Designer**: Jack Davis; **Photographer (cover)**: Will Zehr; **Illustrators**: Gretchen Walters, M.R. Greenberg, and Keith Blomberg; **Printer**: Edwards

Printed in the United States of America 15 14 13 12

Human Kinetics
Web site: www.humankinetics.com

United States: Human Kinetics, P.O. Box 5076, Champaign, IL 61825-5076
800-747-4457
e-mail: humank@hkusa.com

Canada: Human Kinetics, 475 Devonshire Road, Unit 100, Windsor, ON N8Y 2L5
800-465-7301 (in Canada only)
e-mail: orders@hkcanada.com

Europe: Human Kinetics, Units C2/C3 Wira Business Park, West Park Ring Road
Leeds LS16 6EB, United Kingdom
+44 (0) 113 278 1708
e-mail: hk@hkeurope.com

Australia: Human Kinetics, 57A Price Avenue, Lower Mitcham, South Australia 5062
08 8277 1555
e-mail: liahka@senet.com.au

New Zealand: Human Kinetics, P.O. Box 105-231, Auckland Central
09-523-3462
e-mail: hkp@ihug.co.nz

Contents

INTRODUCTION

OBJECTIVES

The reader will be able to:

1. **Identify evidence that the importance of physical activity is becoming more widely recognized.**
2. **Describe some of the barriers preventing physical activity from achieving its potential for improving the health of the overall population.**
3. **Describe how health fitness instructors (HFIs) can promote physical activity for everyone.**
4. **List the general competencies needed by HFIs and personal fitness trainers (PFTs).**

The major thrust of this book is that physical activity is an important and essential element in human health and well-being. The book is written for current and future health fitness instructors (HFIs) and personal fitness trainers (PFTs) who are and will be providing guidance for individuals, communities, and groups so that they can gain the benefits of regular physical activity in a positive and safe environment.

This introduction presents the positive and negative aspects of physical activity. The general requirements needed by fitness professionals are outlined. This framework sets the stage for the detailed information and guidelines contained in the book that are needed to be a competent HFI or PFT.

BEST OF TIMES AND WORST OF TIMES FOR PHYSICAL ACTIVITY PROFESSIONALS

In the 1990s, the importance of physical activity has achieved widespread acceptance by the public, professional organizations, and the medical community. It seems that almost everyone recognizes the overwhelming evidence, accumulated by exercise scientists over the past 5 decades, that points to the importance of regular physical activity to quality of life, health, and prevention and rehabilitation of many health problems. The information at the top of the box on page xii ("The Good News") illustrates this widespread acceptance.

Numerous organizations, conferences, statements, and other indicators prove that health-related professionals are recognizing the importance of a combined nutrition and physical activity message for the health of our society. For example, the Center for Disease Control and Prevention, Division of Adolescent School Health (5), is promoting *Coordinated School Health*, an integrated approach to physical activity, nutrition, mental health, and other aspects of health for school children.

Public recognition of the importance of physical activity for good health is a *major* accomplishment for fitness scholars and professionals who have been conducting and disseminating research findings related to the importance of physical activity for many years. To have so many statements promoting physical activity appear within the space of a few years indicates the excitement being felt by all those involved with physical activity; however, there are many challenges left for HFIs who wish to promote the benefits of physical activity for everyone (see "The Bad News" at the bottom of the box on pages xii-xiii).

1 In Review: Professional groups, such as the American College of Sports Medicine (ACSM) and the American Heart Association (AHA), and governmental agencies, such as the Center for Disease Control and Prevention (CDC), the National Institutes of Health (NIH), and the Surgeon General's Office, have released reports emphasizing the importance of physical activity to good health.

Good News and Bad News for Physical Activity Professionals

THE GOOD NEWS

People know that physical activity is important for good health: Surveys indicate that women and men of all ages, races, and socioeconomic status believe that regular physical activity is important for health.

***Healthy People 2000* activity and fitness objectives:** The *Healthy People 2000* objectives (14) list physical activity and fitness as the first of 22 priority areas.

American Heart Association: The American Heart Association (4) included physical inactivity and low fitness levels as primary risk factors along with smoking, hypertension, and high cholesterol.

NIH Consensus Conference on Physical Activity and Cardiovascular Health: The National Institutes of Health (8) released a Consensus Statement on the importance of physical activity for cardiovascular health.

CDC, Division of Adolescent School Health: The Centers for Disease Control and Prevention, Division of Adolescent School Health issued guidelines for healthy levels of nutrition (6) and physical activity (7) for adolescents.

United States Department of Agriculture and United States Department of Health and Human Services: The revised *Dietary Guidelines for the Nation* (13) includes a statement on the importance of physical activity.

President's Council on Physical Fitness and Sports: The President's Council on Physical Fitness and Sports (10) announced that the Advertising Council adopted a 3-year, multimillion dollar campaign dealing exclusively with fitness and youth.

Office of the Surgeon General: The Office of the Surgeon General released its Report on Physical Activity and Health. The report strongly supports the role of physical activity for good health and prevention of major health problems (16).

THE BAD NEWS

Twenty-four percent of Americans remain sedentary: Although there was a general increase in the number of individuals who participated in physical activity in the 1960s and 1970s, there was little change during the 1980s and early 1990s (12, 15). In 1994, about one out of four Americans was completely sedentary (15).

The public is confused about what physical activity is recommended for health and fitness. The "Exercise Lite" (9) recommendations are often viewed as contradictory, rather than supplementary, to the earlier ACSM recommendations for fitness improvement (1, 2).

The resources allocated for physical activity have lagged far behind money spent for other aspects of health: For example, one estimate of federal funding for the 22 *Healthy People 2000* areas (11) found that physical activity and fitness was 21 out of 22 *Healthy People 2000* areas!

Safe, attractive, and well-supervised facilities for participation in activity are not available for many individuals: Bike and walking trails are an exception rather than a rule in communities. Low-cost recreation programs for the masses are simply not sufficient to accommodate all who could benefit.

Health and physical education in the schools: Health and physical education are low on the priority list for schools and are often among the first curricular components cut during budget crises.

2 **In Review: Resources for and access to safe and supervised quality physical activities lag far behind the position statements on physical activity's importance. The public is confused regarding what exactly *is* recommended for physical activity to improve health and fitness.**

WHAT IS NEEDED TO PROMOTE PHYSICAL ACTIVITY

The obvious need is to have communities, schools, states, and the nation endorse the importance of regular physical activity for the nation's health by working with fitness professionals and allocating resources to encourage everyone to choose activity as part of a healthy lifestyle. Three elements of a strategy to enhance our nation's health through physical activity are clarity, access, and safety.

Clarity

Fitness scholars and professionals must clearly interpret and explain the evidence about the nature of physical activity as it relates to various health, fitness, and performance variables. New evidence must be viewed and interpreted within a clearly articulated model that indicates what type of physical activity is related to which outcomes for particular groups of individuals. In addition, we must become more adept at providing short and simple explanations for the media's use that are accurate and easy to understand. Chapters 1 and 2 deal with this issue.

Access

The issue of access is largely outside our direct control. We must nonetheless work continually with public and private partners to provide an environment that makes regular physical activity available and attractive to people of all ages and every socioeconomic status. This includes good health and physical education programs in the schools for all children and youth; community activity programs that are convenient and open to everyone; and programs at the work site, in preschool programs, and in facilities serving older adults. Qualified fitness professionals are an essential part of these programs.

Safety

We must also advocate that participation in all physical activities takes place in a positive and safe environment. Safe equipment, activities appropriate to each individual's age and fitness level, and careful monitoring of signs and symptoms of participants are all part of a quality program. For example, helmets should be worn for cycling, skating, and other activities; sit-ups in a supine position should be avoided by pregnant women past their fourth month; and older adults should be monitored carefully for any signs of cardiovascular problems.

3 **In Review: HFIs must provide clear guidelines for physical activity recommendations combined with adequate resources so that everyone can participate in quality physical activity in an enjoyable and safe atmosphere.**

ROLE OF THE HEALTH FITNESS PROFESSIONAL

HFIs and PFTs play a very important role because many individuals need help in exercising safely and in achieving higher levels of fitness. The HFI and PFT should be aware of the U.S. Department of Health and Human Service's health objectives for the nation in the year 2000, including specific goals of improved health status, reduced risk factors, increased public awareness, improved services and protection, and improved surveillance and evaluation services. Specifically, goals for the year 2000 include increasing the number of people involved in

- both moderate- and vigorous-intensity exercise,
- muscular strength/endurance and flexibility activities,
- physical education in the schools and fitness programs at work, and
- exercise facilities and programs.

The HFI and PFT educate fitness participants about health, fitness, and performance, and they help in the establishment of healthy lifestyles. The HFI and PFT should be aware of the broad range of factors included in total fitness (see chapters 1 and 2). The main focus of this book and of most of the HFI's activity, however, is on physical activity and physical fitness related to positive health.

To accomplish these responsibilities, the HFI and PFT must possess certain competencies and provide a good role model. This book is meant to provide, in a single source, descriptions of all the knowledge, skills, and abilities needed by the health fitness professional.

Qualifications for Health Fitness Professionals

The health fitness professional must understand a wide variety of fields related to fitness. One of the first of several certification programs for fitness professionals was developed by the ACSM. Following are the general ACSM recommended fields of study for health fitness professionals, specifically, for the exercise leader and the HFI* (3).

- Exercise Physiology
- Emergency Procedures/Safety
- Exercise Programming
- Functional Anatomy and Biomechanics
- Health Appraisal and Fitness Testing
- Human Behavior/Psychology
- Human Development and Aging
- Nutrition and Weight Management
- Pathophysiology/Risk Factors
- Program Administration/Management

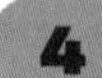

In Review: The role of the HFI and PFT is to help individuals achieve the highest possible fitness levels through a healthy lifestyle. Competencies needed for this role include an understanding of exercise from many perspectives and the ability to implement this knowledge in practical situations.

SOURCE LIST

1. American College of Sports Medicine (ACSM) (1978)
2. ACSM (1990)
3. ACSM (1995)
4. American Heart Association (1992)
5. Center for Disease Control and Prevention (CDC), Division of Adolescent School Health (1995)
6. CDC (1996a)
7. CDC (1996b)
8. National Institutes of Health (1996)
9. Pate et al. (1995)
10. President's Council on Physical Fitness and Sports (PCPFS) (1995a)
11. PCPFS (1995b)
12. Stephens (1987)
13. United States Department of Agriculture (USDA) (1996)
14. USDHHS (1991)
15. USDHHS (1994)
16. USDHHS (1996)

*This information appears on pages 307-334 of *Guidelines for Exercise Testing and Prescription* (5th ed.) by American College of Sports Medicine, 1995, Philadelphia: Williams and Wilkins. Copyright 1995 by Williams & Wilkins. Reprinted by permission.

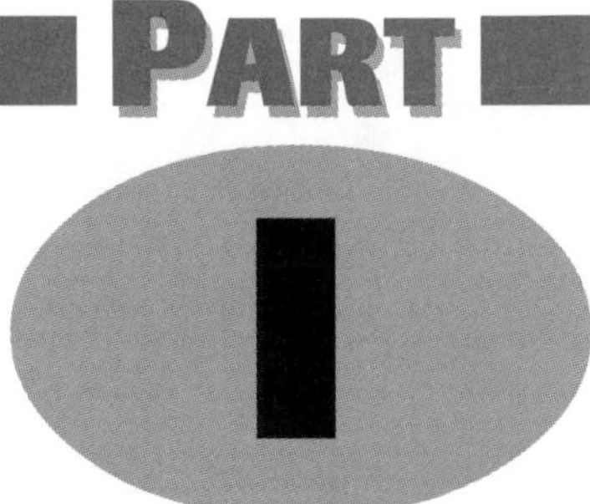

Physical Activity, Fitness, and Health

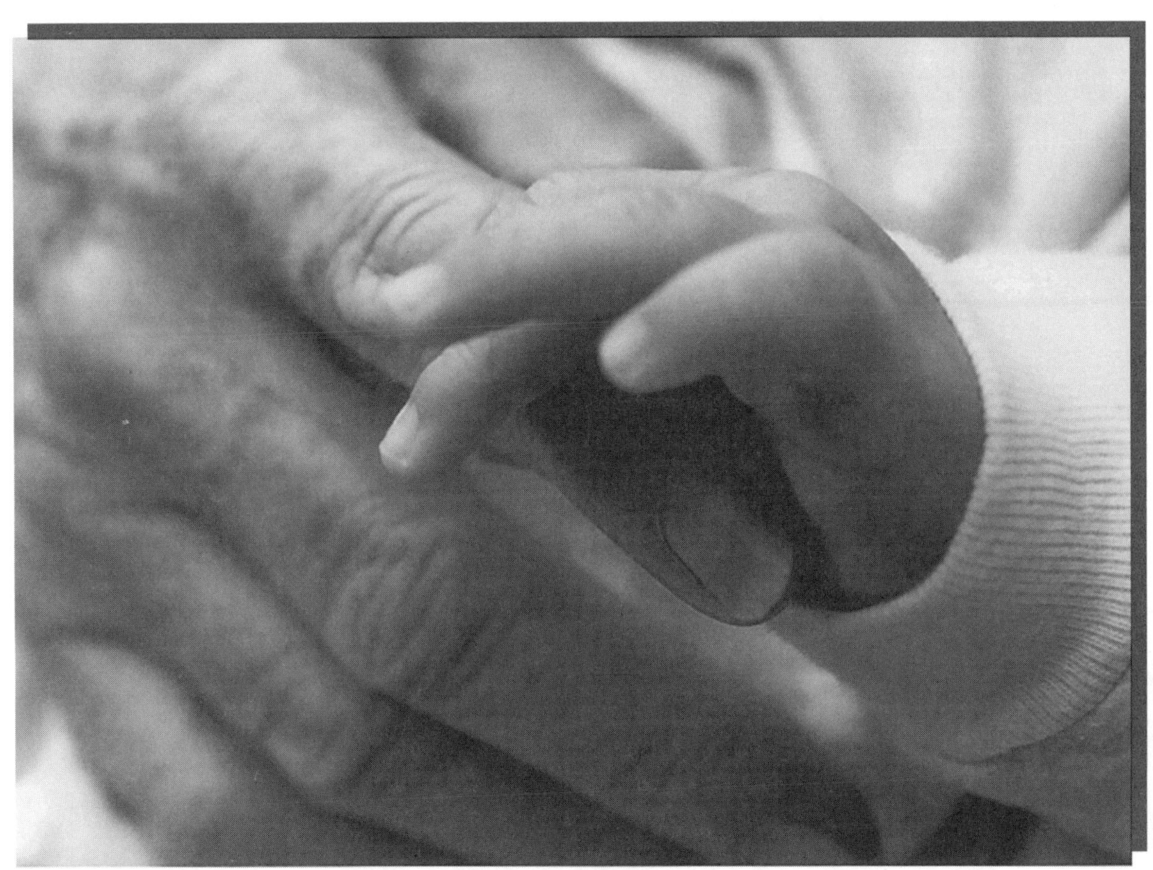

© Photophile/Mark Keller

Part I summarizes the current evidence regarding physical activity and health in chapter 1. Next, it describes the relationships among health, fitness, and performance in chapter 2. Finally, chapter 3 provides a process for screening potential fitness participants and recommends criteria to be used for medical referrals and the development of supervised and unsupervised programs.

CHAPTER

1

Physical Activity and Health

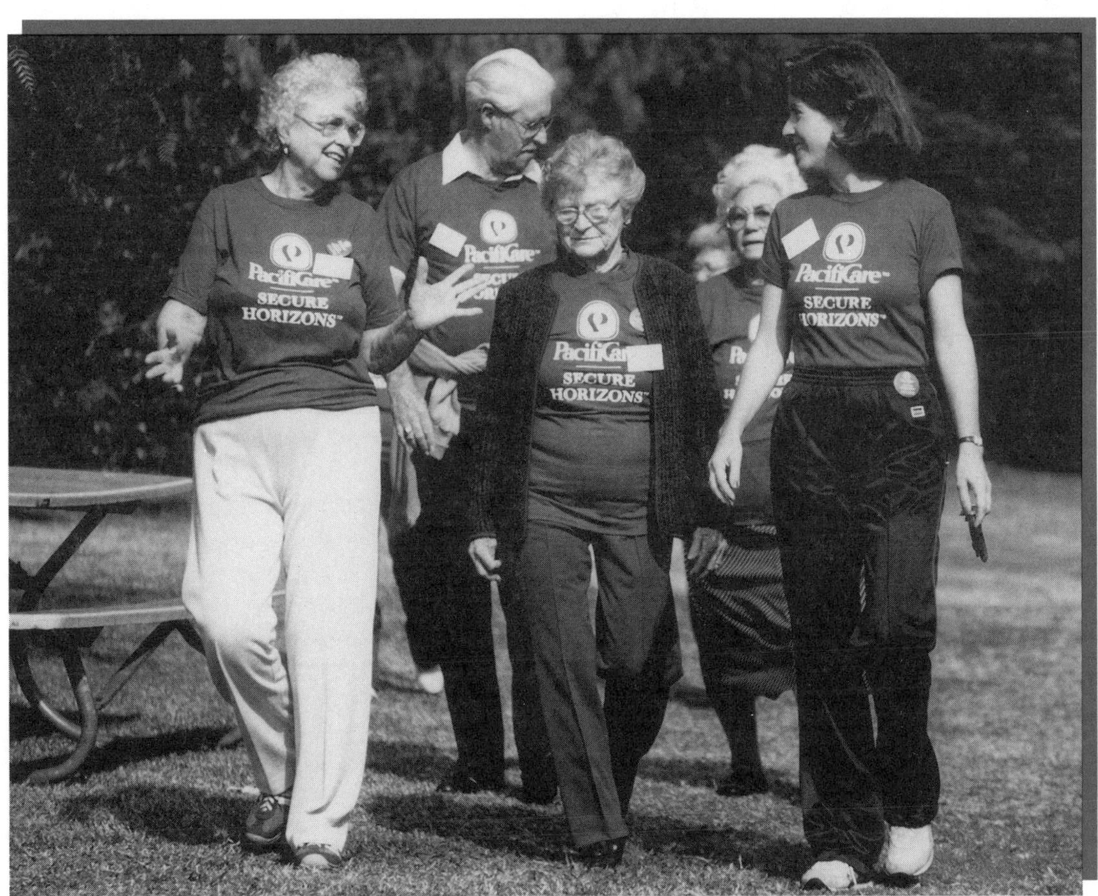

OBJECTIVES

The reader will be able to:

1. **Describe the relationship of physical activity to health.**
2. **Describe the elements of total fitness.**
3. **Understand the role of physical activity in affecting quality of life.**
4. **Describe the goals and behaviors of a healthy life.**
5. **Describe the link between physical activity and lowered risk of premature health problems.**
6. **Understand the pathophysiology of arteriosclerosis and other cardiovascular problems.**
7. **Identify risk factors for coronary heart disease and designate those that may be favorably modified by regular and appropriate physical activity habits.**
8. **Differentiate between the amount and type of exercise required for various health benefits and that required for fitness development.**
9. **Identify the short-term and long-term benefits associated with fitness participation.**
10. **Be aware of the risks associated with exercise participation.**

From the beginning of recorded history, philosophers and health professionals have observed that regular physical activity is an essential part of a healthy life. Hippocrates wrote the following in *Regimen*, about 400 B.C.:

> Eating alone will not keep a man [woman] well; he [she] must also take exercise. For food and exercise, while possessing opposite qualities, yet work together to produce health. . . . And it is necessary, as it appears, to discern the power of various exercises, both natural exercises and artificial, to know which of them tends to increase flesh and which to lessen it; and not only this, but also to proportion exercise to bulk of food, to the constitution of the patient, to the age of the individual. . . . (20, p. 229)

CONNECTIONS BETWEEN PHYSICAL ACTIVITY AND HEALTH

Starting in the 1940s with such fitness pioneers as T. K. Cureton, Bruno Balke, and Peter Karpovich, numerous experimental studies explored the effects of regular physical activity on components of fitness, especially cardiorespiratory fitness and body composition. These studies led to the 1978 American College of Sports Medicine (ACSM) position statement, with Michael Pollock as senior author, concerning the amount and type of physical activity needed to improve fitness (1). Those recommendations, although slightly modified in revised position statements (2, 3), continue to be the gold standard for fitness improvement (see part V). It appeared from these studies that doing a little bit of activity had little effect on cardiorespiratory fitness; in fact, groups assigned to perform less than the ACSM recommendations often were not different from the sedentary control groups.

During the same time frame, epidemiological studies were exploring risk factors for various health problems, especially heart disease. Physical activity, inadequately measured, was a minor part of many of these studies; however, there were several studies that compared more and less active populations, almost always finding less risk among the active individuals. Increasingly, more attention was paid to the role of physical activity in the larger population studies. In addition, a few studies investigated the relationship of fitness level to heart disease and other health problems.

Haskell (14) was one of the first scholars to observe the apparent contradiction of the relationship of physical activity to *fitness* and *health* outcomes. The 1978 ACSM statement was a good summary of findings from the experimental studies on what was needed to make fitness changes over a few months, but the large population studies spanning several years appeared to show that sedentary groups with activity levels below the ACSM recommendations had reduced risk of heart disease and other health problems with low levels of activity. Two of the major population studies had sufficient data to analyze different levels of physical activity (31) and different levels of cardiorespiratory fitness (5) to determine relative risks of heart disease and all-cause mortality. These studies confirmed the earlier observations about the importance of lower levels of activity in terms of reducing the very high risks of completely sedentary groups. Figures 1.1 and 1.2 (17) show the relationship between activity level, fitness level, and risk of coronary heart disease (CHD). The biggest reduction in risk is shown going from the lowest activity or fitness level to a slightly increased level of activity or fitness. These studies also show additional benefit from higher levels of activity and fitness.

Based on these and other studies, the ACSM, Center for Disease Control and Prevention (CDC), and the President's Council on Physical Fitness and Sports (PCPFS) (32) issued a position statement that supplemented the earlier ACSM statement. This later statement proclaimed that sedentary individuals can greatly reduce their risk of developing heart disease and other health problems simply by performing just 30 min of light to moderate activity most days of the week. Additional fitness benefits can result from going beyond that to the 3 to 5 days per week of vigorous aerobic activity specified in the original ACSM position statement, but the greatest boost in improving the health of our nation would come from sedentary individuals beginning to do just a little bit of exercise every day! This position is reflected in the *Healthy People 2000* objectives (39) for both daily moderate and regular vigorous activity. The National Institutes of Health (NIH) Consensus Conference on Physical Activity and Cardiovascular Health (30) drew the same conclusions.

> **1** **In Review: An active lifestyle enhances the quality of life. An increase in total physical activity at low to moderate intensities is associated with a decrease in the risk of heart disease. Regular vigorous physical activity increases cardiorespiratory fitness.**

WHAT WE KNOW ABOUT PHYSICAL ACTIVITY, FITNESS, AND HEALTH

For many people, it would be impossible to describe the highest level of positive, dynamic health without including physical activity. Physical activity is essential to optimal physical and mental health.

Consistent with the link between activity and positive health, a sedentary lifestyle is a major element in poor health for a large number of individuals. Just adding regular physical activity to the lifestyle of individuals who do no activity provides substantial increases in overall health.

Elements Involved in Total Fitness

Although we can recognize individuals who have that special optimal quality of life, it is difficult to describe it in concise and precise terms. Many individuals and groups have used the term **wellness** to emphasize that positive health is much more than simply being free from illness, that there is an added quality to being well. We use the term **total fitness** to try to capture this same concept. Total fitness (also

> **wellness** — Positive health that is more than simply being free from illness. See **total fitness.**
>
> **total fitness** — Optimal quality of life, including social, mental, spiritual, and physical components. Also called wellness, or positive health.

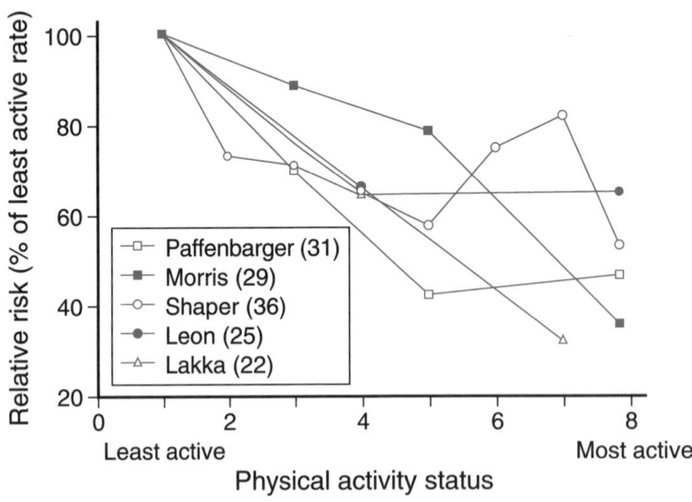

FIGURE 1.1 Physical activity and risk of coronary heart disease.

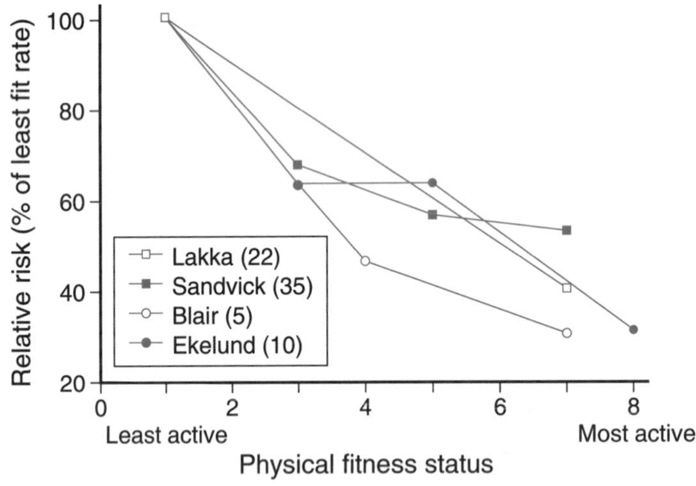

FIGURE 1.2 Physical fitness and risk of coronary heart disease.

called *wellness*, or *positive health*) is a condition reached through striving for optimal quality of life in all aspects of life—social, mental, psychological, spiritual, and physical. This dynamic, multidimensional state has a positive health base and includes individual performance goals. The highest quality of life includes all these components: Mental alertness and curiosity, emotional feelings, meaningful relations with others, awareness and involvement in societal strivings and problems, recognition of the broader forces of life, and the physical capacity to accomplish personal goals with vigor appear to be essential elements of a healthy life. These aspects of total fitness are interrelated; a high level in one of the areas enhances the other areas, and, conversely, a low level in any area restricts the accomplishments possible in other areas. Although physical activity plays a major role in the physical dimension, it can also contribute to learning, relationships, and a sense of our human limitations within the broader perspective. An optimal quality of life requires a person to strive, grow, and develop, but the highest level of fitness may never be achieved. The totally fit person nevertheless continually reaches for the highest quality of life possible.

2 **In Review: Total fitness is striving for the highest level of existence, including mental, psychological, social, spiritual, and physical components. It is dynamic, multidimensional, and related to heredity, environment, and individual interests.**

Heredity

Individuals can achieve fitness goals up to their genetic potential, but it is not possible to establish the relative portion of a person's health or performance that is determined by heredity and development. Even though heredity influences physical activity, fitness status, and health (6), most people can lead healthy or unhealthy lives regardless of their genetic makeup. Thus, genetic background neither dooms a person to poor health nor guarantees a high fitness level.

Environmental Factors

We are born not only with fixed genetic potentials but also into environments that affect our development in many ways. An environment includes physical factors (e.g., climate, altitude, pollution) and social factors (e.g., networks of friends, parental values, characteristics of the workplace) that affect activity, fitness, and health. Some elements, such as nutrition or the air we breathe and water we drink, affect us directly. Other elements, such as the values and behaviors of people we admire, influence our lifestyles indirectly.

Certain aspects of our environments can be controlled—many of the mental and physical activities we do are a matter of choice. However, we are all affected in various ways by our past and current environments. For example, some children have inadequate food as a part of their environments and obviously cannot think about other aspects of fitness until that basic need is fulfilled.

Individual Interests

A major ingredient in total fitness involves individual choices for discretionary use of time. These selected activities are important in two ways: the nature of the activity and preparation for enjoyable participation.

One of the purposes of education is to provide people a positive exposure to a wide variety of activities that enrich life. Thus a well-educated person has many mentally and physically healthy activities from which to choose.

The long-term interests that are developed may require additional preparation for their enjoyment. For example, someone may enjoy reading and tennis as a result of early positive involvement in both. In addition to becoming involved in groups interested in literature, the individual will need to pay attention to proper posture, lighting, and so on while reading. The person will need to develop underlying fitness components and specific skills to continue to enjoy playing tennis.

Quality of Life

The purpose of the opening section of the chapter dealing with global notions of health is to emphasize the point that the importance of physical activity goes beyond whether it can prolong life or prevent heart disease. Later in this chapter we explore the evidence that activity is linked to longevity and reduced risk of heart disease; however, the point here is that regular physical activity would be important for life's quality even if it had no relationship to length of life or premature disease. Several studies have explored the relationship between physical activity and the overall quality of life, including such variables as mental, psychological, and social well-being. Although the type and amount of physical activity essential for global quality of life are not as easily or precisely described, interest in and evidence related to the role that physical activity plays in one's quality of life are increasing (37).

The energy and physical, mental, psychological, and social well-being that can result from appropriate physical activity are reasons enough to promote activity. The reduced risk of developing premature health problems and the potential of a longer life are additional benefits.

3 **In Review: Physical activity is an important ingredient in the quality of life because it increases energy and promotes physical, mental, and psychological well-being in addition to conferring worthy health benefits.**

Goals and Behaviors for a Healthy Life

Health is defined as being alive with no major health problem (also called "apparently healthy"). The two primary health goals are to delay death and to avoid disease. Although these goals do provide a minimum basis for lack of disease, they are

health — Being alive with no major health problem. Also called apparently healthy.

not the optimal goals for total fitness. The primary health goals, displayed below, are desirable first steps, but they fall far short of the optimal level of fitness.

Delaying Death

The death rate for humans is 100%! Death cannot be avoided; but beyond your inherited characteristics, there are some things that you can do to help postpone it for a period of time. Most generally, you can practice a healthy and safe lifestyle in a healthy and safe environment.

Avoiding Disease

Along with delaying death, the other minimum health goal for all of us is to obtain a medical diagnosis that we are free from disease (that we are "apparently healthy"). We try to prevent sickness, illness, and known diseases through awareness, health checks, and healthy habits. You have probably assisted at or attended health fairs that help people identify signs, symptoms, and test scores that might be indicative of possible medical problems.

Positive activities and habits are related to total fitness and low risk of developing major health problems. These behaviors include exercising regularly; maintaining healthy nutrition; getting adequate sleep; relaxing and coping with stressors; practicing safety habits; and abstaining from tobacco, excess alcohol, and nonessential drugs.

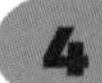

In Review: The primary health goals are to avoid premature death and to avoid preventable disease. Components related to these goals include heredity, environment, habits, and health status. Behaviors that contribute to a healthy life are regular exercise; proper nutrition; adequate sleep; relaxation; and abstinence from tobacco, excess alcohol, and nonessential drugs.

Health Goals, Components, and Behaviors

Goal	Component	Behavior
Delay death	Heredity	
	Healthy habits	Nutrition
		No smoking/drugs
		Limited alcohol
		Relaxation
		Sleep
		Coping with stressors
	Safe habits	Seat belts
		Avoid high risks
	Environment	Clean air and water
Avoid disease	Heredity	
	Prevention	Medical/dental exams
		Immunization
	Aware of symptoms	Check with health provider
	Lower CHD risk	Daily moderate activity
	Nutrition	Balance different foods
		Low fat, cholesterol, salt
		Intake = expenditure
		High complex carbohydrates

PHYSICAL ACTIVITY AND PREVENTION OF PREMATURE HEALTH PROBLEMS

If one lives long enough, health problems will develop, leading to an inability to function independently and eventually causing death. One aspect of an individual's quality of life is to prevent or delay the premature development of these health problems, prolonging the healthy and independent living portions of life. There is evidence that physical activity is related to lower risk of premature development of many health problems including anxiety (23), atherosclerosis (27), back pain (33), cancer (24), chronic lung disease (41), coronary heart disease (15), depression (28), diabetes (12, 13), hypertension (11), obesity (18), osteoporosis (9), and stroke (21). An active lifestyle is also related to estimates of prolonged quality of life (37) and independent living in the elderly (8) and individuals with disabilities (26). In fact, the Surgeon General's Report on *Physical Activity and Health* (40) reviews the evidence relating physical activity to reduced risks of a variety of health problems. Although fewer studies have been done in some health problem-related areas, evidence shows that physical activity may reduce the risks of colon cancer, non-insulin dependent diabetes, osteoporosis, as well as all-cause mortality.

In Review: Regular physical activity helps prevent and delay premature development of a variety of major health problems.

Pathophysiology of Arteriosclerosis and Other Cardiovascular Problems

Cardiovascular problems cause the majority of premature deaths in the United States (40). In addition, many who survive with these problems have severe limitations in their lives. There are many different forms of these heart health problems (refer to source list note 34 for a comprehensive description of the various cardiovascular diseases):

- **Arteriosclerosis**
- **Atherosclerosis**
- **Coronary artery thrombosis**
- **Coronary heart disease (CHD)**
- **Embolism**
- **Heart attack**
- **Hypertension**
- **Myocardial infarction (MI)**
- **Stroke**
- **Thrombosis**

CHD is the single leading cause of premature death in the United States (40). **Cholesterol** is predominant

arteriosclerosis — An arterial disease characterized by the hardening and thickening of vessel walls.

atherosclerosis — A form of arteriosclerosis in which fatty substances are deposited in the inner walls of the arteries.

coronary artery thrombosis — Occlusion of a coronary artery by a blood clot.

coronary heart disease (CHD) — Atherosclerosis of the coronary arteries. Also called coronary artery disease (CAD).

embolism — Sudden obstruction of a blood vessel by a solid body such as a clot carried in the bloodstream.

heart attack — A general term used to describe an acute episode of heart disease; common name for myocardial infarction.

hypertension — High blood pressure. Normally systolic blood pressure exceeds 140 mmHg or diastolic pressure exceeds 90 mmHg in someone who has hypertension.

myocardial infarction (MI)— Death to a section of heart tissue in which the blood supply has been cut off.

stroke — A vascular accident (embolism, hemorrhage, or thrombosis) in the brain, often resulting in sudden loss of body function.

thrombosis — A blood clot in a blood vessel.

cholesterol — A fatty substance in which carbon, hydrogen, and oxygen atoms are arranged in rings.

in the plaques that clog up the arteries. As the coronary arteries become narrowed and hardened, the arteries may not be able to supply the oxygen needed by the heart muscle (myocardium). This inability to supply myocardial oxygen is likely to occur when more oxygen is needed (e.g., during stress or strenuous activity). The resulting imbalance between the need for and supply of oxygen may lead to pain in the chest (angina), neck, jaw, or left shoulder and arm. The narrowed section of the artery may close or become totally occluded, which will lead to a myocardial infarction. (See chapter 3 for standards that define abnormal levels of cholesterol and blood pressure.)

High blood pressure (hypertension) is the most common cardiovascular disease (40). Hypertension is related to CHD and stroke. Stroke is the result of obstructions in or hemorrhages of blood vessels in the brain. It usually results in an abrupt disruption of bodily function and loss of consciousness and may cause partial paralysis. There is some evidence that regular physical activity reduces the risk of stroke.

In Review: In arteriosclerosis and other cardiovascular problems, vessel walls thicken and harden so that they can't deliver enough oxygen to the myocardium.

Primary and Secondary Risk Factors for Cardiovascular Disease

Large-population epidemiological studies of cardiovascular problems have found that several characteristics (**risk factors**) are highly related to the premature development of cardiovascular disease. (See source list note 40 for a comprehensive review of epidemiological studies and risk factors.) Traditionally, health risks have been divided into primary and secondary risk factors. Primary and secondary risk factors for heart disease are presented below.

Primary risk factors are those characteristics that are highly associated with a particular health problem (e.g., heart disease), independent of all other variables. For example, smoking (a primary risk factor) puts an individual at high risk for heart disease even if no other risk factors are present (e.g., the individual is female, young, Caucasian, active, lean, has no family history of heart disease, copes well with stress, and has normal levels of blood pressure and cholesterol). Secondary risk factors, on the other hand, are highly associated with the health problem *only* when other risk factors are present. For example, being under stress (a secondary risk factor), would not put an individual at high risk if no other risk factors were present. Inability to cope with stress does, however, increase the risk of heart disease when other risk factors are present.

Primary and Secondary Risk Factors for Heart Disease

Primary	Secondary
Smoking	Obesity
High total cholesterol[a]	High very low-density cholesterol
High low-density cholesterol	Inability to cope with stress
Low high-density cholesterol	Older age
High blood pressure	African-American
Physical inactivity	Male
Low cardiorespiratory fitness	Family history
Diabetes	High-fat diet
	High fibrinogen

[a]The sum of all forms of cholesterol.

Note. Refer to chapters 3 and 8 for detailed information on the different types of cholesterol and their relationship to risk of heart disease.

Although this distinction has been helpful in the past, the differentiation between primary and secondary is increasingly difficult to maintain. For example, earlier reviews concluded that physical inactivity was a secondary risk factor, and cardiorespiratory fitness was not listed under either category of risk. Later studies (5, 31) have found strong evidence that both physical inactivity and low levels of cardiorespiratory fitness are primary risk factors. Others believe, based on some evidence, that obesity, a high-fat diet, or high fibrinogen are primary rather than secondary risk factors (30). For our purposes, the health fitness instructor (HFI) should know all the risk factors and, more importantly, what individuals need to do to lower their risks of developing health problems.

Alterable and Unalterable Risk Factors

Another way to classify risk factors is to distinguish between inherited risk factors that cannot be altered and unhealthy lifestyle behaviors that can be modified. The risk factors that cannot be altered include the family history of premature cardiovascular disease, gender (men are at greater risk), race (African-Americans having higher risk), and age (the risk increases for all of us as we grow older).

Part of the risk associated with family history and age cannot be changed. The good news, however, is that some of the family history risks can be changed. These alterable family history risks include an unhealthy diet; sedentary lifestyle; smoking; and poor stress-coping behaviors that tend to be transmitted from parents to children. These are the types of behaviors that can be corrected with proper attention throughout life, especially in early childhood.

In terms of aging, many fitness characteristics (e.g., maximum cardiovascular function and amount of body fat) get worse with age; that is, if people from 20 to 80 years of age were tested and the results were plotted against age, a steady deterioration (i.e., decreased cardiovascular function, increased fat) would occur with each decade. This decline, starting in the mid-20s, has been called the *aging curve*. A portion of the deterioration seen in aging curves, however, is caused by older individuals participating in less activity—not by the aging process itself. People who maintain active lifestyles slow down the fitness decline seen in typical aging curves.

Other characteristics that increase risk include smoking, high levels of serum cholesterol, high blood pressure, glucose intolerance, high fibrinogen, obesity, inability to cope with stressors, and low levels of physical activity and cardiorespiratory fitness. Fortunately, many of these characteristics can be favorably altered with healthy habits.

Numerous studies have shown that more active people have a lower risk of heart disease than sedentary individuals; however, in the past, physical inactivity was viewed as less important than control of serum cholesterol, blood pressure, and smoking. Recent studies (5, 31) indicate that both physical activity (such as expending 2000 kcal per week in exercise) and high cardiorespiratory fitness levels (such as being able to go longer on a treadmill test) are major factors related to the prevention of heart disease and all-cause mortality. Physical inactivity and low levels of fitness deserve to be included with the same emphasis as the traditional primary risk factors. Regular exercise also affects many of the CHD risk factors, resulting in an improvement in serum cholesterol levels, blood pressure, glucose tolerance, fibrinogen, and body fat (30). Activity also assists in learning to cope with stressors. See the summary on page 12 of how physical activity affects disease risk factors.

Although these risk factors normally have been linked with some form of cardiovascular disease, many of them are also related to pulmonary (e.g., chronic obstructive pulmonary disease) and metabolic (e.g., diabetes) health problems.

Low-Back Problems

Clinical evidence indicates that several risk factors are associated with **low-back problems** (see chapter 13):

- Lack of abdominal muscle endurance
- Lack of flexibility in the midtrunk and hamstrings
- Poor posture—lying, sitting, standing, and moving
- Poor lifting habits
- Injury of low back

risk factors — A characteristic, sign, symptom, or test score that is associated with increased probability of developing a health problem. For example, people with hypertension have increased risks of developing coronary heart disease.

low-back problems — Strong discomfort in the low-back area, often caused by lack of muscular endurance and flexibility in the midtrunk region, or improper posture or lifting.

Effect of Physical Activity on Risk Factors

Risk factor	Effect of regular physical activity: Improve	May improve	No effect
Older age			X
Smoking		X	
High total cholesterol	X		
High low-density cholesterol	X		
African-American			X
Low high-density cholesterol	X		
Fibrinogen	X		
Male			X
High very low-density cholesterol	X		
Family history			X
High blood pressure	X		
Physical inactivity	X		
Low cardiorespiratory fitness	X		
High-fat diet		X	
Obesity	X		
Diabetes		X	
Inability to cope with stress		X	

- Overuse of low-back muscles
- Inability to cope with stressors

Regular activities that strengthen the abdominal muscles and increase flexibility in the low back and hamstrings are highly recommended for the prevention of low-back problems.

In Review: Some inherited characteristics and behaviors place an individual at higher risk of premature health problems (such as cardiovascular disease and low-back problems) and death. Risk factors of high serum cholesterol levels, high blood pressure, glucose intolerance, high fibrinogen, obesity, and mechanisms for stress reduction can be reduced or eliminated through physical activity.

IMPLICATIONS FOR FITNESS PROFESSIONALS

Fitness professionals need to keep up with the constantly evolving recommendations for health and physical fitness that have direct application for fitness programs and exercise recommendations. Because of the nature of the media's use of brief headlines and TV sound bites that provide only limited and confusing information about the latest fitness recommendations, it is important to help individuals put each new study or report into perspective in terms of the overall recommendations for a healthy life by providing more in-depth explanations.

Exercise Prescription

One of the most controversial and confusing areas for the public is how much and what type of physical activity should be done for health and fitness benefits. One reason for this confusion is that recommendations differ for individuals depending on their current activity levels and their fitness, health, and performance goals. It is not surprising that headlines and 20-s sound bites provide conflicting messages, when one recommendation deals with functional living in the frail elderly, another with making cardiorespiratory improvements in active adults, and yet another on how to train for a marathon. Any set of guidelines for exercise recommendations that does not consider activity status and ultimate goals will add to the confusion.

It is possible to have clear and consistent recommendations for physical activity (see the Activity Pyramid in figure 1.3). The purpose of this section is to provide the basis for physical activity recommendations by including current activity status and indicating different fitness results that may occur. As the past few years have illustrated so clearly, providing exercise recommendations is a dynamic process that should be in tune with new research findings. Thus, while we are confident that the following recommendations are appropriate for the mid-1990s, there is a need to continually review research findings and to periodically update these recommendations.

The three items on pages 14 and 15 show general recommendations for anyone who is not severely ill who wishes to include more physical activity in his or her life, the "Exercise Lite" physical activity recommendations for sedentary individuals to reduce risks of some major health problems, and the traditional recommendations for individuals who are moderately active and desire to obtain additional health and fitness benefits from vigorous activity. Each item includes an activity goal, a fitness goal, screening prior to activity, and recommended activity to meet one's goals. A summary of the recommendations completes the box. Recommendations for individuals who desire to engage in sports are discussed in chapter 2.

8 **In Review: Exercise prescription must consider the individual's current status and desired outcomes. By making some simple changes, everyone can include more physical activity as part of their daily lives. Sedentary individuals should work toward performing at least 30 minutes of daily moderate activity to reduce their risks of heart disease, and moderately active individuals can improve their overall level of fitness by incorporating regular vigorous workouts into their weekly schedules.**

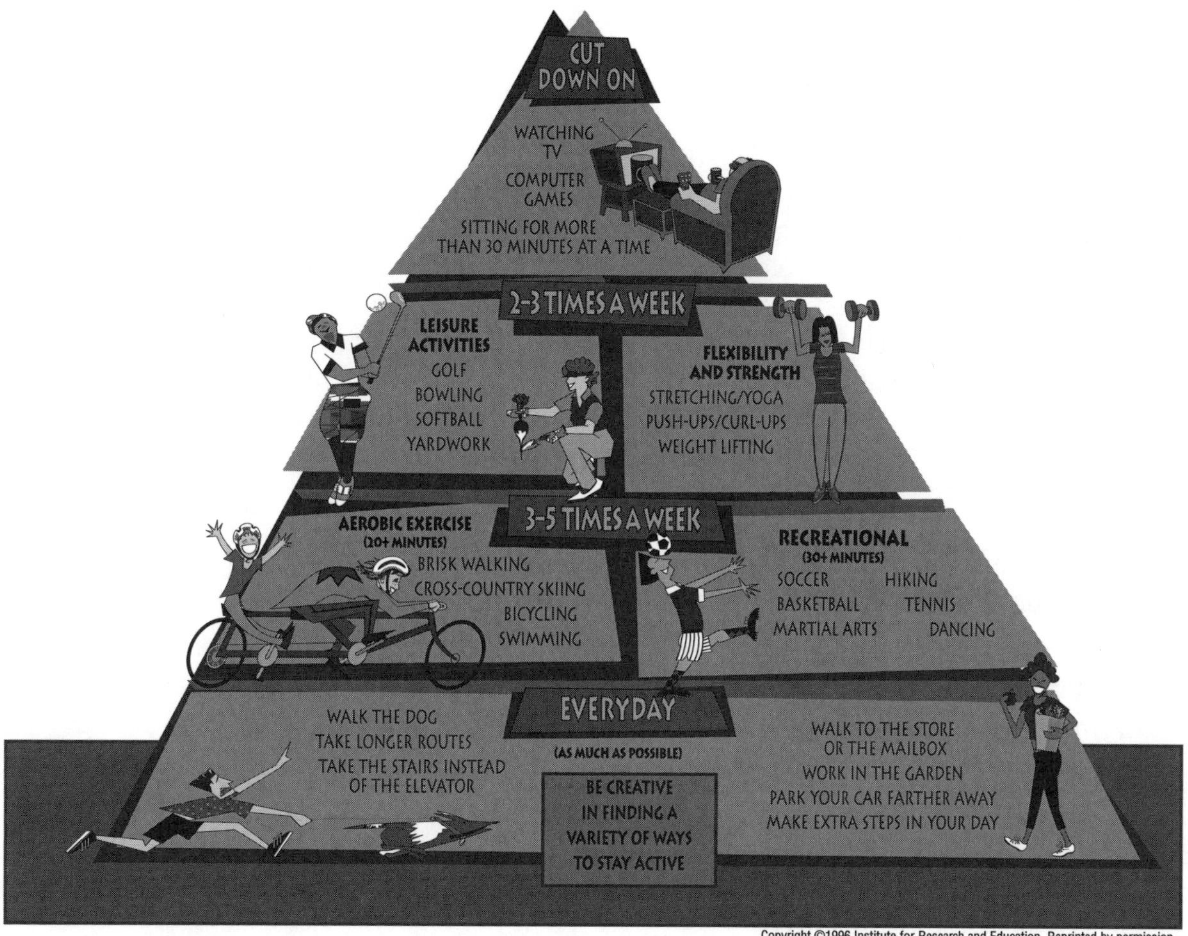

Activity Pyramid.

General Exercise Recommendations and Recommendations for Sedentary and Moderately Active Individuals

Physical activity for everyone

Activity goal:
To include more physical activity as part of daily life.

Fitness goal:
To expend energy (calories) and to enhance functional living.

Screening prior to activity (adapted from the PAR-Q—see chapter 3):
Do you have any of the following symptoms?

Pain or discomfort in your chest, neck, jaw, or arms
Shortness of breath with slight exertion
Dizziness
Ankle swelling
Fast heart rate at rest
Leg pain
Heart murmur
Unusual fatigue with normal activities

If you regularly experience any of the above symptoms, contact a physician. If you are free from these symptoms, you can engage in the following activities with minimal risks.

Recommendations for everyone:
Include physical activity as part of daily routines (e.g., walking rather than riding, taking stairs rather than elevators or escalators, parking at a distance and walking to stores or work, walking around the house and office, gardening, yard work). Lift, push, pull, or carry light to moderately heavy items such as grocery bags, trash, boxes. Include flexibility by moving all joints through a full range of motion at least 3 days per week. Emphasize static stretches for the lower back and thigh area, holding each stretch for 10-30 seconds and doing each one 3-5 times.

"Exercise Lite": Physical activity for sedentary individuals

A sedentary individual is one who does no regular physical activity or is unable to walk more than a few minutes without discomfort or fatigue.

Activity goal:
To perform at least 30 min of daily moderate physical activity.

Fitness goal:
To improve functional living, enhance safety, and reduce risks of heart disease.

Screening prior to activity (adapted from ACSM guidelines [3]):
Do you have any of the following?

Heart condition that a physician told you limits activity
Chest pain during activity
Chest pain during last month when not doing activity

Loss of balance because of dizziness
Loss of consciousness
Bone or joint problem that would be made worse with activity
Prescribed drugs for blood pressure or heart condition
Any other reason why you should not do physical activity

If you answer yes to any of these, see a physician prior to changing your physical activity levels.

Recommended activity:

Perform at least 30 min of walking or related low-impact activity (e.g., cycling, swimming) daily. Start slowly with short, lower-intensity activity and gradually increase the distance and intensity. Also increase physical activity as part of your daily routine (see examples in activities for everyone).

Physical activity for moderately active individuals

A moderately active individual can walk 30 min at a brisk pace without discomfort or fatigue.

Activity goal:

To include regular vigorous physical fitness workouts.

Fitness goal:

To increase levels of physical fitness and quality of life.

Screening prior to activity (adapted from ACSM guidelines [3]):

It is recommended that individuals who meet any of the following conditions have a medical examination and a graded exercise test prior to increasing their physical activity:

Over 40 years of age
Known cardiovascular disease
Any of the symptoms listed on the previous page under screening for everyone
Two or more of the following risk factors: cigarette smoking, high blood pressure, high cholesterol, diabetes, obesity

Recommended activity:

Engage in fitness workouts with the following characteristics:

Aerobic activities—3-5 days per week

200-400 calories (kcal) expended per session (e.g., jog 3 mi, walk 6 mi, cycle 12 mi, swim 3/4 mi)
Vigorous intensity—causes sweating, increased breathing, feels between light and hard work (50%-85% max METs, or 60%-90% of maximum heart rate)
Examples include walking, jogging, cycling, cross-country skiing, stepping
Workout includes a warm-up and cool-down with slow walking and stretching

Muscular strength/endurance exercises—2-3 days per week

Separate exercises for major muscle groups
One set of 8–12 repetitions for each muscle group
Full range of motion
Adhere to specific recommended techniques

(continued)

(continued)

Summary of exercise recommendations

	Sedentary to moderately active	Moderately to vigorously active
Screening	PAR-Q*	ACSM*
Warm-up	5 min	10 min
Flexibility	Daily	3-5 d/wk
Aerobic		
Duration	30 min	20 min
Intensity	Moderate	Vigorous
Frequency	Daily	3-5 d/wk
Muscular strength/endurance		2-4 d/wk
Cool-down	5 min	10 min

*See chapter 3.

Intensity

You'll notice that one of the major differences in the current recommendations relates to **intensity**. There is no universal agreement on definitions of different levels of intensity. Pollock and Wilmore (34) present five categories of exercise intensity from very light to very heavy based on percentage of maximal heart rate (MHR) and oxygen uptake ($\dot{V}O_2max$) and rating of perceived exertion. We are using two categories adapted from the moderate- and vigorous-intensity recommendations of the ACSM, CDC, and PCPFS (32):

- **Moderate intensity**—Activities that use energy three to six times the resting metabolism (3-6 METs—see chapter 7) are moderate-intensity activities. Moderate activity ranges from approximately 40% to 60% of an individual's maximal functional capacity. For most people, that would be walking a mile in 14 to 23 minutes. Moderate-intensity activity causes a slightly increased rate of breathing, and it feels light to somewhat hard; yet individuals doing moderate activity can easily carry on a conversation.
- **Vigorous intensity**—Doing activities at more than six times the resting metabolism (>6 METs) is vigorous-intensity activity, or activity that is above 60% of maximal functional capacity. Walking a mile in less than 14 minutes, jogging, cycling, cross-country skiing, exercising to music, and playing endurance sports (racquetball, soccer, tennis) would all be considered vigorous activity. These activities result in increased rates of breathing and sweating, and feel from somewhat hard to very hard. Vigorous-intensity activity used to meet health and fitness goals need not reach maximal levels; however, vigorous-intensity activities for high-level performance often include maximal-level exertion.

Here are other exercise-related terms that we will use throughout the book:

- **Physical activity** (30)
- **Exercise training** (7, 16)

Benefits of Physical Activity

The long-term benefits of regular activity in terms of health and fitness are well known, including reduced risk of major health problems and improvement in cardiorespiratory function, muscular strength and endurance, flexibility, and reduction of fat. Although we normally focus on the long-term (chronic) effects of regular physical activity, part of the benefit of physical activity is the repeated acute (or short-term) activity. For example, in addition to the reduction in resting blood pressure as a result of

Table 1.1 Short- and Long-Term Benefits of Physical Activity

Variable	Short-term benefits	Long-term benefits
Heart rate	+, then -	- (except max)
Stroke volume		+
Ejection fraction		+
Lactate threshold		+
Fibrinogen	-	-
Fibrinolysis	+	+
Blood pressure	+, then -	-
Oxygen uptake, max		+
Muscle mass		+
Strength/endurance		+
Fat		-
Cholesterol, HDL		+
LDL, VLDL		-
Flexibility		+
Appetite	-	+
Use of leisure time	+	+
Positive mood	+	
Anxiety	-	-
Depression	-	-
Self-esteem		+
Stress	+, then -	-
Overreaction to stress		-

Note. + = increases, - = decreases, HDL = high-density lipoprotein, LDL = low-density lipoprotein, VLDL = very low-density lipoprotein.

chronic activity, there is some additional lowering of blood pressure following each acute bout of exercise. There are positive psychological effects of a single bout of activity, such as a positive mood change following exercise for many individuals. Finally, the time spent in physical activity is *not* being spent in unhealthy behaviors, such as smoking or eating unhealthy snacks. Table 1.1 summarizes some of the acute and chronic effects of physical activity.

9 **In Review: The short- and long-term benefits of physical activity are summarized in table 1.1.**

Exercise-Related Risks

Exercise and fitness tests involve risk of injury, cardiovascular problems, or death. High-intensity exercise and competition in many sports place extreme demands on the cardiovascular system and include increased risk of musculoskeletal injury. In addition, some fitness participants become obsessed with exercise and overtrain, ending up with decreased fitness and frequent injuries.

Moderate-intensity exercise is a very low-risk activity. There is an increased risk of myocardial infarction or sudden death with vigorous exercise, but these risks are still very low. In the general population, it is estimated that there are 7 deaths and 56 myocardial infarctions for every 100 000 exercisers (38). In the postcardiac population, there is one death for every 784 000 patient hr of exercise and one

intensity (of physical activity) — The magnitude of energy required for a particular activity, often referred to in terms of absolute amount of energy expended (e.g., multiples of resting metabolism—METs) or relative to a percentage of one's own maximum (e.g., $\dot{V}O_2$ or HR).

physical activity — Bodily movement produced by skeletal muscles that requires energy expenditure at a level to produce healthy benefits.

exercise training — Structured program of physical activity aimed at achieving some fitness goal.

myocardial infarction for every 294 000 patient hr of exercise (38). Because of the decreased risk of heart disease in active or fit persons, the overall risk of a cardiovascular problem is greater for those who maintain sedentary habits (40).

The risks from exercise testing are also quite low, with 1/1000 risk of a complication requiring hospitalization and 1/10 000 risk of death during or immediately following the test (3).

Exertion-related deaths are uncommon and are generally related to congenital heart defects (e.g., hypertrophic cardiomyopathy, Marfan's syndrome, severe aortic-valve stenosis, prolonged QT syndromes, cardiac conduction abnormalities) or to acquired myocarditis. The NIH Consensus Statement on Physical Activity and Cardiovascular Health (30) recommends that individuals with these conditions remain active but not participate in vigorous or competitive athletics.

The tendency is to deal with the question of risk by identifying various classes of individuals for whom a certain type of medical examination or test is recommended before initiation of an exercise program (see chapter 3). Per Olof Åstrand, a well-known Swedish physiologist, has offered another view. He states that consulting a physician is advisable if there are any doubts about health, but that "there is less risk in activity than in continuous inactivity." He continues, "It is more advisable to pass a careful medical examination if one intends to be sedentary in order to establish whether one's state of health is good enough to stand the inactivity!" (4). This view is consistent with recent evidence that physical activity and a high level of cardiorespiratory fitness are directly related to a lower risk of heart disease and death (30).

10 **In Review: There is some risk of injury, cardiovascular problems, and death with exercise. The health risk of an inactive lifestyle is higher than the risk associated with the kind of fitness activities and tests recommended in this book.**

Case Studies

You can check your answers by referring to appendix A.

1.1

You have just presented a speech on physical fitness to a local service club. One of the members says that he knows of two men who have died in incidents related to exercise during the past 5 years, and he has read that there have been other exercise-related deaths. He has decided that it will be safer to lead a quiet life and not take the risk of exercising. How would you respond?

1.2

A client calls you and complains that he has been deceived by all the exercise recommendations you have given him over the past several years. He just read a report from the Centers for Disease Control and Prevention indicating that a person has to only do moderate exercise (walking) to achieve health benefits. He wants to know if he should continue his vigorous exercise program in which he exercises at his target heart rate for 30 min 3 to 4 times per week, or should he switch to a walking program? How would you respond?

Source List

1. American College of Sports Medicine (ACSM) (1978)
2. ACSM (1990)
3. ACSM (1995)
4. Åstrand & Rodahl (1986)
5. Blair et al. (1989)
6. Bouchard & Perusse (1994)
7. Caspersen, Powell, & Christensen (1985)
8. Chodzko-Zajko (1996)
9. Drinkwater (1994)
10. Ekelund et al. (1988)
11. Fagard & Tipton (1994)
12. Giacca, Shi, Marliss, Zinman, & Vranic (1994)
13. Gudat, Berger, & Lefebvre (1994)
14. Haskell (1984)
15. Haskell (1995)
16. Haskell (1996a)
17. Haskell (1996b)
18. Hill, Drougas, & Peters (1994)
19. Institute for Research and Education (1996)
20. Jones (1953)
21. Kohl & McKenzie (1994)
22. Lakka et al. (1994)
23. Landers & Petruzzello (1994)
24. Lee (1994)
25. Leon et al. (1987)
26. McCartney (1994)
27. Moore (1994)
28. Morgan (1994)
29. Morris et al. (1990)

30. National Institutes of Health (1996)
31. Paffenbarger, Hyde, & Wing (1986)
32. Pate et al. (1995)
33. Plowman (1994)
34. Pollock & Wilmore (1990)
35. Sandvick et al. (1993)
36. Shaper & Wannamethee (1991)
37. Shephard (1996)
38. Thompson & Fahrenbach (1994)
39. United States Department of Health and Human Services (USDHHS) (1991)
40. USDHHS (1996)
41. Whipp & Casaburi (1994)

CHAPTER

2

Physical Fitness and Performance

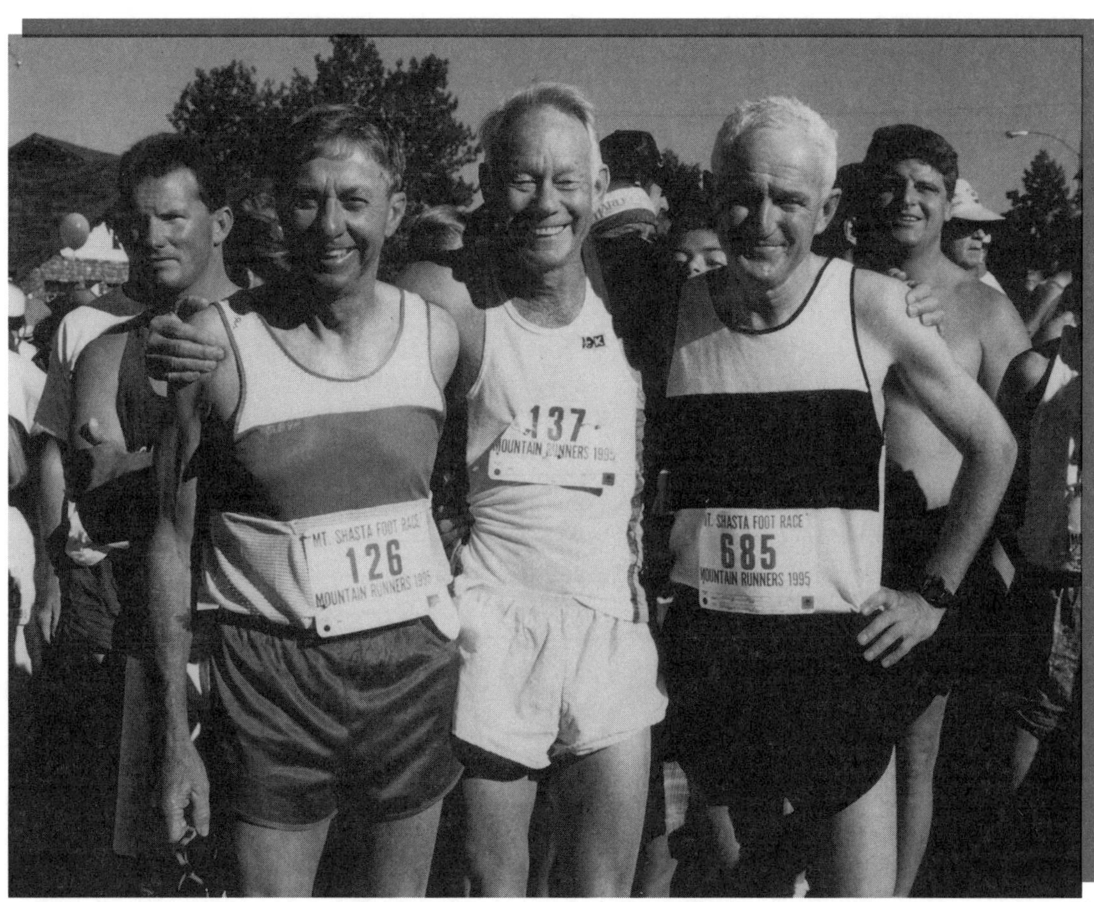

© Photophile/Mark E. Gibson

OBJECTIVES

The reader will be able to:

1. **Describe the goals of fitness and performance.**
2. **Demonstrate an understanding of the components of fitness.**
3. **Define and differentiate among terms related to fitness and performance.**
4. **Define the major components of performance.**
5. **Describe healthy behaviors related to fitness.**
6. **Describe factors related to setting individual fitness goals.**
7. **Explain the role of fitness professionals in encouraging healthy behavior.**

Chapter 1 dealt with the importance of physical activity for total fitness, health, and prevention of premature health problems. It presented the two-prong recommendation for moderate- and vigorous-intensity activity. The first part of the physical activity recommendations emphasizes the importance of sedentary individuals doing some regular low- to moderate-intensity activity for health goals. The second part of the recommendation is to provide vigorous activity (exercise) to enhance fitness benefits and to provide the basis for participation in a variety of performance activities that also enrich life for many individuals. Using recommended definitions, the first chapter dealt with physical activity and health while this chapter explores exercise, physical fitness, and performance. We continue the discussion of activity, fitness, and health by comparing the goals, components, and behaviors related to **physical fitness** (1) and **performance**.

PHYSICAL FITNESS GOALS

The physical fitness goals are to lower risks of developing health problems and to maintain positive physical health. You are undoubtedly familiar with the components of these goals.

To Lower Risks of Developing Health Problems

This goal is an extension of the health goal to avoid disease (chapter 1). Many of the health problems responsible for premature deaths can be prevented with careful screening and preventive action (e.g., immunization). There are still many people in the world who need this basic health care, and medical science can provide this service. The solution to this aspect of health care is finding the resources and political will to make it available to everyone.

In more affluent sectors of societies, where preventive health care is routine, another set of health problems has emerged (e.g., cardiovascular diseases) causing premature death or disability. As seen in chapter 1, physical activity plays a major role in preventing the development of premature health problems.

To Maintain a Physical Well-Being

Many of the same characteristics that lower our risk for developing serious health problems also provide a higher quality of life. In other words, having high levels of functional capacity and optimal levels of body fat help us feel good and have the energy to do things that enrich our lives. In addition, having good muscular endurance and flexibility in the midtrunk area are related to a healthy low back. As people increase their levels of physical fitness, they move toward a better life; whereas decreases in physical fitness lead toward health problems and decreased quality of life.

PERFORMANCE GOALS

The primary performance goals are to complete daily tasks efficiently and to achieve desired levels in selected sports. These goals also involve a number of components.

To Complete Daily Tasks Efficiently

To get through the day efficiently, we must have fundamental motor skills to be able to accomplish various tasks. We must be able to move the body from place to place and push, pull, pick up, carry, and do a number of other tasks requiring use of the hands and arms. Moderate levels of muscular strength and endurance, flexibility, and cardiorespiratory function are essential for these routine tasks. In addition, we need special abilities to perform the unique activities related to work or home.

This goal is also related to the positive health goal of independent functional living. It is an extension of the physical fitness goal of having healthy levels of cardiorespiratory function, relative leanness, muscular strength and endurance, and flexibility.

To Achieve Desired Levels of Sports Performance

Many individuals also engage in selected games, sports, and high-level performance. In addition to high levels of physical fitness, these activities require specific kinds and levels of motor abilities (such as agility, balance, coordination, power, and speed related to the sport) as well as the particular skills of the sport.

1 **In Review: The goals of physical fitness are to have a positive physical health base with a low risk of health problems. Performance goals are to be able to engage in daily tasks with adequate energy and to participate successfully in selected sports.**

COMPONENTS OF PHYSICAL FITNESS AND PERFORMANCE

The components of physical fitness and performance are derived directly from their goals. The physical fitness goals are achieved by doing the types of exercise that improve and maintain cardiorespiratory function, a healthy level of body fat, muscular strength and endurance, and flexibility. The performance goals are enhanced by specific conditioning to achieve and maintain high levels of aerobic and anaerobic energy; muscular strength, endurance, and power; speed; agility; coordination; balance; and sports skills.

Physical Fitness Components

Components of physical fitness are **cardiorespiratory function**, **relative leanness**, **muscular strength and endurance**, and **flexibility**.

Cardiorespiratory function is essential not only for the health and physical fitness goals of preventing premature cardiovascular problems, but also for providing the energy to accomplish other elements of the quality of life. Chapter 4 explains the physiology underlying this component, chapter 11 describes

physical fitness — A set of attributes that people have or achieve relating to their ability to perform physical activity.

performance — The ability to perform a task or sport at a desired level. Also called motor fitness, or physical fitness.

cardiorespiratory function — The ability of the circulatory and respiratory systems to supply fuel during sustained physical activity.

relative leanness — The relative amount of body weight that is fat and nonfat. Also called body composition.

muscular strength — The ability of the muscle to generate the maximum amount of force.

muscular endurance — The ability of the muscle to perform repetitive contractions over a prolonged period of time.

flexibility — The ability to move a joint through the full range of motion without discomfort or pain.

ways to test it, and chapter 14 deals with exercise prescription for improving your cardiorespiratory function.

The importance of healthy levels of body fat relates to numerous health and psychological problems. One of the major negative trends reported in the *Healthy People 2000* objectives (2) is the substantial increase in obesity in all ages since the mid-1980s. This is a complex area involving nutrition, physical activity, and behavior modification covered in chapters 8, 9, and 10.

The activities that improve and maintain muscular strength and endurance appear to be important for bone density, thus helping prevent osteoporosis, a problem of decreasing bone mass that affects older women in particular. Chapter 5 provides the basic anatomy, chapter 12 describes ways to assess strength and endurance, and chapter 15 deals with exercise prescription for increasing strength and endurance.

Midtrunk strength, endurance, and flexibility are essential elements in maintaining a healthy low back. Flexibility and the low-back function are covered in chapters 13 and 16.

2 **In Review: Physical fitness components are cardiorespiratory function, relative leanness, muscular strength and endurance, and flexibility. These fitness elements are related to a higher quality of life and to prevention of major health problems.**

Performance Components

Cardiorespiratory function, body composition, muscular strength and endurance, and flexibility are important for both performance goals. In the first place, modest levels of these fitness components are important to the efficiency with which we can do daily tasks around the home, yard, and at work. Although this is important at all ages, it is a top priority for elderly individuals because it allows them to continue to live independently for a longer period of time.

Second, higher levels of these fitness components also provide the basis for successful participation in a variety of sport and performance activities. Although an individual can attain health and fitness goals by doing non-sporting activities, participation in sports and games provides enjoyable health and fitness supplements. In a small percentage of the population, of course, sports provide professional careers. In addition to the fitness components, each sport has unique demands for energy, body composition, strength, endurance, and flexibility, along with skill requirements specific to each particular sport. Many sports demand high levels of **agility**, **balance**, **coordination**, **power**, and **speed** that are directly related to the sport.

In Review: The definitions on pages 23 and 25 differentiate among terms related to fitness and performance.

Examples of Performance Goals

Because most of this book deals with health and fitness, the following example illustrates the differing needs for the two performance goals. The first performance goal is to complete daily tasks efficiently. Most individuals move their bodies around during the day, doing some bending, lifting, carrying, pushing, and pulling requiring cardiorespiratory function, muscular strength and endurance, and flexibility, movements made easier without excess fat. In addition to those common needs, the particular lifestyle situation adds other needs. Contrast, for example, a computer programmer, a fire fighter, and a parent staying home with an infant. The computer programmer will need some stretching and relaxation activities to prevent low-back and postural problems and can benefit from short activity breaks. The fire fighter is sedentary for most of the time but must be able to respond quickly with near maximal levels of anaerobic energy, muscular strength and endurance, in an adverse environment with heavy equipment. This person must engage in regular vigorous aerobic, anaerobic, and resistance exercise to maintain the conditioning necessary to respond to emergencies. The parent needs flexibility, strength, and endurance to lift and carry the infant and other items through an obstacle course of toys, clothes, and so on, in addition to learning to perform with sleep deprivation.

The second performance goal is to achieve desired levels in selected sports, games, and competitions. Although high fitness levels are desirable as a base, individuals here also have very different needs. Compare, for example, 10K runners, basketball players, and golfers. The runners rely on high levels of aerobic power that comes from lots of distance running,

Recommendations for Vigorously Active Individuals Performing Specific Sports or Work Tasks

A vigorously active individual is able to jog 3 mi at moderate to vigorous intensity (60%-80% maximal oxygen uptake, 70%-85% maximal heart rate) 3-5 times/week without discomfort or undue fatigue.

Activity goal:

To engage successfully in selected work or sport performance activities.

Fitness goal:

To have the underlying levels of fitness and the specific skills needed to be able to perform the tasks at the desired level with minimum risks of health problems or injury.

Screening prior to activity:

If the training involves maximal exertion, a medical examination including a maximal exercise test is recommended.

Recommended activities:

Do fitness activities (listed on page 15 for moderately active) as base.

Add additional training related to specific requirements of sport or activity. You may need to exceed total work, intensity, duration, and/or frequency of fitness workouts.

Develop and maintain skills related to the sport or work tasks.

Be aware of safety concerns in performance.

Increase time for warm-up including moderate-intensity activities directly related to the performance of the sport or work tasks.

with careful stretching before and after. Basketball players depend on a combination of aerobic and anaerobic energy; coordination; and very specific passing, shooting, and defensive skills. Golfers require a moderate cardiorespiratory base, some muscular power, and coordination of a complex skill used in different contexts.

The information above provides recommendations for performance of sports or work tasks similar to the format used in chapter 1 for recommendations for sedentary and moderately active individuals to increase their activity for health and fitness goals. This table extends that idea to those vigorously active individuals who want to engage in sports and endurance performance.

4 In Review: Performance components include a general fitness base. Specific levels of fitness components and unique skills related to the sport or game are needed for performance.

agility — Ability to start, stop, and move the body quickly in different directions.

balance — Ability to maintain a certain posture, or to move without falling.

coordination — Ability to do a task integrating movements of the body and different parts of the body.

power — Ability to exert muscular strength quickly.

speed — Ability to move the whole body quickly.

BEHAVIORS THAT SUPPORT FITNESS AND PERFORMANCE COMPONENTS

The first two sections of this chapter discussed definitions, goals, and components related to physical fitness and performance. To achieve the components of physical fitness, a person must adopt healthy behaviors.

Behaviors that contribute to fitness goals include adopting healthy eating habits; exercising regularly; avoiding smoking, using illegal drugs, and drinking too much alcohol; getting adequate sleep and managing

Area	Goal	Components	Behaviors
Physical fitness	To lower risks of developing health problems	Good inherited characteristics	Wise selection of parents
		Healthy levels of Cholesterol Blood pressure Body fat Glucose tolerance Functional capacity	Healthy diet, low fat and salt; balanced caloric intake and expenditure; regular moderate exercise
		Substance use	No smoking or drug abuse; limited use of alcohol
		Stress	Getting adequate sleep and learning to relax; coping with stressors
	To maintain a physical well-being	Healthy levels of Body fat Functional capacity	Healthy diet, low fat and salt; balanced caloric intake and expenditure; regular vigorous exercise
		Substance use	No smoking or drug abuse; limited use of alcohol
		Stress	Getting adequate sleep and learning to relax; coping with stressors
		Midtrunk flexibility	Static streching of low back and legs
		Abdominal endurance	Abdominal curl-ups
		Flexibility	Static stretching
		Muscular strength and endurance	Resistance exercise

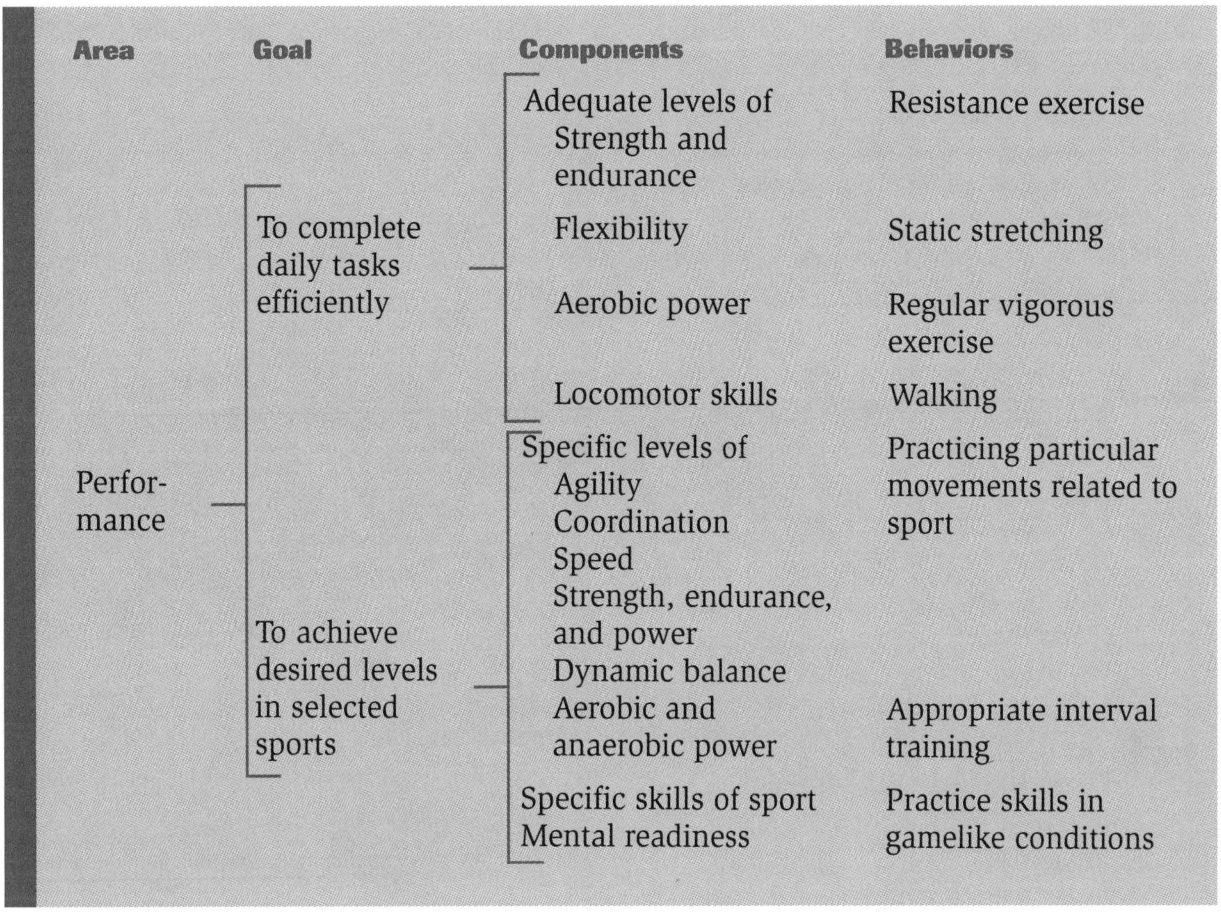

stress; and adopting a stretching and strength training regimen. Performance goals can be reached by adopting healthy behaviors such as developing a resistance training program, using static stretching exercises, participating in regular vigorous exercise, practicing specific sport-related movements, using interval training, and practicing skills in gamelike conditions.

The illustration on pages 26 and 27 summarizes the goals, components, and behaviors for physical fitness and performance.

COMMON BEHAVIORS FOR FITNESS AND HEALTH

Although common behaviors for fitness and health are distinct, they are also interrelated. People who exercise and exhibit other healthy behaviors are more likely to be fit. Achieving fitness standards leads to a healthy, longer life. On the other hand, sedentary existence is related to low levels of fitness and major health problems that shorten life.

We have tried to show both the common and unique elements of health, fitness, and performance in these first two chapters. You have probably noticed that there is some repetition in the behaviors recommended for delaying death, avoiding disease, providing low risk of major health problems, and the development of high levels of positive health. Although individuals need to be educated about signs, symptoms, risk factors, and so on, the major emphasis of a fitness program should be on the behaviors listed on the Health and Fitness Behaviors list (page 28).

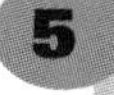

In Review: Although there are some differences between health and fitness goals, there are many recommended behaviors common to both goals. Health and fitness are enhanced with regular exercise and sleep, nutritious diet, no smoking or drug abuse, limited alcohol, ability to cope with stressors, ability to relax, preventive checkups, and safe habits.

Health and Fitness Behaviors

- Regular physical activity
  - Low-intensity activity
  - Moderate-intensity exercise
  - Abdominal curl-ups
  - Static stretching for low-back flexibility
  - Whole-body flexibility and strength/endurance exercise
- Healthy diet
  - Proper proportions of fat, carbohydrates, and proteins
  - Balance between energy expenditure and intake
  - Balance among food groups
  - High levels of complex carbohydrates
  - Low saturated and total fat
  - Low salt
- Substance use
  - No smoking
  - No drugs (except as prescribed by physician)
  - Limited alcohol use
- Stress
  - Learn to cope with stressors
  - Learn to relax
- Regular sleep
- Regular tests for fitness and health
  - Health risk appraisal
  - Healthy habits
  - Fitness status

SETTING FITNESS GOALS

People entering your fitness class or asking you to be their personal trainer have taken an important first step toward improving their fitness levels. It is your responsibility to help them

- understand the components of fitness,
- analyze their current fitness status,
- begin or continue appropriate exercise habits,
- determine other health behaviors that need to be changed, and
- take appropriate steps to change unhealthy behavior.

Chapter 20 suggests ways to help participants start changing unhealthy behaviors.

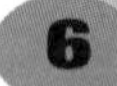

In Review: Information presented in chapters 1 and 2 will help HFIs and personal fitness trainers (PFTs) to assist individuals in setting appropriate health, fitness, and performance goals.

TAKING CONTROL OF PERSONAL HEALTH STATUS

One of the most frustrating and exciting aspects of dealing with current health problems is that individuals can modify their health status and control major health risks. The frustrating aspect is that many people find it difficult to change unhealthy lifestyles. The exciting element is that they *can* gain control of their health. The HFI and PFT are at the cutting edge of health, in much the same way in which the scientist discovering vaccines for major health problems was at the turn of the 20th century. This opportunity to provide assistance to people who wish to alter their unhealthy lifestyles carries the responsibility to make recommendations based on the best evidence available. The HFI and PFT can help people gain control of their lives through an evaluation of their risk factors and behaviors related to health. Chapter 3 examines this type of health appraisal.

7 **In Review: Physical activity professionals live in an exciting time because of the increasing evidence and recognition that regular physical activity is an essential element for the good life. Nevertheless, it will be a worthwhile challenge to motivate people to begin and continue an active lifestyle when there is so much competition for everyone's time.**

CASE STUDY

You can check your answers by referring to appendix A.

2.1

Two people come to you and both say they want to "get in shape." After talking with them, you discover that Fred seems to be free from major health problems, but he hasn't done any regular activity for 20 years. Susan, also apparently healthy, has been jogging and doing exercise to music, 2 to 4 times per week for the past 5 years. She has just joined an adult soccer league and wants to be able to compete at a higher level. How would you help them understand their goals?

SOURCE LIST

1. Caspersen, Powell, & Christensen (1985)
2. United States Department of Health and Human Services (1994)

CHAPTER

3

Health Appraisal

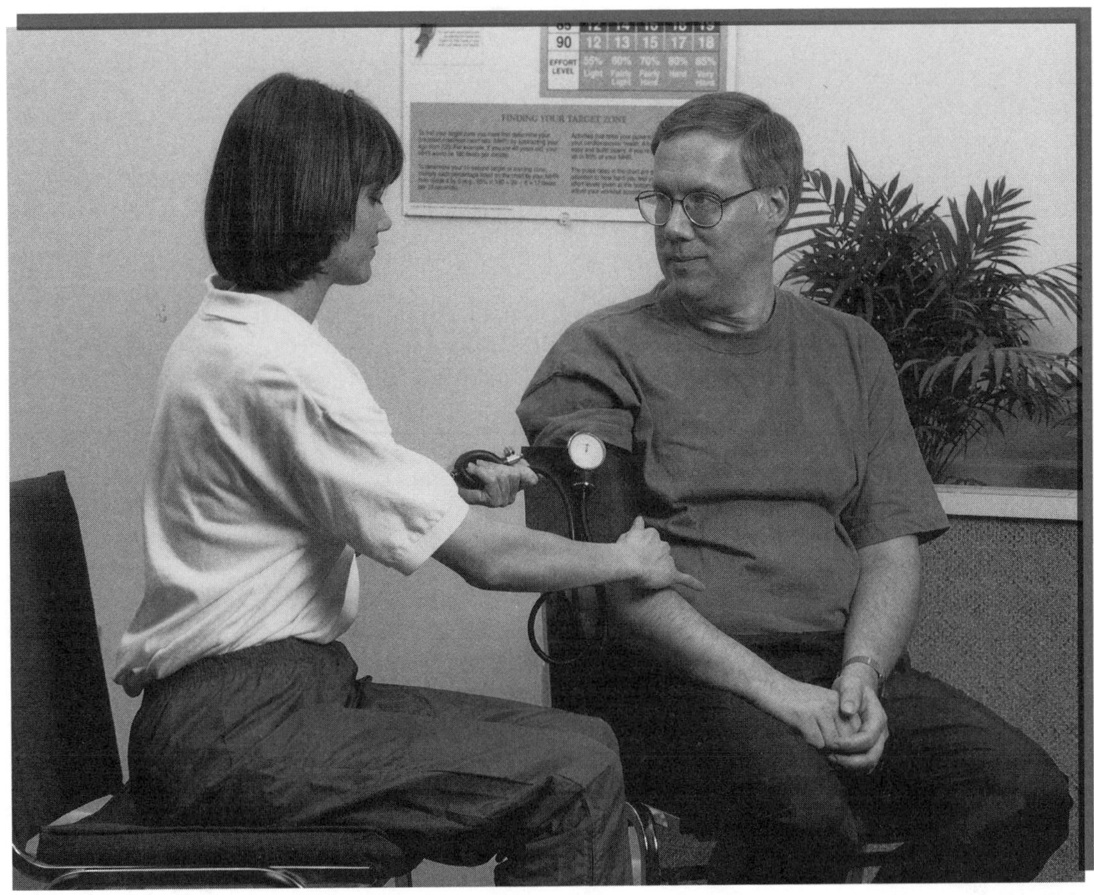

© Chris Brown

The reader will be able to: **OBJECTIVES**

1. Understand the purpose of evaluating the health status of potential fitness participants and identify appropriate instruments for health appraisal.
2. Describe appropriate screening for moderate- and vigorous-intensity exercise.
3. Make recommendations for the type of fitness program participants should develop based on their health status, describe the categories of participants who should receive medical clearance prior to administration of an exercise test or participation in an exercise program, and identify relative and absolute contraindications to exercise testing or participation.
4. List the conditions and test scores that may indicate the need for a supervised program or special attention during exercise.
5. Identify individuals who need educational material.
6. Identify conditions that would require a change in exercise recommendations and describe the signs/symptoms for participants (including special populations) to defer, delay, or terminate the exercise session.

An important responsibility of the health fitness instructor (HFI) or personal fitness trainer (PFT) is to help potential fitness participants determine their current health status. If the person has a major health problem that has been diagnosed and is being treated, then you must rely on guidance from the fitness program director and medical professionals for appropriate fitness programs. If health status has been carefully analyzed by physicians and health professionals and there are no health problems or unhealthy behaviors, then the individual can start or continue a fitness program, making modifications based on their personal interests. Most people, however, are somewhere in between these two extremes. They do not have a known major health problem, but their health status has not been thoroughly checked.

EVALUATING HEALTH STATUS

The HFI or PFT can assist individuals in evaluating their health status by examining five major categories:

- Diagnosed medical problems
- Characteristics that increase the risk of health problems
- Signs or symptoms indicative of health problems
- Lifestyle behaviors related to positive or negative health
- Fitness test results

The health status of the individual is evaluated to provide information to the person concerning health status and healthy and unhealthy behaviors. Health status is also used to make decisions concerning appropriate physical activity recommendations for health and fitness improvement.

Health Status Questionnaire

The Health Status Questionnaire (HSQ) (form 3.1) provides information concerning the first four categories in the list above. Part 1 of the HSQ provides *personal and emergency information* about the individual. You should keep the emergency information readily available in case you need to call the participant's physician or family. Part 2 of the HSQ includes a *medical history* of the participant and her or his family. This information will aid the director of the fitness program in deciding appropriate physical activity and educational programs. Part 3 deals with *behaviors* known to be related to *safety and health*. You might be able to help the participant modify these behaviors for a healthier lifestyle. Part 4 looks at health-related attitudes associated with the healthy life. Individual questions and parts of questions are coded to help the HFI and PFT utilize the information. The key to the codes appears at the end of the HSQ.

Forms and charts are included in the Fitness Participant Handbook, *Fitness Facts* (4). Encourage participants in your fitness program to complete these forms and submit them to you so you can assist them in their programs. (Some of these forms are included in this book for your information and use.)

1 **In Review: Evaluating participants' health status provides the basis for recommended physical activity programs. The HSQ helps appraise medical conditions, characteristics, symptoms, and behaviors.**

Fitness Testing

Testing is the other source of information concerning an individual's health status. Items included in fitness testing are listed in table 3.1. Chapters 6, 9, and 11-13 of this book include detailed recommendations for fitness testing.

People of all ages with varying levels of fitness can be encouraged to engage in moderate-intensity activities without either medical clearance or fitness testing. The walking program found in chapter 17 is a good example of the type of exercise that can be almost universally recommended. The Physical Activity Readiness Questionnaire (PAR-Q) (9) can be used as a simple screening for individuals beginning moderate-intensity exercise. It has been shown to be useful in referring those who need additional medical screening and advice while not excluding the majority of people who will benefit from participation in daily moderate-intensity exercise. The rest of this chapter deals primarily with the screening procedures used for people interested in vigorous-intensity exercise.

The American College of Sports Medicine (ACSM) recommends that all men over 40 years of age and women over 50 years of age have a maximal graded exercise test (GXT), with a physician present, before beginning vigorous-intensity exercise. The maximal GXT, with physician present, is also recommended for those who have a high risk of heart disease. Submaximal tests, without a physician, can be administered by qualified testers to individuals without disease or symptoms to determine cardiorespiratory fitness and to serve as a baseline for exercise prescription. Table 3.2 summarizes the ACSM recommendations (1, table 2-7) concerning who should have medical clearance and submaximal or maximal graded exercise tests prior to participation and who should have medical supervision while taking exercise tests.

The ACSM guidelines are reasonable for people who are planning to begin an exercise program with vigorous intensity, such as jogging, aerobic dance, racquetball, or tennis. There is increasing evidence, however, that regular moderate-intensity activity, such as walking done without any discomfort, has some health benefits with extremely low risk.

Table 3.1 Components of Fitness Testing

Minimum battery	Additional variables
REST	
Heart rate (HR) (beats · min^{-1})	12-lead ECG[a]
Blood pressure (BP) (mmHg)	Blood profile[b]
% fat	Flexibility for specific joints
Waist-to-hip ratio	Pulmonary function
Sit-and-reach (cm)	
SUBMAXIMAL	
HR	ECG
BP	Blood profile
Rating of perceived exertion (RPE)	
MAXIMAL	
BP	$\dot{V}O_2$max
RPE	Blood profile
Time to max (min)	ECG
Functional capacity (METs)	Modified pull-ups (no. up to 25)
Curl-ups (no. up to 35)	

[a]ECG abnormalities are medically evaluated to determine appropriate referral or placement.
[b]Includes total cholesterol, HDL cholesterol, triglycerides, and glucose. See ACSM, 1995 (1), table 3.7, p. 37 for other blood variables.

FORM 3.1

Health Status Questionnaire

Instructions

Complete each question accurately. All information provided is confidential if you choose to submit this form to your fitness instructor.

Part 1. Information about the individual

1. ______________________________ ______________
   Social Security number Date
2. ______________________________ ______________
   Legal name Nickname
3. ______________________________ ______________
   Mailing address Home phone
   ______________________________ ______________
   Business phone
4. *EI* ______________________________ ______________
   Personal physician Phone
   ____
   Address
5. *EI* ______________________________ ______________
   Person to contact in emergency Phone
6. Gender (circle one): Female Male (*RF*)
7. *RF* Date of birth: ______________________________
   Month Day Year
8. Number of hours worked per week: Less than 20 20-40 41-60 Over 60
9. *SLA* More than 25% of time spent on job (circle all that apply)
   Sitting at desk Lifting or carrying loads Standing Walking Driving

Part 2. Medical history

10. *RF* Circle any who died of heart attack before age 50:
    Father Mother Brother Sister Grandparent
11. Date of
    Last medical physical exam: ______________
    Year
    Last physical fitness test: ______________
    Year
12. Circle operations you have had:
    Back *SLA* Heart *MC* Kidney *SLA* Eyes *SLA* Joint *SLA* Neck *SLA*
    Ears *SLA* Hernia *SLA* Lung *SLA* Other ______________________

FORM 3.1

13. Please circle any of the following for which you have been diagnosed or treated by a physician or health professional:

Alcoholism *SEP*
Anemia, sickle cell *SEP*
Anemia, other *SEP*
Asthma *SEP*
Back strain *SLA*
Bleeding trait *SEP*
Bronchitis, chronic *SEP*
Cancer *SEP*
Cirrhosis, liver *MC*
Concussion *MC*
Congenital defect *SEP*
Diabetes *SEP*
Emphysema *SEP*
Epilepsy *SEP*
Eye problems *SLA*
Gout *SLA*
Hearing loss *SLA*
Heart problem *MC*
High blood pressure *RF*
Hypoglycemia *SEP*
Hyperlipidemia *RF*
Infectious mononucleosis *MC*
Kidney problem *MC*
Mental illness *SEP*
Neck strain *SLA*
Obesity *RF*
Phlebitis *MC*
Rheumatoid arthritis *SLA*
Stroke *MC*
Thyroid problem *SEP*
Ulcer *SEP*
Other ________________

14. Circle all medicine taken in last 6 months:

Blood thinner *MC*
Diabetic *SEP*
Digitalis *MC*
Diuretic *MC*
Epilepsy medication *SEP*
Heart rhythm medication *MC*
High blood pressure medication *MC*
Insulin *MC*
Nitroglycerin *MC*
Other ________________

15. Any of these health symptoms that occurs frequently is the basis for medical attention. Circle the number indicating how often you have each of the following:

5 = Very often
4 = Fairly often
3 = Sometimes
2 = Infrequently
1 = Practically never

a. Cough up blood *MC*
1 2 3 4 5

b. Abdominal pain *MC*
1 2 3 4 5

c. Low-back pain *MC*
1 2 3 4 5

d. Leg pain *MC*
1 2 3 4 5

e. Arm or shoulder pain *MC*
1 2 3 4 5

f. Chest pain *RF MC*
1 2 3 4 5

g. Swollen joints *MC*
1 2 3 4 5

h. Feel faint *MC*
1 2 3 4 5

i. Dizziness *MC*
1 2 3 4 5

j. Breathless with slight exertion *MC*
1 2 3 4 5

k. Palpitation or fast heart beat *MC*
1 2 3 4 5

l. Unusual fatigue with normal activity *MC*
1 2 3 4 5

Part 3. Health-related behavior

16. *RF* Do you now smoke? Yes No

17. *RF* If you are a smoker, indicate number smoked per day:

Cigarettes: 40 or more 20-39 10-19 1-9
Cigars or pipes only: 5 or more or any inhaled Less then 5, none inhaled

(continued)

FORM 3.1 *(continued)*

18. *RF* Do you exercise regularly? Yes No
19. How many days per week do you accumulate 30 minutes of moderate activity?

    0 1 2 3 4 5 6 7 days per week
20. How many days per week do you normally spend at least 20 minutes in vigorous exercise?

    0 1 2 3 4 5 6 7 days per week
21. Can you walk 4 miles briskly without fatigue? Yes No
22. Can you jog 3 miles continuously at a moderate pace without discomfort? Yes No
23. Weight now: __________ lb. One year ago: __________ lb. Age 21: __________ lb.

Part 4. Health-related attitudes

24. *RF* These are traits that have been associated with coronary-prone behavior. Circle the number that corresponds to how you feel:

    6 = Strongly agree
    5 = Moderately agree
    4 = Slightly agree
    3 = Slightly disagree
    2 = Moderately disagree
    1 = Strongly disagree

    I am an impatient, time-conscious, hard-driving individual.

    1 2 3 4 5 6
25. List everything not already included on this questionnaire that might cause you problems in a fitness test or fitness program:

Code for Health Status Questionnaire

The following code will help you evaluate the information in the Health Status Questionnaire.

EI = Emergency Information—must be readily available.
MC = Medical Clearance needed—do not allow exercise without physician's permission.
SEP = Special Emergency Procedures needed—do not let participant exercise alone; make sure the person's exercise partner knows what to do in case of an emergency.
RF = Risk Factor for CHD (educational materials and workshops needed).
SLA = Special or Limited Activities may be needed—you may need to include or exclude specific exercises.

OTHER (not marked) = Personal information that may be helpful for files or research.

Physical Activity Readiness Questionnaire

Name of participant ______________________

Date ______________________

PAR Q & YOU

PAR-Q is designed to help you help yourself. Many health benefits are associated with regular exercise, and the completion of PAR-Q is a sensible first step to take if you are planning to increase the amount of physical activity in your life.

For most people physical activity should not pose any problem or hazard. PAR-Q has been designed to identify the small number of adults for whom physical activity might be inappropriate or those who should have medical advice concerning the type of activity most suitable for them.

Common sense is your best guide in answering these few questions. Please read them carefully and check (√) the ☐ YES or ☐ NO opposite the question if it applies to you.

YES	NO	
☐	☐	1. Has your doctor ever said you have heart trouble?
☐	☐	2. Do you frequently have pains in your heart and chest?
☐	☐	3. Do you often feel faint or have spells of severe dizziness?
☐	☐	4. Has a doctor ever said your blood pressure was too high?
☐	☐	5. Has your doctor ever told you that you have a bone or joint problem such as arthritis that has been aggravated by exercise or might be made worse with exercise?
☐	☐	6. Is there a good physical reason not mentioned here why you should not follow an activity program even if you wanted to?
☐	☐	7. Are you over age 65 and not accustomed to vigorous exercise?

If You Answered

YES to one or more questions

If you have not recently done so, consult with your personal physician by telephone or in person BEFORE increasing your physical activity and/or taking a fitness appraisal. Tell your physician what questions you answered YES to on PAR-Q or present your PAR-Q copy.

programs

After medical evaluation, seek advice from your physician as to your suitability for

- unrestricted physical activity starting off easily and progressing gradually;
- restricted or supervised activity to meet your specific needs at least on an initial basis. Check in your community for special programs or services.

NO to all questions

If you answered PAR-Q accurately, you have reasonable assurance of your present suitability for

- A GRADUATED EXERCISE PROGRAM—a gradual increase in proper exercise promotes good fitness development while minimizing or eliminating discomfort.
- A FITNESS APPRAISAL—Canadian Standardized Test of Fitness (CSTF).

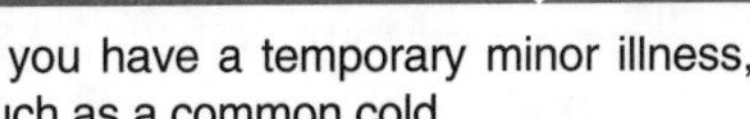

postpone

If you have a temporary minor illness, such as a common cold.

Developed by the British Columbia Ministry of Health. Conceptualized and compared by the Multidisciplinary Advisory Board on Exercise (MABE).

Reference PAR-Q Validation Report British Columbia Ministry of Health 1978.
Produced by the British Columbia Ministry of Health and The Department of National Health and Welfare.

Table 3.2 ACSM Recommendations for (A) Medical Examination and Exercise Testing Prior to Participation and (B) Physician Supervision of Exercise Tests

A. Medical examination and clinical exercise test recommended prior to:

	Apparently healthy		Increased risk*		Known disease†
	Younger‡	Older	No symptoms	Symptoms	
Moderate exercise§	No‖	No	No	Yes	Yes
Vigorous exercise¶	No	Yes#	Yes	Yes	Yes

B. Physician supervision recommended during exercise test:

	Apparently healthy		Increased risk*		Known disease†
	Younger‡	Older	No symptoms	Symptoms	
Submaximal testing	No‖	No	No	Yes	Yes
Maximal testing	No	Yes#	Yes	Yes	Yes

*People with two or more risk factors or one or more signs or symptoms.
†People with known cardiac, pulmonary, or metabolic disease.
‡Younger implies ≤ 40 years for men, ≤ 50 years for women.
§Moderate exercise as defined by an intensity of 40% to 60% $\dot{V}O_2max$; if intensity is uncertain, moderate exercise may alternately be defined as an intensity well within the individual's current capacity, one which can be comfortably sustained for a prolonged period of time, that is, 60 min, which has a gradual initiation and progression, and is generally noncompetitive.
‖A "No" response means that an item is deemed "not necessary." The "No" response does not mean that the item should not be done.
¶Vigorous exercise is defined as exercise intense enough to represent a substantial cardiorespiratory challenge or if it results in fatigue within 20 min.
#A "Yes" response means that an item is recommended. For physician supervision, this suggests that a physician is in close proximity and readily available should there be an emergent need.
Reprinted from American College of Sports Medicine 1995.

Regular medical examinations are encouraged for everyone. Obviously, seeing a physician is appropriate whenever there are special medical problems. Table 3.3 presents guidelines for the frequency of medical examinations recommended by the National Conference on Preventive Medicine (8).

2 **In Review:** **Moderate-intensity exercise can be recommended for anyone who has self-screened with the PAR-Q. All aspects of health status—medical problems, health-related characteristics, signs, symptoms, behaviors, and fitness tests—should be evaluated prior to vigorous-intensity exercise. Graded exercise tests are recommended as the first part of a fitness program.**

Table 3.3 Recommended Frequency of Medical Exams

Age	Frequency of medical examination
0 to 1	At least 4 times
2, 5, 8, 15, 18, 25	At each age listed
35 to 65	Every 5 years
Over 65	Every 2 years

MAKING DECISIONS BASED ON HEALTH STATUS

Health status information, informed consent of the potential participant, and the goals and interests of the individual are all part of making decisions about appropriate physical activities. The following guidelines based on health status must be tempered with consideration of your interaction with participants regarding their long-term goals and interests. We discuss the decision-making process in terms of a structured fitness program/center; however, the same guidelines can be used by PFTs working with individuals.

Making Fitness Program Decisions

A fitness program might not use all of the items on the HSQ—the program director should decide what items are relevant for a specific fitness program. Each item on the HSQ is coded to help you identify emergency information and the items that are related to major health problems or require special attention (see HSQ Code). The health status form and fitness testing allow the fitness program director to recommend one of the following actions concerning the person's request to enter a fitness program:

- Denial of request for entry to fitness program and/or immediate referral for medical attention
- Admission to one of the following fitness programs:

  Medically supervised exercise

  Exercise carefully prescribed and supervised by an exercise leader

  Vigorous-intensity exercise

  Any unsupervised physical activity
- Educational information, workshops, or professional help

The fitness director needs to decide whether a potential fitness participant should get medical clearance before beginning a fitness program. The standards in this area are changing. In the 1960s and 1970s it was recommended that everyone get a complete medical examination prior to beginning a fitness program. Three factors, however, have caused that standard to change. First, it is increasingly recognized that being active is healthier than being inactive. Second, there is increasing evidence that beginning a good fitness program involves a very low risk of health problems for the vast majority of people. And third, the expense of time and money cannot be justified for healthy individuals—medical examinations are needed more for individuals with known or suspected health problems.

Each fitness program should determine its policy with regard to medical clearance and testing before beginning an exercise program. The ACSM recommendations (1) (table 3.2) can serve as guidelines for the development of policy.

Guidelines for Determining Necessary Supervision

The box on pages 40-41 summarizes the criteria for determining the level of supervision needed by an individual in or beginning a physical activity program. This section discusses the criteria more thoroughly. Selecting specific test scores as an indication of high, moderate, or low risk is somewhat arbitrary. In most cases, it would be more accurate to view the variable as going from low to high risk. For example, it is better to have lower total cholesterol (the sum of all forms of cholesterol). Although 240 mg/dl has been set as a high-risk level, a person with 239 mg/dl is not really different from someone with 242 mg/dl. Nor is a person with 202 mg/dl really different from someone with 198 mg/dl, even though 200 mg/dl is set as a target goal. We should encourage everyone to decrease their total cholesterol; as it decreases, they will have lower risk. There is nothing magical about getting below 240 mg/dl or 200 mg/dl—these are only goals that have been set along the continuum of high to low risk.

Note that the values listed for medical referral and for supervised programs are guidelines to be used along with other information by the individual and fitness program director. For example, the risk of the same total cholesterol would be viewed differently for people with different levels of HDL-C (high-density lipoprotein cholesterol). Some of the variables may be influenced by pretest activities and reaction to the testing situation itself (especially in the person who is not accustomed to being tested). Borderline scores, especially at rest and during light work, should be replicated before medical referral. For example, if a high resting heart rate or blood pressure is measured, it may have been due to the participant having eaten, smoked, or participated in physical exercise just before the test. Was the person anxious about taking the test itself? Were there unusual conditions during the test (e.g., lots of people, noise)? The individual should relax for a few minutes, be reassured about the purpose and safety of the test, and then be measured again. On the other hand, a test session might be scheduled for another day. If the questionable test result is repeated, the program director may refer that individual to a physician.

Conditions and Test Score Criteria for Physical Activity Decisions

Basis for medical referral

Conditions

Breathlessness with slight exertion
Cirrhosis
Concussion
Cough up blood
Current medication for heart, blood pressure, or diabetes
Faintness or dizziness
Heart operation, disease, or problem
Pain in the abdomen, leg, arm, shoulder, or chest
Phlebitis
Stroke
Swollen joints

Test scores[a]

Resting HR > 100 bpm
Resting SBP > 160 mmHg
Resting DBP > 100 mmHg
% fat > 40 female; > 30 male
Cholesterol > 240 mg/dl
Cholesterol/HDL > 5
Triglycerides > 200 mg/dl
Fasting glucose > 120 mg/dl
Vital cap < 75% predicted
FEV_1 < 75%

Basis for a supervised program

Conditions (currently under control)[b]

Alcoholism
Allergy
Anemia
Asthma
Bleeding trait
Bronchitis
Cancer
Colitis
Diabetes
Emphysema
Epilepsy
Hypoglycemia
Mental illness
Peptic ulcer
Pregnancy
Thyroid problem

Test scores[c]

Hypertension 140-155/90-95 mmHg
Hyperlipidemia (cholesterol) 240-255 mg/dl
Cholesterol/HDL 4.5-4.8
Obesity 32%-38% female; 25%-28% male
Waist-to-hip ratio > 0.8 female; > 0.9 male
Smoking > 20 cigarettes/day
Exercise < 1.5 hr/week at or above moderate intensity

Basis for special attention

Conditions

Arthritis
Back, eye, joint, lung, or neck operations
Eye problems
Gout
Hearing loss
Hernia
Lengthy time spent driving, lifting, sitting, or standing
Low-back pain

Test scores

Values of risk factors approaching those in supervised programs	% fat < 15% or > 30% females; < 6% or > 25% males[d]
Any of the reasons for stopping a maximal test that occur at light to moderate work	Curl-ups < 10
Max RPE < 5 (15 on 6-20 scale)	Sit-and-reach < 15 cm
Max METs < 8	Modified pull-ups < 5
Max $\dot{V}O_2$ < 30	Push-ups < 10

Note. Any condition or test value that causes the person or the HFI to be concerned for the person's health or safety is the basis for medical referral. FEV_1 = forced expiratory volume in 1 s; RPE = rating of perceived exertion.

[a]Any of these individual scores would be the basis for referral. A person might also be referred if more than one test score approached these values.

[b]Severe or uncontrolled levels should be referred for medical attention.

[c]Persons with higher scores should be referred for medical attention.

[d]Participants who have either too little fat or too much fat may have health problems that need special attention. If there is any question, refer them to the program director.

There may be other factors that would cause a person with the characteristics we have listed under "supervised" programs to be medically referred (e.g., multiple risk factors close to the referral value). Or the medical consultant may recommend that someone in our "referral" category be in the supervised program, based on a recent medical examination or conversation with the personal physician. Programs with excellent and accessible medical and emergency personnel may want to use higher values for referral than a program that is isolated from medical and emergency facilities. It is recommended that each program, in consultation with its medical advisors, establish its own standards.

Medical Referral

All people indicating illness, characteristics, or symptoms coded MC (medical clearance) in the HSQ are referred to appropriate medical personnel. With permission of the appropriate physician, the individual can be placed in a medically supervised, or HFI-supervised, fitness program. The items that fall into those categories, as well as the test scores from the fitness tests that would be the basis for medical referral, are shown in the box on pages 40-41.

The values selected for medical referral or supervised programs are somewhat arbitrary, but they are based on the recommendations of experts in these areas. All of the variables (with the exception of high heart rate) have been listed as risk factors for CHD at these levels. The values for medical referral are considered very high (with substantial risk of CHD). The "minimal" level indicating problems in these areas (with greater risk of CHD than normal values) are reflected in our values for supervised programs.

A high resting heart rate (HR) indicates severe stress, which may have a physical or emotional base. Extreme amounts of fat put the individual at high risk for a variety of health problems (see chapter 9). A high level of serum glucose is related to diabetes. High blood pressure has been the subject of numerous reports and conferences. For example, the fifth report of the Joint Committee on Detection, Evaluation, and Treatment of High Blood Pressure (5) identifies mild, moderate, and severe hypertension as systolic blood pressure of 140, 160, or 180 mmHg, respectively; with diastolic blood pressure of 90, 100, or 110 mmHg as mild, moderate, or severe hypertension, respectively. These values are based on repeat measurements.

The role of serum lipids in the atherosclerotic process has been extensively investigated. Cholesterol and triglycerides are carried in the blood stream in lipoproteins, with the following subdivisions:

- **Very low-density lipoproteins (VLDL)**—High levels are a high risk of CHD.
- **Low-density lipoprotein cholesterol (LDL-C)**—This is the form of cholesterol that is responsible for the buildup of plaque in the inner walls of the arteries (atherosclerosis). Thus, high levels of LDL-C are related to a high risk of CHD.
- **High-density lipoprotein cholesterol (HDL-C)**—This form of cholesterol protects against the development of CHD, in that it helps transport cholesterol to the liver, where it is eliminated. Thus, *low* levels of HDL-C are related to a high risk of CHD.
- **Total cholesterol**—Because LDL-C is usually the primary factor in the total amount, a high level of total cholesterol is also a risk factor for CHD.
- **Total cholesterol/HDL-C ratio**—High ratios of total cholesterol to HDL-C are indicative of a high risk of CHD.

The second report of the National Cholesterol Education Program (3) selected 200 mg/dl and below as desirable total cholesterol, with 240 mg/dl and higher as high risk. LDL-C levels 160 mg/dl and over are high risk, with 130 mg/dl and below being low risk. HDL-C values 35 mg/dl and below are considered a high risk for CHD. Values of 5 or over for the total cholesterol/HDL-C ratio are high risk, whereas values less than 3.5 are low risk (7). In addition, the ACSM (1) lists HDL-C greater than 60 mg/dl (1.6 mmol/L) as a *negative* risk factor for CHD.

Pulmonary function is frequently evaluated as a part of the screening aspect of a fitness program. Although many of these variables change little during a typical fitness program, the HFI or PFT can provide a service to participants by suggesting that people with low values participate in additional testing. The following aspects of pulmonary function should be tested:

- **Vital capacity (VC)**—A person whose VC is less than 75% of the value predicted for her or his age, gender, and height should be referred to a physician for further testing.
- **Forced expiratory volume in 1 s (FEV_1)**—A person who can expel less than 75% of his or her VC in 1 s should be referred to a physician. See ACSM (1) for evaluation of pulmonary function tests.

3 **In Review: Based on evaluation of their health status, HFIs can advise people to seek medical attention, begin moderate-intensity exercise, or participate in vigorous-intensity exercise with or without supervision. The items listed in the box on pages 40-41 for medical referral or supervised programs are guidelines to be used with other information on the individual in making a decision concerning safe and appropriate physical activity. Individuals with medical conditions or characteristics, symptoms, behaviors, or test scores that place them at a high risk for major health problems should have medical clearance before increasing their level of physical activity.**

Supervised Program

The conditions and test scores listed in the box on pages 40-41 may be the basis for medical referral if they are severe; however, individuals with mild or moderate levels can participate in moderate-intensity exercise or in carefully supervised fitness programs. A person indicating items on the HSQ coded SEP (special emergency procedure) or with risk factors for CHD (coded RF) can be placed in a carefully supervised fitness program, with the necessary emergency procedures readily available, or participate in moderate-intensity exercise with education about what to do in case of an emergency. It is important that the program director determine whether any of the participants have these or other conditions that might affect their ability to exercise.

Numerous conditions and fitness test scores call for special or limited activities. Your recommended adaptation of activities will be based on common sense regarding the condition, talking with the participant about how to deal with the situation, and consulting with the fitness director or physician about appropriate limitations. You should encourage these individuals to include special activities aimed at improving the fitness component(s) for which they obtained the low score(s).

Although we recommend that all fitness participants be screened prior to participation in a vigorous-intensity exercise program, we know that exercise leaders are often in a position to lead vigorous-intensity exercise (such as an aerobic dance class) for people who have not been screened. A simple checklist (see form 3.3, Checklist for Walk-In, Vigorous-Intensity Exercisers) can be done either by each individual prior to exercise (in writing or orally), or by the exercise leader asking for answers from the group as the first part of the exercise session.

We suggest that you refer all those who answer yes to any of these questions to the director of the fitness program prior to exercise. The director should decide whether to make a medical referral, recommend moderate-intensity exercise, or allow participation in the vigorcus-intensity supervised program. For example, individuals who have been active in the past without problems may be allowed in the exercise program even if they have high cholesterol or smoke, whereas previously sedentary individuals with the same risk factors might be directed to a walking and stretching program.

4 **In Review: Individuals with moderate risk of major health problems or conditions that require special attention or emergency procedures may be directed to physical activities under supervision by a qualified instructor or medical personnel. Exercise leaders who have unevaluated individuals in a group program should include some screening as part of the class.**

Unsupervised Program

People without any of the problems coded under MC, SEP, or RF in the HSQ can participate in an **unsupervised program** and be admitted to any of the fitness activities offered by a fitness center. If they have not been active in the past few months, it is recommended that they begin with moderate-intensity activities; but they will be able to progress quickly to other activities of interest and greater intensity.

Education

The HSQ and fitness test results also provide the fitness leader with information about needed education and workshops. All people with risk factors (RF) for CHD should be given information about their increased risk. Sufficient evidence allows you to indicate areas of potential health problems, assist individuals in becoming aware of the risk characteristics that cannot be changed, and help people to change those health-related behaviors that can be modified. Chapter 20 provides information to assist the fitness leader in using behavior modification for desired behavior changes. There are also a number of questions on the HSQ indicating a need for education in terms of exercise, nutrition, alcohol, smoking, or stress management. This information will be useful for the program director in deciding what workshops and educational materials should be offered to the participants.

In Review: Individuals who have moderate risk of CHD, conditions that might be affected by exercise, or borderline fitness scores should receive education about their problems and know what to do in emergencies.

CHANGE OF HEALTH/ FITNESS STATUS

This chapter has dealt with the initial screenings and the resulting decisions concerning appropriate fitness programs. The HFI and PFT need to understand that people who are in exercise programs may have changes in their health/fitness status that require a change in their program. One of the purposes of periodic testing is to determine whether people should be reassigned to different programs.

very low-density lipoproteins (VLDL) — Mainly triglycerides. A secondary risk factor for CHD.

low-density lipoprotein cholesterol (LDL-C) — A plasma protein containing relatively more cholesterol and triglycerides and less protein.

high-density lipoprotein cholesterol (HDL-C) — A plasma lipid-protein complex containing relatively more protein and less cholesterol and triglycerides.

total cholesterol — The sum of all forms of cholesterol.

total cholesterol/HDL-C ratio — One of the best ways to determine risk of CHD in terms of cholesterol.

vital capacity (VC) — The amount of air that can be expelled from the lungs after a maximal inspiration.

forced expiratory volume in 1 s (FEV_1) — The ratio of the volume of air expelled in 1 s compared to the total VC.

unsupervised program — A group of fitness activities conducted without qualified fitness personnel. For people with a low risk of health problems.

FORM 3.3

Checklist for Walk-In, Vigorous-Intensity Exercisers

_______ Yes	_______ No	Have, or have had, cardiovascular disease (i.e., heart problems)
_______ Yes	_______ No	Have pains or pressure in the left or midchest area, neck, or left shoulder or arm at rest or in response to exertion
_______ Yes	_______ No	Often feel faint or have spells of dizziness
_______ Yes	_______ No	Experience extreme breathlessness after mild exercise
_______ Yes	_______ No	Have high blood pressure
_______ Yes	_______ No	Have high cholesterol
_______ Yes	_______ No	Smoke more than a pack of cigarettes a day
_______ Yes	_______ No	Am over 60 years of age and not accustomed to vigorous exercise
_______ Yes	_______ No	Have bone or joint problems that would interfere with or be aggravated by exercise
_______ Yes	_______ No	Have two or more of the following (check, which ones): a. Family history of premature coronary heart disease b. Obesity c. Type A behavior with stressful occupation and/or lifestyle d. Diabetes
_______ Yes	_______ No	Have a medical condition not mentioned here that might need special attention in an exercise program
_______ Yes	_______ No	Taking medication for a cardiorespiratory problem

It is common for individuals to make improvements that will safely allow additional exercise options as part of their fitness programs. In other cases, negative changes might occur that need your attention. For example, if an individual in an unsupervised program develops chronic symptoms such as pain in the chest or legs during exercise, he or she should be referred to a physician, retested, or placed in the supervised program, depending on the severity of the problem. Temporary symptoms such as unusual fatigue may suggest a modification of the exercise (e.g., lowering the arms to lower heart rate) or a temporary deferment of the exercise session.

There are reasons to discontinue a vigorous-intensity exercise program, including severe psychological, medical, or drug- or alcohol-abuse problems that are not responding to therapy, or problems that are aggravated by activity (6).

There are other reasons to temporarily defer exercise, including excessive heat, humidity, or pollution; sunburn; overindulgence in food, alcohol, stimulating beverages, or drugs such as decongestants, bronchodilators, or atropine; dehydration; or anything that causes unusual discomfort with exercise. Exercise should be deferred with major changes in resting blood pressure or emotional problems (adapted from 2 and 6).

6 **In Review: The HFI should be alert to temporary or chronic conditions, such as the ones discussed in this section, that will change an individual's health status, resulting in an increase or decrease in exercise options, a postponement of exercise, a reevaluation of the degree of supervision needed during exercise, or a medical referral.**

Case Studies

You can check your answers by referring to Appendix A.

3.1

You are teaching an exercise-to-music class open to the public. Everyone in the class answered no to all the questions on the checklist for walk-in, vigorous-intensity exercisers, except for one obese woman who answered that she becomes breathless after mild exercise. When you talk to her, it is obvious that she does not know her blood pressure or cholesterol levels. She has never done any fitness or sport activities and cannot climb a flight of stairs or walk two blocks without getting out of breath. She has been reading about the importance of exercise and decided that she should become active. What advice would you give her?

3.2

An African-American male letter carrier for the post office, age 42, has just signed up for the fitness program. He appears to be a little nervous. According to his HSQ, he can engage in unsupervised exercise. You are checking his resting HR and BP prior to a GXT and measure HR = 110 and BP = 180/86. What would you do?

3.3

John is a 50-year-old white male, and is employed as an executive with a large computer firm. He is responsible for the marketing of new computer systems in a very competitive environment. He is married and has three children, ages 14, 18, and 22. He feels the financial pressures associated with college bills, and the need to keep up with the neighbors. His father died of a heart attack last year at age 72; his mother is 70 and suffered a stroke 3 months after her husband's death. John smokes a pack of cigarettes a day and, recently, he experienced dizziness when climbing stairs. He decided to get a physical exam. The following values were obtained: resting BP = 148/96 mmHg; total cholesterol = 198 mg/dl; HDL-C = 25 mg/dl; glucose = 90 mg/dl; ht = 70 in.; wt = 198 lb; % fat = 32%.

a. List his risk factors.
b. What kind of nonpharmacological intervention programs do you think his physician might recommend?

Source List

1. American College of Sports Medicine (1995)
2. American Heart Association (1987a)
3. Expert Panel on Detection, Evaluation, and Treatment of High Blood Cholesterol in Adults (1993)
4. Franks & Howley (1989a)
5. Joint Committee on Detection, Evaluation, and Treatment of High Blood Pressure (1993)
6. Painter & Haskell (1988)
7. Pollock & Wilmore (1990)
8. Sharkey (1990)
9. Shephard (1988)

PART

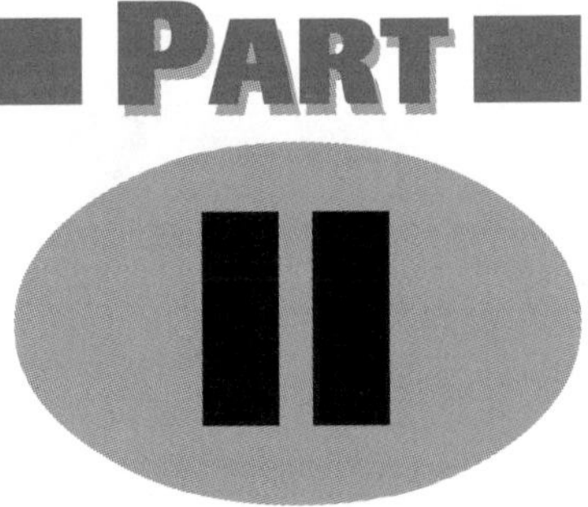

Scientific Foundations of Physical Activity and Fitness

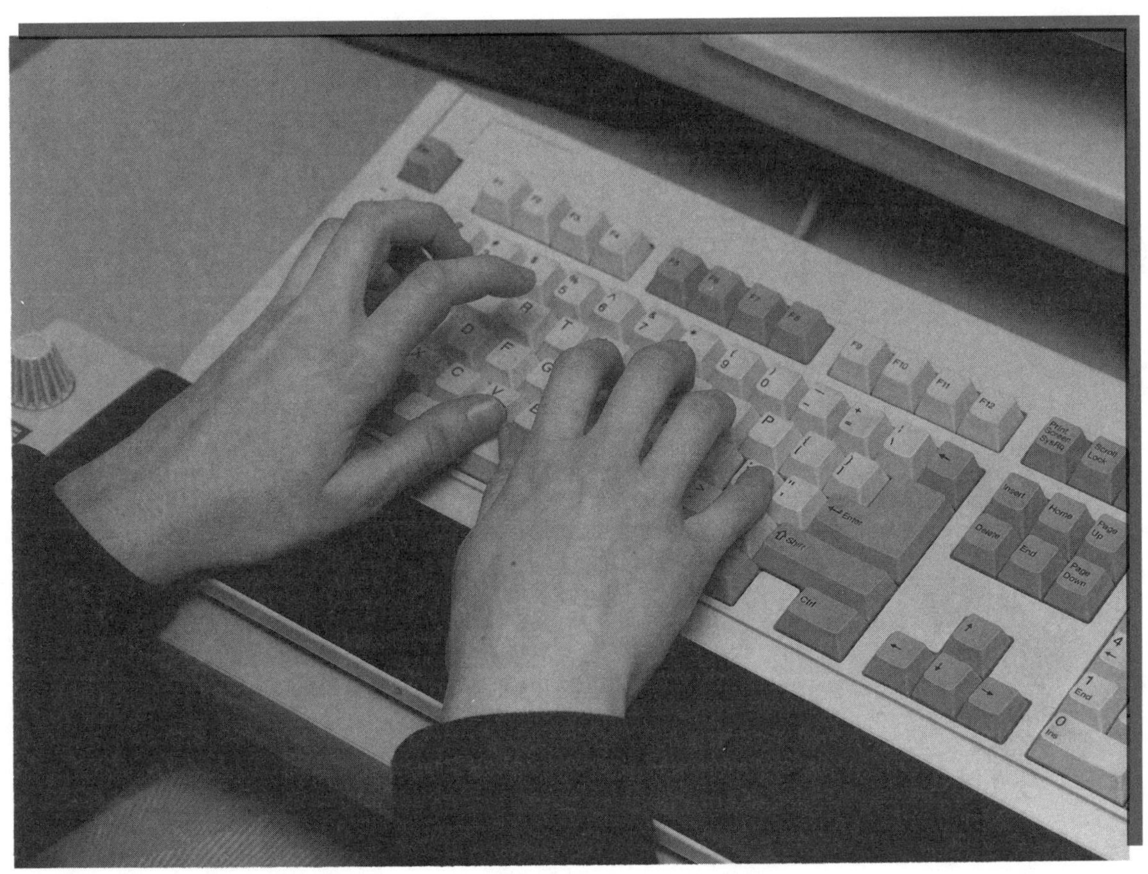

Part II provides the basic scientific foundation for understanding the structure and function of the human body, how to measure and evaluate fitness levels, and how to determine energy expenditure. Chapter 4 covers the basic concepts of energy, muscle function, and the physiological response to acute and chronic physical activity. Differences due to gender, type of exercise, and temperature are described. Chapter 5 reviews the bones, joints, and muscles of the body and how they are used biomechanically in common physical activities. Chapter 6 describes evaluation concepts and how they can be applied to fitness testing. Specific instructions are given for calibrating common exercise equipment. Chapter 7 provides the basis for determining the energy expenditure of a variety of physical activities.

CHAPTER 4

Exercise Physiology

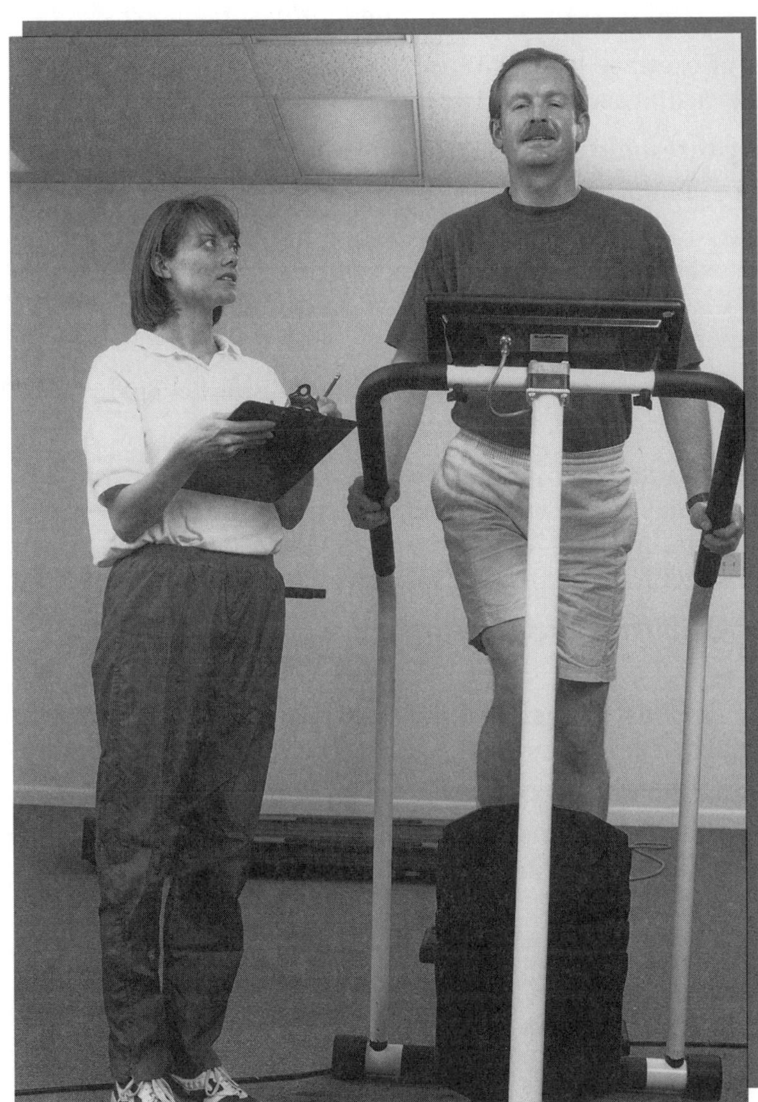

© Chris Brown

The reader will be able to:

OBJECTIVES

1. Indicate the methods by which muscle produces energy aerobically and anaerobically and evaluate the importance of each type of energy production in fitness and sport activities.
2. Describe the structure of skeletal muscle and the sliding-filament theory of muscle contraction.
3. Describe the power, speed, endurance, and metabolism of the different types of muscle fibers.
4. Describe tension development in terms of twitch, summation, and tetanus, and describe the role of recruitment of muscle fiber types in exercise of increasing intensities.
5. Describe the various fuels for muscle work and the effect of exercise intensity and duration on the respiratory exchange ratio.
6. Describe the means by which ATP is supplied to the muscle during the transition from rest to steady-state work and the effects of training on those responses.
7. Describe the effect of types of exercise tests, training, heredity, gender, age, altitude, carbon monoxide, and cardiovascular and pulmonary diseases on $\dot{V}O_2$max.
8. Describe how the ventilatory threshold and the lactate threshold are indicators of fitness as well as predictors of performance in endurance events.
9. Explain the changes in heart rate, stroke volume, cardiac output, and oxygen extraction during a graded exercise test and the effect of training on those responses. Link the variation in $\dot{V}O_2$max in the population to differences in maximal cardiac output and oxygen extraction.
10. Describe the changes in systolic blood pressure and the double product during a graded exercise test and how they differ for arm and leg work.
11. Summarize the effects of endurance training on muscle, metabolic and cardiovascular responses to submaximal work, and $\dot{V}O_2$max. Describe the effect of reduced training or cessation of training on $\dot{V}O_2$max, and the degree to which endurance training effects are specific to the muscles involved in the training.
12. Describe how men and women differ in their cardiovascular responses to graded exercise.
13. Contrast the cardiovascular responses measured during dynamic exercise with those measured during isometric exercise or heavy-resistance training exercises.
14. Contrast the importance of the different mechanisms for heat loss during heavy exercise and during submaximal exercise in a hot environment. Describe the effect of training in a hot and humid environment on heat tolerance.

Health fitness instructors (HFIs) and personal fitness trainers (PFTs) need to know the basic aspects of exercise physiology in order to prescribe appropriate activities, deal with weight loss concerns, and explain to participants what happens as a result of training or when exercise is done in a hot and humid environment. This chapter can't possibly cover the extensive detail found in an exercise physiology text; instead we summarize major topics and, where possible, apply the discussion to exercise testing and exercise prescription. We refer the interested reader to the exercise physiology texts listed at the end of this chapter (2, 6, 20, 39, 46, 61).

RELATIONSHIP OF ENERGY AND WORK

Energy is what makes a body go. Several kinds of energy exist in biological systems: electrical energy in nerves and muscles; chemical energy in the synthesis of molecules; mechanical energy in the contraction of a muscle to move an object; and thermal energy, derived from all of these processes, that helps to maintain body temperature. The ultimate source of the energy for biological systems is the sun. The radiant energy from the sun is captured by plants and used to convert simple atoms and molecules into carbohydrates, fats, and proteins. The sun's energy is trapped within the chemical bonds of these food molecules.

For the cells to use this energy, the foodstuffs must be broken down in a manner that conserves most of the energy contained in the bonds of the carbohydrates, fats, and proteins. In addition, the final product must be in a form that can be used by the cell—adenosine triphosphate, or ATP. Cells use ATP as the primary energy source for biological work, whether electrical, mechanical, or chemical. ATP is a molecule that has three phosphates linked together by high-energy bonds. When the bond between the phosphates is broken, energy is released and may be used by the cell. At this point the ATP has been reduced to a lower energy state: adenosine diphosphate (ADP) and inorganic phosphate (P_i).

$$ATP \rightarrow ADP + P_i + \text{energy for work}$$

When a muscle is doing work, ATP is constantly being broken down to ADP and P_i. The ATP must be replaced as fast as it is being used if the muscle is to continue to generate force. The muscle cell has a great capacity to replace ATP under a wide variety of circumstances, from a short, quick dash to a marathon. Edington and Edgerton (16) devised a logical approach to this topic of supplying energy for muscle contraction. They divided the energy sources into immediate, short-term, and long-term sources of ATP (energy).

Immediate Sources of Energy

The very limited amount of ATP stored in a muscle might meet the energy demands of a maximal effort lasting about 1 s. **Creatine phosphate (CP)**, another high-energy phosphate molecule stored in the muscle, is the most important immediate source of energy. CP can donate its phosphate molecule (and the energy therein) to ADP to make ATP, allowing the muscle to continue to develop force.

$$CP + ADP \rightarrow ATP + C$$

This reaction takes place as fast as the muscle forms ADP. Unfortunately, the CP store in muscle lasts only 3 to 5 s when the muscle is working maximally. This process does not require oxygen and is one of the **anaerobic** (without oxygen) mechanisms for producing ATP. CP would be the primary source of ATP during a shot put, a vertical jump, or the first seconds of a sprint.

Short-Term Sources of Energy

As the muscle store of CP decreases, the cell begins to break down muscle glycogen (the muscle glucose [a simple sugar] store) to produce ATP at a very high rate. This process is called **glycolysis**, and it does not require oxygen (like the breakdown of CP, it too is an anaerobic process).

creatine phosphate (CP) — A high-energy phosphate compound that represents the primary immediate anaerobic source of ATP at the onset of exercise. Important in all-out activities lasting a few seconds.

anaerobic — Energy supplied without oxygen, causing an oxygen debt. Creatine phosphate and glycolysis supply ATP when oxygen is not present.

glycolysis — The metabolic pathway producing ATP from the anaerobic breakdown of glucose. The short-term source of ATP that is important in all-out activities lasting less than 2 min.

Muscle glycogen → 2 lactic acid + 3 ATP

Glycolysis allows the muscle to continue doing intense work but only for a limited period of time. An end product of glycolysis is lactic acid; as exercise continues, lactic acid accumulates in the muscle cells and the blood. This accumulation of acid in the muscle slows down the rate at which the glycogen can be broken down and may actually interfere with the mechanism involved in muscle contraction. Supplying ATP via glycolysis has its obvious shortcomings, but it does allow a person to run at high rates of speed for short distances. This short-term source of energy is of primary importance in events involving maximal work of about 2 or 3 min.

Long-Term Sources of Energy

The long-term source of energy involves the production of ATP from a variety of fuels, but this method requires the utilization of oxygen (it is **aerobic**). The primary fuels include muscle glycogen, blood glucose, plasma free fatty acids, and intramuscular fats. These molecules are broken down so they can transfer the energy contained in their chemical bonds to a site in the cell where ATP is synthesized. Most of these reactions occur in the **mitochondria** of the cell, where oxygen is used.

Carbohydrates and fats + O_2 → ATP

ATP production via aerobic mechanisms is slower than from the immediate and short-term sources of energy, and during submaximal work it may be 2 or 3 min before the ATP needs of the cell are completely met by this aerobic process. One reason for this lag is the time it takes for the heart to increase the delivery of oxygen-enriched blood to the muscles at the rate needed to meet the ATP demands of the muscle. The aerobic production of ATP is the primary means of supplying energy to the muscle in maximal work lasting more than 2 to 3 min and for all types of submaximal work.

Interaction of Exercise Intensity, Duration, and Energy Production

The proportion of energy coming from the anaerobic sources (immediate and short-term energy) is very much influenced by the intensity and duration of the activity. Figure 4.1 shows that during an all-out activity lasting less than 1 min (e.g., a 400-m dash), the muscles obtain most of the ATP from anaerobic sources. In a 2- to 3-min maximal effort, approximately 50% of the energy comes from anaerobic sources and 50% comes from aerobic sources; in a 10-min maximal effort, the anaerobic component drops to 15%. Thus the anaerobic component is considerably less than 15% in a typical submaximal training session.

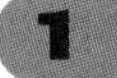

In Review: ATP is supplied at a high rate by the anaerobic processes: creatine phosphate breakdown and glycolysis. Anaerobic energy production is important in short explosive events (e.g., shot put) and in athletic competitions requiring maximal effort for less than 3 min. ATP is supplied during prolonged exercise by the aerobic metabolism of carbohydrates and fats in the mitochondria of the muscle. This is the primary means of supplying energy to the muscle in maximal work lasting more than 2 to 3 min and all submaximal work.

UNDERSTANDING MUSCLE STRUCTURE AND FUNCTION

Exercise means movement, and movement requires muscle action. To discuss human physiology related to exercise and endurance training, we must start with skeletal muscle, the tissue that converts the chemical energy of adenosine triphosphate (ATP) to mechanical

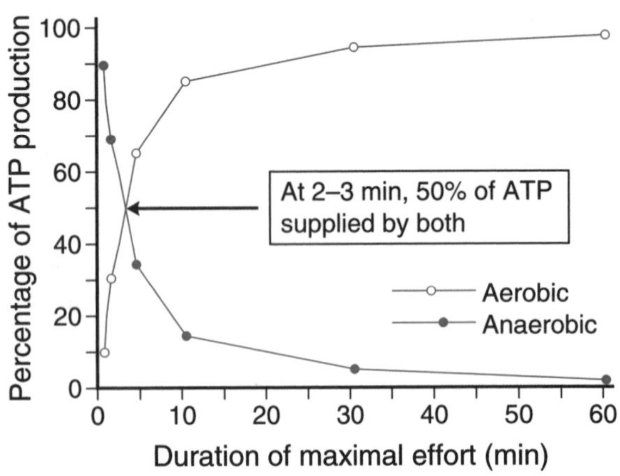

FIGURE 4.1 Percentage of contribution to total energy supply during maximal work of various durations (45).

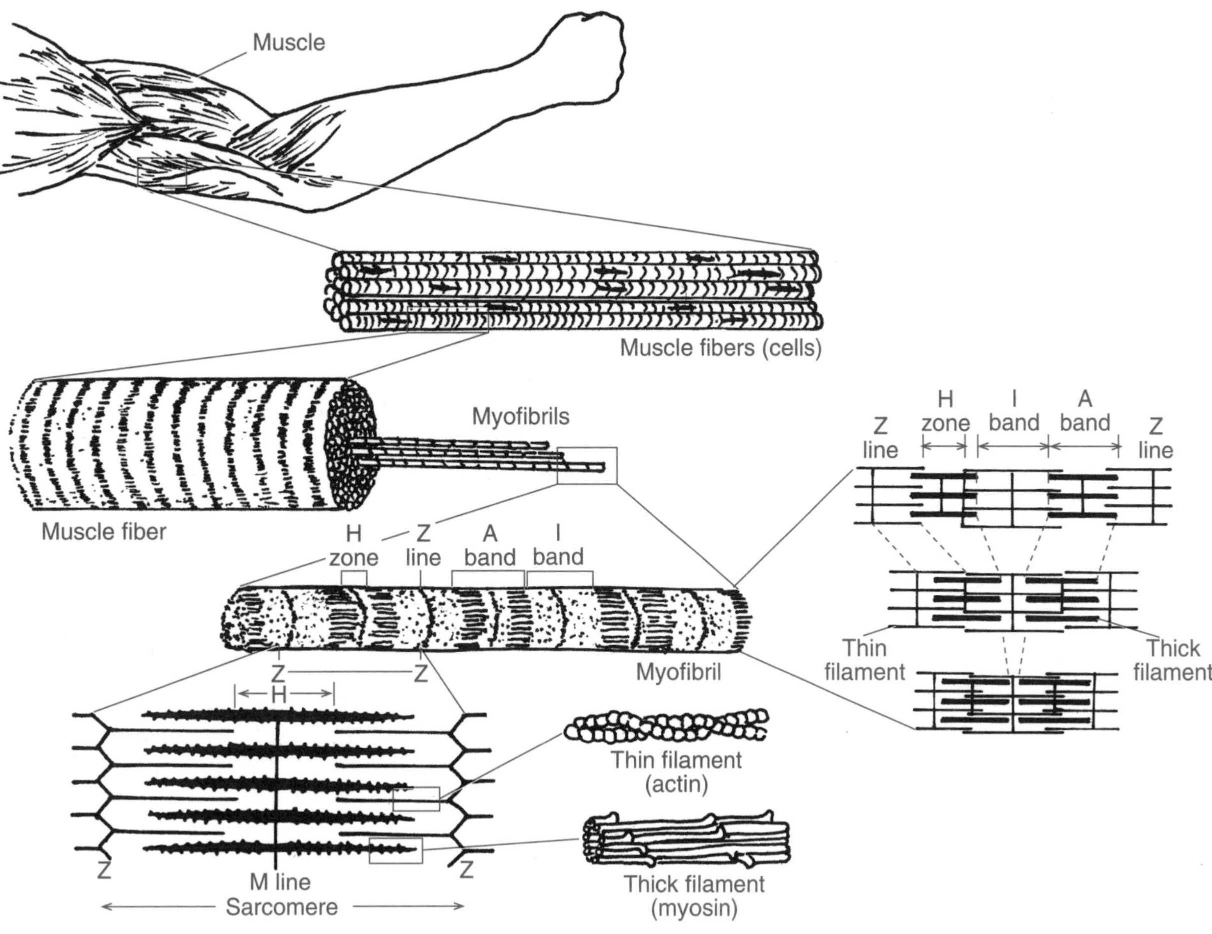

FIGURE 4.2 Levels of fibrillar organization within a skeletal muscle, and changes in filament alignment and banding pattern in a myofibril during shortening.
Reprinted, by permission of McGraw-Hill, from Vander, Sherman, and Luciano, 1980, *Human physiology (3rd ed.)*.

work. How does a muscle do this? We begin with a presentation of the structure of skeletal muscle.

Figure 4.2 shows the structure of skeletal muscle, from the intact muscle to the smallest functional unit. A **muscle fiber** is a cylindrical cell that has repeating light and dark bands, giving it the name *striated muscle*. The striations are due to a more basic structural component called the **myofibril**, which runs the length of the muscle. Each myofibril is composed of a long series of **sarcomeres**, the fundamental unit of muscle contraction. Figure 4.2 shows the sarcomere to be composed of the thick

aerobic — Processes in which energy (ATP) is supplied when oxygen is utilized while a person is working.

mitochondria — Cellular organelles responsible for the generation of energy (ATP) through the aerobic system.

muscle fiber — Muscle cell. Contains myofibrils that are composed of sarcomeres; uses chemical energy of ATP to generate tension, which, when greater than the resistance, results in movement.

myofibril — Found inside muscle fibers and composed of a long string of sarcomeres; the basic unit of muscle contraction.

sarcomeres — The basic units of muscle contraction. Contain actin and myosin; tension is developed as the myosin cross bridges pull the actin toward the center of the sarcomere.

filament **myosin** and the thin filament **actin** and is bounded by connective tissue called the **Z line** (60).

An enlargement of two sarcomeres in Figure 4.2 shows the **A band**, **I band**, and **H zone**, and the changes that take place when the sarcomere goes from the resting state to the contracted state. The I band is composed of actin and is bisected by the Z line, and the A band is composed of myosin and actin. According to the **sliding-filament theory** of muscle contraction, the thin actin filaments slide over the thick myosin filaments, pulling the Z lines toward the center of the sarcomere. In this way the entire muscle shortens, but the contractile proteins *do not* change size. How does the muscle release the energy in ATP to make this happen?

If ATP is the energy supply, then an ATPase (an enzyme) must exist in muscle to split ATP and release the potential energy contained within its structure. The ATPase is found in an extension of the thick myosin filament, the **cross bridge**, which also possesses the ability to bind to actin. Figure 4.3 shows the interaction of ATP, the cross bridge, and actin that leads to the shortening of the sarcomere (60).

Because all of the components needed for muscle contraction are present (ATP, actin, myosin), why aren't the cross bridges always moving and the muscle always in the state of contraction? At rest there are two proteins associated with actin that block the interaction of myosin with actin: **troponin,** which has the capacity to bind calcium, and **tropomyosin**. Figure 4.4 shows that when a muscle is depolarized (excited) by a motor nerve, the action potential spreads over the surface of the muscle fiber and enters the fiber through special channels called **transverse tubules** (shown as #1 in the figure). Once inside the muscle fiber, this wave of depolarization spreads over the **sarcoplasmic reticulum (SR)**, a membrane that surrounds the myofibril, and calcium is released from the SR into the sarcoplasm (#2 in the figure). When the calcium binds with troponin, the tropomyosin aligns the binding site on actin so the myosin cross bridge can interact with it (#3 in the figure). The formation of **actomyosin** releases the energy, the cross bridge that is bound to actin moves, and the sarcomere shortens (#4 in figure). This sequence is repeated as long as there is calcium present and the muscle has ATP to replace what is used. Muscle relaxation is achieved when the calcium is pumped back into the sarcoplasmic reticulum and troponin and tropomyosin

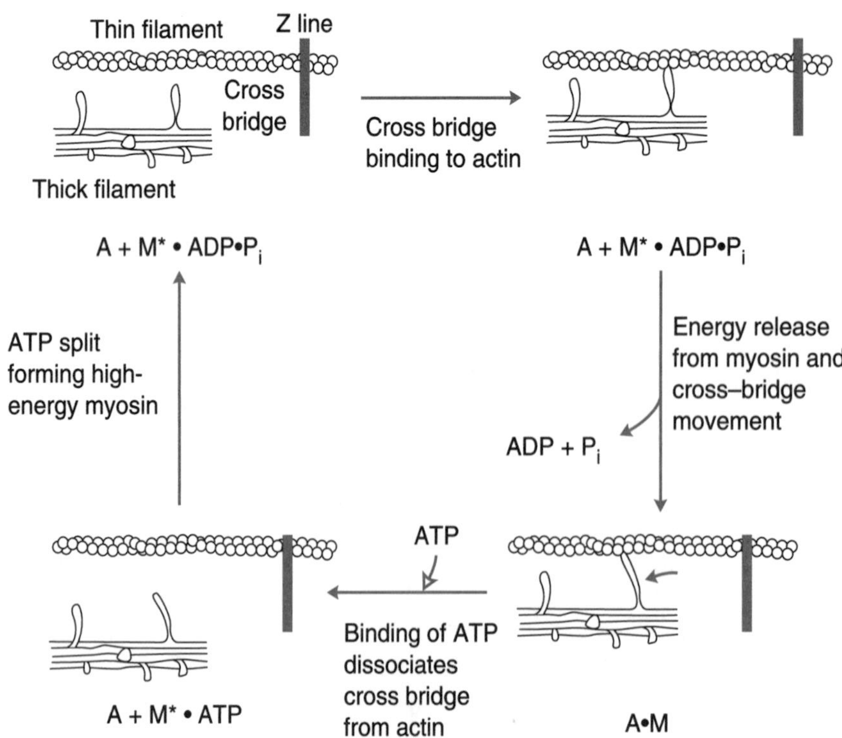

FIGURE 4.3 Chemical and mechanical changes during the four stages of a single cross-bridge cycle. Start reading the figure at the lower left.

Reprinted, by permission of McGraw-Hill, from Vander, Sherman, and Luciano, 1985, *Human physiology (4th ed.)*.

can again block the interaction of actin and myosin (#5 and #6 in figure) (60). The muscle needs ATP for cross-bridge movement, to pump the calcium back to the SR, and for the maintenance of the resting membrane potential that allows the muscle to be depolarized.

2 **In Review: Muscle contraction occurs when ATP is split to form a high-energy myosin-ATP cross bridge; the myosin-ATP cross bridge binds to actin and energy is released; the cross bridge moves and pulls actin toward the center of the sarcomere; finally, ATP binds to and releases the cross bridge from actin to start the process over again. Calcium release from the sarcoplasmic reticulum blocks inhibitory proteins (troponin and tropomyosin) and allows the cross bridge to bind to actin to initiate movement of the cross bridge. Relaxation occurs when calcium is pumped back into the sarcoplasmic reticulum and ATP binds to the cross bridge.**

Muscle Fiber Types and Performance

Muscle fibers vary in their abilities to produce ATP by the different aerobic and anaerobic mechanisms described earlier in the chapter. Some muscle fibers contract quickly and have an innate capacity to produce great amounts of force, but they fatigue quickly. These muscle fibers produce most of their ATP by creatine phosphate breakdown and glycolysis, and they are termed **fast glycolytic (FG)**, or **Type IIb**, fibers. Other muscle fibers contract slowly and produce only small amounts of force, but they have great resistance to fatigue. These fibers produce most of their ATP aerobically in the mitochondria and are called **slow oxidative (SO)**, or **Type I**, fibers. They have many mitochondria and a relatively large number of capillaries helping to deliver oxygen to the mitochondria. Lastly, there is a fiber with a combination of Type I and Type IIb characteristics. It is a fast-contracting muscle fiber that not only produces a great force when stimulated, but it also possesses a resistance to fatigue because of its large number of mitochondria and capillaries. These fibers are

myosin— A thick contractile protein in sarcomeres that can bind actin and split ATP to generate cross-bridge movement and the development of tension.

actin — Thin protein constituent of the sarcomere; binds to myosin to form cross bridges to facilitate muscle contraction.

Z line — The connective tissue of a sarcomere, the basic unit of muscle contraction.

A band — Portion of the sarcomere composed of myosin and actin; the length of the A band remains constant during muscle shortening.

I band — An area of the sarcomere that is bisected by the Z line and is composed of actin; the I band decreases during muscle shortening as the actin slides over the myosin.

H zone — The mid-area of the sarcomere containing only myosin.

sliding-filament theory — The theory that muscular tension is generated when the actin in the sarcomere slides over the myosin due to the action of the myosin cross bridges.

cross bridge — Part of myosin filament that binds to actin, releasing energy that results in the shortening of the sarcomere.

troponin — Binds calcium released from the sarcoplasmic reticulum and works with tropomyosin to allow the myosin cross bridge to interact with actin and initiate cross-bridge movement.

tropomyosin — A protein in muscle that regulates muscle contraction; works with troponin.

transverse tubules— Connects the sarcolemma (muscle membrane) to the sarcoplasmic reticulum; action potentials move down the transverse tubule to cause the sarcoplasmic reticulum to release calcium to initiate muscle contraction.

sarcoplasmic reticulum (SR) — The network of membranes that surround the myofibril; stores calcium needed for muscle contraction.

actomyosin — The active form of myosin that can release the energy contained in the cross bridge.

Type IIb or fast glycolytic (FG) fiber — A fast-contracting muscle generating great tension; produces energy by anaerobic metabolism and fatigues quickly.

Type I or slow oxidative (SO) fiber — A slow-contracting fiber generating a small amount of tension with most of the energy coming from aerobic processes; active in light to moderate activities and possesses great endurance.

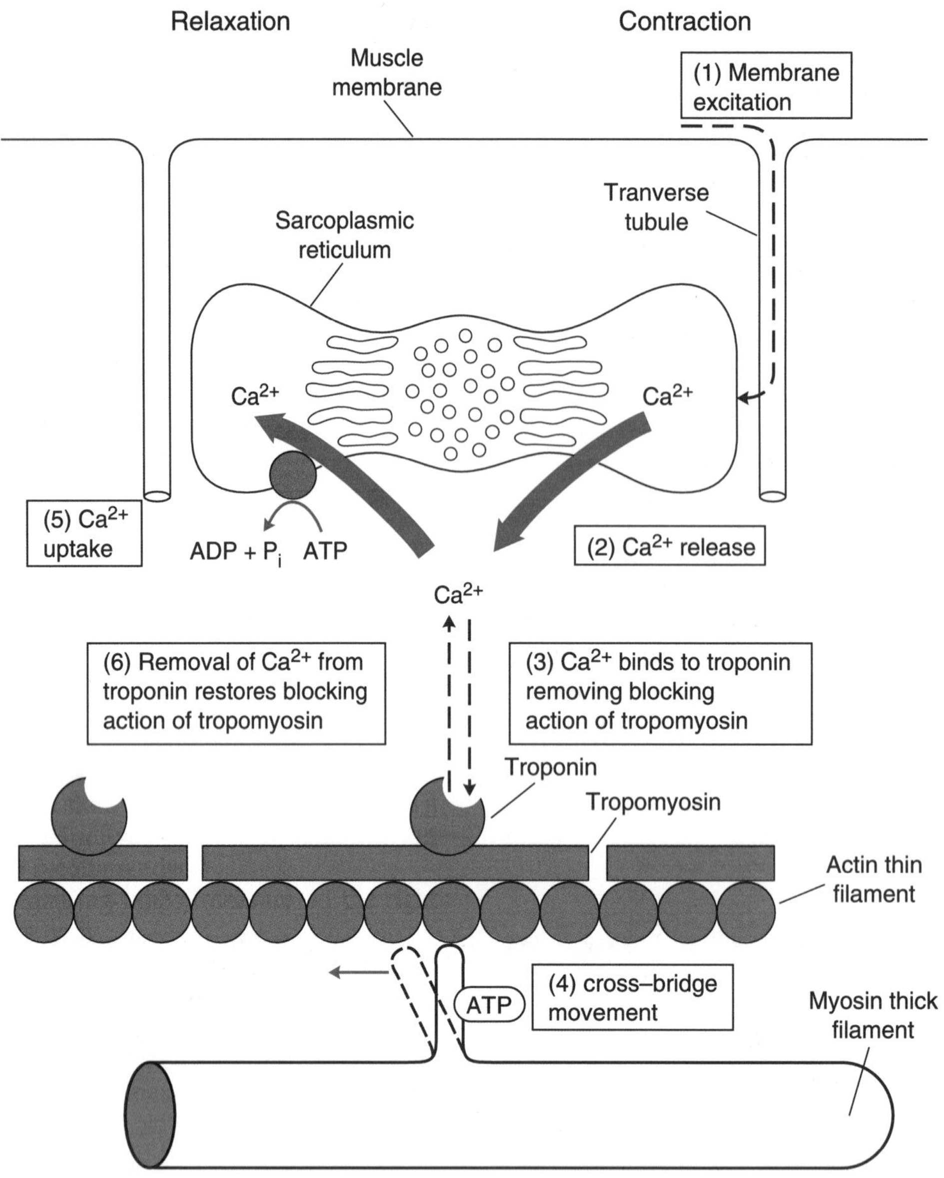

FIGURE 4.4 Role of calcium in muscle excitation-contraction coupling.
Reprinted, by permission of McGraw-Hill, from Vander, Sherman, and Luciano, 1985, *Human physiology (4th ed.)*.

called **fast oxidative glycolytic (FOG)**, or **Type IIa**, fibers.

3 **In Review: Muscle fibers differ in speed of contraction, force, and resistance to fatigue. Type I fibers are slow, have low force, and are fatigue resistant. Type IIa fibers are fast, have high force, and are fatigue resistant. Type IIb fibers are fast twitch, have high force, and are fatigable.**

Muscle Fiber Types: Genetics, Gender, and Training

In the average male and female, about 52% of the muscle fibers are Type I, with the fast-twitch fibers divided into approximately 33% Type IIa and approximately 13% Type IIb (53, 54). There is great variation, however, in the distribution of fiber types in the overall population. On the basis of studies comparing identical to fraternal twins, the distribution of fast and slow fibers seems to be genetically fixed. In addition, fast-twitch fibers cannot be converted to slow-twitch fibers, and vice versa, with endurance training programs (3). In contrast, the capacity of the muscle fiber to produce ATP aerobically (its oxidative capacity) seems to be easily altered by endurance training. In fact, in some elite endurance athletes Type IIb fibers can't be found; they have been converted to the oxidative version, Type IIa (53). The increase in mitochondria and capillaries in endurance-trained muscles allows an individual to meet ATP demands via the aerobic processes, with less glycogen depletion and lactate formation (28).

Tension (Force) Development in the Muscle

The tension, or force, generated by a muscle depends on more than the fiber type. When a single threshold-level stimulus excites a muscle fiber, a single, low-tension twitch results, a brief contraction followed by relaxation. If the frequency of stimulation is increased, the muscle fiber can't relax between stimuli, and the tension of one contraction is added on to the previous one. This is called **summation**. A further increase in the frequency of stimulation results in the contractions fusing together into a smooth, sustained, high-tension contraction called **tetanus**. The force of contraction is dependent on more than just the frequency of stimulation; it is dependent also on the degree to which the muscle fibers contract simultaneously (synchronous firing) and the number of muscle fibers recruited. This latter factor is the most important.

Figure 4.5 shows the order of recruitment of the different muscle fiber types as the intensity of exercise increases. The order is from the most to the least oxidative, from the slowest fiber to the fastest (Type I → Type IIa → Type IIb) (51). Consequently, at higher work rates when the Type IIb fibers are being recruited, there is a greater chance of producing lactic acid. Although chronic light exercise (less than 40% $\dot{V}O_2$max) recruits and causes a training effect in only the Type I fibers, exercise beyond 70% $\dot{V}O_2$max involves all fiber types. This has important implications in the specificity of training and the potential for transferring training effects from one activity to another. Obviously, if you don't use a muscle fiber, it can't become "trained."

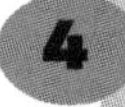

In Review: Muscle tension is dependent on the frequency of stimulation leading to a tetanus contraction, the synchronous firing of muscle fibers, and the recruitment of muscle fibers. The order of recruitment of muscle fibers is from the most to the least oxidative. Light exercise uses Type I muscle fibers, moderate exercise requires the recruitment of Type IIa fibers. Both favor the aerobic metabolism of carbohydrates and fats. Heavy exercise requires the involvement of Type IIb fibers that favor anaerobic glycolysis which increases the likelihood of lactate production.

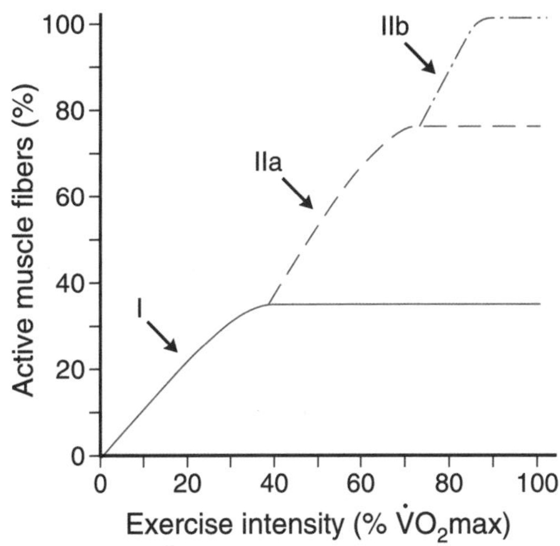

FIGURE 4.5 Order of muscle fiber type recruitment in exercise of increasing intensity.
Reprinted, by permission of McGraw-Hill, from Sale, 1987, Influence of exercise and training on motor unit activation. In *Exercise and sport sciences reviews*, vol. 15, edited by Pandolf.

Type IIa or fast oxidative glycolytic (FOG) fiber — A fast-contracting muscle generating great tension that can produce energy aerobically as well as anaerobically; adds to Type I fiber's tension as exercise intensity increases.

summation — The additive effect of force generated during repetitive muscle contractions without complete muscle relaxation between contractions.

tetanus — Increase in skeletal muscle tension in response to very high-stimulation frequencies. The resulting contractions fuse together into a smooth, sustained, high-tension contraction.

METABOLIC, CARDIOVASCULAR, AND RESPIRATORY RESPONSES TO EXERCISE

A primary task of the HFI or PFT is to recommend physical activities that increase or maintain cardiorespiratory function. Activities that demand the production of energy (ATP) by aerobic mechanisms automatically cause the circulatory and respiratory systems to deliver oxygen to the muscle to meet the demand. The selected aerobic activities must be strenuous enough to challenge the cardiorespiratory systems to cause them to improve. This crucial link between aerobic activities and cardiorespiratory function provides the basis for much of exercise programming. The following sections present a summary of selected metabolic, cardiovascular, and respiratory responses to submaximal work and to a graded exercise test taken to maximum. We begin with a discussion of how oxygen uptake is measured.

Measuring Oxygen Uptake

How does oxygen get to the mitochondria? Oxygen enters the lungs when a person inhales; it then diffuses from the alveoli of the lungs into the blood. Oxygen is bound to hemoglobin in the red blood cells, and the heart delivers the oxygen-enriched blood to the muscles. Oxygen then diffuses into the muscle cells to the mitochondria where it is used (consumed) in the production of ATP. How is oxygen consumption measured during exercise?

Oxygen consumption ($\dot{V}O_2$) is measured by subtracting the volume of oxygen exhaled from the volume of oxygen inhaled.

$$\dot{V}O_2 = \text{volume } O_2 \text{ inhaled} - \text{volume } O_2 \text{ exhaled}$$

In the classic approach to measuring $\dot{V}O_2$ the subject breathes through a two-way valve that allows room air (containing 20.93% O_2 and 0.03% CO_2) to be inhaled into the lungs while directing exhaled air to a meteorological balloon, or Douglas bag (see figure 4.6). A volume meter measures the L of air inhaled per min, which is called the **pulmonary ventilation**. The exhaled air contained in the meteorological balloon is analyzed for its oxygen and carbon dioxide content, and the oxygen consumption (uptake) is calculated by simply multiplying the volume of air breathed by the percentage of oxygen extracted. Oxygen extraction is the percentage of oxygen extracted from the inhaled air, the difference between the 20.93% O_2 in room air and the percent O_2 in the meteorological balloon.

The following example indicates the general steps used to calculate $\dot{V}O_2$—the exact procedure is discussed in appendix B.

$$\dot{V}O_2 = \text{Pulmonary ventilation } (L \cdot min^{-1}) \cdot O_2 \text{ extraction}$$

If ventilation = 60 L · min^{-1}, and exhaled O_2 = 16.93%, then

$$\dot{V}O_2 = 60\ L \cdot min^{-1} \cdot (20.93\%\ O_2 - 16.93\%\ O_2)$$

$$\dot{V}O_2 = 60\ L \cdot min^{-1} \cdot 4.00\%\ O_2 = 2.4\ L \cdot min^{-1}$$

Carbon dioxide (CO_2) is produced in the mitochondria and diffuses out of the muscle into the venous blood where it is carried back to the lungs. There it diffuses into the alveoli and, in this example, is exhaled into the meteorological balloon. Carbon dioxide production ($\dot{V}CO_2$) can be calculated as described for the $\dot{V}O_2$.

If ventilation = 60 L · min^{-1}, and exhaled CO_2 = 3.03%, then

$$\dot{V}CO_2 = 60\ L \cdot min^{-1} \cdot (3.03\%\ CO_2 - 0.03\%\ CO_2)$$

$$\dot{V}CO_2 = 60\ L \cdot min^{-1} \cdot 3.00\%\ CO_2 = 1.8\ L \cdot min^{-1}$$

The ratio of CO_2 production [$\dot{V}CO_2$] to oxygen consumption [$\dot{V}O_2$] at the cell is called the **respiratory quotient (RQ)**. Because $\dot{V}CO_2$ and $\dot{V}O_2$ are measured at the mouth rather than at the tissue, this ratio is

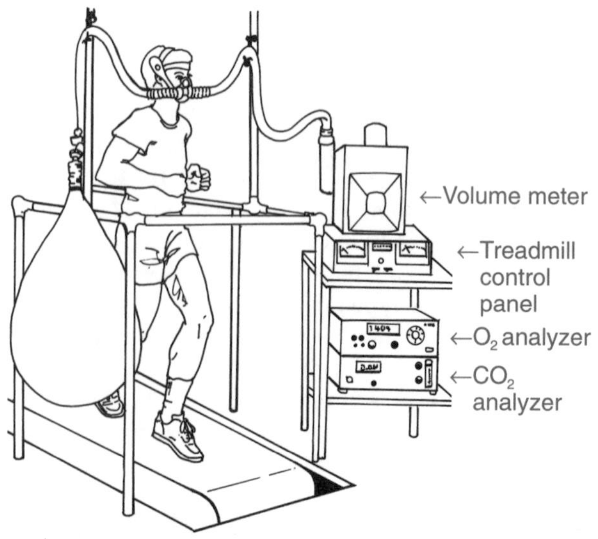

FIGURE 4.6 Conventional equipment involved in the measurement of oxygen uptake.

Respiratory Exchange Ratios for Carbohydrate and Fat

For glucose

$$C_6H_{12}O_6 + 6\ O_2 \rightarrow 6\ CO_2 + 6\ H_2O + \text{energy}$$

$$R = \frac{6\ CO_2}{6\ O_2} = 1.0$$

For palmitate (a fatty acid)

$$C_{16}H_{32}O_2 + 23\ O_2 \rightarrow 16\ CO_2 + 16\ H_2O + \text{energy}$$

$$R = \frac{16\ CO_2}{23\ O_2} = 0.7$$

called the **respiratory exchange ratio (R)**. R is an important measure in that it can tell us what type of fuel is being used during exercise (see the next section).

$$R = \dot{V}CO_2 \div \dot{V}O_2$$

Using the values already calculated,

$$R = 1.8\ L \cdot min^{-1} \div 2.4\ L \cdot min^{-1} = 0.75$$

Fuel Utilization During Exercise

In general, protein contributes less than 5% to total energy production during exercise, and for the purpose of our discussion it will be ignored (46). This leaves carbohydrate (muscle glycogen and blood glucose, which is derived from liver glycogen) and fat (adipose tissue and intramuscular fat) as the primary fuels for exercise. The ability of the respiratory exchange ratio to provide good information about the metabolism of fats and carbohydrates during exercise is due to the following observations about the metabolism of fats and glucose.

When R = 1.0, 100% of the energy is derived from carbohydrates, 0% from fat; when R = 0.7, it is the reverse. When R = 0.85, approximately 50% of the energy is derived from carbohydrates and 50% from fat. For the measurement to be correct, the subject must be in a steady state. If lactic acid is increasing in the blood, the plasma bicarbonate HCO_3^- buffer store will react with the acid (H^+) and produce CO_2, which is exhaled as we are stimulated to hyperventilate:

$$H^+ + HCO_3^- \rightarrow H_2CO_3 \rightarrow H_2O + CO_2$$

This CO_2 is not the result of the aerobic metabolism of carbohydrate and fat, and when the CO_2 is exhaled it will result in an overestimation of the true value of R. During strenuous work when Type IIb fibers are recruited, lactic acid is produced, driving R over 1.0.

Effect of Exercise Intensity on Fuel Utilization

Figure 4.7 shows the changes in R during progressive work up to $\dot{V}O_2$max. In the progressive test, R increases at about 40% to 50% $\dot{V}O_2$max, indicating that Type IIa fibers are being recruited and carbohydrates (CHO) are becoming a more important fuel source. This has an adaptive advantage—the muscle obtains about 6% more energy from each liter of O_2 when carbohydrates are used (5 kcal · L^{-1}) compared to when fat is used (4.7 kcal · L^{-1}).

The carbohydrate fuels for muscular exercise include muscle glycogen and blood glucose. Muscle glycogen is the primary carbohydrate fuel for heavy

oxygen consumption ($\dot{V}O_2$) — The rate at which oxygen is utilized during a specific level of an activity; oxygen uptake.

pulmonary ventilation — The number of L of air inhaled or exhaled per min.

respiratory quotient (RQ) or respiratory exchange ratio (R) — The ratio of the volume of carbon dioxide produced to the volume of oxygen utilized during a given period of time ($\dot{V}CO_2/\dot{V}O_2$).

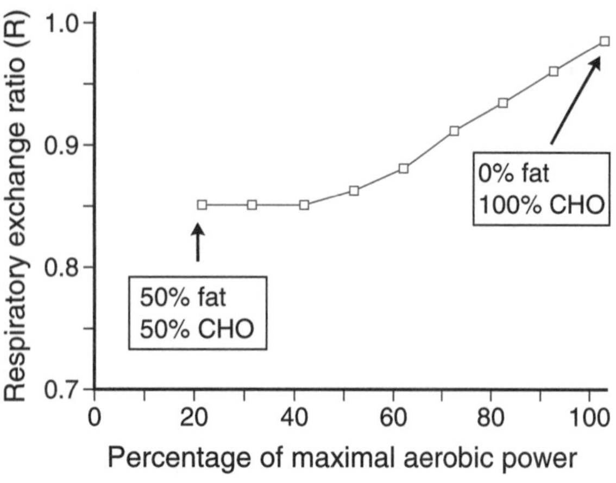

FIGURE 4.7 Changes in the respiratory exchange ratio with increasing exercise intensity (2).

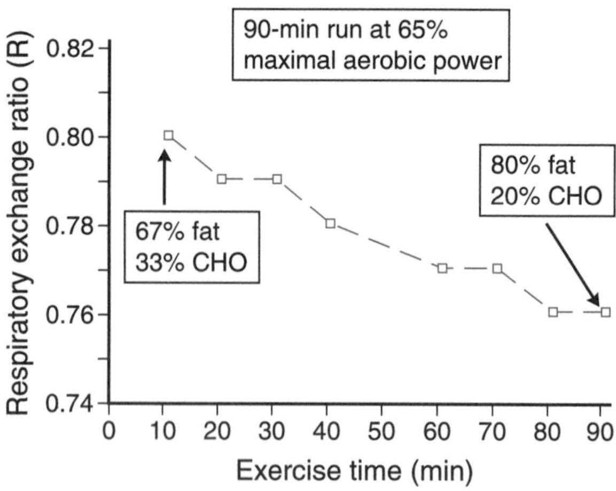

FIGURE 4.8 Changes in the respiratory exchange ratio during prolonged steady-state exercise (47).

exercise lasting less than 2 hr, and inadequate muscle glycogen results in premature fatigue (9). As muscle glycogen is used during prolonged heavy exercise, blood glucose becomes more important in supplying the carbohydrate fuel. In heavy exercise lasting 3 hr or more, blood glucose provides almost all the carbohydrate used by the muscles. Therefore, heavy exercise is limited by the availability of carbohydrate fuels, which must be either stored in abundance prior to exercise (muscle glycogen) or replaced through ingestion of carbohydrate drinks during exercise (blood glucose) (8).

Effect of Exercise Duration on Fuel Utilization

Figure 4.8 shows the change in R during a 90-min test at 60% to 70% of the subject's $\dot{V}O_2$max (47). R decreases over time, indicating a greater reliance on fat as a fuel. The fats are derived from both intramuscular fat stores and adipose tissue, which releases free fatty acids into the blood to be carried to the muscle. This increased use of fat spares the remaining carbohydrate (CHO) stores and extends the time to exhaustion.

Effect of Diet and Training on Fuel Utilization

The type of fuel used during exercise is dependent on diet. It has been demonstrated clearly that a high-carbohydrate diet increases the muscle glycogen content and extends the time to exhaustion, compared to an average diet (31). Furthermore, the capacity of the muscle to increase its glycogen store is increased if strenuous exercise is performed prior to eating the high-carbohydrate diet (31, 57). Finally, during prolonged heavy exercise carbohydrate drinks help to maintain the blood glucose concentration and extend the time to fatigue (8).

Endurance training results in an increase in the number of mitochondria in the muscles involved in the training program. This increases the capacity of the muscle to use fat as a fuel and the ability to process the available carbohydrate aerobically. This results in a sparing of the carbohydrate store and a reduction in lactate production, both of which favorably influence performance (28).

5 **In Review: The respiratory exchange ratio (R) can be used as an index of fuel use during exercise. When R = 1.0, 100% of the energy is derived from carbohydrate; when R = 0.7, 100% of the energy is derived from fat. When lactic acid is increasing in the blood during heavy exercise, the acid is buffered by plasma bicarbonate. This causes CO_2 to be produced and invalidates the use of R as an indicator of fuel use during exercise. As exercise intensity increases, the R increases, indicating that carbohydrates become more important in generating ATP. During prolonged exercise, the R decreases over time, indicating that fat is being used more and carbohydrates are being spared.**

Transition From Rest to Steady-State Work

Some readers might mistakenly assume from the discussion of the immediate, short-, and long-term sources of energy that these various sources of ATP are used in distinct activities and do not work together to allow a person to make the transition from rest to exercise. When an individual steps onto a treadmill belt moving at a velocity of 200 m · min^{-1} (7.5 mi · hr^{-1}), the ATP requirement increases from the low level needed to stand alongside the treadmill to the new level of ATP required by the muscles to run at 200 m · min^{-1}. This change in the ATP supply to the muscle must take place in the first step onto the treadmill. Failure to do so results in the individual drifting off the back of the treadmill. What energy sources supply ATP during the first minutes of work?

Oxygen Uptake

The cardiovascular and respiratory systems cannot instantaneously increase the delivery of oxygen to the muscles to completely meet the ATP demands by aerobic processes. In the interval between the time a person steps onto the treadmill and the time his or her cardiovascular and respiratory systems deliver the correct amount of oxygen, the immediate and short-term sources of energy supply the needed ATP. The volume of oxygen "missing" in the first few minutes of work is the **oxygen deficit** (figure 4.9). Creatine phosphate supplies some of the needed ATP, and the anaerobic breakdown of glycogen to lactic acid provides the rest until the oxidative mechanisms meet the ATP requirement. When the oxygen uptake levels off during submaximal work, the oxygen uptake value is said to represent the **steady-state oxygen requirement** for the activity. At this point the ATP need of the cell is being met by the production of ATP with oxygen in the mitochondria of the muscle on a "pay as you go" basis.

When the individual stops running and steps off the treadmill, the ATP need of the muscles that were involved in the activity drops suddenly back toward the resting value. The oxygen uptake decreases quickly at first and then more gradually approaches the resting value. This elevated oxygen uptake in recovery from exercise is called the oxygen repayment, **oxygen debt**, or excess post-exercise oxygen consumption (EPOC) (figure 4.9). In part, the elevated oxygen uptake is being used to make additional ATP to bring the CP store of the muscle back to normal (remember that it was depleted somewhat at the onset of work). Some of the "extra" oxygen taken in during recovery from exercise is used to pay the ATP requirement for the higher heart rate and breathing during recovery (compared to rest). A small part of the oxygen repayment is used by the liver to convert a portion of the lactic acid produced at the onset of work into glucose (46).

If an individual reaches the steady-state oxygen requirement earlier during the first minutes of work, she or he incurs a smaller oxygen deficit. This results in less CP depletion and the production of less lactic acid. Endurance training speeds up the kinetics of oxygen transport; that is, it decreases the time needed to reach a steady state of oxygen uptake. People in poor condition, as well as people with cardiovascular or pulmonary disease, take longer to reach the steady-state oxygen requirement. As a result, they incur a larger oxygen deficit and must produce more ATP by the immediate and short-term sources of energy at the onset of work (24, 44).

Heart Rate and Pulmonary Ventilation

The link between the cardiorespiratory responses to work and the time it takes to reach the steady-state oxygen requirement should be no surprise. Figure 4.10 shows the typical heart rate and pulmonary ventilation responses to a submaximal run test. The shape of the curve in each case resembles the curve for oxygen uptake described earlier.

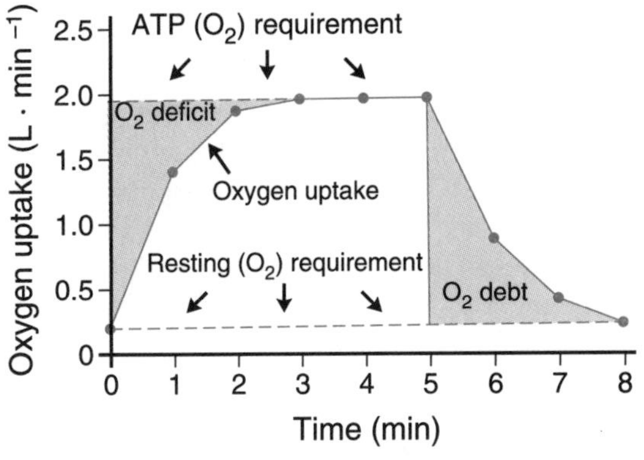

FIGURE 4.9 Oxygen deficit and oxygen debt (repayment) during a 5-min run on a treadmill.

oxygen deficit — The difference between the steady-state oxygen requirement of a physical activity and the measured oxygen uptake.

steady-state oxygen requirement — When the oxygen uptake levels off during submaximal work, the oxygen uptake value is said to represent the steady-state oxygen requirement for the activity.

oxygen debt — The amount of oxygen used during recovery from work that exceeds the amount needed for rest.

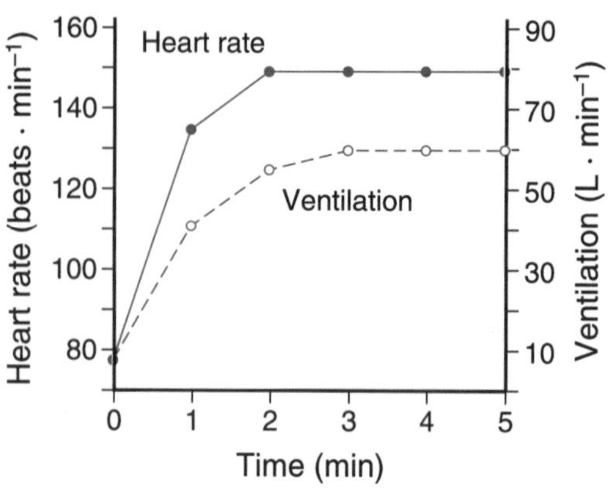

FIGURE 4.10 Heart-rate and pulmonary-ventilation responses during a 5-min run on a treadmill.

In addition, the muscle has something to do with the lag in the oxygen-uptake response at the onset of work. An untrained muscle has relatively few mitochondria available to produce ATP aerobically and also has relatively few capillaries per muscle fiber to bring the oxygen-enriched arterial blood to those mitochondria. Following an endurance training program both of these factors increase, so the muscle can produce more ATP aerobically at the onset of work. The result is a reduction in lactic acid production at the onset of work and a lowering of the blood lactic acid concentration for a fixed submaximal work rate following an endurance training program (24, 28, 44).

6 **In Review: At the onset of submaximal exercise, the $\dot{V}O_2$ does not increase immediately (oxygen deficit), and some of the ATP must be supplied anaerobically by CP and glycolysis. At the end of exercise the $\dot{V}O_2$ remains elevated for some time to (a) replenish CP stores, (b) support the energy cost of the elevated heart rate and breathing, and (c) synthesize glucose from lactic acid. With training the oxygen deficit is reduced due to a more rapid increase in $\dot{V}O_2$ at the onset of work, allowing the steady-state oxygen requirement to be reached more quickly.**

GRADED EXERCISE TEST (GXT)

A clear link exists between oxygen consumption and cardiorespiratory fitness because oxygen delivery to tissue is dependent on lung and heart function. One of the most common tests used to evaluate cardiorespiratory function is a graded exercise test (GXT) in which the individual exercises at progressively increasing work rates until maximum work tolerance is reached. During the test the individual may be monitored for cardiovascular variables (ECG, heart rate, blood pressure), respiratory variables (pulmonary ventilation, respiratory frequency), and metabolic variables (oxygen uptake, blood lactic acid level). The manner in which an individual responds to the GXT gives important information about cardiorespiratory function.

Oxygen Uptake and Maximal Aerobic Power

Oxygen uptake, measured as described earlier, is expressed per kilogram of body weight to facilitate comparisons between people and for the same person over time. The $\dot{V}O_2$ value in liters per minute is simply multiplied by 1000 to convert the $\dot{V}O_2$ to ml · min⁻¹; that value is divided by the subject's body weight in kilograms to yield a value expressed in milliliters per kilogram per minute.

$$\dot{V}O_2 = 2.4\ L \cdot min^{-1} \cdot 1000\ ml \cdot L^{-1}$$
$$= 2400\ ml \cdot min^{-1}$$

For a 60-kg subject,

$$2400\ ml \cdot min^{-1} \div 60\ kg = 40\ ml \cdot kg^{-1} \cdot min^{-1}$$

Figure 4.11 shows a GXT conducted on a treadmill in which the speed is constant (3 mi · hr⁻¹) and the grade changes 3% every 3 min. With each stage of a GXT the oxygen uptake increases to meet the ATP demand of the work rate. Also, the individual incurs a small oxygen deficit at each stage as the cardiovascular system tries to adjust to the new demand placed on it by the increased work rate.

It has been shown that apparently healthy individuals reach the steady-state oxygen requirement by 1.5 min or so of each stage of the test up to moderately heavy work (42, 43). People who have low cardiorespiratory fitness or cardiovascular and pulmonary diseases may not be able to reach the expected values in the same amount of time and might incur larger oxygen deficits with each stage of the test. The oxygen uptake measured at various stages of the test on these latter individuals would be lower than expected because they could not reach the expected steady-state demands of the test at each stage.

Toward the end of a GXT, a point is reached at which the work rate changes (i.e., the grade on the

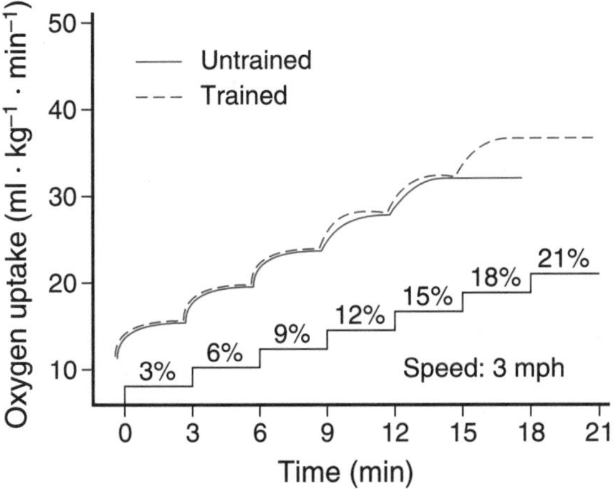

FIGURE 4.11 Oxygen uptake responses to a graded exercise test (36).

treadmill is increased) but the oxygen uptake does not. In effect, the limits of the cardiovascular system to transport oxygen to the muscle have been reached. This point is called **maximal aerobic power**, or **maximal oxygen uptake ($\dot{V}O_2$max).** A complete leveling off in the oxygen consumption is not seen in all cases because it requires the individual to work one stage past the actual point at which $\dot{V}O_2$max is reached. This requires the subject to be highly motivated. In some GXT protocols the "plateau" in oxygen uptake is judged against the criteria of less than 2.1 ml · kg^{-1} · min^{-1} increase in $\dot{V}O_2$ from one stage to the next (59). Other criteria for having achieved $\dot{V}O_2$max include an R greater than 1.15 (32) and a blood lactate concentration greater than 8 mmol · L^{-1}, about 8 times the resting value (1). These and other criteria have been used alone and in combination to increase the likelihood that the individual has really achieved $\dot{V}O_2$max (30). Participation in a 10- to 20-week endurance training program causes an increase in $\dot{V}O_2$max. If this trained person were to retake the GXT, he or she would reach the steady state sooner at light to moderate work rates and then go one stage further into the test, at which time the greater $\dot{V}O_2$max is measured.

Maximal aerobic power is the greatest rate at which the body (primarily muscle) can produce ATP aerobically. It is also the upper limit at which the cardiovascular system can deliver oxygen-enriched blood to the muscles. Thus maximal aerobic power is not only a good index of cardiorespiratory fitness, it is also a good predictor of performance capability in aerobic events such as distance running, cycling, cross-country skiing, and swimming. In the apparently healthy person, maximal aerobic power is usually understood as the quantitative limit at which the cardiovascular system can deliver oxygen to tissues. This usual interpretation must be tempered by the mode of exercise (test type) used to impose the work rate on the individual subject.

Test Type

For the average person, the highest value for maximal aerobic power is measured when the subject completes a GXT involving uphill running. A GXT conducted at a walking speed usually results in a $\dot{V}O_2$max value 4% to 6% below the graded running value, and a test on a cycle ergometer may yield a value 10% to 12% lower than the graded running value (18, 40, 41). Lastly, if a subject works to exhaustion using an arm ergometer, then the highest oxygen-uptake value is less than 70% of that measured with the legs (21). Knowledge of these variations in maximal aerobic power is helpful in making recommendations about the intensity of different exercises needed to achieve target heart rate (THR). At any given submaximal work rate, most physiological responses (heart rate, blood pressure, and blood lactic acid) are higher for arm work than for leg work (21, 56). Maximal aerobic power is influenced by more than the type of test used in its measurement. Other factors include endurance training, heredity, gender, age, altitude, pollution, and cardiovascular and pulmonary disease.

Training and Heredity

Typically, endurance training programs increase $\dot{V}O_2$max by 5% to 25%, with the magnitude of the change depending primarily on the initial level of fitness. A person with a low $\dot{V}O_2$max makes the largest percentage change as a result of a training program. Eventually a point is reached where further training does not increase $\dot{V}O_2$max. It has been demonstrated that approximately 40% of the extremely high values of maximal aerobic power

maximal aerobic power or **maximal oxygen uptake ($\dot{V}O_2$max)** — The maximal rate at which oxygen can be used by the body during maximal work; related directly to the maximal capacity of the heart to deliver blood to the muscles. Expressed in L · min^{-1} or ml · kg^{-1} · min^{-1}.

found in elite cross-country skiers and distance runners are related to a genetic predisposition for having a superior cardiovascular system (4). Because typical endurance training programs may increase $\dot{V}O_2$max by only 20% or so, it is unrealistic to expect a person with a $\dot{V}O_2$max of 40 ml · kg^{-1} · min^{-1} to increase the value to 80 ml · kg^{-1} · min^{-1}, a value measured in some elite cross-country skiers and distance runners (52). On the other hand, those who do severe interval training can achieve gains of 44% in $\dot{V}O_2$max (23).

Gender and Age

Women have $\dot{V}O_2$max values about 15% lower than men's; that difference exists across ages 20 to 60 years. The 15% difference between men and women is an average difference, and a considerable overlap in $\dot{V}O_2$max values exists in these populations (2). The aging effect indicates a gradual but systematic 1%-per-year reduction in $\dot{V}O_2$max in most people. Given that the average person becomes heavier and more sedentary with age, some of the decrease in $\dot{V}O_2$max is as much a reflection of these changes as it is a specific outcome of the aging process. In fact, evidence indicates that individuals who remain active and maintain their body weight show half the decrease in $\dot{V}O_2$max over the years (33, 34, 35).

Altitude and Pollution

$\dot{V}O_2$max decreases with increasing altitude. At 7400 ft (2300 m) $\dot{V}O_2$max is only 88% of the sea-level value. This decrease in $\dot{V}O_2$max is due primarily to the reduction in the arterial oxygen content that occurs as the oxygen pressure decreases with increasing altitude. With the lower arterial oxygen content at high altitudes, the heart must pump more blood per minute to meet the oxygen needs of any task. As a result, the heart rate response is higher at submaximal intensities when performed at higher altitudes (29).

Carbon monoxide, produced from the burning of fossil fuel as well as from cigarette smoke, binds readily to hemoglobin and can decrease oxygen transport to muscles. The critical concentration of carbon monoxide in blood needed to decrease $\dot{V}O_2$max is 4.3%. After that, there is approximately a 1% decrease in $\dot{V}O_2$max for every 1% increase in the carbon monoxide concentration in the blood (48).

Cardiovascular and Pulmonary Diseases

Cardiovascular and pulmonary diseases decrease $\dot{V}O_2$max by diminishing the delivery of oxygen from the air to the blood and reducing the capacity of the heart to deliver blood to the muscles. Patients with cardiovascular disease have some of the lowest $\dot{V}O_2$max (functional capacity) values, but they also experience the largest percentage changes in $\dot{V}O_2$max in endurance training programs. Table 4.1 shows common values for $\dot{V}O_2$max in a variety of populations (2, 20).

Table 4.1 Maximal Aerobic Power Measured in Healthy and Diseased Populations

Population	$\dot{V}O_2$max (ml · kg^{-1} · min^{-1}) Men	Women
Cross-country skiing	82	66
Distance runners	79	62
College students	45	38
Middle-age adults	35	30
Postmyocardial infarction patients	22	18
Severe pulmonary-diseased patients	13	13

Note. Data compiled from Åstrand and Rodahl 1986, Fox, Bowers, and Foss 1993, and the Fort Sanders Cardiac Rehabilitation Program.

In Review: Maximal oxygen uptake, $\dot{V}O_2$max, is the greatest rate at which O_2 can be delivered to working muscles during dynamic exercise. $\dot{V}O_2$max is influenced by heredity and training, decreases about 0.5 to 1.0% per year as we age, and is about 15% lower in women compared to men of the same age. $\dot{V}O_2$max is lower at high altitude, and carbon monoxide decreases $\dot{V}O_2$max due to its ability to bind to hemoglobin and limit oxygen transport. Cardiovascular and pulmonary diseases negatively affect $\dot{V}O_2$max; however, large improvements can be attained through endurance training for individuals with cardiovascular disease.

Blood Lactic Acid and Pulmonary Ventilation

Lactic acid produced by a muscle is released into the blood. Figure 4.12 shows that during a GXT, blood lactate concentration changes little or not at

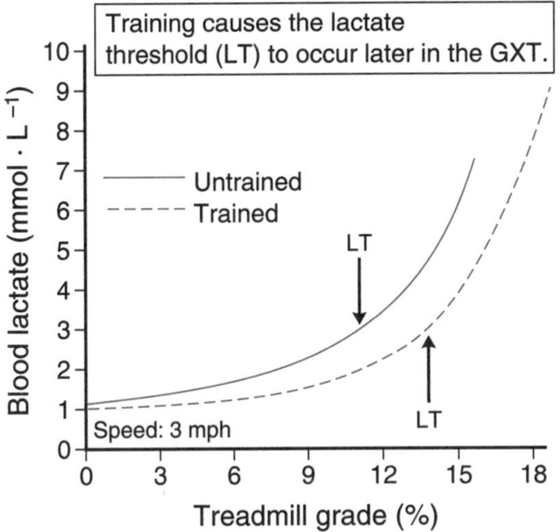

FIGURE 4.12 Changes in the blood lactic acid (lactate) concentration during a graded exercise test. LT indicates lactate threshold (17).

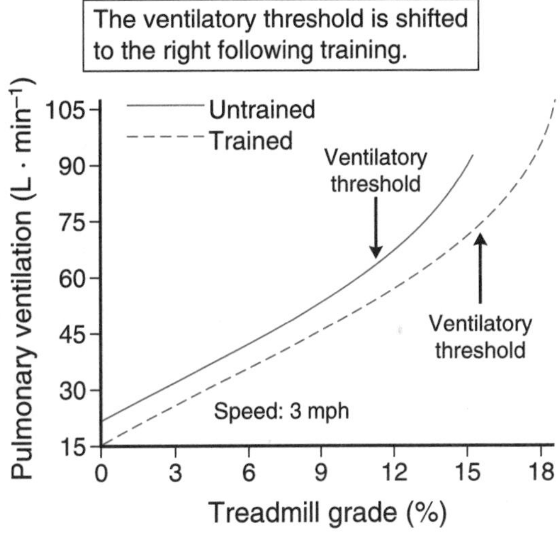

FIGURE 4.13 The pulmonary ventilation response to a graded exercise test. (The ventilatory threshold is shown with an arrow.)

all at the lower work rates; the lactate is metabolized as fast as it is produced (5). As the GXT increases in intensity, a point is reached at which the blood lactate concentration suddenly increases. The work rate at which the lactate concentration suddenly increases is called the **lactate threshold**. It is also called the **anaerobic threshold,** but because several conditions other than an oxygen lack (hypoxia) at the muscle cell can result in lactate production and release into the blood, lactate threshold is the preferred term. An endurance training program causes an increase in the mitochondria number of the trained muscles, allowing the aerobic metabolism of carbohydrates and the use of more fat as fuel. As a result, when the subject takes the GXT again, less lactate is produced and the lactate threshold occurs at a later stage of the test. The lactate threshold is a good indicator of endurance performance and has been used to predict performance in marathon races (58).

Pulmonary ventilation is the volume of air inhaled or exhaled per minute and is calculated by multiplying the frequency (f) of breathing by the tidal volume (TV), the volume of air moved in one breath. For example,

$$\text{Ventilation } (\text{L} \cdot \text{min}^{-1}) = \text{TV } (\text{L} \cdot \text{breath}^{-1}) \cdot \text{f (breaths} \cdot \text{min}^{-1})$$

$$30\ (\text{L} \cdot \text{min}^{-1}) = 1.5\ \text{L} \cdot \text{breath}^{-1} \cdot 20\ \text{breaths} \cdot \text{min}^{-1}.$$

Pulmonary ventilation increases linearly with work rate until 50% to 80% of $\dot{V}O_2$max, at which point a relative **hyperventilation** results (see figure 4.13). The inflection point in the pulmonary ventilation response is called the **ventilatory threshold.** The ventilatory threshold has been used as a noninvasive indicator of the lactate threshold and as a predictor of performance (15, 45). The increase in pulmonary ventilation is mediated by changes in the frequency of breathing (from about 10 to 12 breaths · min^{-1} at rest to 40 to 50 breaths · min^{-1} during maximal work) and the tidal volume (from 0.5 L · breath^{-1} at rest to 2 to 3 L · breath^{-1} in maximal work). Endurance training programs result in a lower pulmonary ventilation during submaximal work; the ventilatory threshold

lactate threshold — The point during a graded exercise test at which the blood lactate concentration suddenly increases; a good indicator of the highest sustainable work rate.

anaerobic threshold — The sudden increase in lactic acid in the blood during a graded exercise test. *See also* **lactate threshold**.

hyperventilation — A level of ventilation beyond that needed to maintain the arterial carbon dioxide level; can be initiated by a sudden increase in the hydrogen ion concentration due to lactic acid production during a progressive exercise test.

ventilatory threshold — The intensity of work at which the rate of ventilation sharply increases.

occurs later into the GXT. The maximal value for pulmonary ventilation tends to change in the direction of $\dot{V}O_2max$.

> **8** **In Review:** **The point at which the blood lactic acid concentration and the pulmonary ventilation suddenly increase during a GXT is called the lactate and ventilatory thresholds, respectively. The lactate and ventilatory thresholds are good predictors of performance in endurance events (e.g., 10k runs, marathons).**

Heart Rate

Once the heart rate reaches about 110 beats · min^{-1}, it increases linearly with each work rate in a GXT until the maximal heart rate is reached. The dashed line on the graph in figure 4.14 shows the influence of a training program on the subject's heart rate response at the same work rates. The lower heart rate at submaximal work rates is a beneficial effect because it decreases the oxygen needed by the heart muscle. Maximal heart rate shows no change or is slightly reduced as a result of an endurance training program.

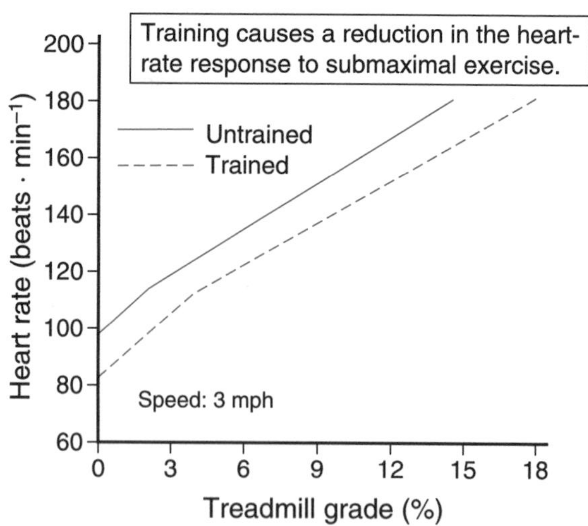

FIGURE 4.14 The heart rate response to a graded exercise test (17).

Stroke Volume

The volume of blood pumped by the heart per beat (ml · $beat^{-1}$) is called the stroke volume (SV). For individuals doing work in the upright position (cycling, walking), stroke volume increases in the early stages of the GXT until about 40% $\dot{V}O_2max$ is reached and then levels off (see figure 4.15). Consequently, heart rate is the sole factor responsible for the increased flow of blood from the heart to the working muscles for work rates greater than 40% $\dot{V}O_2max$. This is what makes the heart rate a good indicator of the metabolic rate during exercise; it is linearly related to exercise intensity from light to heavy exercise. One of the primary effects of an endurance training program is an increase in stroke volume at rest and during work; this is due, in part, to an increase in the volume of the ventricle, without any change in ventricle-wall thickness (17). This increases the **end diastolic volume**, the volume of blood in the heart just before contraction. So even if the same fraction of blood in the ventricle is pumped per beat (**ejection fraction**) following endurance training, the heart pumps more blood *per minute* at the same heart rate.

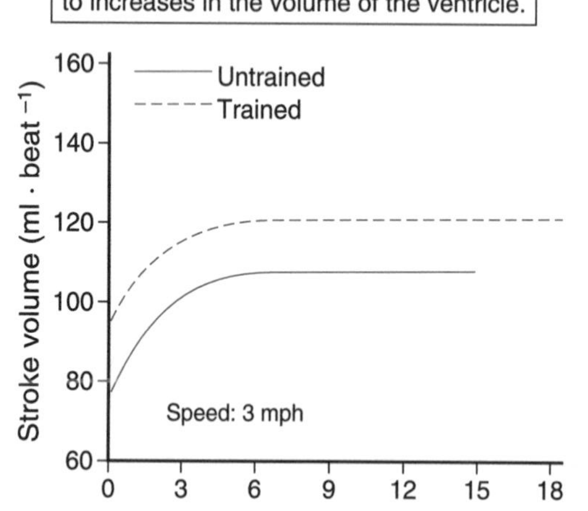

FIGURE 4.15 The stroke volume response to a graded exercise test (17).

Cardiac Output

Cardiac output (liters per minute) is the volume of blood pumped by the heart per minute and is calculated by multiplying the heart rate (beats · min^{-1}) by the stroke volume (ml · $beat^{-1}$).

Cardiac output (Q) = heart rate · stroke volume
= 60 beats · min^{-1} · 80 ml · $beat^{-1}$
= 4800 ml · min^{-1} or 4.8 L · min^{-1}

Cardiac output increases linearly with work rate. Generally, the cardiac output response to light and moderate work is not affected by an endurance training program. What is changed is the manner in which the cardiac output is achieved, with a lower heart rate and a higher stroke volume.

The maximal cardiac output (highest value reached in a GXT) is the most important cardiovascular variable determining maximal aerobic power because the oxygen-enriched blood (carrying about 0.2 L O_2 per liter of blood) must be delivered to the muscle for the mitochondria to use. If a person's maximal cardiac output is 10 L · min^{-1}, only 2 L O_2 would leave the heart for the tissues per minute (i.e., 0.2 L O_2 per liter of blood times a cardiac output of 10 L · min^{-1} = 2 L O_2 · min^{-1}). A person with a maximal cardiac output of 30 L · min^{-1} would deliver 6 L O_2 per minute to the tissues. One of the effects of an endurance training program is an increase in the maximal cardiac output and thus the delivery of oxygen to the muscles (see figure 4.16). This increase in maximal cardiac output is matched by an increase in the capillary number in the muscle to allow the blood to move slowly enough through the muscle to maintain the time needed for oxygen to diffuse from the blood to the mitochondria (53). The increase in maximal cardiac output accounts for 50% of the increase in maximal oxygen uptake that occurs in previously sedentary individuals who engage in endurance training programs (50).

In the normal population the major variable influencing the maximal cardiac output is the stroke volume. Differences in maximal cardiac output and maximal aerobic power that exist between females and males, between trained and untrained individuals, and between the world-class endurance athlete and the average person can be explained to a large degree on the basis of differences in maximal stroke volume. This is shown in table 4.2, where $\dot{V}O_2$max varies by a factor of 3 among three distinct groups, while maximal heart rate is almost the same for all three groups. Clearly, maximal stroke volume is the primary factor related to the differences that exist among individuals in $\dot{V}O_2$max.

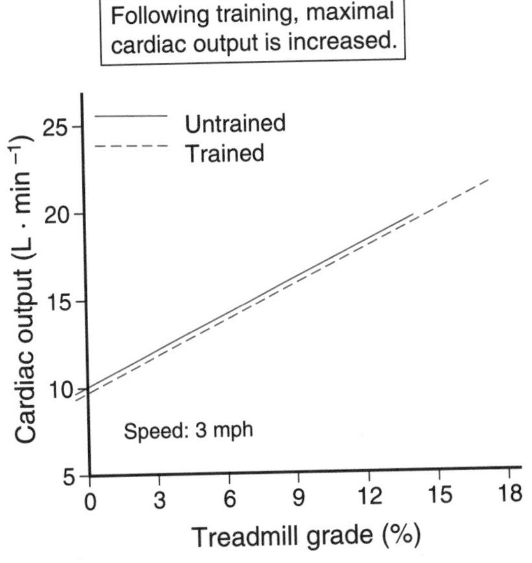

FIGURE 4.16 The cardiac output response to a graded exercise test (17).

end diastolic volume — The volume of blood in the heart just prior to ventricular contraction; a measure of the stretch of the ventricle.

ejection fraction — The fraction of the end diastolic volume ejected per beat (stroke volume divided by end diastolic volume).

Table 4.2 Maximal Values of $\dot{V}O_2$max, Heart Rate, Stroke Volume, and (a-$\bar{v}$) Oxygen Difference in 3 Groups Having Very Low, Normal, and High Maximal $\dot{V}O_2$max

Group	Max $\dot{V}O_2$ (L · min^{-1})	=	Heart rate (beats · min^{-1})	×	Stroke volume (ml · beat^{-1})	×	(a-$\bar{v}$) Oxygen difference (ml · L^{-1})
Mitral stenosis	1.60	=	190	×	50	×	170
Sedentary	3.20	=	200	×	100	×	160
Athlete	5.20	=	190	×	160	×	170

Note. From L. Rowell, "Circulation," *Medicine and Science in Sports*, 1 pp. 15-22, 1969, © by the American College of Sports Medicine.

Oxygen Extraction

Two factors determine the oxygen uptake at any time: the volume of blood delivered to the tissues per min (cardiac output) and the volume of oxygen extracted from each liter of blood. Oxygen extraction is calculated by subtracting the oxygen content of mixed venous blood (as it returns to the heart) from the oxygen content of the arterial blood. This is called the arteriovenous oxygen difference, or the $(a\text{-}\bar{v})O_2$ difference.

$$\dot{V}O_2 = \text{cardiac output} \cdot (a\text{-}\bar{v})O_2 \text{ difference}$$

$$\text{At rest, cardiac output} = 5\text{ L} \cdot \text{min}^{-1}$$

$$\text{arterial oxygen content} = 200\text{ ml } O_2 \text{ per liter of blood (ml} \cdot \text{L}^{-1})$$

$$\text{mixed venous oxygen content} = 150\text{ ml } O_2 \cdot \text{L}^{-1}$$

$$\dot{V}O_2 = 5\text{ L} \cdot \text{min}^{-1} \cdot (200 - 150\text{ ml } O_2 \cdot \text{L}^{-1})$$

$$\dot{V}O_2 = 5\text{ L} \cdot \text{min}^{-1} \cdot 50\text{ ml } O_2 \cdot \text{L}^{-1}$$

$$\dot{V}O_2 = 250\text{ ml} \cdot \text{min}^{-1}$$

The $(a\text{-}\bar{v})O_2$ difference is a measure of the ability of the muscle to extract oxygen, and it increases with exercise intensity. The ability of a tissue to extract oxygen is a function of the capillary-to-muscle-fiber ratio and the number of mitochondria in the muscle fiber. Endurance training programs increase all of these factors, leading to an increase in the maximal capacity to extract oxygen in the last stage of the GXT (53). This increase in the $(a\text{-}\bar{v})O_2$ difference accounts for about 50% of the increase in $\dot{V}O_2$max that occurs with endurance training programs in previously sedentary individuals (50).

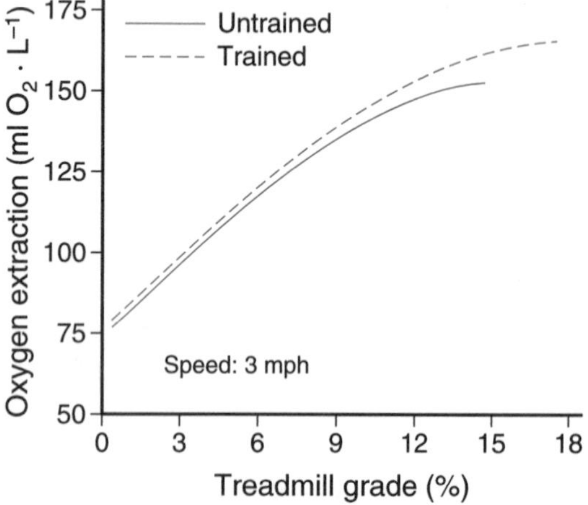

FIGURE 4.17 The changes in oxygen extraction (difference between the oxygen content of arterial blood and the mixed venous blood in the right heart) during a graded exercise test (17).

9 In Review: During acute exercise, heart rate increases linearly with work rate once a heart rate of 110 beats · min^{-1} has been achieved. During exercise in the upright position stroke volume increases until an intensity of about 40% $\dot{V}O_2$max is reached. Cardiac output (HR x SV) increases linearly with work rate. Following an endurance training program, heart rate is lower and stroke volume is higher at rest and during submaximal work; and maximal cardiac output is increased, due to an increase in maximal stroke volume, with no change or a slight decrease in maximal heart rate. Variations in $\dot{V}O_2$max across the population are due primarily to differences in maximal stroke volume. Fifty percent of the increase in $\dot{V}O_2$max due to training is a result of an increase in maximal stroke volume; the other 50% is due to an increase in oxygen extraction.

Blood Pressure

Blood pressure is dependent on the balance between cardiac output and the resistance the blood vessels offer to blood flow (total peripheral resistance). The resistance to blood flow is altered by the constriction or dilation of blood vessels called **arterioles,** located between the artery and the capillary.

$$\text{Blood pressure} = \text{Cardiac output} \cdot \text{Total peripheral resistance}$$

Blood pressure is sensed by **baroreceptors** in the arch of the aorta and in the carotid arteries. If there is a change in blood pressure, signals from the baroreceptors go to the cardiovascular control center in the brain, which in turn alters cardiac output or the diameter of arterioles. For example, when a person who has been lying in the supine position suddenly stands, blood pools in the lower extremities, stroke volume falls and, with it, blood pressure. If blood pressure is not restored, blood flow to the brain will be reduced and the person might faint. The baroreceptors monitor this fall in blood pressure, and the cardiovascular control center simultaneously increases the heart rate and reduces the diameter of the arterioles (to increase total peripheral resistance) to try to return blood pressure to normal values. During exercise, the arterioles dilate in the active muscle to increase blood flow and meet metabolic demands. This dilation is matched with a constriction of arterioles in the liver, kidneys, and gastrointestinal tract and an increase in heart rate and stroke volume as already mentioned. These coordinated changes maintain blood pressure.

Blood pressure is monitored at each stage of a GXT. Figure 4.18 shows that **systolic blood pressure (SBP)** increases with each stage until maximum work tolerance is reached. At that point, systolic pressure might decrease. A fall in systolic pressure with an increase in work rate is used as one of the indicators of maximal cardiovascular function and can aid in determining the end point for an exercise test. **Diastolic blood pressure (DBP)** tends to remain the same or decrease during a GXT. An increase in diastolic blood pressure toward the end of the test is an indicator that a person's functional capacity has been reached. Endurance training programs result in a reduction in the blood pressure responses at fixed submaximal work rates.

Two factors that determine the oxygen demand (work) of the heart during aerobic exercise are the heart rate and the systolic blood pressure. The product of these two variables is called the **rate-pressure product**, or the **double product**, and is proportional to the myocardial oxygen demand (i.e., the volume of oxygen needed by the heart muscle per minute to function properly). Factors that decrease the heart rate and blood pressure responses to work increase the chance that the coronary blood supply to the heart muscle will adequately meet the oxygen needs of the heart. Endurance training decreases the heart rate and blood pressure responses to fixed submaximal work tasks and is seen as protective against any diminished blood supply (ischemia) to the myocardium. Drugs are also used to reduce heart rate and blood pressure responses to try to reduce the work of the heart (see chapter 22).

When a person does the same rate of work with the arms as with the legs, the heart rate and blood pressure responses are considerably higher during the arm work. This is shown in figure 4.19, in which the rate-pressure product is plotted for various levels of arm and leg work. Given that the load on the heart and the potential for fatigue is greater for arm work, it is clear that an HFI should choose activities that use the large-muscle groups of the legs; this would result in lower heart rate and blood pressure responses and in reduced perception of fatigue (21, 56).

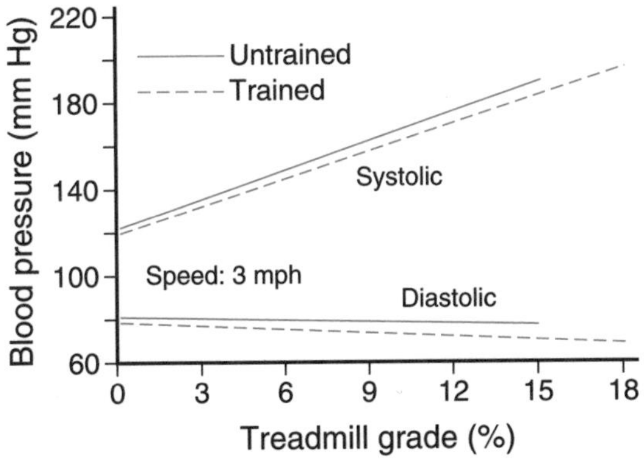

FIGURE 4.18 The systolic and diastolic blood pressure responses to a graded exercise test.

10 **In Review: Systolic blood pressure increases with each stage of a GXT, while diastolic pressure remains the same or decreases. The work of the heart is proportional to the product of the heart rate**

arterioles — Blood vessels between the artery and the capillary; responsible for regulation of blood flow and blood pressure.

baroreceptors — Receptors that monitor arterial blood pressure.

systolic blood pressure (SBP) — The pressure exerted on the vessel walls during ventricular contraction, measured in millimeters of mercury by the sphygmomanometer.

diastolic blood pressure (DBP) — The pressure exerted by the blood on the vessel walls during the resting portion of the cardiac cycle, measured in millimeters of mercury by a sphygmomanometer.

rate-pressure product — The product of heart rate and systolic blood pressure; indicative of the oxygen requirement of the heart during exercise. Also called the **double product**.

double product — The product of the heart rate and systolic blood pressure; indicative of the heart's oxygen requirement during exercise. Also called the **rate-pressure product**.

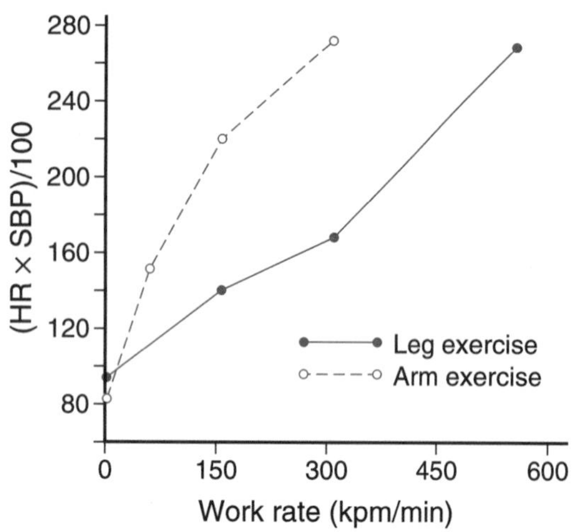

FIGURE 4.19 Rate-pressure product at rest and during arm and leg exercise.
Adapted from Schwade, Blomqvist, and Shapiro 1977.

and the systolic blood pressure. Training lowers both, making it easier for the coronary arteries to meet the oxygen demand of the heart. Heart rate and blood pressure are higher during arm work compared to leg work at the same work rate.

EFFECTS OF ENDURANCE TRAINING AND DETRAINING ON PHYSIOLOGICAL RESPONSES TO EXERCISE

Many observations have been made about the effects of endurance training on various physiological responses to exercise. This section tries to show how some of the effects of endurance training are interrelated.

- *Endurance training increases the number of mitochondria and capillaries in muscle, causing all active fibers to become more oxidative.* This effect is manifested by the increase in the Type IIa fibers and a decrease in Type IIb fibers. These changes increase the endurance capacity of the muscle by using fat for a greater percentage of energy production, sparing the muscle glycogen store and reducing lactate production. This causes the lactate threshold to be shifted to the right, and performance times in endurance events to improve.
- *Endurance training decreases the time it takes to achieve a steady state in submaximal exercise.* This results in a reduction in the oxygen deficit and less reliance on creatine phosphate and anaerobic glycolysis for energy.
- *Endurance training causes an increase in the volume of the ventricle, with no changes in ventricle-wall thickness.* This accommodates an increase in the end diastolic volume, such that more blood is pumped out per beat. The increased stroke volume is accompanied by a decrease in heart rate during submaximal work, so the cardiac output remains the same. The oxygen needs of the tissues are met with less work by the heart.
- *Maximal aerobic power increases with endurance training, the increase being inversely related to the initial $\dot{V}O_2max$.* In formerly sedentary individuals, about 50% of the increase in $\dot{V}O_2$max is due to an increase in maximal cardiac output, a change brought about by an increase in maximal stroke volume, given that maximal heart rate either remains the same or is decreased slightly. The other 50% of the increase in $\dot{V}O_2$max is due to an increase in oxygen extraction at the muscle, shown by an increase in the $(a\text{-}\bar{v})O_2$ difference. This occurs as a result of an increase in the number of capillaries in the trained muscle to allow the arterial blood to flow slowly enough for the oxygen to diffuse to the mitochondria.

Transfer of Training

The training effects that have been discussed are observed only when trained muscles are used in the exercise test. Although this may appear obvious for the decrease in blood lactate that is due, in part, to the increase in the mitochondria of the trained muscles, it is also the cause for the changes that occur in the heart rate response to submaximal work following the training program. Figure 4.20 shows the results of repeated submaximal exercise tests conducted on individuals who trained only one leg on a cycle ergometer for 13 days. The heart rate response to a GXT using the trained leg decreased as expected. At the end of the 13 days of training the untrained leg was now subjected to the same exercise test. The heart rate responded as if a training effect had not occurred. The point of this is to indicate that part of the reason the heart rate response to submaximal

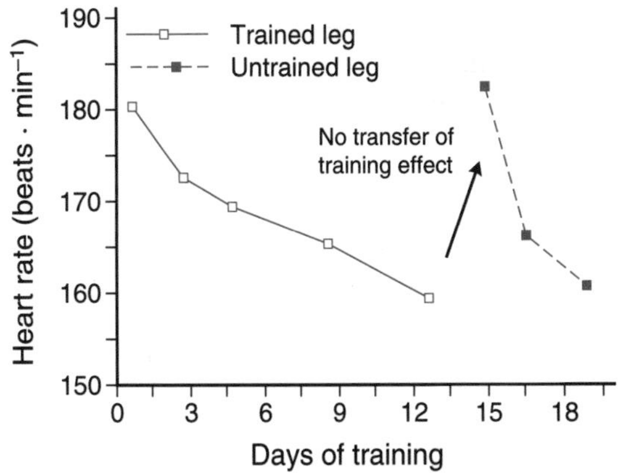

FIGURE 4.20 Lack of transfer of training effect (7).

exercise decreases as a result of the training program is due to signals coming back from the trained muscles (7, 50). This has important implications for training programs, in that being fit and responding in a trained fashion (lower lactate production, lower heart rate, more fat use) are related to doing the exercise test with the same muscle groups involved in the training. The probability of some carryover of the training effect to another activity is dependent on the degree to which the new activity uses the muscles that are already trained.

Detraining

How fast is a training effect lost? A number of investigations have explored this question by having subjects either reduce or completely cease training. Maximal oxygen uptake is usually used as the principal measure to evaluate changes due to detraining, but an individual's response to a submaximal work rate has also been used to track these changes over time.

Cessation of Training

The following study used subjects who had trained for 10± 3 years and agreed to cease training for 84 days (13). They were tested on days 12, 21, 56, and 84 of the detraining period. Figure 4.21 shows that $\dot{V}O_2max$ decreased 7% within the first 12 days of detraining. (Remember that $\dot{V}O_2max$ = cardiac output · $(a\text{-}\bar{v})O_2$ difference.) The decrease in $\dot{V}O_2max$ was due entirely to a decrease in maximal cardiac output because the maximal oxygen extraction [$(a\text{-}\bar{v})O_2$ difference] was unchanged. In turn, the decrease in maximal cardiac output was due entirely to a decrease in maximal stroke volume because maximal heart rate actually increased during the

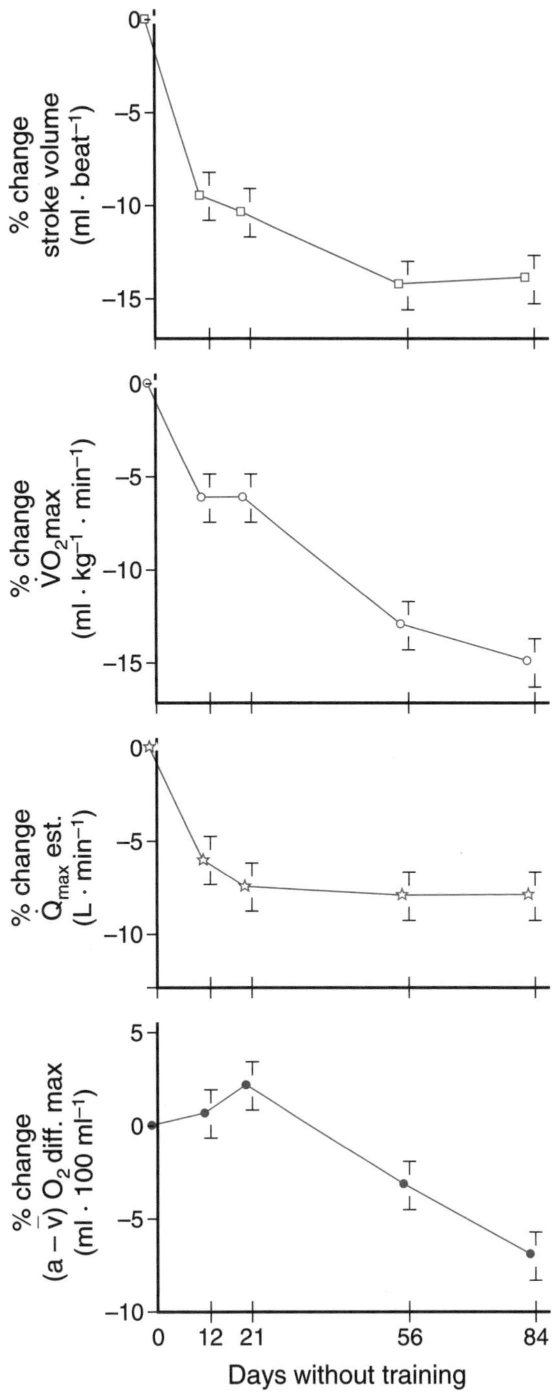

FIGURE 4.21 Effects of detraining upon percentage changes in stroke volume during exercise, maximal O_2 uptake, or $\dot{V}O_2max$, maximal cardiac output or $\dot{Q}_{max}$ est, and maximal arteriovenous O_2 difference, or $(a\text{-}\bar{v})$ O_2 difference max.
Adapted from Coyle 1984.

period of no training. A subsequent study showed that the reduced stroke volume was due to a reduction in plasma volume that occurred in the first

12 days of no training (11). In contrast, the decrease in $\dot{V}O_2max$ that occurred between days 21 and 84 was due to a decrease in the maximal oxygen extraction [$(a-\bar{v})O_2$ difference] because maximal cardiac output was unchanged (see figure 4.21). This decrease in oxygen extraction appeared to be due to a reduction in the number of mitochondria in the muscle, given that the number of capillaries surrounding each muscle fiber was unchanged (10).

The same subjects also completed a standard (fixed work rate) submaximal exercise test during the 84 days of no training (12). Figure 4.22 shows that heart rate and blood lactic acid responses to this work test increased throughout the period of detraining. The higher responses are related to the fact that the same work rate required a greater percentage of $\dot{V}O_2max$ because the latter variable was decreasing throughout the period of detraining. The magnitude of change in heart rate and blood lactic acid responses to this submaximal work bout, however, make them very sensitive indicators of the training state of an individual.

Reduced Training

To evaluate the effect of a reduction in training, Hickson and colleagues (25, 26, 27) first trained subjects for 10 weeks to cause an increase in $\dot{V}O_2max$. The training program was conducted 40 min per day, 6 days per week. Three days involved running at near maximum intensity for 40 min; the other 3 days required six 5-min bouts at near-maximum intensity on a cycle ergometer, with a 2-min rest between work bouts. Subjects expended about 600 kcal per day of exercise, or 3600 kcal per week. At the end of this 10-week training program the subjects were divided into groups that trained at either a one-third or a two-third reduction in the previous frequency (4 and 2 days per week, respectively), duration (26 and 13 min per day, respectively), or intensity (a one-third or two-thirds reduction in work done or distance run per 40-min session). Data collected on the maximal treadmill tests showed that the reduction in duration from 40 to 26 or 13 min, or a reduction in frequency from 6 to 4 or 2 days per week, did not affect $\dot{V}O_2max$. In contrast, $\dot{V}O_2max$ was clearly decreased when the intensity of training was reduced by either one third or two thirds. What is interesting is that the subjects were able to maintain $\dot{V}O_2max$ when the total exercise done per week was reduced from 3600 kcal to 1200 kcal in the two-thirds reduced frequency and duration group; but they were not able to maintain $\dot{V}O_2max$ when the intensity was reduced, even though the subjects were still expending about 1200 kcal per week. This points to the importance of the exercise intensity in maintaining $\dot{V}O_2max$ and confirms that it takes less exercise to maintain than to achieve a specific level of $\dot{V}O_2max$.

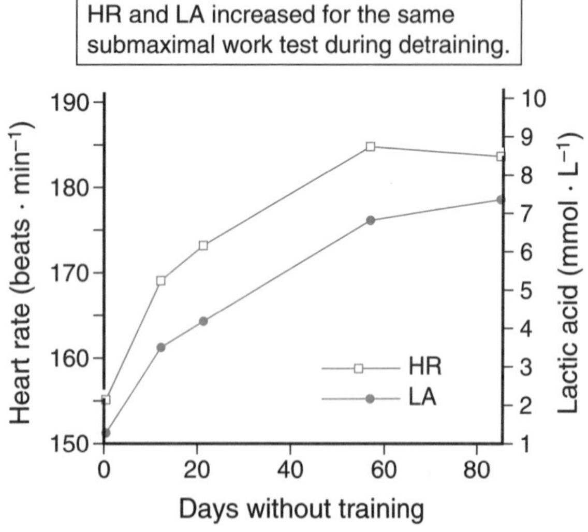

FIGURE 4.22 Changes in the heart rate and blood lactic acid concentration responses to a standard exercise test taken during 84 days of detraining (12).

11 In Review: Endurance training increases the ability of a muscle to use fat as a fuel and spare carbohydrate; decreases the time it takes to achieve a steady state during submaximal work; increases the size of the ventricle; and increases $\dot{V}O_2max$ due to increases in stroke volume and oxygen extraction. Endurance training effects (lower heart rate, lower blood lactate) do not "transfer" when untrained muscles are used to perform the work. Maximal oxygen uptake decreases with cessation of training. The initial decrease is due to a decrease in stroke volume and, later, to a reduction in oxygen extraction. Maximal oxygen uptake can be maintained by doing intense exercise, even when exercise duration and frequency are reduced.

CARDIOVASCULAR RESPONSES TO EXERCISE FOR FEMALES AND MALES

Generally, little or no difference exists between boys and girls in $\dot{V}O_2max$ or in their cardiovascular responses to submaximal exercise. During puberty, differences between girls and boys appear and are related to the female's higher percentage of body fat, lower hemoglobin, and smaller heart size relative to body weight (2). These latter factors also affect a woman's cardiovascular responses to submaximal work. For example, if an 80-kg male were walking on a 10% grade on a treadmill at 3 mi · hr^{-1}, the $\dot{V}O_2$ would be 2.07 L · min^{-1} or 25.9 ml · kg^{-1} · min^{-1}. The heart rate might be 140 beats · min^{-1} for this person. If he had to now carry a backpack weighing 15 kg, the $\dot{V}O_2$ expressed per kg would not change (25.9 ml · kg^{-1} · min^{-1}), but the total oxygen requirement would increase 389 ml · min^{-1} (i.e., 15 kg · 25.9 ml · kg^{-1} · min^{-1}) to carry the 15-kg load. His heart rate would obviously be higher with this load than without, even though the $\dot{V}O_2$ expressed per kilogram of body weight is the same. Likewise, performance in the 12-min run test to evaluate maximal aerobic power was decreased by 89 m when body weight was experimentally increased to simulate a 5% gain in body fat (14). When a postpubescent woman walks on a treadmill at a given grade and speed, her heart rate is higher than a comparable male's heart rate because of the additional fat weight she carries. The lower hemoglobin and smaller relative heart size also cause the heart rate to be higher at the same oxygen uptake expressed per unit of body weight.

The differences between males and females in the cardiovascular response to submaximal work becomes more exaggerated when work is done on a cycle ergometer where a given work rate demands a similar $\dot{V}O_2$ in liters per min, independent of gender or training. As previously mentioned, the average woman has less hemoglobin and a smaller heart volume compared to the average male. To deliver the same volume of oxygen to the muscles, the woman must have a higher heart rate to compensate for the smaller stroke volume and must have a slightly higher cardiac output to compensate for the lower hemoglobin concentration (2). These differences between women and men in the cardiovascular responses to cycle ergometry are shown in figure 4.23.

12 **In Review: At the same work rate, or $\dot{V}O_2$, women respond with a higher heart rate to compensate for a lower stroke volume. The cardiac output is slightly higher to compensate for the lower hemoglobin level (and oxygen content) of the arterial blood.**

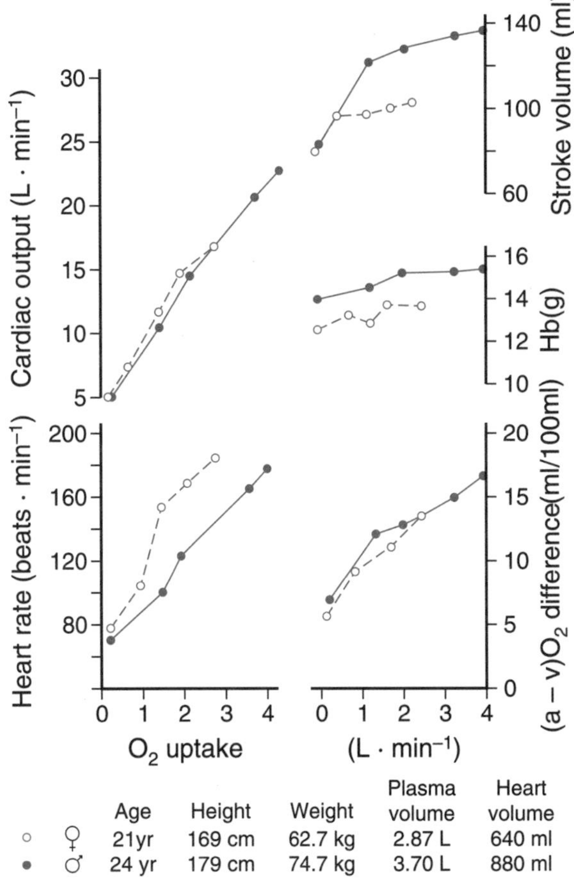

FIGURE 4.23 The cardiovascular responses of well-trained men and women to cycle ergometry exercise. Adapted, by permission of McGraw-Hill, from Åstrand and Rodahl, 1986, *Textbook of work physiology (3rd ed.)*.

CARDIOVASCULAR RESPONSES TO ISOMETRIC EXERCISE AND WEIGHT LIFTING

Most endurance exercise programs use dynamic activities involving large-muscle masses to place loads on the cardiorespiratory system. The previous summary of the physiological responses to a GXT indicates the rather proportional nature of the cardiovascular load to the exercise intensity. But this is not necessarily the case for activities that fall into the strength training category, in which a person can have a disproportionately high cardiovascular load relative to the exercise intensity. In the previous discussion of cardiovascular responses to a GXT, a progressive rise in the heart rate and systolic blood pressure responses was observed with each stage of the test. Figure 4.24 shows the heart rate and blood

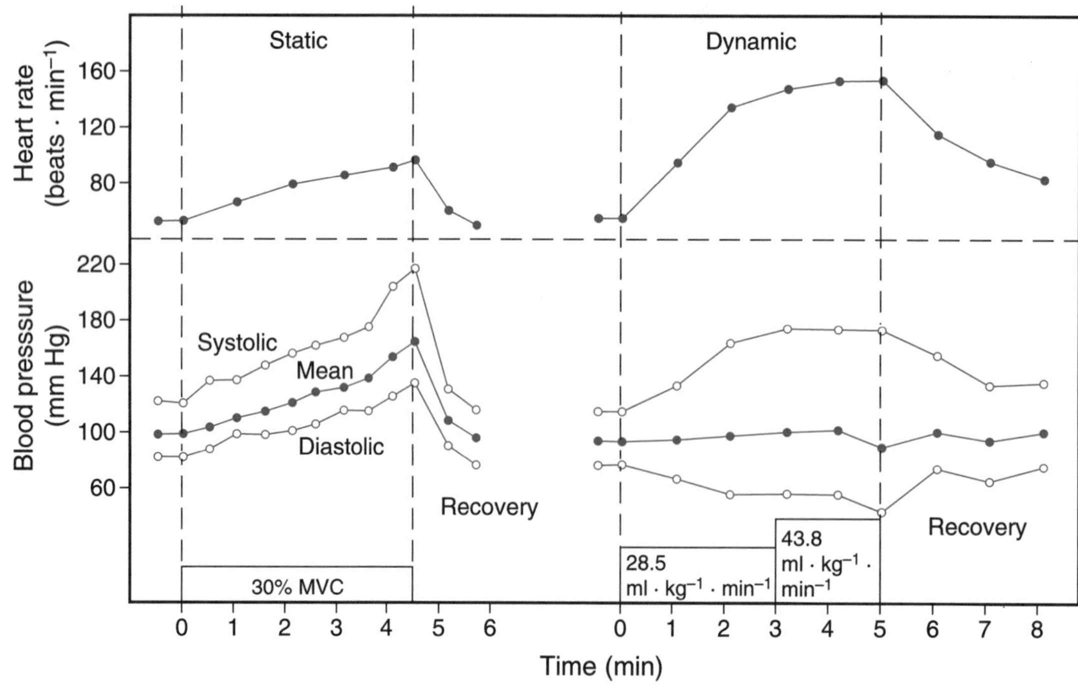

FIGURE 4.24 Comparison of the heart rate and blood pressure responses to a fatiguing, sustained hand-grip contraction at 30% of maximal voluntary contraction strength (30% MVC) and an exhausting treadmill test.
Adapted from Lind and McNichol 1967.

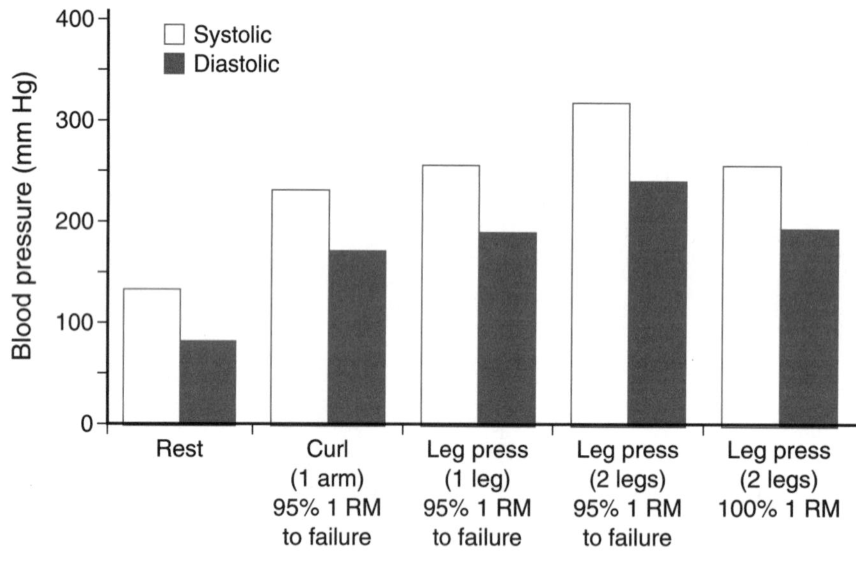

FIGURE 4.25 Blood pressure responses during weight lifting. (RM = repetition maximum.) (38)

pressure response to an isometric exercise test (sustained handgrip) at only 30% maximal voluntary contraction strength and to a treadmill test using two exercise intensities. The most impressive change during the sustained handgrip is in blood pressure; the systolic and diastolic pressures increase over time, and the magnitude of the systolic pressure exceeds 220 mmHg. This kind of exercise places an additional load on the heart and is not recommended in strength training programs for older adults or people with heart disease (37).

Dynamic, heavy-resistance exercises can also cause extreme blood pressure responses. Figure 4.25 shows the peak blood pressure response achieved during exercises done at 95% to 100% of the maximum weight that could be lifted one time (1-RM, or repetition maximum). Note that both systolic and diastolic blood pressures are elevated, with average values exceeding 300/200 mmHg for the two-leg leg press done to fatigue. The elevation in pressure was believed to be due to the compression of the arteries by the muscles, a reflex response due to the "static" component associated with near-maximal dynamic lifts, and the Valsalva maneuver, which can cause, independently, an elevation of blood pressure (38). Another study reported peak values of about 190/140 mmHg for exercises of 50%, 70%, and 80% of 1-RM done to fatigue in novice and untrained lifters. Body builders responded with lower pressures, indicating a cardiovascular adaptation to weight training (19).

13 **In Review: Isometric exercise and heavy-resistance training exercise cause very high blood pressure responses compared to those measured during dynamic endurance exercise.**

REGULATING BODY TEMPERATURE

Under resting conditions the body's core temperature is 37 °C, and there is a balance between heat production and heat loss. Heat production mechanisms include the basal metabolic rate, shivering, work, and exercise. When exercise is done, the mechanical efficiency is about 20% or less, which means that 80% or more of the energy production ($\dot{V}O_2$) is converted to heat. For example, if you are working on a cycle ergometer at a rate requiring a $\dot{V}O_2$ of 2.0 L · min^{-1}, your energy production is about 10 kcal · min^{-1}. At 20% efficiency, 2 kcal · min^{-1} goes to do work, and 8 kcal · min^{-1} is converted to heat. If most of this added heat is not lost, core temperature might rise quickly to dangerous levels. How does the body lose excess heat?

Heat-Loss Mechanisms

Heat is lost from the body by four processes. In **radiation**, heat is transferred from the surface of one object to the surface of another, with no physical contact between the objects. Heat loss depends on the temperature gradient, that is, the temperature difference between the surfaces of the objects. When a person is seated at rest in a comfortable environment (21°C to 22°C), about 60% of body heat is lost through radiation to cooler objects. **Conduction** is the transfer of heat from one object to another by direct contact, and, like radiation, conduction is dependent on a temperature gradient. When we sit on cold marble benches, we lose heat from our bodies by conduction. **Convection** is a special case of conduction in which heat is transferred to air (or water) molecules, which become lighter and rise away from the body to be replaced by cold air (or water). Heat loss can be increased by increasing the movement of the air (or water) over the surface of the body. For example, a fan enhances heat loss by placing more cold air molecules into contact with the skin. It should be clear that all of these heat-loss mechanisms can be heat-gain mechanisms as well. We gain heat from the sun by radiation across 93 million miles of space, and we gain heat by conduction when we sit on hot sand at the beach because the sand temperature is greater than skin temperature. Similarly, if a fan were to place more hot air (warmer than skin temperature) into contact with the skin, we would gain, not lose, heat. Heat gained from the environment is added to that generated by exercise and puts an additional strain on heat-loss mechanisms.

The last heat-loss mechanism is the evaporation of sweat. **Sweating** is the process of producing a watery solution over the surface of the body. **Evaporation** is a process in which liquid water is converted

radiation — The process of losing heat from the surface of one object to the surface of another object; the heat loss is dependent on a temperature gradient between the surfaces of the objects.

conduction — The transmission of energy, heat, electricity, or sound. For example, conduction is the passage of electrical currents and nerve impulses through body tissues.

convection — Special case of conduction related to heat loss. Heat is transferred to air or water which become less dense and rise, carrying heat away from the body.

sweating — The process of moisture coming through the pores of the skin from the sweat glands, usually as a result of heat, exertion, or emotion.

evaporation — Conversion from the liquid to the gaseous state by means of heat, as in evaporation of sweat; results in the loss of 580 kcal per liter of sweat evaporated.

to a gas. This conversion requires about 580 kcal of heat per liter of sweat evaporated. The heat for this comes from the body, and thus, the body is cooled. At rest, about 25% of heat loss is due to evaporation, but during exercise it becomes the primary mechanism for heat loss.

Evaporation is dependent on the **water vapor pressure gradient** between the skin and the air and is not directly dependent on temperature. The water vapor pressure of the air is dependent on the **relative humidity** and the **saturation pressure** at that air temperature. For example, the relative humidity can be 90% in winter; but because the saturation pressure of cold air is low, on such a day the water vapor pressure of the air is also low, and you can see water vapor rising from your body following exercise. In warm temperatures, however, the relative humidity is a good indicator of the water vapor pressure of the air. If the water vapor pressure of the air is too high, sweat will not evaporate; and sweat that does not evaporate does not cool the body (46).

Body Temperature Response to Exercise

Figure 4.26 shows that during exercise in a comfortable environment the core temperature increases to a level proportional to the relative intensity (% $\dot{V}O_2$max) of the exercise and then levels off (52). The gain in body heat that occurs early in exercise triggers the heat-loss mechanisms discussed in the preceding section. After 10 to 20 min heat loss equals heat production, and the core temperature remains steady (22). What are the most important heat-loss mechanisms during exercise?

Heat Loss During Exercise

Exercise intensity and environmental temperature have major impacts on which heat-loss mechanism is primarily responsible for maintaining the core temperature during exercise. When a person participates in a series of progressively more difficult exercise tests in an environment that allows heat loss by all the mechanisms just mentioned, the contribution that convection and radiation make to overall heat loss is modest This is due to the fact that the temperature gradient between the skin and the room is not altered much during exercise; consequently the rate of heat loss is relatively constant. To compensate for this, evaporation picks up when heat loss by convection and radiation levels off, and it is responsible for most of the heat loss in heavy exercise (figure 4.27).

If a person performs steady-state exercise in an environment in which the temperature is increasing, the role that evaporation plays becomes even more important. Figure 4.28 shows that as environmental temperature increases, the gradient for heat loss by convection and radiation decreases, and, with it, the rate of heat loss by these processes also decreases. As a result, evaporation must compensate to maintain core temperature.

An important insight to be gained from this discussion is that in strenuous exercise or hot environments, evaporation is the most important process for losing heat and maintaining body temperature in the safe range. It should be no surprise, then, that

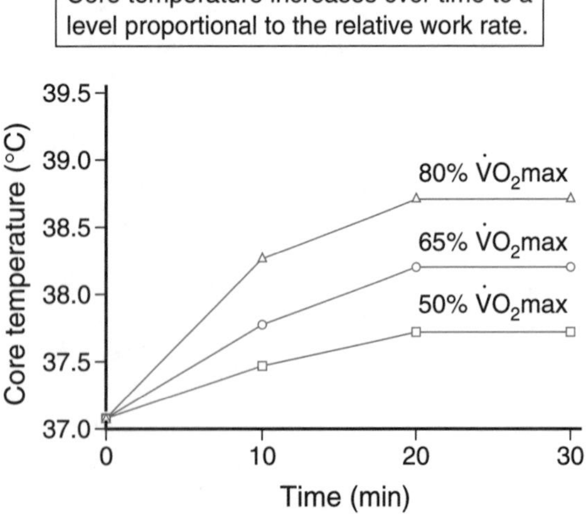

FIGURE 4.26 Core temperature response to exercise (54).

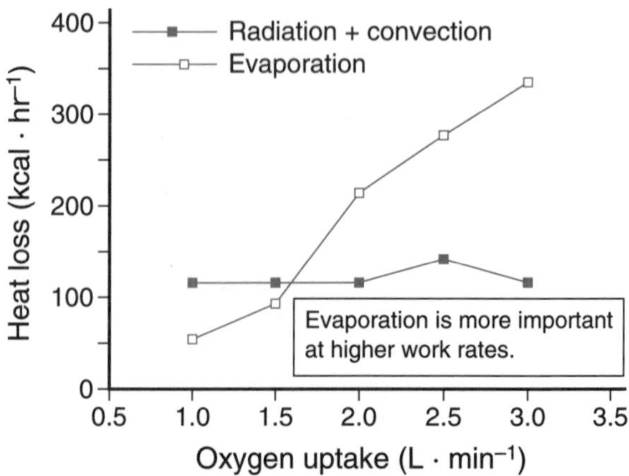

FIGURE 4.27 Importance of evaporation as a heat loss mechanism as exercise intensity increases (2, p. 595).

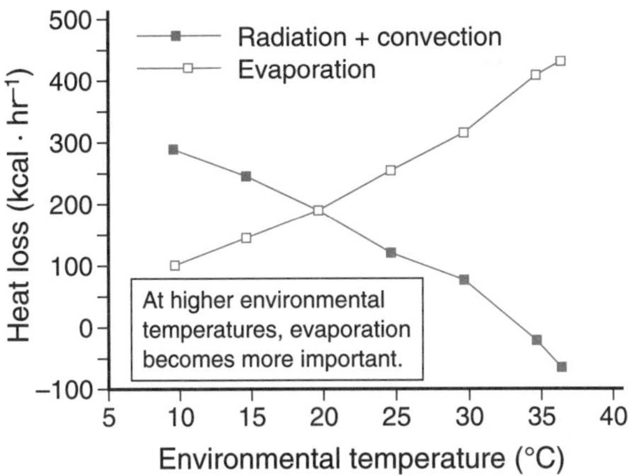

FIGURE 4.28 Importance of evaporation as a heat loss mechanism during exercise as environmental temperature increases (2, p. 598).

factors that affect sweat production (such as dehydration) or that interfere with the evaporation of sweat (such as impermeable clothing) are causes for concern. Chapter 14 provides the specifics on how to deal with heat and humidity when prescribing exercise, and chapter 21 provides important information on preventing and treating heat-related disorders.

Training in a hot and humid environment for as little as 7 to 12 days results in specific adaptations that lead to improved heat tolerance and, as a result, the trained individual's body temperature is lower during submaximal exercise (22). Adaptations that lead to improved heat tolerance include

- an increase in plasma volume,
- an earlier onset of sweating,
- a higher sweat rate,
- a reduction in salt loss in sweat, and
- reduced blood flow to the skin.

14 **In Review: Heat can be lost from the body by radiation and convection when a temperature gradient exists from the skin to the environment; however, evaporation is the primary mechanism of heat loss during high-intensity exercise or during exercise in a hot environment. Body temperature increases during submaximal exercise and achieves a new level proportional to the exercise intensity. Acclimatization to heat can be achieved in 7 to 12 days of training in a hot and humid environment and improves one's ability to exercise safely.**

Case Studies

You can check your answers by referring to appendix A.

4.1

A female competitive distance runner takes a graded exercise test (GXT) on a motor driven treadmill in which the speed of the run increases 0.5 mi · hr^{-1} each minute, with the test starting at 5 mi · hr^{-1}. Blood samples for lactic acid determination were obtained each minute, and the lactate threshold was found to occur at the 8 mph stage of the test. Unfortunately, no one at the testing center knew what this meant relative to performance, and she has come to you for help. What would you tell her?

4.2

A client with whom you have been working retakes a maximal GXT following 10 wk of endurance training and finds his heart rate lower at each stage of the test. He is bothered by this because he thought his heart would be stronger and beat more times per min. What would you tell him to help him understand what happened?

4.3

A female client is bothered by the fact that elite women runners who train as hard as elite male runners don't achieve the same performance times in distance races. She wants to know why, and has come to you for the answer. How would you respond?

water vapor pressure gradient — The tendency for water to evaporate is dependent on the gradient between the water vapor pressure on the skin and the water vapor pressure in the air.

relative humidity — A measure of the dryness of the air; the ratio of the amount of water vapor in the air to the maximum the air can hold at that temperature times 100%.

saturation pressure — Water vapor pressure that exists at a particular temperature when the air is saturated with water.

SOURCE LIST

1. Åstrand (1952)
2. Åstrand & Rodahl (1977, 1986)
3. Bassett (1994)
4. Bouchard et al. (1986)
5. Brooks (1985)
6. Brooks, Fahey, & White (1996)
7. Claytor (1985)
8. Coggan & Coyle (1991)
9. Costill (1988)
10. Coyle (1988)
11. Coyle, Hemmert, & Coggan (1986)
12. Coyle, Martin, Bloomfield, Lowry, & Holloszy (1985)
13. Coyle et al. (1984)
14. Cureton et al. (1978)
15. Davis (1985)
16. Edington & Edgerton (1976)
17. Ekblom, Åstrand, Saltin, Stenberg, & Wallstrom (1968)
18. Faulkner, Roberts, & Conway (1971)
19. Fleck & Dean (1987)
20. Fox, Bowers, & Foss (1993)
21. Franklin (1985)
22. Gisolfi & Wenger (1984)
23. Hickson, Bomze, & Holloszy (1977)
24. Hickson, Bomze, & Holloszy (1978)
25. Hickson, Foster, Pollock, Galassi, & Rich (1985)
26. Hickson, Kanakis, Davis, Moore, & Rich (1982)
27. Hickson & Rosenkoetter (1981)
28. Holloszy & Coyle (1984)
29. Howley (1980)
30. Howley, Bassett, & Welch (1995)
31. Hultman (1967)
32. Issekutz, Birkhead, & Rodahl (1962)
33. Kasch, Boyer, Van Camp, Verity, & Wallace (1990)
34. Kasch, Wallace, & Van Camp (1985)
35. Kasch, Wallace, Van Camp, & Verity (1988)
36. Katch & McArdle (1977)
37. Lind & McNicol (1967)
38. MacDougall, Tuxen, Sale, Moroz, & Sutton (1985)
39. McArdle, Katch, & Katch (1996)
40. McArdle, Katch, & Pechar (1973)
41. McArdle & Magel (1970)
42. Montoye, Ayen, Nagle, & Howley (1986)
43. Nagle, Balke, Baptista, Alleyia, & Howley (1971)
44. Powers, Dodd, & Beadle (1985)
45. Powers, Dodd, Deason, Byrd, & McKnight (1983)
46. Powers & Howley (1997)
47. Powers, Riley, & Howley (1980)
48. Raven (1974)
49. Rowell (1969)
50. Rowell (1986)
51. Sale (1987)
52. Saltin (1969)
53. Saltin & Gollnick (1983)
54. Saltin, Henriksson, Nygaard, Anderson, & Janssen (1977)
55. Saltin & Hermansen (1966)
56. Schwade, Blomqvist, & Shapiro (1977)
57. Sherman (1983)
58. Tanaka & Matsuura (1984)
59. Taylor, Buskirk, & Henschel (1955)
60. Vander, Sherman, & Luciano (1980, 1985)
61. Wilmore & Costill (1994)

CHAPTER

5

Functional Anatomy and Biomechanics

Jean Lewis

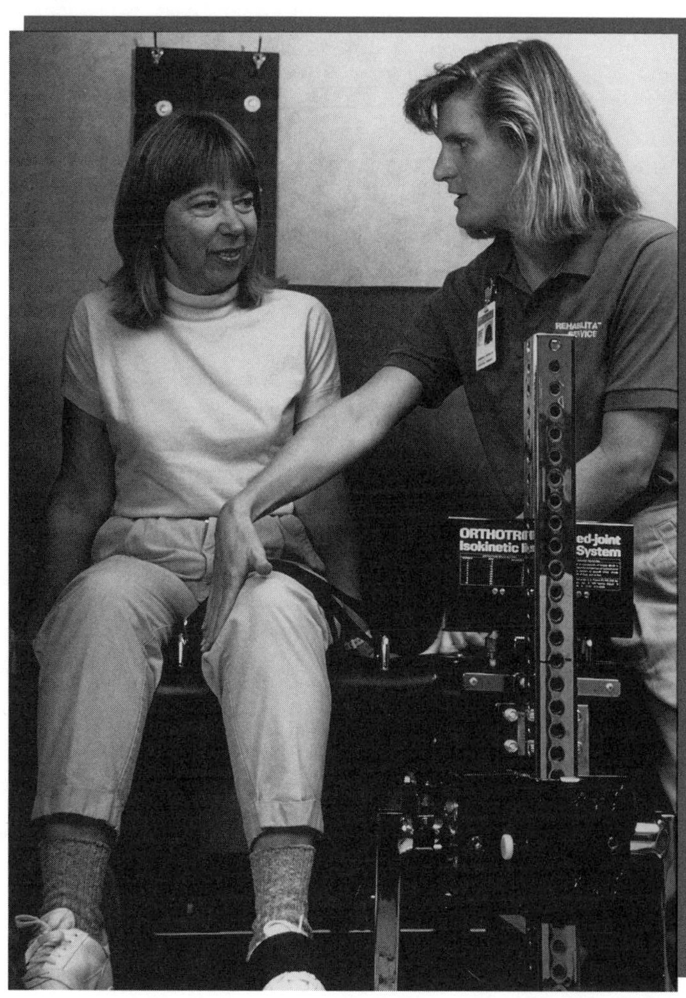

OBJECTIVES

The reader will be able to:

1. **Describe the general structure of long bones.**
2. **Identify the major bones of the skeletal system and classify them by shape.**
3. **Describe the process of ossification of long bones.**
4. **Distinguish between synarthrodial, amphiarthrodial, and diarthrodial joints, both structurally and functionally, and identify the structures of a diarthrodial joint.**
5. **List the factors that determine range and direction of motion at the joints.**
6. **Name and demonstrate the movements possible at each joint.**
7. **Describe forces that can cause joint movement and that can resist movement caused by another force.**
8. **Describe the gross structure of a muscle.**
9. **Explain how muscle tension can be increased.**
10. **Describe the phases of a ballistic movement including the type of muscle contraction.**
11. **Explain the differences between concentric, eccentric, and isometric muscle contractions.**
12. **Describe the roles of muscles.**
13. **List the major muscles in each muscle group, and identify the major actions and joint(s) of involvement of the following muscles: trapezius, serratus anterior, deltoid, pectoralis major, latissimus dorsi, biceps brachii, brachialis, triceps brachii, flexor and extensor carpi radialis and ulnaris, rectus abdominis, external oblique, erector spinae, gluteus maximus, gluteus medius, iliopsoas, rectus femoris, the three vasti muscles, the three hamstring muscles, tibialis anterior, soleus, and gastrocnemius.**
14. **Cite specific errors that occur during exercise for the vertebral column, lumbosacral joints, and knee joint.**
15. **Analyze locomotion, throwing, cycling, jumping, and swimming for the movements and muscle involvement.**
16. **Describe good lifting techniques.**
17. **Describe the three factors that determine stability and identify the interrelationships among line of gravity, base of support, balance, and stability, and describe the practical applications of these interrelationships during physical activity.**
18. **Describe torque and its relationship to muscle contractions.**
19. **Describe how an exerciser can change body segment positions to alter the resistive torque.**

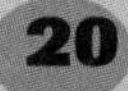 20 **Explain how the mechanical principles of rotational inertia and angular momentum have application to movement.**

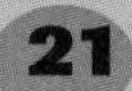 21 **Discuss the common errors seen in locomotion and throwing and striking.**

A knowledge of the bones, joints, and muscles; an understanding of the involvement of muscle forces and other forces; and the ability to apply biomechanical principles to human movement are essential for the health fitness instructor (HFI). With this knowledge and understanding the instructor will be better equipped to lead and direct physical activity in a safe manner for participants seeking the health-related effects of exercise. This knowledge will also help the instructor earn the respect of clients, who will view the instructor as a professional in the field, rather than a technician who may know what to do and how but not *why*. This chapter is but a summary; for detailed presentations of these topics see the references (1-9) at the end of this chapter.

UNDERSTANDING SKELETAL ANATOMY

Most of the 200 distinct bones in the human skeleton are involved in producing movement. Their high mineral component gives them rigidity; the protein component makes them resistant to tension. The two types of bone tissue are (a) compact tissue, which is the dense, hard, outer layer of bone, and (b) spongy, or cancellous tissue, which has a latticelike structure to allow greater structural strength along the lines of stress at a reduced weight. Bones are often divided into four classifications according to their shapes: long, short, flat, and irregular.

Long Bones

The long bones, found in the limbs and digits, serve primarily as levers for movement. Each long bone consists of the **diaphysis**, or shaft, which is made up of thick, compact bone around the hollow medullary cavity; the expanded ends, or **epiphyses**, composed of spongy bone with a thin, outer layer of compact bone; the **articular cartilage**, a thin layer of hyaline cartilage covering the articulating surfaces (the surfaces of a bone that meet or come into contact with another bone to form a joint) that provides a friction-free surface and helps absorb shock; and the **periosteum**, a fibrous membrane covering the entire bone (except where the articular cartilage is present) that serves as an attachment site for many muscles. (See figure 5.1.)

 1 **In Review: The structures of a long bone include the diaphysis, or shaft; the epiphyses, or expanded ends; the periosteum, which covers the bone except at the articulating surfaces; and the articular cartilage that covers the articulating surfaces to provide a friction-free surface and help absorb shock.**

Short, Flat, and Irregular Bones

In addition to long bones, the skeleton is made up of short bones, flat bones, and irregular-shaped bones (see figure 5.2).

The tarsals (ankle) and carpals (wrist) are the short bones. Their composition (spongy bone with a thin outside layer of compact bone) provides greater strength, but their cubic shape decreases their movement potential.

The flat bones, such as the ribs, ilia, and scapulae, serve primarily as broad sites for muscle attachments and, in the case of the ribs and ilia, to enclose cavities and protect internal organs. These bones are also spongy and covered with a thin layer of compact bone.

The ischium, pubis, and vertebrae are irregular shaped bones that serve special purposes such as

diaphysis — The shaft of a long bone.

epiphyses — The ends of long bones.

articular cartilage — Cartilage covering bone surfaces that articulate (meet or come into contact) with other bone surfaces.

periosteum — The connective tissue surrounding all bone surfaces except the articulating surfaces.

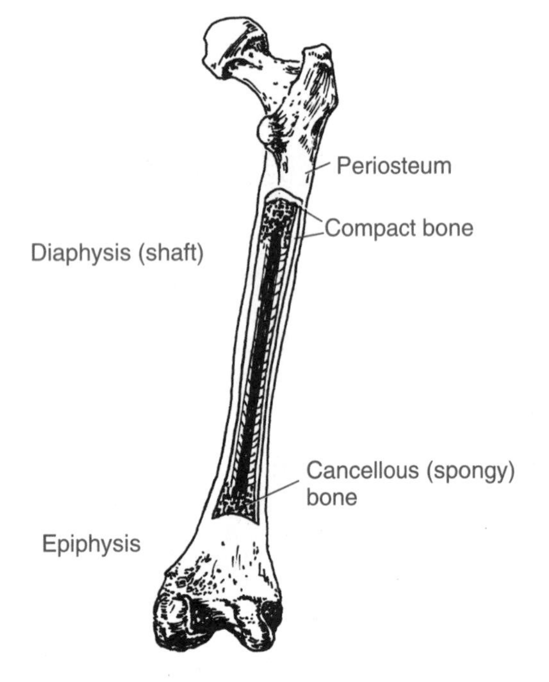

FIGURE 5.1 The femur, an example of a long bone.

protecting internal parts and supporting the body in addition to being sites for muscle attachments.

In Review: Figure 5.2 shows the major skeletal bones, long bones, short bones, flat bones, and irregular bones classified by shape. Each particular type of bone has a specific structure and purpose.

Ossification of Bones

The skeleton begins as a cartilaginous structure, which is gradually replaced by bone (**ossification**). This process begins at the diaphysis of long bones (in centers of ossification) and spreads toward the epiphyses. The **epiphyseal plates** between the diaphyses and epiphyses are the growth areas where the cartilage is replaced by bone; bone growth in length and width continues until the epiphyseal plates are completely ossified. During growth, additional cartilage is laid down to eventually be replaced

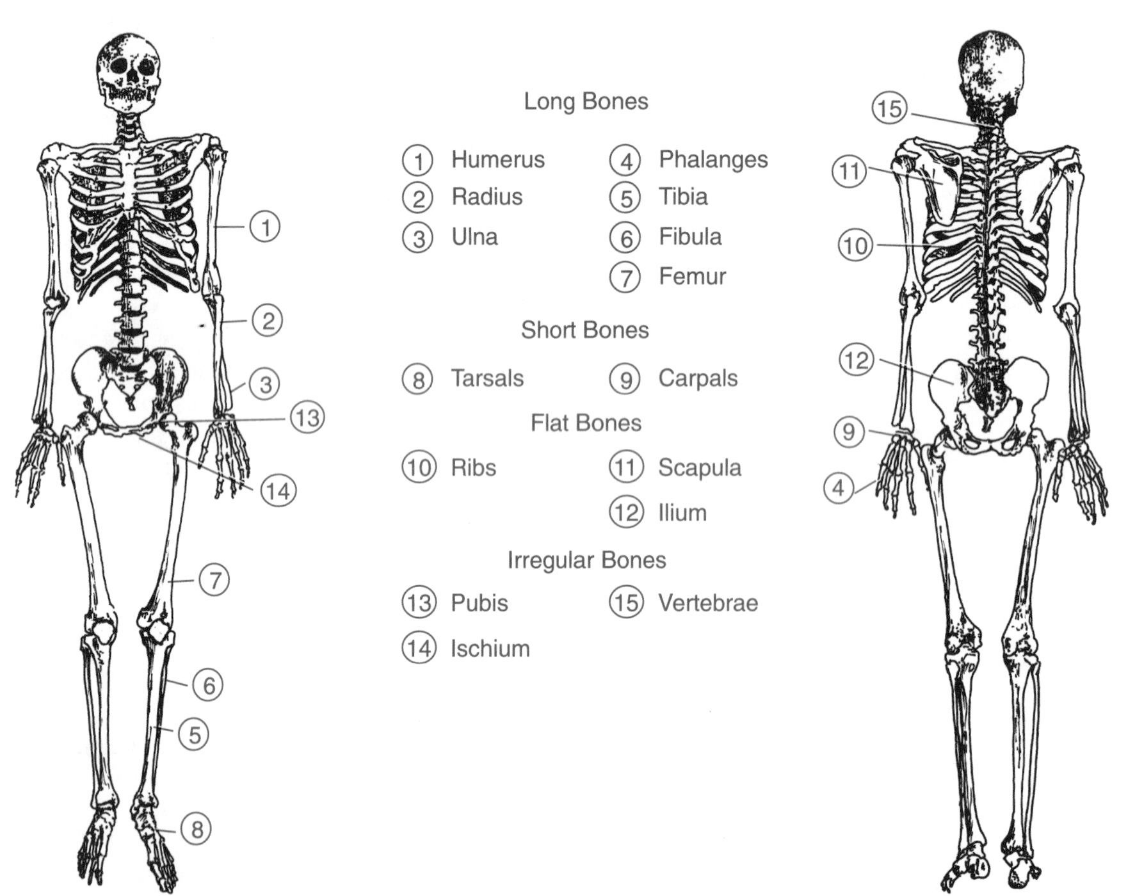

FIGURE 5.2 Front and back view of the human skeleton, with bones classified by shape.

by bone. When no further cartilage is produced, and the cartilage present is replaced by bone, growth ceases. Other secondary centers of ossification develop in the epiphyses and in some bony protuberances, such as the tibial tuberosity and the articular condyles of the humerus. Short bones have one center of ossification. Dates of closure vary. Although bone fusion at some centers of ossification may occur by puberty or earlier, most of the long bones do not have complete ossification until the late teens. Premature closing, which results in a shorter bone length, can be caused by trauma, abnormal stresses, malnutrition, and drugs.

3 **In Review: Ossification is the replacement of cartilage with bone. Generally, bone growth is completed by the late teens.**

STRUCTURE AND FUNCTION OF THE JOINTS

Joints, the places where bones meet or articulate, are often classified according to the amount of movement that can take place at those sites. The classifications are synarthrodial, amphiarthrodial, and diarthrodial joints. The **synarthrodial joints** are the immovable joints. The bones merge into each other and are bound together by fibrous tissue that is continuous with the periosteum. The sutures, or the lines of junction, of the cranial (skull) bones are prime examples of this type of joint. The **amphiarthrodial** (or **cartilaginous**) **joints** allow only slight movement in all directions. Usually a fibrocartilage disk separates the bones, and movement can occur only by deformation of the disk. Examples of these joints are found in the tibiofibular joints and the sacroiliac joints and between the bodies of the vertebrae of the spine. **Ligaments**, which are tough, fibrous bands of connective tissue, connect the bones to each other, not only in this type of joint but also in all joints.

Diarthrodial (or **synovial**) **joints** (see figure 5.3) are freely movable joints that allow a variety of movement direction and range; therefore, most of the joint movements during physical activity occur at diarthrodial joints. The diarthrodial joints are the most common and include most joints of the extremities. Strong and fairly inelastic ligaments, along with connective and muscle tissue that crosses the joint, are responsible for maintaining the stability of the joint. Diarthrodial joints have distinct physical characteristics that also differentiate them from the other types of joints. The articulating surfaces of the bones are covered by articular cartilage, a type of hyaline cartilage that reduces friction and acts somewhat as a shock absorber. Each joint is enclosed by an **articular capsule**, a ligamentous structure that may be fairly thin in spots or thick enough to be considered separate ligaments. The **synovial membrane** lines the inner surface of the capsule. It secretes synovial fluid into the **joint cavity**, the space enclosed by the articular capsule, to bathe (or lubricate) the joint to allow for ease of movement.

Normally, the joint cavity is small and therefore contains little synovial fluid, but an injury to the joint can result in an increased secretion of synovial fluid and resulting swelling. Some diarthrodial joints, such as the sternoclavicular, distal radioulnar, and knee joints, also have a partial or complete fibrocartilage disk between the bones to aid in the absorption of shock and, in the case of the knee, to give

ossification — The replacement of cartilage by bone.

epiphyseal plates — The sites of ossification in long bones.

synarthrodial joints — Immovable joints.

amphiarthrodial joints — A type of joint that allows only slight movement in all directions. Also called the cartilaginous joints.

ligament — The connective tissue that attaches bone to bone.

diarthrodial joints — A type of freely moving joint characterized by its synovial membrane and capsular ligament. Also called synovial joints.

articular capsule — A ligamentous structure that encloses a diarthrodial joint.

synovial membrane — The inner lining of the joint capsule; secretes synovial fluid into the joint cavity.

joint cavity — The space between bones enclosed by the synovial membrane and articular cartilage.

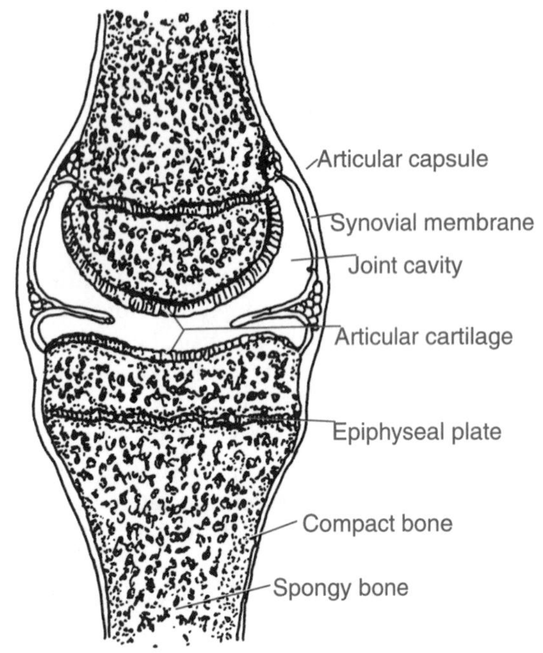

FIGURE 5.3 A diarthrodial or synovial joint.

greater stability to the joint. The partial, semilunar-shaped disks between the femur and tibia at the knee are called **menisci**.

To reduce frictional rubbing that occurs as the lengths of tendons change during muscle contraction, tendons are often surrounded by tendinous sheaths—cylindrical, tunnel-like sacs lined with synovial membrane. For example, the two proximal tendons of the biceps brachii muscle pass through these tunnels in the bicipital groove of the humerus. **Bursae**, or sacs of synovial fluid that lie between muscles, tendons, and/or bones, also reduce friction between the tissues and act as shock absorbers. Many bursae are found around the shoulder, elbow, hip, and knee. Bursitis, or the inflammation of a bursa, can be caused by repeated friction or mechanical irritation, or as a result of inflammatory or degenerative conditions of the tendons.

4 **In Review: The types of joints are synarthrodial, which do not allow movement; amphiarthrodial, which allow only slight movement; and diarthrodial, or synovial, joints, which are characterized functionally by their wide range of movement and structurally by the presence of articular cartilage, an articular capsule, synovial membrane, and synovial fluid within the joint cavity.**

FACTORS THAT DETERMINE DIRECTION AND RANGE OF MOTION

Most of the movement at a joint is rotary in nature: The bone moves around a fixed axis, the joint. The structures of the bones at and near their articulating ends largely determines both the direction and the range of movement. Ball-and-socket joints, which are found at the hip and shoulder, allow a wide range of movement in all directions; but a hinge joint, such as the elbow joint, restricts both direction and range of movement because bone impinges on bone. The length of the ligaments, and to a lesser extent their **elasticity**, or ability to lengthen (stretch) passively and return to their normal length, are also factors in range of movement. For example, the iliofemoral ligament at the anterior hip joint is a strong but short ligament that prohibits much hip hyperextension. Elasticity can be changed by appropriate exercise; the amount of elasticity is determined by the amount and type of physical activity in which an individual engages.

5 **In Review: The potential range and direction of motion is related to the shape of the articulating ends of the bones, the length of ligaments, and the elasticity of connective tissue.**

Specific Joint Movements

Specific terminology is used to describe the direction of movement at the different joints. The anatomical position (standing with arms at sides and turned so the palm of the hand faces forward) serves as a point of reference. Although different terminology may be used for specific joints, **flexion** in general is anterior or posterior movement from the anatomical position that brings two bones together, **extension** is the return from flexion, and **hyperextension** is the continuation of extension past the anatomical position. **Abduction** is the movement of a bone laterally from the anatomical position; **adduction**, the return back toward the anatomical position. **Rotation** occurs when the bone spins around its longitudinal axis so that its surface faces a different direction.

Shoulder Girdle

This joint complex includes the articulations between the sternum and clavicle and between the clavicle and scapula. Rotary joint movement occurs at those articulations, but the movement terms *elevation, depression, abduction, adduction*, and *upward* and *downward rotation* describe the resulting movements of the scapulae. (See figure 5.4.) Abduction, adduction, and scapular elevation and depression can all occur without shoulder joint movement but may enhance it. Upward and downward rotation can occur only when the humerus is moved upward, outward, and downward. If the scapulae cannot rotate upward, the arms cannot be elevated sideways above the horizon (beyond 90°).

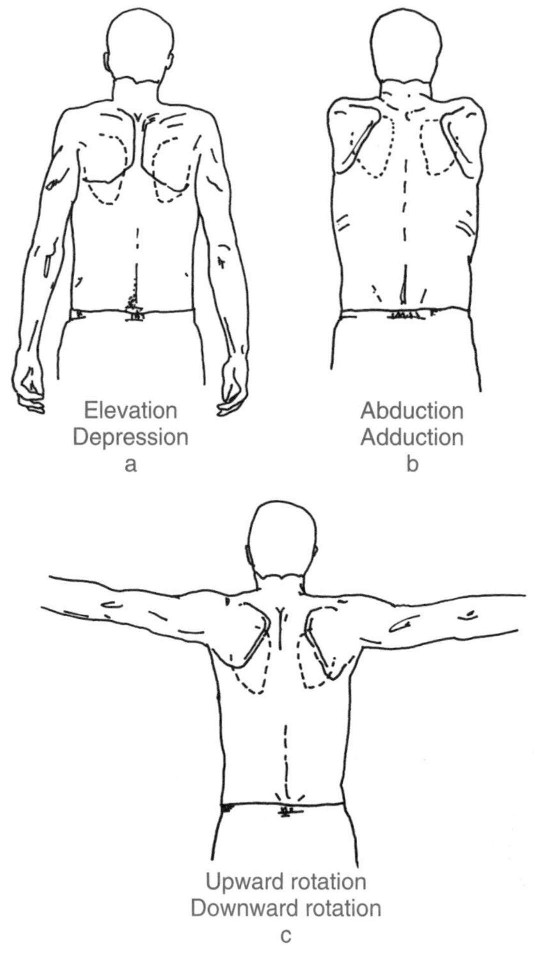

FIGURE 5.4 Movements of the scapulae.

Shoulder Joint

Because of its ball-and-socket structure, the shoulder joint can move in all directions—flexion; extension; hyperextension; abduction; adduction; lateral (outward, away from the midline) and medial (inward, toward the midline) rotation; and circumduction, which is the circular movement of the arm in a wide arc. Horizontal extension and horizontal flexion are movements of the arm parallel to the ground. (See figure 5.5.)

Scapula movements can enhance shoulder-joint movements. As the arm flexes or horizontally flexes, scapula abduction can move the hand out farther in front. Scapula adduction can allow the arm to move back more during hyperextension and horizontal extension. Elevation of the scapula can allow the hand to reach higher. Medial rotation may be accompanied by scapula abduction; lateral rotation, by scapula adduction.

Elbow Joint

Sometimes referred to as the humeroulnar joint for the bones involved in elbow-joint movement, the elbow joint allows only flexion and extension because of its bony arrangement. (See figure 5.6.) The ability of some individuals to hyperextend the elbow joint is due to the shape of the articulating surfaces.

menisci — Partial, semilunar-shaped disks between the femur and tibia and the knee.

bursae — Fibrous sacs lined with synovial membrane that contain a small quantity of synovial fluid. Bursae are found between tendon and bone, skin and bone, and between muscle and muscle. Their function is to facilitate movement without friction between these surfaces.

elasticity — Ability of ligaments and tendons to lengthen passively and return to their resting length.

flexion — Anterior or posterior movement that brings two bones together.

extension — Increasing the angle at a joint, such as straightening the elbow.

hyperextension — A continuation of extension past the anatomical position.

abduction — Movement of a bone laterally away from the anatomical position.

adduction — The return back to the anatomical position from the abducted position.

rotation — The movement of a bone around its longitudinal axis.

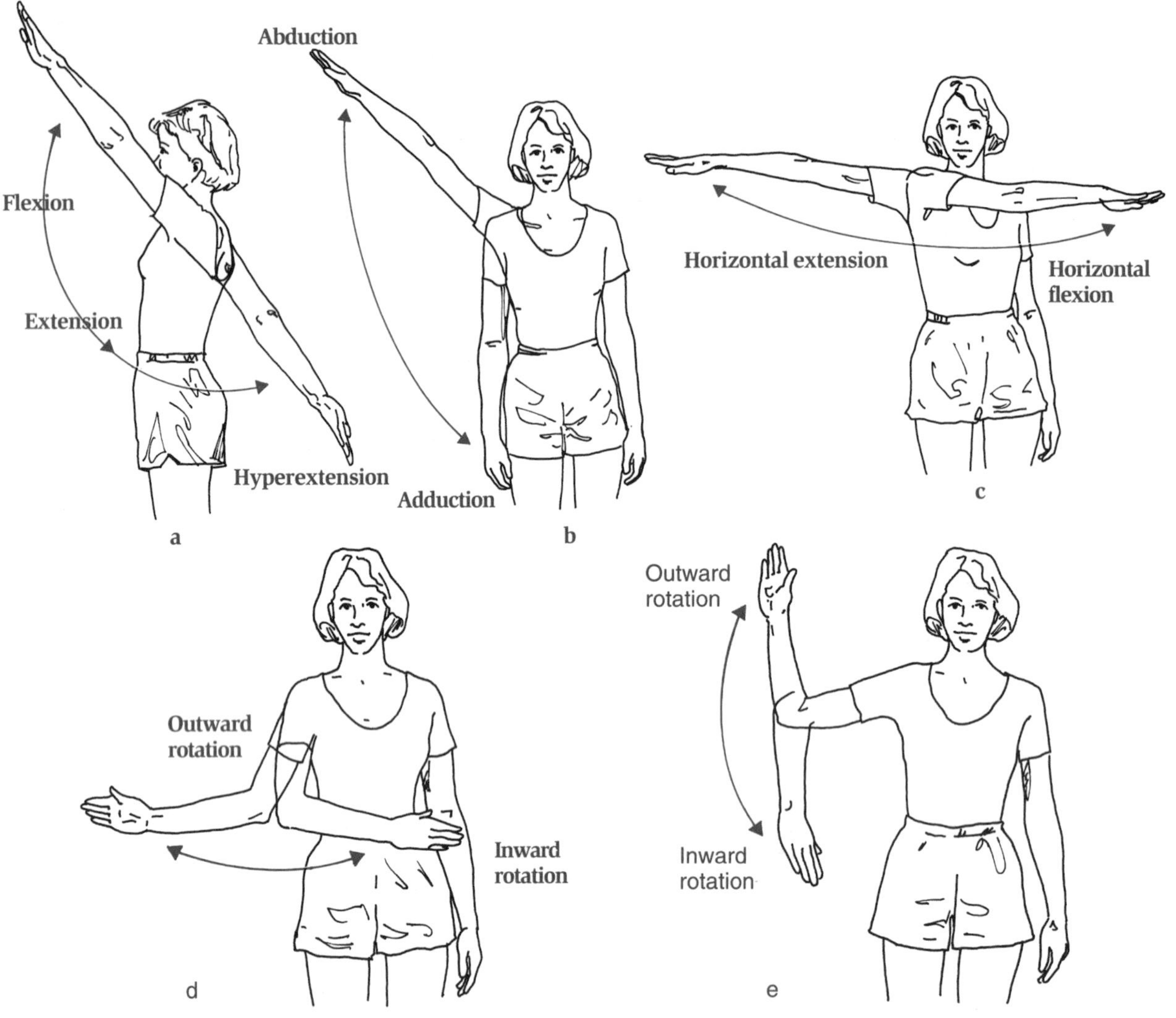

FIGURE 5.5 Movements of the shoulder joint.

Radioulnar Joints

Pronation and supination are the movements of the radius around the ulna in the lower arm. (See figure 5.7.) Although the wrist is not involved in these movements, the position of the radioulnar joints can be identified by the direction in which the palm of the hand is facing. When the arms are hanging down alongside the trunk, the palm faces forward in the supinated position and toward the back in the pronated position. In the supinated position, the radius and ulna are parallel to each other; in the pronated position, the radius lies across and on top of the ulna. Pronation combined with shoulder-joint medial rotation, and supination combined with shoulder-joint lateral rotation, move the hand around the midline even farther.

Wrist Joint

Movement at the wrist joint can occur in two planes of direction: flexion, extension, and hyperextension; and abduction (sometimes referred to as radial flexion) and adduction (ulnar flexion). (See figure 5.8.)

Metacarpophalangeal and Interphalangeal Joints

The second through the fifth metacarpophalangeal joints allow flexion and extension, and abduction and adduction of the fingers. The MP joint of the thumb allows only flexion and extension, but it is the only digit that also allows movement at the carpometacarpal joint (which gives the thumb its movement ability). All the interphalangeal (IP) joints of the fingers and toes only flex and extend.

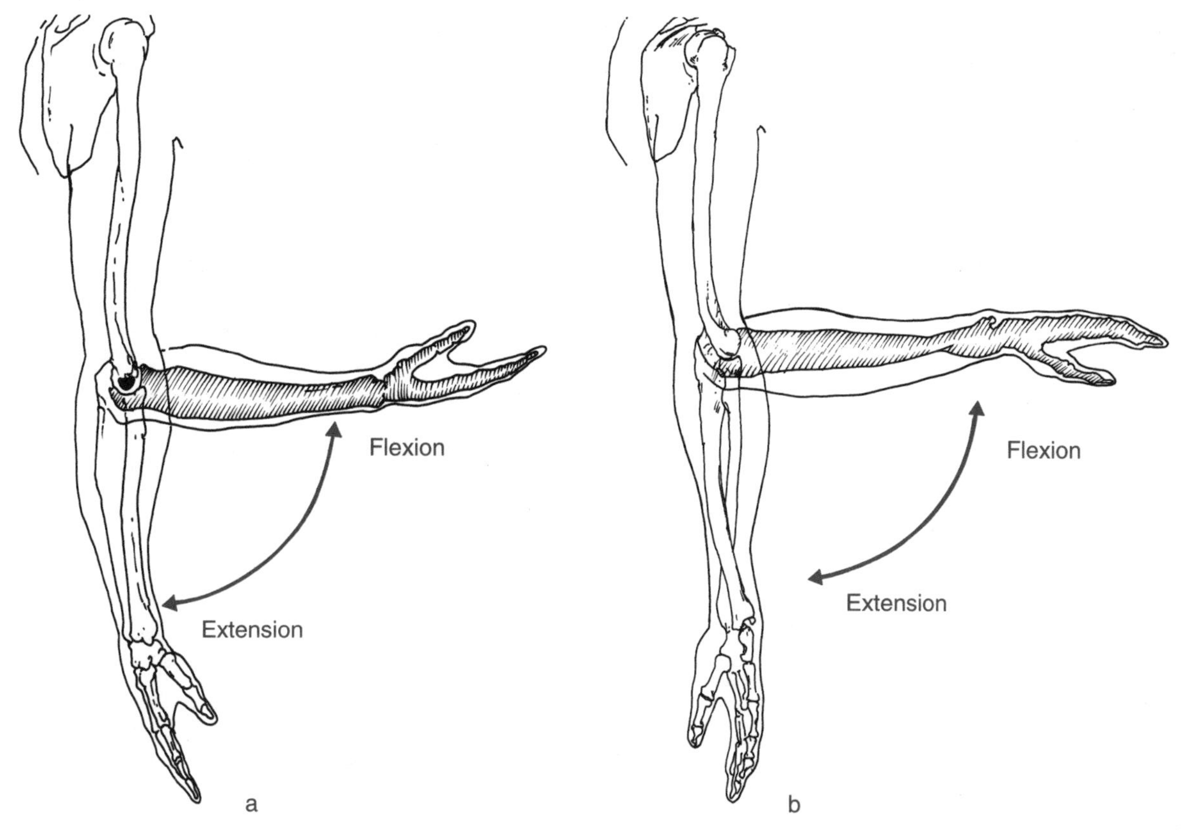

FIGURE 5.6 Movements of the elbow joint.

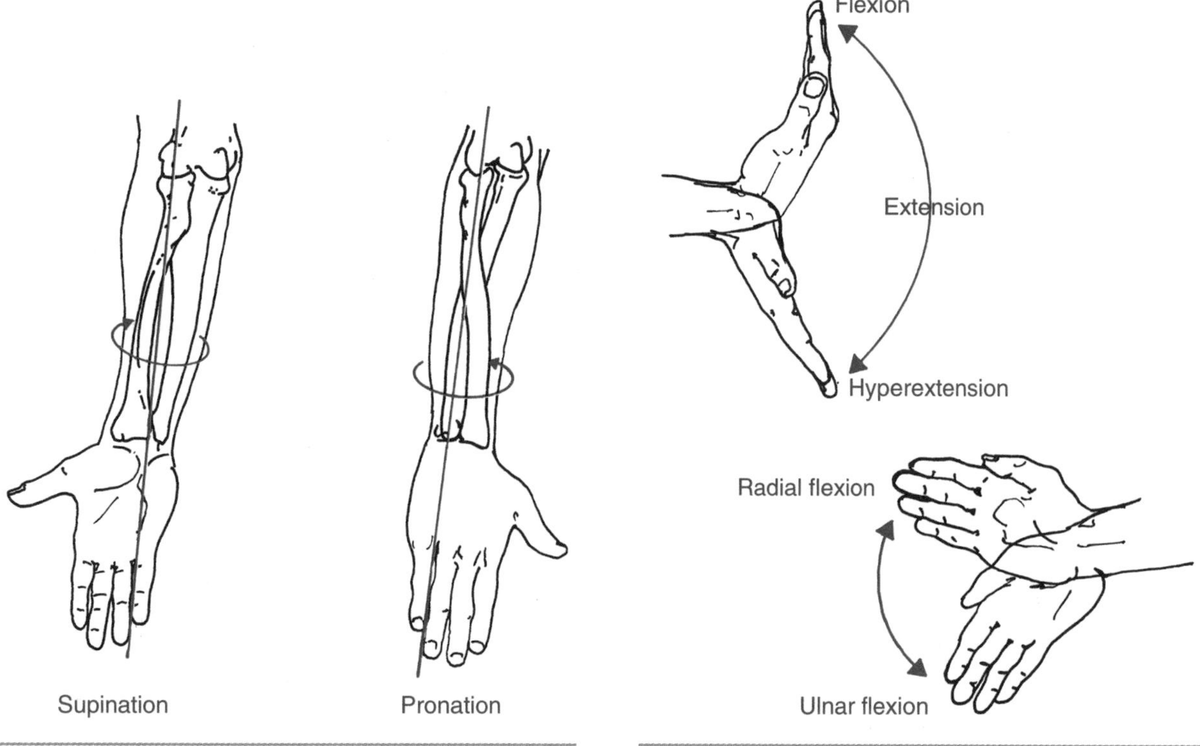

FIGURE 5.7 Movements of the radioulnar joints.

FIGURE 5.8 Movements of the wrist joint.

Vertebral Column

Movements of the trunk—flexion, extension, hyperextension, lateral flexion, and rotation—occur at all the joints of the vertebral column. (See figure 5.9.)

Lumbosacral Joint: Pelvis Movement

The tilts of the pelvis (see figure 5.10) occur mainly at the joint formed by the fifth lumbar vertebra and the pelvis. The reference point for the direction of the tilts is the iliac crest. As the crest moves forward and down, the pelvis is going toward a forward, or anterior, pelvic tilt; as the crest rotates toward the back, the pelvis has a backward, or posterior, tilt. The anterior pelvic tilt is usually accompanied by a hyperextension of the lumbar vertebrae; a backward tilt by a flattening out of the lumbar vertebrae.

Hip Joint

The hip joint structure is similar to the shoulder joint, a ball-and-socket arrangement; and the same movements are possible. (See figure 5.11.) Because of the deepness of the socket and the tightness of the ligaments at the hip joint, range of motion at this joint,

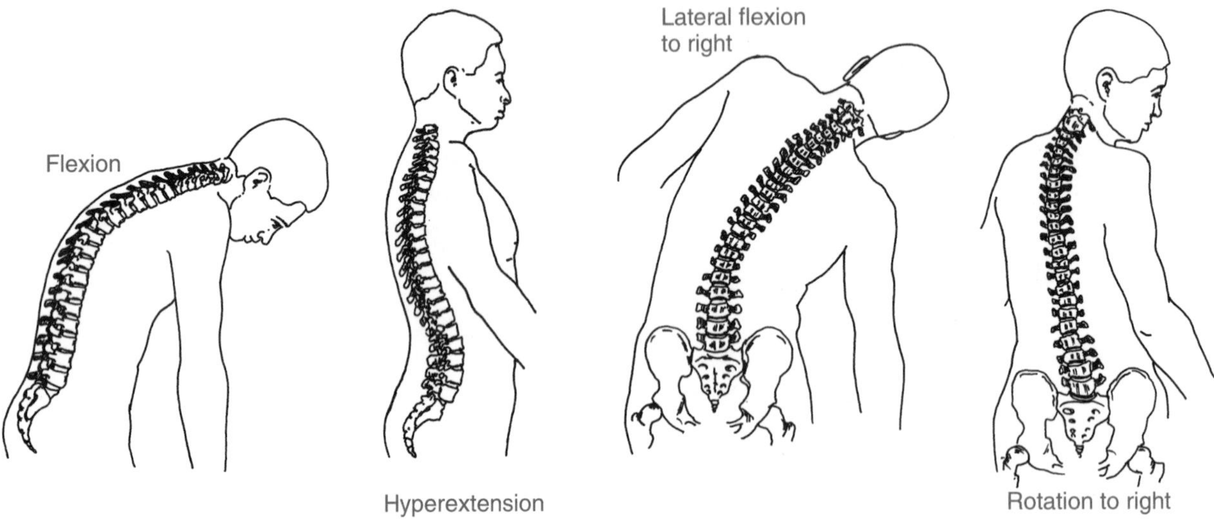

FIGURE 5.9 Movements of the vertebral column.

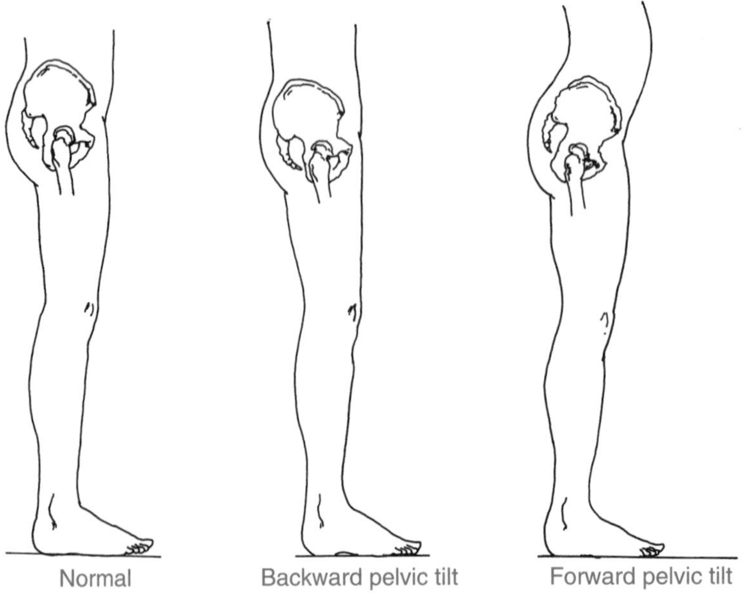

FIGURE 5.10 Movements of the lumbosacral joint.

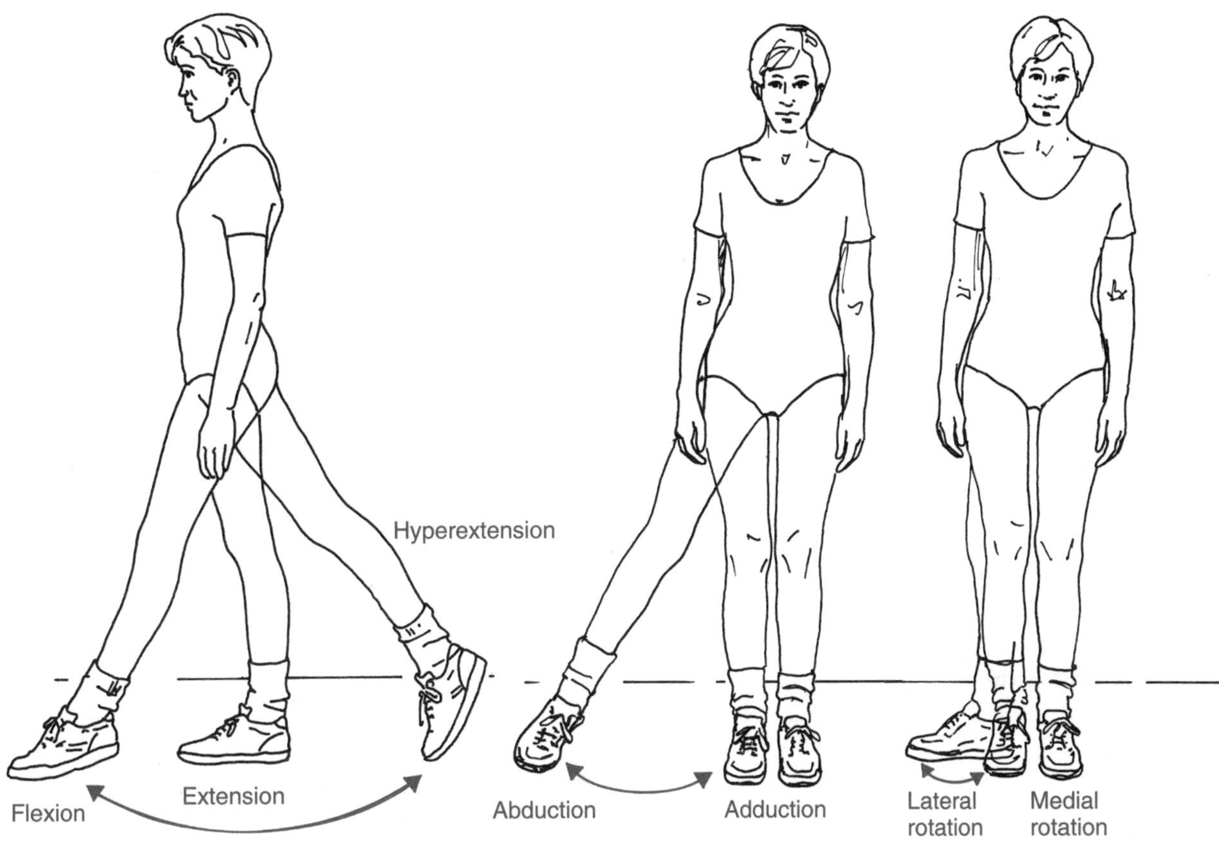

FIGURE 5.11 Movements of the hip joint.

especially for hyperextension, is less than at the shoulder joint. True hip abduction is also limited to about 45° by bony impingement. The leg can be lifted higher only by rotating the hip laterally.

Knee Joint

Flexion and extension are the major movements at the knee. Although some hyperextension may be possible, it should be avoided. (See figure 5.12.) When the knee is in a flexed position, a limited amount of rotation, abduction, and adduction is possible.

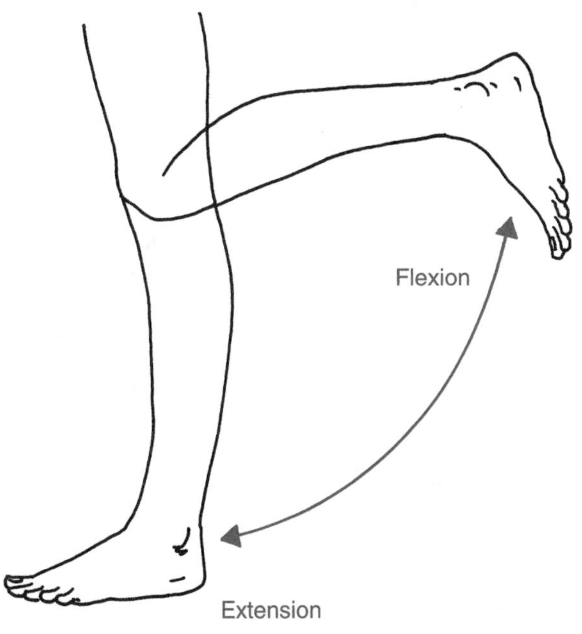

FIGURE 5.12 Movements of the knee joint.

Ankle Joint

Also called the talocrural joint, the ankle is limited to movement in one plane only. Plantar flexion (pointing the toes downward) is still sometimes referred to as extension; dorsiflexion (flexing the toes back), as flexion. (See figure 5.13.)

Intertarsal Joints

The sideways movements of the foot occur between the different tarsal joints in the foot. (See figure 5.14.) Inversion can be considered a combination of

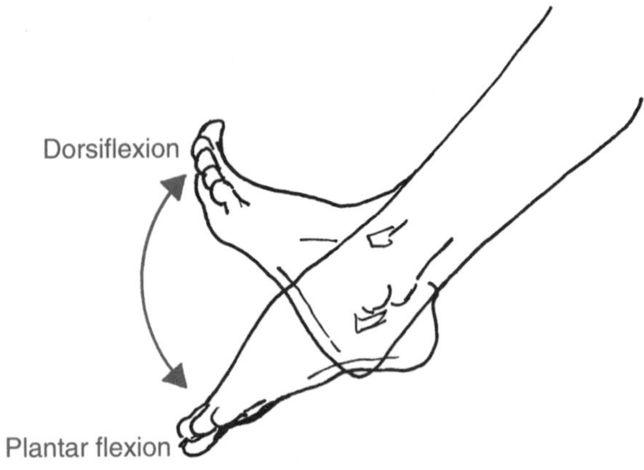

FIGURE 5.13 Movements of the ankle joint.

pronation and adduction; eversion, a combination of supination and abduction.

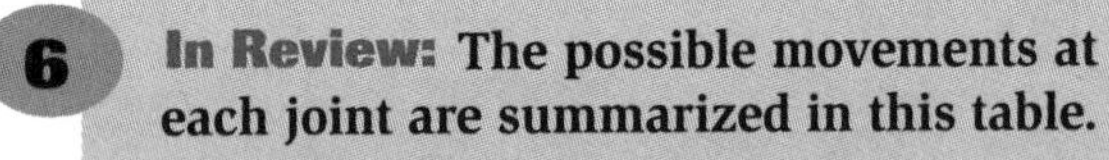

6 In Review: The possible movements at each joint are summarized in this table.

Joint	Movements
Shoulder girdle	Elevation, depression; abduction, adduction; upward rotation, downward rotation
Shoulder joint	Flexion, extension, hyperextension; abduction, adduction; medial rotation, lateral rotation; horizontal flexion, horizontal extension
Elbow joint	Flexion, extension
Radioulnar joint	Pronation, supination
Wrist joint	Flexion, extension, hyperextension; radial flexion, ulnar flexion
Metatarsophalangeal joints	Flexion, extension; abduction, adduction
Vertebral column	Flexion, extension, hyperextension; lateral flexion; rotation
Lumbosacral joint	Forward pelvic tilt, backward pelvic tilt
Hip joint	Flexion, extension, hyperextension; abduction, adduction; medial rotation, lateral rotation
Knee joint	Flexion, extension
Ankle joint	Plantar flexion, dorsiflexion
Intertarsal joint	Eversion, inversion

Forces Related to Joint Movement

Several **forces** can act on the bones. These forces can cause, resist, or even prevent movement at the joints.

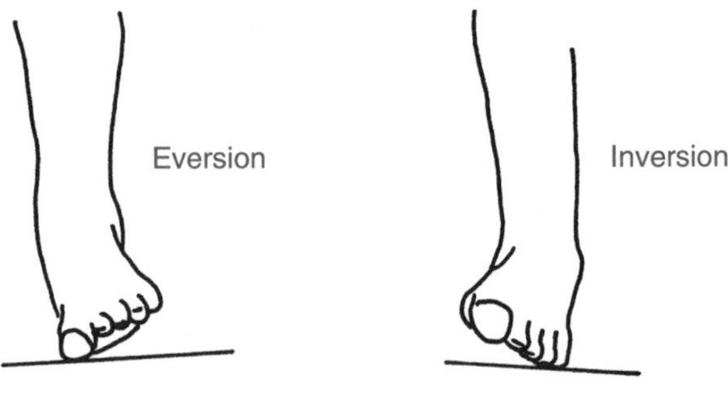

FIGURE 5.14 Movements of the intertarsal joints.

Forces That Cause Movement

Joint movement is primarily caused by either a muscle-shortening contraction or gravitational pull, although other forces, such as another person pushing or pulling on a body part, may also cause joint movement. Whether a muscle contraction will cause the movement depends upon the force of that contraction and the amount of resistance from the other forces.

Forces That Resist or Prevent Movement Caused by Another Force

The same forces that can cause movement also act to resist or prevent movement. Joint movement caused by gravity can be resisted or decelerated by eccentric muscle contraction (causes a lengthening of the muscle; see the section on eccentric contraction later in the chapter). Gravity always resists movement occurring in the direction away from the earth. Other forces that can resist movement include internal tissue restriction by tight ligaments and tendons, exercise bands, hydraulic or air pressure devices on resistance training equipment, and water.

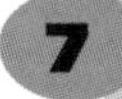

7 In Review: Forces that can both cause and resist joint movements include muscle contraction and gravity.

VOLUNTARY (SKELETAL) MUSCLE

A skeletal muscle, which is involved in joint movements, consists of thousands of muscle fibers (e.g., the brachioradialis has approximately 130 000 fibers; the gastrocnemius has over 1 million) and connective tissue. Each fiber is enclosed by the connective tissue endomysium. The **fasciculi**, or bundles of fibers grouped together, are surrounded by the **perimysium**; and the entire muscle is enclosed by the **epimysium**. The **tendon** is the passive part of the muscle made up of the elastic connective tissues. Each muscle is attached either to the bone itself; to the periosteum of the bone; or to deep, thick fascia by tendons and the perimysium and epimysium connective tissues. The sizes and the shapes of the tendons vary and depend upon their functions and the shape of the muscle itself. Some tendons (e.g., the hamstring muscle tendons found at the sides of the posterior knee and the Achilles tendon) are obvious and significant parts of the entire muscle length, but other muscles such as the supraspinatus and infraspinatus (muscles that abduct and rotate the arm) seem to lie directly on the bone with no observable tendon. Many of the distal attachments (attachments farthest away from the body part being moved) that are usually found on bones that show the largest movements have a more defined tendinous structure than the proximal attachments (attachments nearest to the body part being moved). Broad and flat tendons, such as the proximal tendinous sheath of the latissimus dorsi, are called **aponeuroses**. Refer to figure 5.15 for anterior and posterior views of surface muscles. Other muscles lie underneath the surface muscles.

8 In Review: The structures associated with muscle include fasciculi, perimysium, epimysium, tendons, and aponeuroses.

Muscle Contraction

Each muscle fiber is innervated, or receives its stimulus, by a branch of a motor neuron. The functional organization, or **motor unit**, consists of a single motor neuron and its branches and all the muscle fibers innervated by that motor neuron. With a sufficiently strong stimulus, each muscle fiber within that motor unit contracts maximally; muscular tension increases as a result of the stimulation of more motor units (**recruitment**) or an increased rate of stimulation (summation). A muscle that has as its primary purpose a strength or power movement (as does the gastrocnemius) rather than a delicate movement (as does any of the finger muscles), has a large number of muscle fibers and also has many muscle fibers per motor unit. When a muscle develops tension, or contracts, it tends to shorten toward the middle, pulling on all of its bony attachments. Whether the bone(s) of attachment move as a result of that contraction depends upon the amount of the force of the contraction and the resistance to that movement from other forces. Muscles contract in three major ways: concentric contractions, eccentric contractions, and isometric contractions.

In Review: The motor unit consists of a single motor neuron and its branches and all the muscle fibers innervated by that motor neuron. Muscular tension is increased by recruitment and summation.

Concentric Contraction

A **concentric contraction** occurs when a muscle contracts forcibly enough to actually shorten. This shortening pulls the bones of attachment closer to each other, causing movement at the joint. Figure 5.16 illustrates elbow flexion against gravity as a result of a concentric contraction: The muscles responsible for the flexion are able to contract with sufficient force to shorten, which pulls the lower arm toward the humerus. Although the pull is on all the bones of attachment, usually only the bone

force — Any push or pull that tends to cause movement.

fasciculi — Bundles of muscle fibers surrounded by perimysium.

perimysium — The connective tissue surrounding fasciculi within a muscle.

epimysium — The connective-tissue sheath surrounding a muscle.

tendon — A band of tough, inelastic, fibrous connective tissue that attaches muscle to bone.

aponeuroses — Broad, flat, tendinous sheaths attaching muscles to each other.

motor unit — The functional unit of muscular contraction that includes a motor nerve and the muscle fibers that its branches innervate.

recruitment — Stimulation of additional motor units to increase the strength of a muscle contraction.

concentric contraction — A shortening of the muscle; causes movement at the joint

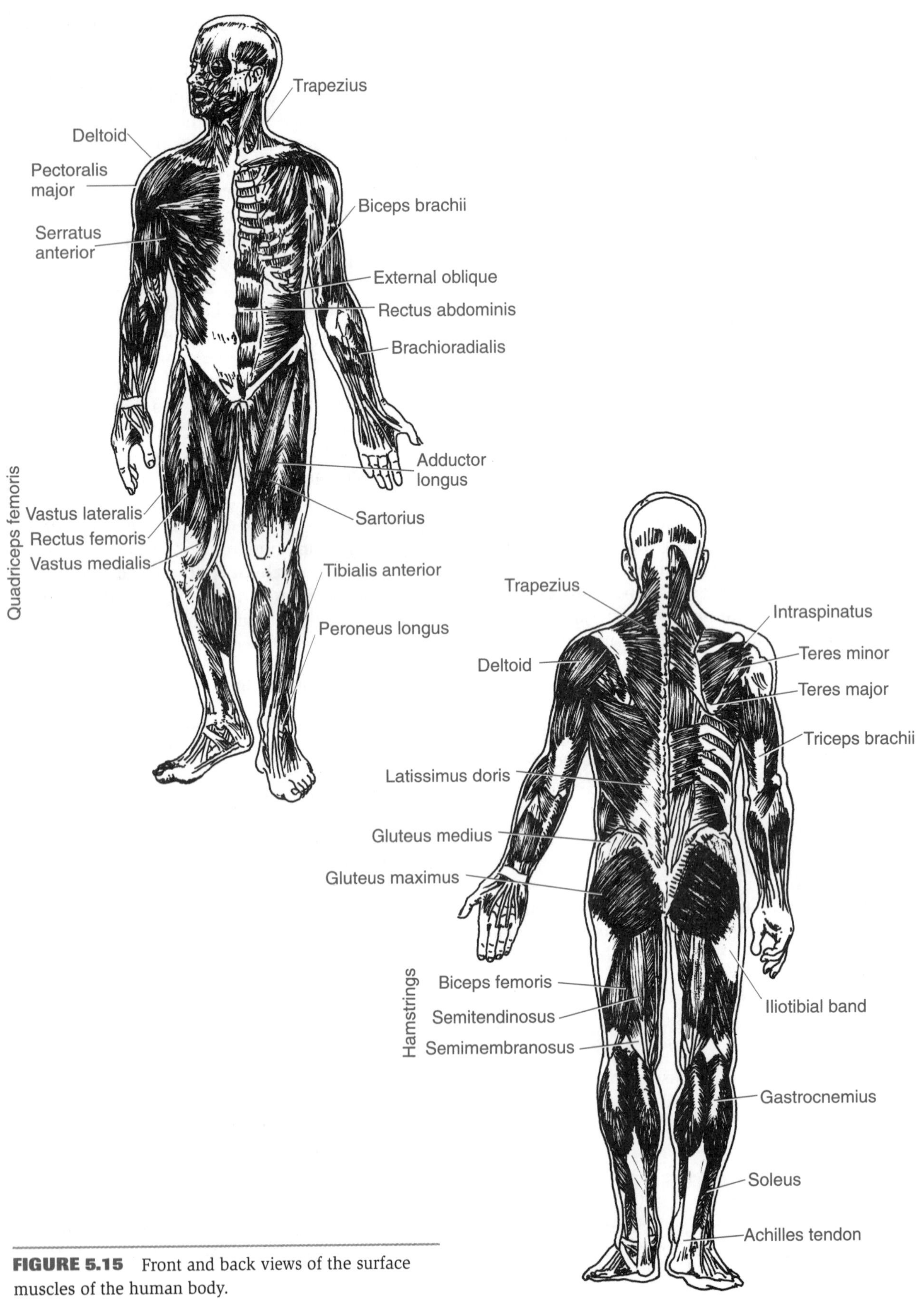

FIGURE 5.15 Front and back views of the surface muscles of the human body.

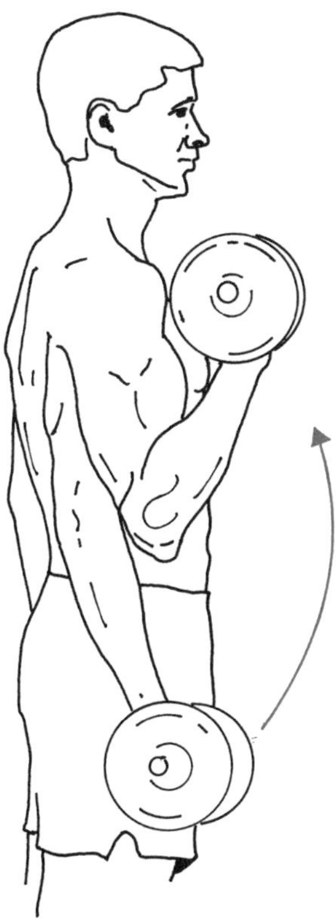

FIGURE 5.16 Concentric contraction by the elbow flexors.

farthest from the trunk (e.g., a limb) will move in a concentric contraction. To stand up from a semisquat position, there must be extension at the hip joints and knee joints, but gravity is resisting that extension. The muscles must develop sufficient force to overcome the gravitational force; if sufficient force is developed, the muscle will shorten in a concentric contraction, pulling on the bones to cause extension. Resistance training with free weights uses gravitational pull as the resistance; the use of pulleys changes the direction of the gravitational pull, offering resistance to movement in other directions. Although gravity is not a factor in water, the water itself resists movement in all directions.

To exercise muscles by using gravity as the resisting force, the movements must be done in the direction opposite the pull of gravity (i.e., away from the earth). Arm abduction from a standing position is a movement opposite the pull of gravity, so a concentric contraction is required by the muscles that will pull the humerus into the abducted position. Movements such as shoulder horizontal flexion and extension (see figure 5.5) executed from a standing position occur parallel to the ground and therefore are not resisted by gravity. Internal tissue friction is the only resistance, but concentric contraction by the muscles responsible for these movements is still necessary. During these movements, gravity is still trying to draw the arm toward the earth, but it is not interfering with the horizontal movement. To perform horizontal flexion and extension against the resistance of gravity, the performer must get into a position in which the movements are away from the pull of gravity. To horizontally extend the shoulder joints against gravity, the performer can be lying prone on a bench or floor, or, by standing with the trunk flexed at the hip. Horizontal flexion against gravity can be done from a supine position on the floor.

A concentric contraction is also necessary for a rapid movement, regardless of the direction of another force. When an external force could cause the desired movement without any muscular contraction, but too slowly, concentric contractions produce the desired speed. An example of this is seen in the arm movements during the second count of a jumping jack, when the arms adduct from their abducted position: Gravity would adduct the arms, but concentrically contracting muscles cause the movement to occur much more quickly.

A muscle that is very effective in causing a certain joint movement is a prime mover, or **agonist**. Assistant movers are muscles that are not as effective for the same movement. For example, the peroneus longus and brevis are prime movers for eversion of the intertarsal joints, but they can offer only a little assistance in plantar flexion of the ankle joint. During a concentric contraction, muscles that act opposite to the muscles causing the concentric contraction, the **antagonist** muscles, are basically passive and lengthen as the agonists shorten in contraction. For example, for elbow flexion to occur against the pull of gravity, the muscles responsible for elbow flexion are contracting concentrically; the antagonists, or the muscles responsible for elbow extension, relax and lengthen passively during the movement. In some fitness activities, such as aerobic dance, however, the antagonist muscles can be contracted to offer more resistance to the concentrically

agonist muscle — A muscle that is very effective in causing a certain joint movement. Also called the prime mover.

antagonist — A muscle that causes movement at a joint in a direction opposite to that of the joint's **agonist** (prime mover).

contracting muscles. This resistance is done by having all the muscles contracted (such as a body builder's pose) during the movements.

Eccentric Contraction

An **eccentric contraction** occurs when a muscle generates tension that is not great enough to cause movement but instead acts as a brake to control the speed of movement caused by another force. (See figure 5.17.) The muscle exerts force, but its length increases. Arm abduction requires a concentric contraction of muscles; gravity will adduct the arm back down to the side. To adduct the arm more slowly than gravity, the same muscles that contracted concentrically to abduct the arm now contract eccentrically to control the speed of the lowering arm. Eccentric contractions may also occur when a muscle's maximum effort still is not great enough to overcome the opposing force; movement will be caused by that force in spite of the maximally contracting muscle, which is still lengthening. An example of this would be if someone, with the elbow joint flexed to a 90° position, were handed a heavy weight. The exerciser tries to flex the elbow joint or even maintain the position but lacks the strength to do so. The elbow joint extends despite the efforts to flex it. Muscles antagonist to the eccentrically contracting muscles passively shorten during the movement.

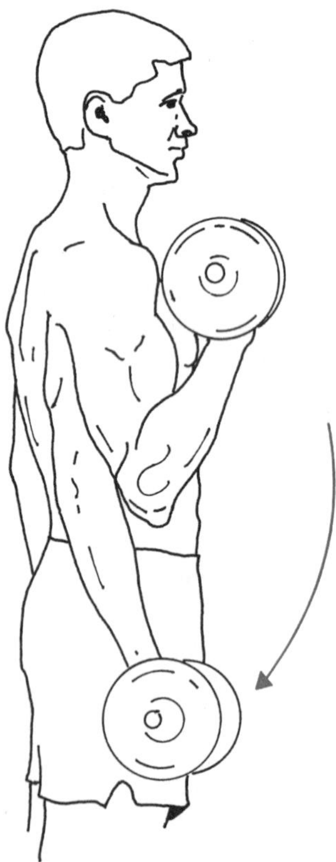

FIGURE 5.17 Eccentric contraction by the elbow flexors.

Ballistic Movements and Muscle Contraction

A **ballistic**, or fast, **movement** occurs when resistance is insignificant, as in throwing a ball, and requires a burst of concentric contractions to initiate the movement. Once movement has begun, the muscles that contracted to cause the movement basically shut down; any further contraction slows the movement. Other muscles actively guide the movement in the appropriate direction. Eccentric contractions of muscles that are antagonist, or opposite, to the muscles that initiated the movement decelerate and eventually stop the movement. For example, one of the most important movements in the actual throwing motion is medial rotation of the shoulder joint. The muscles responsible for medial rotation concentrically contract quickly to begin the throwing motion. After the ball is released, the muscles responsible for lateral rotation contract eccentrically to slow and eventually stop the movement; this is called the follow-through. The reverse is true for the windup, or preparation for the actual throw. All of this occurs in an exceedingly short period of time.

The exercise jumping jacks requires repeated ballistic movements in which opposing muscles come into play. The arm movements require concentric contraction by the agonist muscles to initiate the rapid movement. Once the movement is initiated, these muscles basically shut down. To stop the abduction movement and initiate the arm movement in the opposite direction, muscles antagonistic to those that concentrically contracted to initiate the movement come into play. They contract eccentrically to decelerate the movement, and then contract concentrically to initiate the next arm movement (adduction).

10 **In Review: A ballistic movement is a rapid movement that begins with the agonist muscles contracting concentrically to initiate movement; then "coasting," in which there is minimal muscle activity; and lastly, follow-through with an eccentric contraction of the antagonist muscles to decelerate the movement.**

Isometric Contraction

During an **isometric**, or static, **contraction**, the muscle exerts a force that counteracts an opposing force. The muscle length does not change, so no movement occurs, and the joint position is maintained. The contractile part of the muscle shortens, but the elastic connective tissue lengthens proportionately; no overall change in the entire muscle length occurs. Holding the arm in an abducted position or maintaining a semi-squat position requires an isometric contraction, producing just enough muscle force to counteract the pull of gravity and resulting in no movement. The effort involved in trying to move an immovable object (e.g., pushing against a wall) is another example of isometric contractions; although the amount of muscular force can be maximal, no joint movement will occur. (See figure 5.18.)

Quad sets, a rehabilitation exercise in which the knee extensor muscles are contracted with the knee already in the extended position, provide another example of a static contraction. A backward pelvic tilt desired during some exercises is maintained by isometric contraction of the abdominal muscles after they have contracted concentrically to tilt the pelvis backward. During all resistance exercises that involve the arms and/or legs, the trunk muscles should be contracted isometrically for stabilization of the trunk to help prevent injury.

11 **In Review: A concentric contraction, which results in a shortening of the muscle and therefore a pulling on the bones of attachment, is necessary if joint movement is to be in a direction opposite another force, such as gravity, and rapid, regardless of the direction of any other forces. An eccentric contraction, which results in a lengthening of the muscle, controls the velocity of movement caused by another force. An isometric contraction, which results in no change in the length of a muscle, prevents movement.**

Roles of Muscles

As previously mentioned in the discussion of muscular contractions, muscles can act in several ways and have several functions. They can cause movement (concentric contraction), decelerate movement caused by another force (eccentric contraction), or

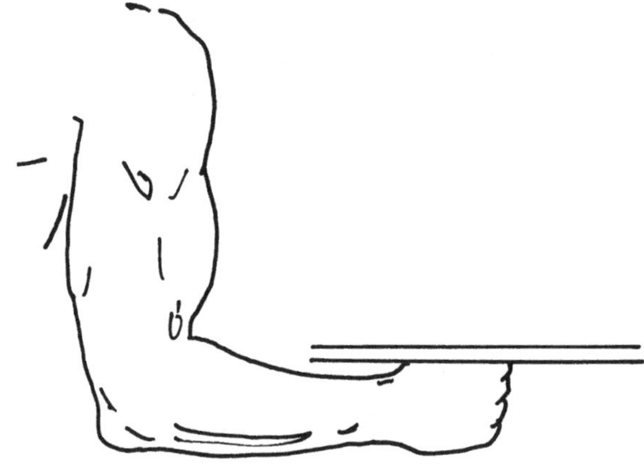

FIGURE 5.18 Isometric contraction by the elbow flexors.

prevent movement (isometric contraction). Muscles may also contract isometrically to stabilize or prevent an undesirable body-segment movement. For example, during a push-up exercise, gravity tends to cause hyperextension of the vertebral column and hip joint. Isometric contraction of the abdominal muscles prevents this sagging; contracting the abdominal muscles stabilizes the trunk in its proper position.

Another function of the muscle is to counteract an undesirable action caused by the concentric contraction of another muscle. The concentric contraction of most muscles causes more than one movement at the same joint, or movement at more than one joint. If only one of those movements is intended, another muscle would contract to prevent the undesirable movement. For example, concentric contraction of the upper trapezius fibers would cause elevation and some adduction of the scapula. If only adduction were desired, the lower trapezius fibers, which cause depression and adduction,

eccentric contraction — A lengthening of the muscle during its contraction; controls speed of movement caused by another force.

ballistic movement — A rapid movement with three phases: an initial concentric muscle contraction by agonists to begin movement, a coasting phase, and a deceleration by the eccentric contraction of the antagonist muscles.

isometric contraction — A muscle contraction in which the muscle length is unchanged; the muscle exerts a force that counteracts an opposing force. Also called a static contraction.

contract to neutralize the undesirable elevation to avoid unnecessary discomfort. In this example, the different fibers of the trapezius are neutralizing the unwanted action and helping the desired action. The biceps brachii muscle causes elbow flexion and radioulnar supination; for only flexion to occur with biceps brachii contraction, the pronator teres also contracts to counteract the supination.

Muscles also act to guide movements initiated or caused by other muscles. During activities against a great resistance, such as lifting free weights, muscles are contracting to help maintain balance or proper direction of the movement. After muscle force has initiated a ballistic movement, other muscles can help guide the movement in the proper direction.

12 **In Review: The major roles of the muscles are to cause movement (concentric contraction) regardless of an opposing force, decelerate or control the speed of movement (eccentric contraction) caused by another force, and prevent movement (isometric contraction). Other muscle functions include counteracting an undesirable action caused by the concentric contraction of another muscle and guiding movements initiated or caused by another muscle.**

Muscle Groups

A **muscle group** includes all of the muscles that cause the same movement at the same joint. The group is named for the joint where the movement takes place and the common movement that is caused by the concentric contraction of those muscles. The elbow flexors, for example, are a muscle group composed of the specific muscles responsible for flexion at the elbow joint when the muscles contract concentrically. Table 5.1 on pages 98-99 lists the muscles that are prime (and assistant) movers of the muscle groups. Note that a movement being observed at a joint does not necessarily involve the muscle group for the movement that is occurring. The muscle group responsible for the opposite action may be contracting eccentrically to control the movement. For example, the elbow flexor muscle group exerts force to flex the elbow joint during the elbow curl exercise. To return to the starting position, the pull of gravity extends the joint to the original position, but the elbow flexor muscle group is still exerting force to control the speed of that movement with eccentric contractions. To maintain the elbow in a flexed position requires an isometric contraction by those same elbow flexors.

Specific muscles that cause more than one action at a joint or cause movement at more than one joint belong to more than one muscle group. For example, the flexor carpi ulnaris muscle belongs in both the wrist flexor and wrist adductor muscle groups. The biceps brachii is part of the elbow flexor and radioulnar supinator muscle groups.

13 **In Review: A muscle group includes all the muscles that cause a specific movement at a specific joint. Table 5.1 lists the muscles in each muscle group, including the major actions that occur at each joint.**

TIPS FOR EXERCISING MUSCLE GROUPS AND SOME COMMON EXERCISE MISTAKES

Many of the errors in exercise and movement result from a lack of knowledge rather than a lack of muscular strength or coordination. By applying basic knowledge, an exerciser can perform better and more safely. This section offers specific tips and things to be aware of for each major muscle group.

Shoulder-Girdle and Shoulder-Joint Complex

Movement can be enhanced and more muscles involved if a deliberate effort is made to incorporate shoulder-girdle movements with shoulder-joint movements. Optimal involvement of these muscles can be achieved in the following exercises and movements:

- *Forward reaching*. Flexion can be accompanied by scapula abduction if the exerciser reaches the fingertips as far forward as possible.
- *Push-up*. At the completion of a push-up, the scapulae can be abducted to raise the chest a little bit more off the floor.
- *Overhead reaching*. Normally, some scapulae elevation is involved when the arm is overhead. A conscious effort to reach as high as possible will involve the scapulae elevators more; con-

versely, a deliberate attempt to keep the shoulders down for a "long neck" look requires concentric contraction by the scapulae depressors.

- *Sideward arm reaching.* During shoulder-joint horizontal extension in movement or a specific exercise, the arm can be moved farther back with scapula adduction.

Elbow and Radioulnar Joints

Flexion against a resistance requires contraction of the flexor muscles at the elbow joint. The position of the radioulnar joints, whether the arm is supinated or pronated, does not affect the involvement of the elbow-joint muscles. The degree to which these muscles are strengthened, however, is affected by supination and pronation—a good point to remember when instructing participants on how to do curls. Normally, elbow flexion with the radioulnar joint in a pronated position (reverse curls) is a weaker movement because the biceps brachii muscle cannot contract as strongly as when the radioulnar joints are in a supinated position. (The distal tendon of the biceps brachii muscle is wrapped around the radius somewhat in the pronated position, which diminishes its pulling force.) The brachialis muscle, though, is not affected by the radioulnar joint position because it is attached to the ulna, which is the nonmoving bone in radioulnar joint movements. Furthermore, the brachioradialis muscle can contract with more force when the radioulnar joint is in a semipronated, semisupinated position. None of the elbow extensor muscles is affected by the radioulnar joint positions, but the radioulnar joint position will affect the amount of weight that may be pressed (moved) on the lat machine because of the limitation of the strength of the wrist muscles. Tricep push-downs, when the elbow extension occurs with the radioulnar joints in the pronated position, require the wrist flexors to stabilize the wrist joint; triceps pull-downs (supinated position) utilize the wrist extensors, which are usually much weaker than the flexors. If an exerciser wanted to concentrate more on building the elbow extensors, tricep push-downs should be done.

Wrist Joint

The wrist muscles during wrist flexion and extension curl exercises are affected by the position of the radioulnar joints. Gravity acts as a resistance for wrist flexion when the radioulnar joints are in the supinated position and resistance for extension when the radioulnar joints are in the pronated position. Remind exercise participants that the position of the radioulnar joints affects which wrist muscles are strengthened during these exercises.

Vertebral Column and Lumbosacral Joints

In general, neither neck hyperextension nor hyperflexion is desirable. The same pairs of muscles that flex and extend can be strengthened or stretched, one side at a time, by cervical lateral flexion and rotation. The instructor should ask participants to tilt or turn the head from side to side rather than to bend the neck forward or back. Although hyperextension may not be contraindicated for the young, no benefits can be gained and it teaches bad habits.

Many exercises require appropriate positioning of the lumbosacral joint and lumbar vertebrae and contractions by the abdominal muscles for either movement or stabilization. An abdominal curl-up or crunch exercise should begin with a backward pelvic tilt that is maintained throughout the curl-up and return movement. If there is any indication that a backward pelvic tilt cannot be maintained, or if the exerciser feels tightness or an ache in the lumbar area, the exercise should be stopped. If the problem is inadequate strength to maintain the backward tilt position, the exercise should be modified to one that requires less abdominal muscle strength, one that the exerciser has sufficient abdominal strength to do correctly.

A full curl-up, in which the exerciser comes up to a sitting position, requires hip flexion by the hip flexor muscles during the last stages of the exercise. Initially, the abdominal muscles contract concentrically to tilt the pelvis backward and then to flex the vertebral column. Once the flexion is achieved, these muscles contract isometrically to keep the pelvis tilted backward and the trunk in a flexed position. There is a "sticking point" that can be felt by the exerciser during a full curl-up. This occurs when the trunk flexion is complete and the hip flexors begin to bring the trunk to an upright position. Doing partial curl-ups or crunches will help eliminate the role of the hip flexors and focus solely on strengthening the abdominals.

muscle group— A group of specific muscles that are responsible for the same action at the same joint.

Table 5.1 Muscles That Are Prime Movers (and Assistant Movers)

Joint	Prime movers (and assistant movers)
Shoulder girdle	Abductors—serratus anterior, pectoralis minor Adductors—middle fibers of trapezius, rhomboids (upper and lower fibers of trapezius) Upward rotators—upper and lower fibers of trapezius, serratus anterior Downward rotators—rhomboids, pectoralis minor Elevators—levator scapulae, upper fibers of trapezius, rhomboids Depressors—lower fibers of trapezius, pectoralis minor
Shoulder joint	Flexors—anterior deltoid, clavicular portion of pectoralis major (short head of biceps brachii) Extensors—sternal portion of pectoralis major, latissimus dorsi, teres major (posterior deltoid, long head of triceps brachii, infraspinatus/teres minor) Hyperextensors—latissimus dorsi, teres major (posterior deltoid, infraspinatus, teres minor) Abductors—middle deltoid, supraspinatus (anterior deltoid, long head of biceps brachii) Adductors—latissimus dorsi, teres major, sternal portion of pectoralis major (short head of biceps brachii, long head of triceps brachii) Lateral rotators—infraspinatus*, teres minor* (posterior deltoid) Medial rotators—pectoralis major, subscapularis*, latissimus dorsi, teres major (anterior deltoid, supraspinatus*) Horizontal flexors—both portions of pectoralis major, anterior deltoid Horizontal extensors—latissimus dorsi, teres major, infraspinatus, teres minor, posterior deltoid
Elbow joint	Flexors—brachialis, biceps brachii, brachioradialis (pronator teres, flexor carpi ulnaris and radialis) Extensors—triceps brachii (anconeus, extensor carpi ulnaris and radialis)
Radioulnar joint	Pronators—pronator quadratus, pronator teres, brachioradialis Supinators—supinator, biceps brachii, brachioradialis
Wrist joint	Flexors—flexor carpi ulnaris, flexor carpi radialis (flexor digitorum superficialis and profundus) Extensors and hyperextensors—extensor carpi ulnaris, extensor carpi radialis longus and brevis (extensor digitorum) Abductors (radial flexors)—flexor carpi radialis, extensor carpi radialis longus and brevis (extensor pollicis) Adductors (ulnar flexors)—flexor carpi ulnaris, extensor carpi ulnaris
Lumbosacral joint	Forward pelvic tilters—iliopsoas (rectus femoris) Backward pelvic tilters—rectus abdominus, internal oblique (external oblique, gluteus maximus)
Spinal column (thoracic and lumbar areas)	Flexors—rectus abdominus, external oblique, internal oblique Extensors and hyperextensors—erector spinae group Rotators—internal oblique, external oblique, erector spinae, rotatores, multifidus Lateral flexors—internal oblique, external oblique, quadratus lumborum, multifidus, rotatores (erector spinae group)
Hip joint	Flexors—iliopsoas, pectineus, rectus femoris (sartorius, tensor fascia latae, gracilis, adductor longus and brevis) Extensors and hyperextensors—gluteus maximus, biceps femoris, semitendinosus, semimembranosus Abductors—gluteus medius (tensors fascia latae, iliopsoas, sartorius) Adductors—adductor brevis, adductor longus, gracilis, pectineus (adductor magnus) Lateral rotators—gluteus maximus, the six deep lateral rotator muscles (iliopsoas, sartorius) Medial rotators—gluteus minimus, gluteus medius (tensor fascia latae, pectineus)
Knee joint	Flexors—biceps femoris, semimembranosus, semitendinosus (sartorius, gracilis, gastrocnemius, plantaris) Extensors—rectus femoris, vastus medialis, vastus lateralis, vastus intermedius

Joint	Prime movers (and assistant movers)
Ankle joint	Plantar flexors—gastrocnemius, soleus (peroneus longus, peroneus brevis, tibialis posterior, flexor digitorum, flexor hallucis longus) Dorsiflexors—tibialis anterior, extensor digitorum longus, peroneus tertius (extensor hallucis longus)
Intertarsal joint	Inverters—tibialis anterior, tibialis posterior (extensor and flexor hallucis longus, flexor digitorum longus) Everters—extensor digitorum longus, peroneus brevis, peroneus longus, peroneus tertius

*Rotator cuff muscles.

The exercise called leg lifts is considered to be an abdominal exercise, but inadequate instruction is often given as to how to perform it correctly. From a supine position on the floor, the legs are lifted and held up by concentric and then isometric contraction of the hip flexors. Some of the hip flexor muscles also pull the lumbosacral joint into a forward-tilted position. It is the role of the abdominal muscles to prevent that forward tilt and to maintain a flattened lumbar spine and posterior pelvic tilt. The backward pelvic tilt should precede the hip flexion; and, as in the case of the curl-up exercise, if the proper tilt cannot be maintained, the exercise should not be done in that fashion.

There is also a tendency for the pelvis to tilt forward during overhead arm movements from a standing position. This can be prevented by keeping the arms in front of the ears and by flexing the knees slightly.

When weights are lifted from a supine position, as in the bench press, there is a tendency to hyperextend the lumbar spine and tilt the pelvis forward. Although this can allow the exerciser to lift a somewhat heavier weight, it does not increase the work of the arm and chest muscles, and it puts the lower back into a compromising position. Bench presses are best done with the hips and knees in a flexed position and feet on the bench or a bench extension. Upright presses are best done seated with the back supported.

Hip Joint

A common error during side-lying leg raises to exercise the hip abductor muscles is the attempt to move the foot as high as possible. Because the range of motion for true abduction is limited (about 45°), the exerciser often rotates the top leg laterally, which turns the foot out and allows it to go higher. However, this rotation changes the muscle involvement more to the hip flexor muscles. To exercise the primary abductor muscles, the leg should not be rotated; the toes should face forward, not up. Turning the feet out comes from lateral rotation of the hips; there should be no attempt to rotate the knee or the ankle joints.

In backward leg movements to strengthen the gluteus muscles, hyperextension is limited primarily by the tightness of the hip ligaments. A leg can appear to be more hyperextended if it is accompanied by a forward pelvic tilt. The exerciser should be cautioned to keep the pelvis in its proper neutral position, even though some apparent hyperextension is lost.

A common exercise position is standing with feet shoulder-width apart. The exerciser should have the feet turned slightly outward (from hip lateral rotation). Too much rotation is potentially dangerous. During any squatting or standing movement, the knee should be directly over the foot (not in front of the foot) to prevent strain to the lateral and medial knee ligaments. Although the knee can be kept over the foot even in the toed-out position during a squat, some individuals have a tendency to let the knees move toward the inside of the feet. It is easier to determine whether the knee position is a correct one when the feet are almost parallel to each other. During the squat, the exerciser should be able to see the big toe on each foot.

Knee Joint

Hyperflexion can strain and stretch knee ligaments and put pressure on the menisci; therefore, a full squat that creates an angle at the knee joint of less than 90°, especially with additional weights, should not be attempted, nor should sitting on the lower legs. During any lunging movements or forward-back stride positions in which the front knee is in a flexed position, the knee should be over or in back of the foot, not in front. Any knee position that puts a twisting pressure on the knee-joint structures should also be avoided. The hurdler position, with one leg out to the back and side with a flexed knee should be avoided; that leg should also be in front.

Ankle Joint

If the squat exercise is performed with the heels of the feet resting on a low block, the soleus muscles are exercised more than they would be if the feet were flat. This "heels up" position shortens the gastrocnemius muscles even more (they already are shortened by the flexed knee positions) limiting their ability to generate force. The soleus muscles, which do not cross the knees, aren't shortened to the extent that it affects the force generation. The gastrocnemius muscles are weaker, so more of the work is done by the soleus muscles. To increase the force production of the gastrocnemius muscles, the squat could be done with the balls of the feet on the block. A mountain climber would especially benefit from this because it mimics the knee and ankle joint positions in climbing.

Intertarsal Joints

Walking on the insides or outsides of the foot should never be done. Not only does this stress the knees, it can cause ankle sprains. A better way of exercising the invertors and evertors is to walk back and forth, instead of up and down, a ramp or hill.

14 **In Review: The following situations should be avoided during exercise for the vertebral column and lumbosacral joints:**

- **Backward pelvic tilt is not maintained during the abdominal crunch.**
- **Hip flexion precedes backward pelvic tilt in the curl-up and leg lifts.**
- **Pelvis tilts forward during overhead arm movements from a standing position.**
- **Lumbar spine is hyperextended during weight lifting from a supine position.**

Errors to avoid during exercise for the knee include these:

- **Knee moves in front of the foot during lunging and squatting movements.**
- **Twisting pressure is applied to the knee during stretches and exercises.**

MUSCLE GROUP INVOLVEMENT IN SELECTED ACTIVITIES

Human movement is caused or controlled by muscle forces. The following sections briefly analyze the involvement of muscle groups in some common physical activities.

Walking, Jogging, and Running

Jogging can be looked at as a modification of walking; and running, as a fast jog. The different phases and the muscle-group involvement in walking, jogging, and running are similar, but more forceful muscle contractions are needed to increase speed. The three basic phases are the push-off, the recovery of the push-off leg, and the landing.

The push-off is accomplished by the concentric contraction of the hip hyperextensors; the talocrural plantar flexors; and, to a lesser extent, the foot metatarsophalangeal flexors. (See the back leg in figure 5.19.) Because the knee of the back leg is almost in the extended position at push-off, little work is done by the knee extensors to help propel the body forward. The gluteus maximus muscle may assume a greater role in the hip hyperextension as speed increases. Medial rotation takes place at the hip joint; but because the foot is fixed on the ground, this movement is seen at the pelvis.

At the beginning of the recovery phase, the hip flexors contract concentrically to begin the forward leg swing. This is basically a ballistic movement, so the momentum initiated by the hip flexors continues the motion. The knee flexors bend the knee at the beginning of hip flexion, the extensors initiate the straightening of the knee, and the flexors then work eccentrically to control the knee extension at the end of the recovery phase. The talocrural joint is dorsiflexed to clear the foot from the ground and prepare for the landing. (See the recovery leg in figure 5.19.) Running speed is a product of stride length and stride frequency. To increase both factors in running, the hip is flexed to a greater extent and with a much greater velocity. (See figure 5.20, the recovery leg.)

Just prior to landing, the hip extensors contract eccentrically to decelerate the forward leg swing. On contact, the knee extensors contract eccentrically to cushion the impact. The heel should touch the ground first during walking and jogging; as running speed increases, the ball of the foot or the entire

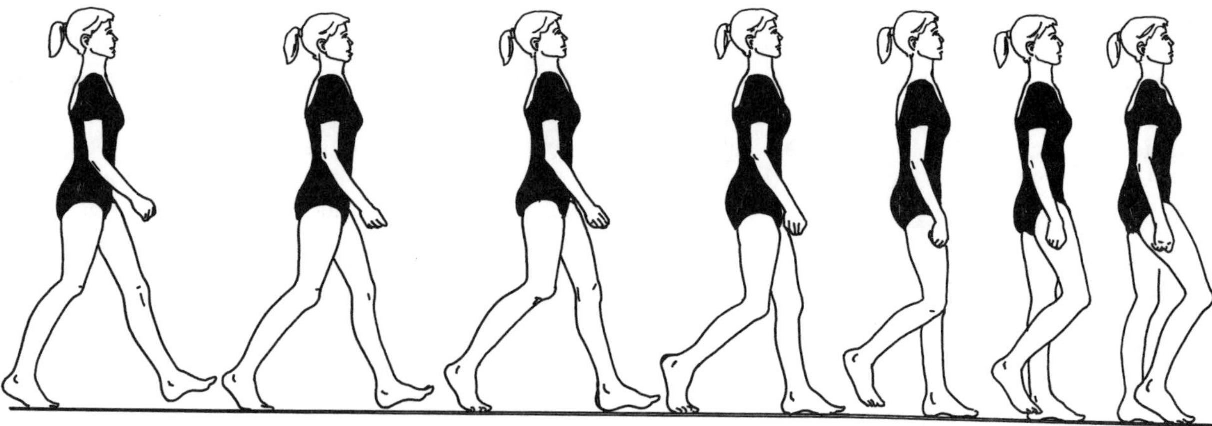

FIGURE 5.19 Walking movements.

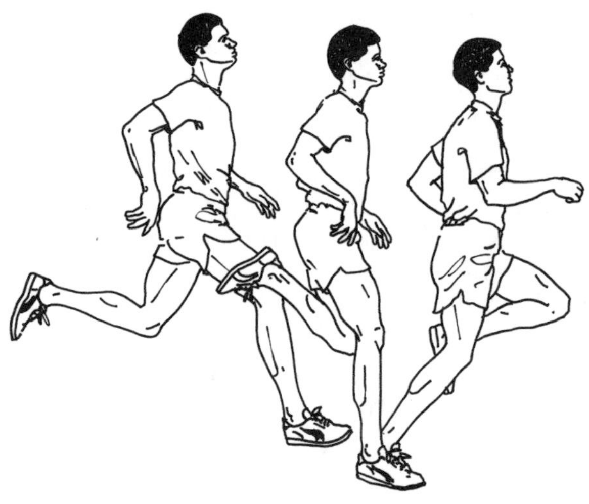

FIGURE 5.20 Running movements.

foot may make contact. During the landing phase in walking and jogging, the talocrural dorsiflexors contract eccentrically to control the speed of movement of the ball of the foot to the ground.

The arm swing requires shoulder flexion and extension to hyperextension. As speed increases, the swing becomes more vigorous, and there is more elbow flexion. For the greatest efficiency, the arms should move in an anterior/posterior direction. To increase the upper limb muscle involvement for exercise, a walker can exaggerate the flexion and hyperextension movements or can abduct and adduct or horizontal flex and extend the shoulder joint.

Walking or running up an incline elicits a greater force of contraction from the gluteus maximus muscle at the hip and from the knee extensors. The talocrural dorsiflexors are more active immediately before landing to position the talocrural joint to conform with the angle of the incline. Because the talocrural joint is in a more dorsiflexed position, the plantar flexors begin contracting during push off from a more stretched position. For these reasons, hill climbing requires greater flexibility in the plantar flexors, especially the soleus muscle, and greater strength in the dorsiflexors. There is also more eccentric contraction by the knee extensors during landing in downhill than in uphill running. As a result, these muscle groups are more apt to become fatigued and be sore afterward.

Jogging in place requires the talocrural plantar flexors to propel the body upward; they work more than any of the other lower extremity muscle groups in this activity. The knee extensors are primarily active in eccentric contraction to cushion the landing. During walking and jogging, the heel is the first part of the foot to make contact with the surface, but in jogging in place, the ball of the foot touches first. The plantar flexors therefore are also active during the landing, contracting eccentrically to control the speed and amount of dorsiflexion. It is better to have sufficient dorsiflexion so the heel touches the ground briefly rather than to always stay up on the toes, which can put quite a strain on the plantar flexors. Additional muscles can be involved with the execution of movements with the leg immediately after push-off and before the foot lands again: hip flexion with flexed or extended knee, hip hyperextension with flexed or extended knee, hip abduction/adduction, hip lateral rotation along with hip and knee flexion that brings the foot to the front of the trunk, and medial rotation with knee flexion that brings the foot behind and to the side of the trunk.

Cycling

The main force in cycling comes from the hip and knee extensor muscles during the downward push. With toe clips, the rider can use the hip and talocrural dorsiflexors to help return the pedal to the up position, if she or he makes a conscious effort to do so.

Jumping

The hip and knee extensors, followed by the talocrural plantar flexors, forcibly contract to propel the body upward. The lean of the trunk primarily determines the angle of takeoff. The trunk extends, and the arms flex from a hyperextended position just before the leg action. If the reach height of the arms is important as in a jump ball in basketball or a tennis smash, the scapulae elevate. During the landing, the hip and knee extensors and the talocrural plantar flexors contract eccentrically.

Overarm Throwing

There are three phases in throwing: the windup, or preparation; the execution, or actual throw; and the follow-through, or recovery. (See figure 5.21.)

In preparation for throwing, there is a weight shift to the back foot, a medial rotation of the back leg (because the leg is fixed to the ground, rotation is seen at the pelvis), trunk rotation and some lateral flexion and hyperextension, shoulder lateral rotation, some horizontal extension of the throwing arm accompanied by the adduction of the scapula, flexion of the elbow, and hyperextension of the wrist. The movements of the throwing arm are all ballistic. The lateral rotation at the shoulder is remarkably fast and powerful. Toward the end of the windup, the medial rotators begin to eccentrically contract to decelerate the rotation in preparation for the actual throw. (See figure 5.21.)

The weight shift forward is the initial movement in the throwing pattern. This is accomplished by the hip abductors, hyperextensors, and lateral rotators; the talocrural plantar flexors; and the intertarsal everters of the back leg. The front hip rotates laterally. The trunk then flexes laterally in the direction opposite that of the windup and rotates, beginning at the lumbar area and continuing through the thoracic vertebrae, and then flexes. There is a forcible medial rotation of the shoulder, along with scapula abduction. Although there is some horizontal flexion, most of the force of the shoulder in an overhand throw comes from this medial rotation. The

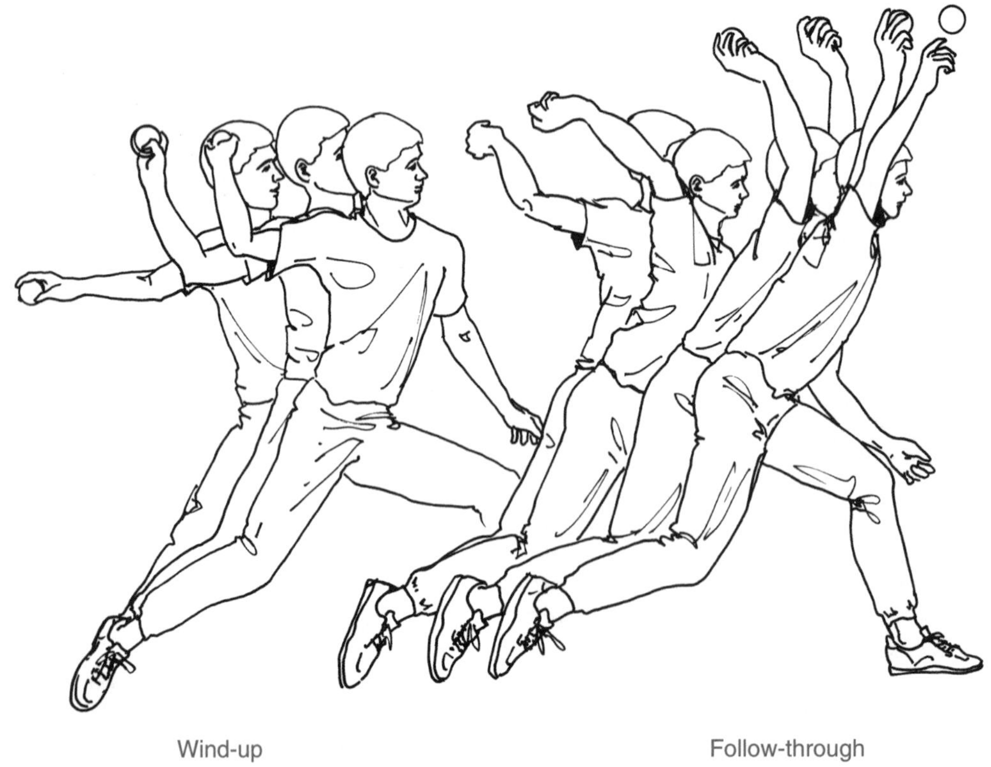

FIGURE 5.21 Overarm throwing movements.

elbow extends, and the wrist moves toward flexion. Depending upon the desired spin on the ball, the radioulnar pronators and the wrist abductors or adductors may also be involved.

Because the actions at the shoulder and elbow joints are vigorous ballistic movements, the shoulder lateral rotators and horizontal extensors contract eccentrically to decelerate the movements; the elbow flexors contract eccentrically to prevent elbow hyperextension.

Swimming and Exercise in Water

Swimming is a unique activity because the water medium offers resistance to movements of submerged body parts in all directions and at all speeds. Exercises or movements performed in water demand concentric contractions. Gravity is not a factor in water, so less stress is put on the weight-bearing joints.

15 **In Review: The movements and muscle involvement for locomotion, throwing, cycling, jumping, and swimming are summarized here:**

Muscle group	Movement task
Hip extensor	Locomotion—push-off; cycling; jumping; swimming—front crawl, back crawl, sidestroke
Talocrural plantar flexor	Locomotion—push-off, landing; jumping
Hip flexor	Locomotion—recovery; swimming—front crawl, back crawl, sidestroke
Knee flexor	Locomotion—recovery
Talocrural dorsiflexor	Locomotion—recovery
Knee extensor	Locomotion—landing; cycling; jumping
Shoulder-joint medial and lateral rotators	Throwing
Elbow flexor	Throwing
Elbow extensor	Throwing
Trunk flexor	Throwing
Trunk rotator	Throwing
Shoulder-girdle downward rotator	Swimming—front crawl, back crawl
Shoulder-girdle abductor	Swimming—back crawl, sidestroke lead arm
Shoulder-girdle adductor	Swimming—front crawl, breast stroke
Shoulder-joint extensors	Swimming—front crawl
Anterior shoulder-joint muscles	Swimming—back crawl, sidestroke lead arm
Posterior shoulder-joint muscles	Swimming—sidestroke trail arm, breast stroke
Hip abductors	Swimming—breast stroke
Hip adductors	Swimming—breast stroke

Lifting and Carrying Objects

The weight to be lifted from the ground should be located close to the lifter's spread feet; the lifter squats, keeping the trunk as erect as possible. The actual lifting should be accomplished by the legs rather than spine or arm action. Proper lifting is begun by moving the trunk to a position as perpendicular to the floor as possible and then tilting the pelvis backward and keeping the abdominal muscles contracted; the knee extensors along with the hip extensors then contract concentrically. The lift should be slow, not jerky. (See figure 5.22.) Insufficient leg strength can result in an incorrect lifting technique. The weight should be carried close to the body, with the trunk assuming a position that allows the line of gravity to fall well within the area of the base. The trunk lateral flexors are more active when the weight

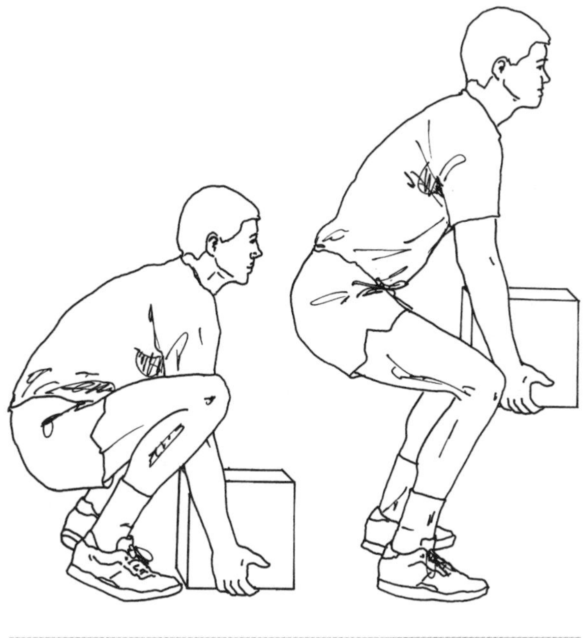

FIGURE 5.22 Lifting technique.

is carried on one side; the extensors are more active when the weight is in front of the body; and when the weight is carried across the top of the back, as in backpacking, the abdominals are more active.

16 **In Review: The steps in proper lifting are to place the feet close to the object, move the vertebral column to an upright position perpendicular to the floor, tilt the pelvis backward, and slowly extend the hips and knees while contracting the abdominals.**

BASIC MECHANICAL CONCEPTS RELATED TO HUMAN MOVEMENT

Knowledge of the laws and principles of mechanics is also important to the understanding of human movement. Some of these basic but important concepts are described next.

Achieving Stability

For an individual to maintain balance, his or her line of gravity must fall within the area of the base of support. In figure 5.23, frame A illustrates the area of the base of support in a standing position with feet together; frame B, with feet apart and forward and back.

Stability, or the ease with which balance can be maintained, is proportional to the distance from the line of gravity to the outer limits of the base that is farthest from a potentially upsetting force. Figure 5.24 compares more stable positions with less stable positions. A wide base of support usually, but not necessarily, ensures greater stability. From a feet-apart position, if one leans so that the line of gravity falls directly over one foot and a pushing force is applied in the same direction of the lean, there is less stability than if the feet were together but with the line of gravity falling over the edge of the foot closer to the applied force.

The degree of stability is also indirectly proportional to the height of the center of gravity, which is below the naval, (the pelvis) above the base; the lower the center of gravity above the base, the greater the force needed to upset the stability. The degree of stability is also directly proportional to the weight of the body. With all other factors being equal, a heavy person is more stable than a lighter one.

Stability may be increased by moving the feet apart to widen the base of support and by flexing the knees and hips to lower the center of gravity. During standing exercises that require some degree of balance, stability can also be aided by having a nearby object such as a wall or chair to hold or push against if necessary. Many exercises can also be executed from a sitting position which increases the base and lowers

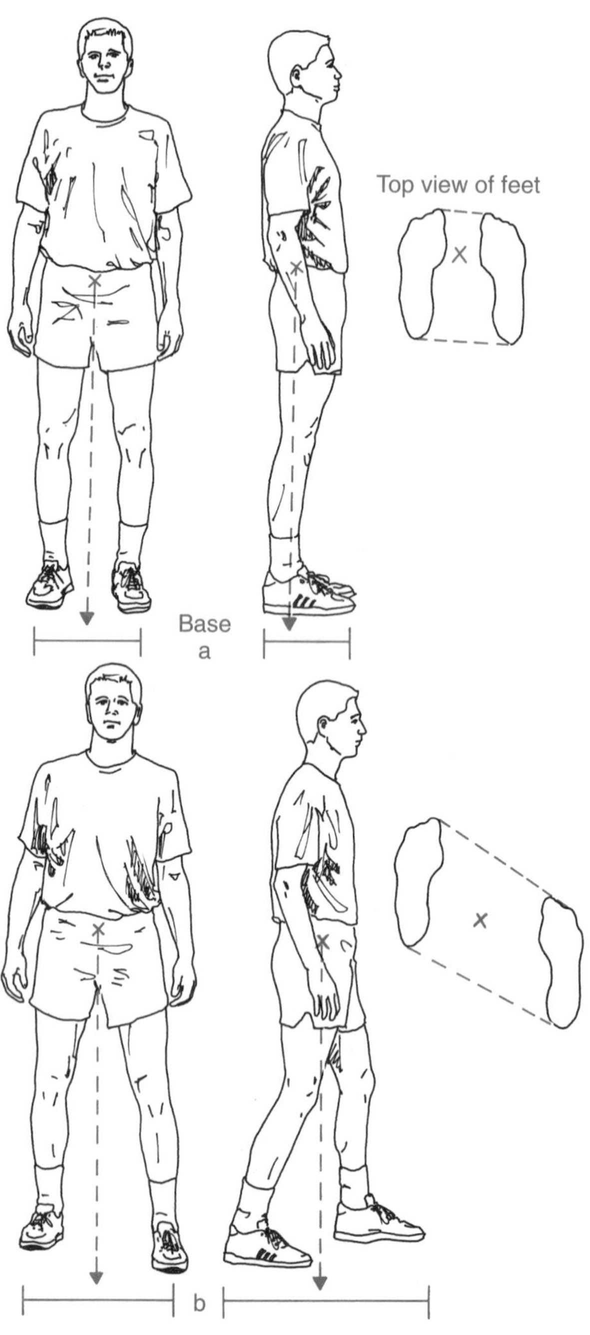

FIGURE 5.23 Bases of support.

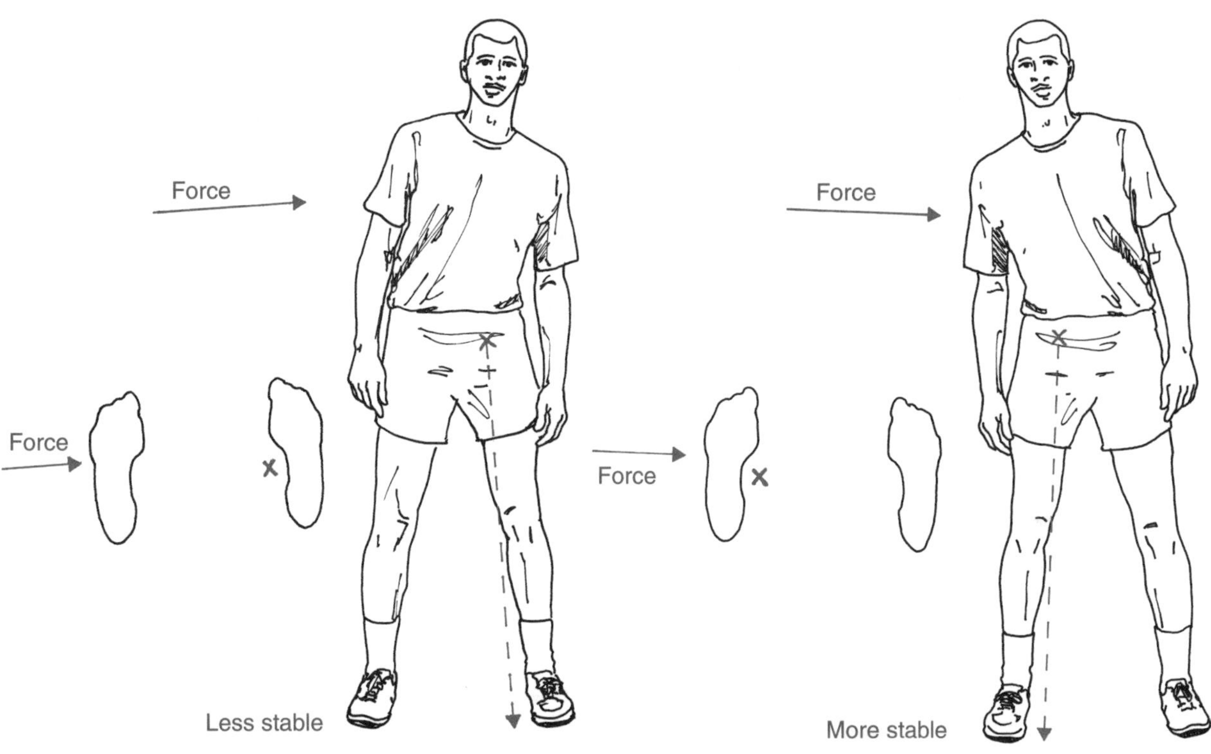

FIGURE 5.24 Relationship between line of gravity and outer limits of base of support.

the center of gravity. To help maintain stability against a potentially upsetting force, the weight should be shifted toward that force. When locomotion is going to occur, a position close to instability is attained by shifting the line of gravity closer to the outer limits of the base (which is the area of the push-off foot in walking, or the hands in a track start position) in the direction of the intended movement. During locomotion as the line of gravity moves outside the limits of the base, a new base is established when the other foot lands, and stability is maintained. If something prevents the foot from establishing a new base, stability is lost. A basketball guard, in taking a charge from a forward, will fall down quicker and easier if the guard is in an unstable position—standing fairly erect with feet side by side instead of front and back, and weight on heels—at the collision (it will hurt more however).

17 **In Review: Stability in humans is directly proportional to the distance of the line of gravity from the limits of the base, indirectly proportional to the height of the center of gravity above the base, and directly proportional to the weight of the body. For stability in a standing position, the knees should be flexed to lower the center of gravity, the feet apart in the direction of an oncoming force to increase the distance of the line of gravity to the outer limits of the upsetting force and the weight of the body (line of gravity) shifted toward the force.**

Torque

A force is any push or pull that tends to cause movement. The effect produced when a force causes rotation is called **torque (T)**. It is the product of the magnitude of the force (F) and the **force arm (FA)**,

stability — The ease with which balance is maintained.

torque (T) — The effect produced by a force causing rotation; the product of the force and length of the **force arm**.

force arm (FA) — Perpendicular distance from the axis of rotation to the direction of the application of that force causing movement.

which is the perpendicular distance from the axis to the direction of the application of that force. Algebraically, torque can be expressed as

$$T = F \times FA$$

When two opposing forces are acting to produce rotation in opposite directions, one of the forces is often designated as the **resistance force (R)**; its force arm, the **resistance arm (RA)**. When considering the torque produced by sufficient muscle force to cause movement against gravity or some other external force, F and FA are designated for the muscle, R and RA for the gravitational or other opposing force.

Applying Torque to Muscle Contraction

Muscle contraction can be considered the force; the FA is the perpendicular distance from the joint (axis) to the direction of the force from its point of application (where the muscle attaches to the bone being moved). Figure 5.25 illustrates the direction of pull of the biceps brachii muscle on the radius; the force arm is the perpendicular distance from the elbow joint to this line of force. If the muscle insertion were closer to the joint, the same force would produce less torque because of the shorter force arm; to produce the same torque, more muscle force must be produced.

Torque is also affected by joint position. Figure 5.26 again shows the direction of pull by the biceps brachii but with the elbow in a less flexed position.

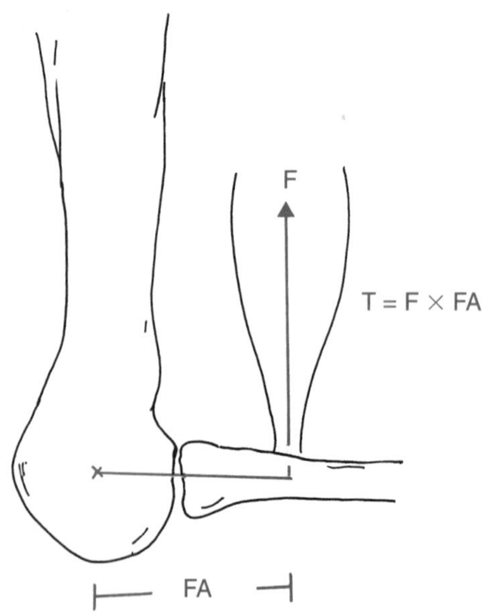

FIGURE 5.25 Force (F) and force arm (FA) of biceps brachii muscle.

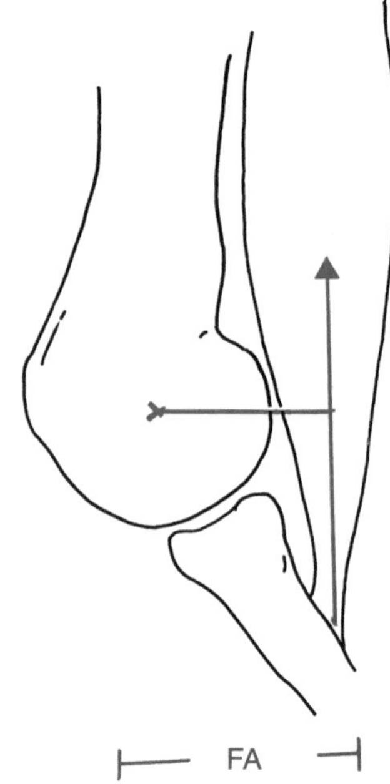

FIGURE 5.26 Effect of a less flexed position of the elbow joint on the force arm of the biceps brachii.

This results in a shorter force arm, so the same muscle force produces less torque at that joint angle.

Torque Resulting From Other Forces

The force from gravitational pull is treated as a resistance force. The resistive force (R) produced by gravity pulling on a body part is the mass of the object; the resistance arm (RA) is the perpendicular distance from the axis of rotation to the point of the object that represents its center of gravity. The torque is the product of the resistive force and the resistance arm. Figure 5.27 illustrates the torque produced as a result of gravity acting on the arm. The torque opposing limb movements can be increased by adding weight to increase both the magnitude of force and the length of the resistance arm, or by adjusting the weight further from the axis. The resistance arm of a force applied by someone pushing or pulling on a limb is the perpendicular distance from the axis to the point of application of the push or pull.

For muscle contraction to cause movement of a bone, the muscle force must produce a torque greater than the opposing or resistance torque; the muscle contraction is concentric. A greater resistance torque results in movement, and the muscle contracts eccentrically. Technically, it can be argued that the muscle force during an eccentric contraction should be considered the resistance, and the external force

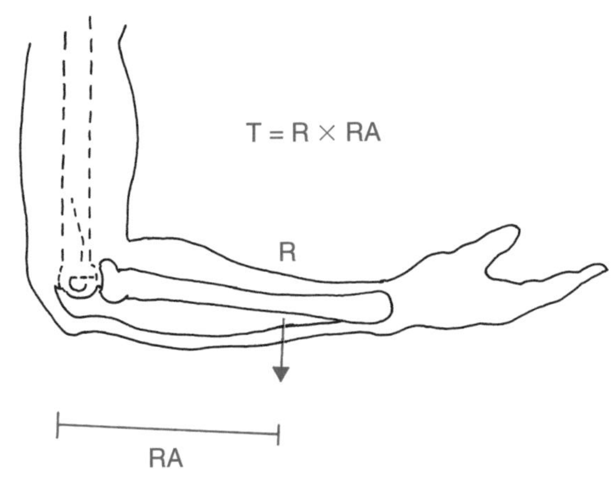

FIGURE 5.27 Resistance (R) and resistant arm (RA) of lower arm.

causing the movement, the force. When the muscular torque equals the resistance torque, no movement occurs; the muscle is contracting isometrically.

> 18 **In Review: Torque can be expressed algebraically as T = F x FA, for the torque that produces the movement, or T = R × RA, for the torque that is opposing the movement. A concentric contraction produces a torque that is greater than the resistive torque. An eccentric contraction produces a torque that is less than the opposing torque. An isometric contraction produces a torque that is the same as the opposing torque.**

Applying Torque to Exercising

Knowledge of torques can be used to modify exercises for different individuals. The amount of muscular contraction necessary during the exercise can be modified to fit an individual's needs by altering the amount of resistance or the resistance arm, or both, to change the resistive torque. For example, resistive torque can be increased with the use of external weights, which would therefore require stronger muscle contractions. The resistance torque can also be changed by altering the position of the body parts. Figure 5.28 shows an exerciser making modifications to reduce the necessary muscle force by not using the weight, to reduce both the resistive force and the resistance arm, and flexing the elbow to reduce the length of the resistance arm.

The arm position during a curl-up exercise determines the length of the resistance arm and therefore the amount of resistance torque against which the abdominal muscles have to work. Arms may be held at the sides of the body to bring the upper body mass closer to the axes of rotation to reduce the necessary muscle force; arms can be put overhead with hands on the scapulae or straight out to increase the resistive torque, therefore increasing the required muscle force. It is important to

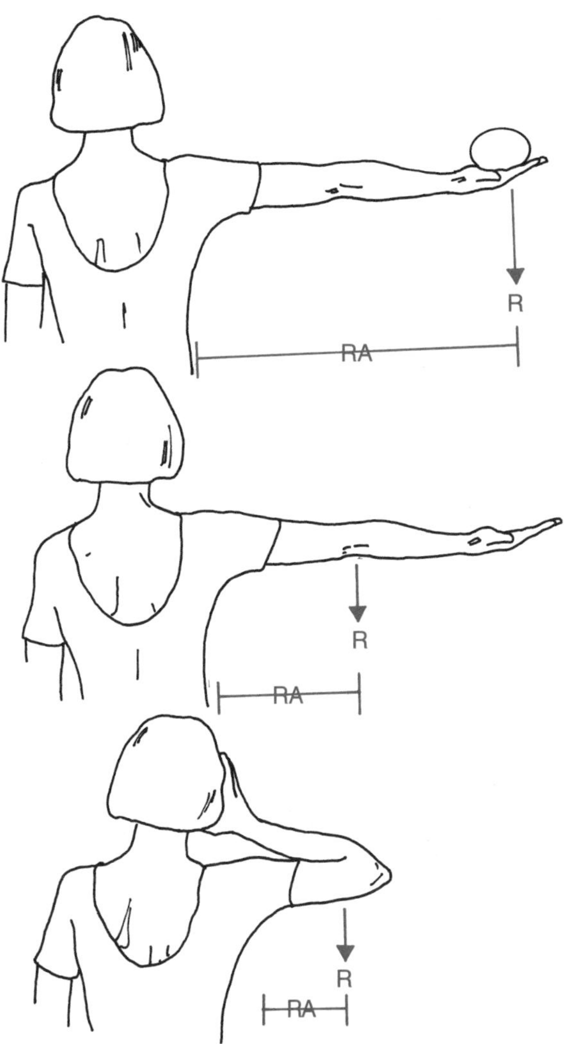

FIGURE 5.28 Modifications of resistive torque.

> **resistance force (R)** — The opposing force that is resisting another force.
>
> **resistance arm (RA)** — Perpendicular distance from the axis of rotation to the direction of the application of that force resisting movement.

realize that modifications to lessen the resistance torque do not necessarily make the exercise "easy" for all individuals. If an exerciser with a lower strength level finds the resistive torque too great to overcome for a sufficient number of repetitions, the limb positions can be altered to reduce the torque against which the muscles have to work; but this individual is still working as hard as a stronger individual who did not have to reduce the resistive torque.

19 **In Review: The torque that resists limb movements can be altered by increasing or decreasing the amount of the resistive force and changing the position of the resistive force relative to the joint to change the resistance arm.**

Rotational Inertia

Rotational inertia (also referred to as the moment of inertia), or the reluctance of a body segment or segments to rotate around an axis or a joint, is dependent on the body's mass and the distribution of that mass around the joint. A leg, for example, has more rotational inertia than an arm, not only because of its heavier mass but also because its mass is concentrated a greater distance away from its axis. A softball bat held by its fat end has less rotational inertia than if it were grasped in the usual manner.

The rotational inertia of body segments before or during movement is dependent on the mass of the segments, which cannot be changed, and the distribution of the mass around the joints, which can be manipulated to result in a change of the rotational inertia. For example, an arm with elbow, wrist, and fingers extended has a greater rotational inertia than an arm with elbow, wrist, and fingers flexed; a leg with extended knee and ankle has more inertia than if the knee were flexed and the ankle dorsiflexed. The amount of muscular force necessary to cause rapid limb movement is proportional to the rotational inertia of the limb to be moved. During jogging, in which speed of running is not a factor, the knee of the recovery leg is flexed to reduce the leg's rotational inertia around the hip joint. Less muscular force is needed to swing the recovery leg forward, thus the possibility of local fatigue of the hip flexor muscles is reduced. In sprinting, the quicker the recovery leg is brought forward, the faster the running speed. Powerful contractions of the hip flexors, along with a greater knee flexion, results in the recovery leg coming through sooner with increased overall speed. Another example of rapid movement to which this principle can be applied is in jumping jacks. Keeping the elbow flexed reduces the rotational inertia. This results in either the reduction of the amount of muscle force by the shoulder abductor and adductor muscle groups to maintain a certain cadence or, if maximum muscle force is still applied, faster movements.

Angular Momentum

Angular momentum, or the quantity of angular motion, is expressed as the product of the rotational inertia, which is determined by both the mass of the moving part and the distribution of the mass around the joints and the angular velocity. A moving body part possesses angular momentum; the faster it is moving and the greater its rotational inertia, the greater the angular momentum. The amount of force necessary to change angular momentum is proportional to the amount of the momentum.

Applying Angular Momentum to Exercising

The concept of angular momentum can be applied to ballistic limb movements during exercise. A fast-moving body segment is decelerated by eccentric muscle contractions; the faster the movement, the greater the mass, or the greater the desired deceleration, the greater the muscle force that must be applied. Care must be taken when rapid ballistic limb movements are performed, especially with added weights. A large amount of momentum may be generated, and considerable muscle strength may be required to decelerate and eventually stop the movement.

Transfer of Angular Momentum

Transfer of angular momentum from one body segment to another can be achieved by stabilizing the initial moving body part at a joint, which will result in angular movement of another body part. For example, in performing a curl-up exercise for the trunk flexors, flinging the arms forward from an overhead position or the elbows from alongside the head results in a transfer of their momentum to the trunk. This decreases the amount of muscular contraction needed by the trunk flexors, and makes the exercise seem easier but the abdominal flexors do not work as hard. A jump with a turn in the air can be better achieved if the arms are swung forcibly across the body in the intended direction of the spin just before takeoff.

20 **In Review: Rotational inertia during fast limb movements can be decreased by moving the mass of the limb closer to the axis or joints. The amount of angular momentum is dependent on the rotational inertia and angular velocity of a moving body segment. The amount of eccentric force necessary to decelerate the angular velocity of a body segment is proportional to the amount of the angular momentum of the body segment. Angular momentum can be transferred from one body segment to another by stabilizing the initial moving body part at a joint.**

COMMON MECHANICAL ERRORS DURING LOCOMOTION, THROWING, AND STRIKING

Success in activities depends in part on the proper execution of movements. Some of the more common errors that violate the laws of mechanics to some degree are discussed in the next sections.

Errors in Locomotion

Some beginning joggers have a tendency to run "stiff legged," or with insufficient knee flexion of the recovery leg. This results in a greater rotational inertia of the leg; the hip flexor muscles exert more force than if the knee were more flexed to bring the mass of the leg closer to the hip axis.

Another potential problem is direction of the arm and leg movements. All movements should be executed in the anterior and posterior directions. Swinging the hands across the trunk rotates the upper trunk; in reaction, the lower trunk rotates in the opposite direction. The recovery leg may also tend to rotate medially at the hip; this swings the recovery foot to the outside. The touchdown foot should land in a forward-backward direction and not pointed to the outside. Sometimes runners are not aware of this tendency, and a suggestion for them to "toe in" somewhat when landing will result in the correct foot alignment.

Some joggers and runners propel themselves too high off the ground during the airborne phase; this results in a shorter stride length. Although the length of time the body is airborne may be the same as when running with less loft, less horizontal distance is covered.

Overstriding, in which the line of gravity from the runner's center of gravity falls in front of the touchdown foot, will decelerate the running speed. No propulsion force against the ground for forward movement can take place until the line of gravity is over and ahead of the foot. Understriding, in which the line of gravity falls well in back of the foot at touchdown, results in a shorter period of time during which the propulsion muscles can work.

Errors in Throwing and Striking

A ball is thrown for accuracy, speed, or distance, which depends in part on the speed of the ball when it leaves the hand. The speed of the ball in the hand just before release is the speed of the ball immediately after it leaves the hand. The more joints that can be involved in the throwing motions, the greater the speed of the ball when it is released. Proper throwing and striking techniques are the same for females and males. Most throwing problems that result in low velocity, such as pushing the ball rather than throwing it, stem from a lack of sufficient trunk rotation or from poor timing of this rotation with the shoulder-joint movements. The thrower should rotate the trunk and hips during the windup so that the pelvis is sideways to the intended direction of the throw and the shoulders rotated even more to the back. As the hips and then the different sections of the spinal column rotate back to begin the execution of the throw, the arm lags behind. This sets up for a whiplike action of the arm and allows an adequate length of time for the important medial rotation. Without this trunk rotation, the resulting inadequate arm rotation produces a pushing motion

rotational inertia — Reluctance to rotate; proportional to the mass and distribution of the mass around the axis.

angular momentum — The quantity of rotation. Angular momentum is the product of the rotational inertia and the angular velocity.

transfer of angular momentum — Transfer of **angular momentum** from one body segment to another can be achieved by stabilizing the initial moving part at a joint.

during the throw. The vertebral column also has to rotate in a wavelike fashion, with the thoracic vertebrae being the last to rotate.

The same sequence of motion applies to striking events, such as tennis and badminton stroking and softball batting. A common fault in learning how to serve a tennis ball or smash a birdie is insufficient trunk rotation. It is easier to hit an object without trunk rotation, but the impact of the racket on the projectile will not be as great. In batting, a common error is the lack of fluid timing between the different body segment movements. The hip, trunk, and arm movements follow one another so the bat is moving with great velocity upon contact with the ball. Beginners often stop one motion before beginning the next.

21 **In Review: Common mechanical errors in locomotion include running "stiff legged," "toeing out," swinging the arms across the trunk, overstriding, understriding, and lifting too high off the ground. The most common mechanical errors in throwing and striking are insufficient trunk rotation and poor timing among the trunk, hip, and arm movements.**

Case Studies

You can check your answers by referring to appendix A.

5.1

You are supervising the resistance training area when you hear a lot of clanging noise coming from the seated leg press area. You discover that the exerciser at that machine is not controlling the descent of the weights. You suggest that he slowly return the weights rather than just letting them drop. He asks you for the reason for the suggestion—he doesn't see any benefit in a controlled return other than that it is not as noisy. What do you tell him?

5.2

Alice wants to know why she can move a heavier weight when she does wrist curls with her palms up than with her palms down; and why she can do more pull-ups with her palms facing her than with her palms away. How would you explain both to her?

5.3

José complains that his lower back aches somewhat when he reaches overhead while standing in place during the cool-down portion of an aerobics class. What would you suggest he do during this movement to prevent the aching?

Source List

1. Gowitzke & Milner (1988)
2. Gray (1994)
3. Hall (1995)
4. Hamill & Knutzen (1995)
5. Hay & Reid (1988)
6. Kreighbaum & Barthels (1996)
7. Luttgens, Deutsch, & Hamilton (1992)
8. Rasch (1989)
9. Thompson (1994)

CHAPTER

6

Measurement and Evaluation

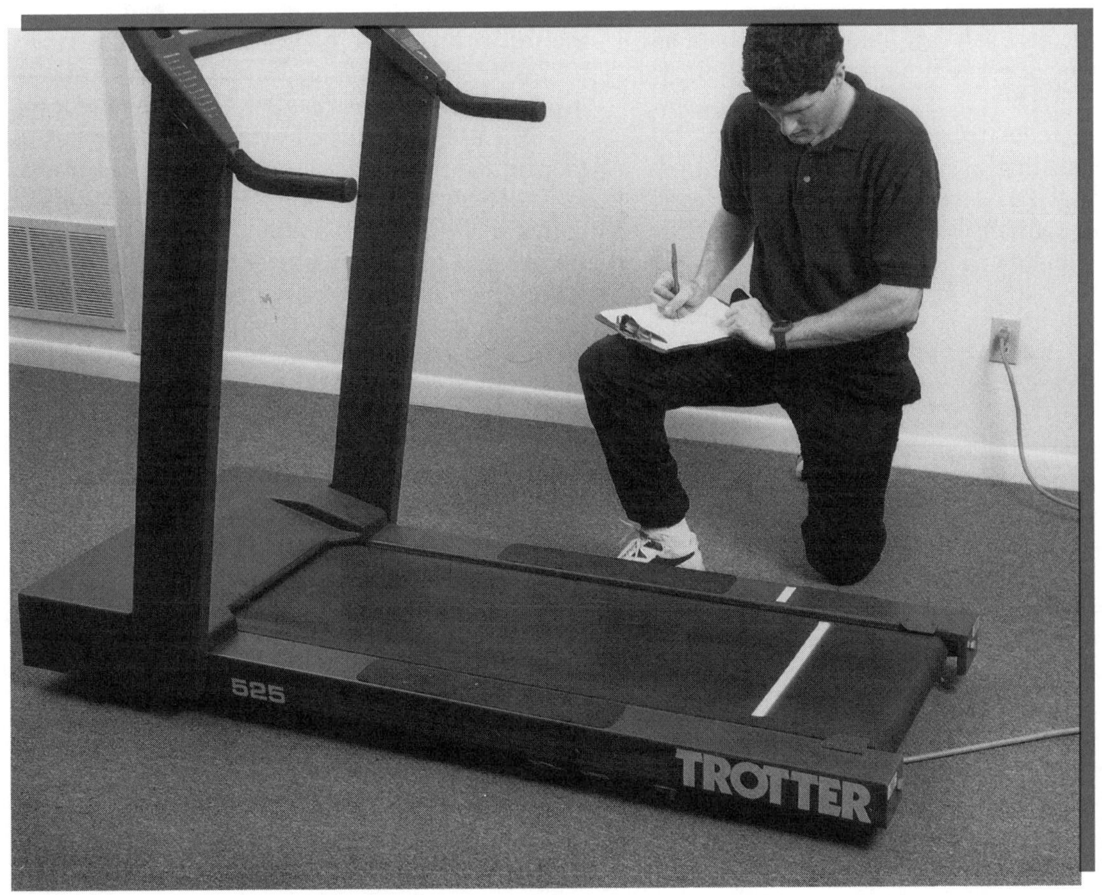

© Chris Brown

OBJECTIVES

The reader will be able to:

1. **Describe the components and types of validity.**
2. **Explain ways to improve the accuracy of test scores.**
3. **Describe how to interpret fitness test scores.**
4. **Describe ways to use test results in a fitness program.**
5. **Calibrate a motor driven treadmill.**
6. **Calibrate a cycle ergometer.**
7. **Calibrate a sphygmomanometer.**

Fitness programs combine knowledge from several areas of exercise science to create a tailored, goal-oriented, and safe program. Other chapters present information based on exercise physiology, anatomy, biomechanics, and exercise psychology. This chapter summarizes aspects of measurement and evaluation that are related to fitness testing. Chapters 9 and 11-13 describe specific tests for body composition, cardiorespiratory function, muscular strength and endurance, and flexibility.

ESTABLISHING VALIDITY

The most important question to raise about a test concerns the test's **validity**: Does the test measure the characteristic I'm interested in evaluating? The two key components of validity are consistency and relevance. Consistency includes the **reliability** of the test results as well as the objectivity of the testers. If the test is repeated without a change in the fitness of the person being tested and the same results are obtained, it is reliable. If different people administer or score the test and they obtain the same results, the test reflects **objectivity**.

Although a test could be reliable and objective and still not be valid, tests that are unreliable or lack objectivity cannot be valid. Once the consistency of the test is ensured, there are four major ways to determine whether the test measures what it is supposed to measure: content, criterion, predictive, and construct validity. **Content validity** indicates that the test seems to be good based on logic, expert testimony, and widespread use. **Criterion validity** involves having an externally valid criterion for the test. For example, underwater weighing serves as the criterion measure for validating skinfold assessment of body fatness. With **predictive validity**, the criterion is measured at some point in the future. For example, risk factors for coronary heart disease (CHD) have been validated with a criterion that is measured in the future (i.e., actual development of CHD). **Construct validity** is provided by showing that a test responds in the ways one would expect based on theoretical understanding of that characteristic. For example, step tests have some validity because people who are physically active score better than inactive people.

1 **In Review: The most important question to ask about a test is whether it measures the characteristics in which you are interested. To do so, a test must give consistent results (reliability), even with different testers (objectivity). A test should have evidence that it is related to the selected characteristic (validity) in terms of expert opinion, comparison with good tests of the same variable, ability to predict future outcomes, and theoretical support.**

The fitness tests recommended in this book have been shown to be reliable and objective when carefully administered by trained professionals. Maximal oxygen uptake and fat percentage estimation by underwater weighing are considered valid tests (and are often used as the "gold standards" for cardiorespiratory fitness and relative leanness, respectively). They have been recommended and used by experts in numerous research investigations and fitness programs (content validity). The tests recommended in chapters 9 and 11-13 also have content validity in that experts in the fitness field use and recommend them. In addition, the endurance run and skinfold fat tests have criterion validity because they are highly related (correlated) with maximal oxygen uptake and underwater weighing, respectively (1). There is some construct validity for all of the tests because they have been shown to be related to other tests of the same variable, they improve with the type of physical conditioning thought to improve the characteristic, and performance on these tests changes with changes in training states.

TIPS FOR INCREASING THE ACCURACY OF TESTING

Fitness leaders can do a number of things to obtain more accurate results (i.e., less error) from testing:

- Properly prepare the person being tested.
- Organize the testing session.
- Attend to details.

Accuracy of testing can be improved by carefully preparing the person being tested and having the tester be precise in an organized testing session. Preparing the individual being tested is part of organizing the test session. In addition to the items just listed, the fitness tester will want to ensure that everything is ready to test individuals accurately and efficiently (see form 6.1, the Fitness Testing Preparation Checklist).

The most fundamental thing a tester can do to improve the accuracy of the testing situation is to pay close attention to all the fine points of assessment. Preparing the subject, organizing the testing situation, and collecting the data with precision can be accurately completed only when the tester attends to each aspect of the test protocol.

In Review: The best test results are found with people who are prepared and who understand what test procedures are going to be used. The participant should practice any unusual or novel aspects of the test beforehand. The HFI should check to determine that the participant has complied with pretest instructions in terms of rest, food, drink, drugs, proper clothing, and exercise and that the individual is physically and mentally prepared to take the test. The HFI should also thoroughly prepare and organize the testing session and collect the data in a precise fashion.

validity — Evaluation of a test to determine if it measures what it is supposed to measure. Validity includes test consistency (reliability) and tester consistency (objectivity). Validity is determined by logic (content), comparison with a valid test (criterion), ability to accurately predict (predictive), and theoretical means (construct).

reliability — The degree to which the same test score will be achieved on separate administrations of a test.

objectivity — When different people administer or score the test, and they obtain the same results.

content validity — Indicates that the test seems to be good based on logic, expert testimony, and widespread use.

criterion validity — Evidence that a test has a high relationship to a valid criterion test. For example, underwater weighing serves as the criterion measure for validating skinfold assessment of body fatness.

predictive validity — The criterion test is measured at some point in the future. For example, risk factors for coronary heart disease (CHD) have been validated with a criterion that is measured in the future (i.e., actual development of CHD).

construct validity — Evidence that a test responds in the ways one would expect based on theoretical understanding of that characteristic.

FORM 6.1

Fitness Testing Preparation Checklist

Is the individual ready?

Be sure the person being tested

1. Has read and understands the test procedures ☐
2. Has signed informed consent form ☐
3. Has practiced the test and is comfortable with it ☐
4. Understands the starting and stopping procedures ☐
5. Understands expectations before, during, and after the test ☐
6. Has complied with all pretest instructions concerning ☐
   A. Rest
   B. Food and drink
   C. Smoking and drugs
   D. Clothes and shoes
7. Does not have any illness or injury ☐
8. Is not on medication (except as planned with physician) ☐
9. Has had a proper warm-up ☐

Is the tester ready?

Attend to each of these items before beginning a testing session:

1. Test(s) to be administered determined for each person ☐
2. Equipment in working order and calibrated ☐
3. Score sheet(s) and other supplies ready ☐
4. Testing assistants clearly understand responsibilities ☐
5. Testing assistants checked out on tasks they are to do ☐
6. Timing and sequence of testing set ☐
7. Starting and stopping instructions clear to tester and subjects ☐
8. Subjects ready for test ☐
9. Emergency equipment and procedures ready ☐
10. Warm-up consistent for all ☐
11. Posttest activities and responsibilities set ☐
12. Temperature, humidity, and barometric pressure recorded and within acceptable limits ☐
13. Testing areas clean, set up, and ready for testing ☐
14. Atmosphere is calm, private, and relaxed ☐

Reprinted from Franks and Howley 1989.

USING TEST SCORES IN A FITNESS PROGRAM

Fitness testing has many uses in a fitness setting, from prescribing exercise to refining programs. Health fitness professionals must know how to interpret test scores and provide feedback to all program participants.

Interpreting Test Scores

What does a body weight of 180 lb reflect? It may mean this: The person really weighs 183 lb, he or she just lost 1 lb of water weight in a workout, the scales weigh 3 lb light, and we have misread the scale 1 lb heavy.

Any observed test result includes **true score** plus **error**. The error may be caused by equipment, environment, psychological factors, and inconsistency of the subject or the tester. Some of the error may be constant (which can be corrected with a set number) or random (which cannot be predicted or corrected). In the body-weight example, the scale error could have been corrected by adding 3 lb to the observed weight; but the tester error could not be predicted, in that the scale might have been read as light one time and heavy the next. One reason several trials are taken for a test is based on the assumption that the random errors will average out; thus if you were to take the average of three body weights, it would reduce the effect of random error.

One way to deal with variability is to use the **standard deviation,** an indication of the variability of test scores based on the difference of each score from the **mean**. The mean is the average. So if a large number of 20-year-old women were tested, one might find that the mean maximal heart rate was 200 beats · min^{-1}. If you looked at each individual's maximal heart rate, you would find a large number that had maximal heart rates within a few beats of 200 and a few women who had maximal heart rates several beats above or below 200. In the case of maximal heart rate, the standard deviation is about 11 beats · min^{-1} for different ages (10). In a normal distribution, standard deviation includes a set percentage of people:

- Mean plus and minus 1 standard deviation = 68% of group
- Mean plus and minus 2 standard deviations = 95% of group
- Mean plus and minus 3 standard deviations = 99% of group

In the example of maximal heart rate, you would expect to find 68% of 20-year-old women with maximal heart rates between 189 and 211 beats · min^{-1} (mean of 200 beats · min^{-1} plus one standard deviation of 11 beats · min^{-1} = 211 beats · min^{-1}; mean of 200 beats · min^{-1} minus one standard deviation of 11 beats · min^{-1} = 189 beats · min^{-1}), 95% between 178 and 222 beats · min^{-1} (mean plus and minus two standard deviations, or 22 beats · min^{-1}), and almost all 20-year-old women with a maximal heart rate between 167 and 233 beats · min^{-1} (mean plus and minus 3 standard deviations, or 3 × 11 = 33 beats · min^{-1}).

Two conclusions can be drawn from the variability of fitness tests. First, when carefully used, fitness tests can give accurate estimates of fitness components. Second, fitness test results are approximations of the fitness components. Thus we can differentiate among cardiorespiratory fitness (CRF) levels of 14, 9, and 6 METs but would not be able to pinpoint differences between 8.6 and 9.4 METs (see chapter 7).

How to Explain Test Scores to Participants

You can help participants evaluate their fitness test scores by doing the following (6, 7, 12):

- Emphasize health status rather than comparison with others.
- Emphasize change rather than current status.
- Provide specific recommendations based on the test data and your understanding of the individual.

true score — For any measurement the observed test result is made up of the true score plus any **error**.

error — An inaccurate score that can result from the testing environment, the equipment, normal variation of the person, and the tester. Some of the error may be constant (which can be corrected with a set number) or random (which cannot be predicted or corrected).

standard deviation — An indication of the variability of test scores based on the difference of each score from the group average.

mean — The average score.

Emphasize Criterion Health Status

One common approach is to compare the fitness participant with people of the same gender and similar age (e.g., "On the 1.5-mi-run test, you were better than 60% of the people your age and gender."). Although individuals may ask for this type of feedback, it is probably the least useful in terms of fitness. Much of the individual comparison with others is based on heredity and early experience. There are limits to how much change can be made even with a great deal of effort. It is unfortunate that many people in fitness programs try to use the "performance" model of being number one. The emphasis should not be on who can run the fastest or who has the lowest cholesterol, but rather on helping all people understand and try to obtain and maintain healthy levels of cardiorespiratory fitness, body composition, and low-back function. Thus, in the first testing session, the feedback should be based on whether people meet desirable health standards rather than on what percentage of the population they could "beat" on a test. This is the approach we have used throughout this book.

We have set fitness standards for people based on what is needed for good health. For example, we would like all women to have from 16% to 25% body fat, and children and men, from 7% to 18% (see chapter 9). It doesn't matter what percentage of the population is currently in that range. What does matter is that if people have less fat than the lower limit of the range, they have health risks associated with having too little fat, and if they have more fat than the upper limit of the range, their risks of developing (or making worse) major health problems increases. The fitness leader should encourage all participants to try to reach and maintain the health standards for cardiorespiratory fitness (CRF), body composition, and low-back function. Health standards for field tests (see chapters 9 and 11-13 for details of the tests) for different ages are presented in table 6.1. Standards for maximal oxygen uptake are given in chapter 11. Although it is common for individuals to perform at lower levels on fitness tests as they get older, it is not healthy to decrease CRF, gain fat, or reduce midtrunk flexibility and abdominal muscle endurance. Therefore, we expect performance times (e.g., time needed to win a 10K race) to decrease, but the minimal fitness standards are the same for adults of all ages. It should be noted that more research is needed to be able to refine these standards; as we find out more about the relationship between test scores and positive health some of these standards may need to be modified.

Focus on Improvement and Goal Setting

The most important question for a fitness participant is not what her or his health status is at this moment in life, but rather what it will be 6 months, 2 years, or 20 years from now. In this way, the person is encouraged to deal with her or his status compared to health standards and can set reasonable, desirable, and achievable goals for the next testing period.

Another way that test results can be used is to help individuals meet specific goals. It may be that the health standards are not appropriate or reasonable for an individual. For example, the mile-run standards cannot be used for people who are swimming for their fitness workouts or for individuals who use wheelchairs. However, individual goals for covering a certain distance in the water or in a wheelchair can be established. Or the fitness leader may want to set intermediary goals for an individual who is very unfit. For example, it would be discouraging to discuss mile-run standards for a person who can only walk a quarter of a mile without stopping. The initial goal for that person may be to work up to being able to walk a mile without stopping. As indicated in chapter 20, it is important to set goals and subgoals to help people begin and continue healthy behaviors.

Recognize Healthy Behaviors

Fitness and lifestyle behaviors (such as getting adequate exercise, nutrition, and rest; avoiding substance abuse; coping with stress) and fitness test scores are interrelated. The fitness leader should emphasize fitness *behaviors*. It is more important for people to begin and continue regular physical activity than to reach a certain level on a graded exercise test. Likewise, it is more important for people to develop healthy eating habits than to have a certain percentage of body fat. By emphasizing healthy behaviors, HFIs can recognize people for their efforts; and in the long run this will be the best way to improve their fitness test scores. An overemphasis on test scores can discourage some participants. Two good examples that recognize physical activity behavior are the Canadian *Active Living Fitness Program* (5) and the President's Council on Physical Fitness and Sports' *Presidential Sports Award* program (11). Both programs provide awards for individuals who do various physical activities for a certain number of hours, thus rewarding the behavior rather than some fitness test result.

Table 6.1 Fitness Test Standards

Test item	Age (yr)[b] 6-9	10-12	13-15	16-30	31-50	51-70
			Mi run (min)			
Males						
Good	14	12	11	10	10	10
Borderline	16	14	13	12	12	12
Needs work	≥18	≥16	≥15	≥14	≥14	≥14
Females						
Good	14	12	13	12	12	12
Borderline	16	14	15	14	14	14
Needs work	≥18	≥16	≥17	≥16	≥16	≥16
			Percent body fat (%)			
Males						
Good	7-18	7-18	7-18	7-18	7-18	7-18
Borderline	22	22	22	22	22	22
Needs work	< 5	< 5	< 5	< 5	< 5	< 5
	> 25	> 25	> 25	> 25	> 25	> 25
Females						
Good	7-18	7-18	16-25	16-25	16-25	16-25
Borderline	22	22	27	27	27	27
Needs work	< 5	< 5	< 14	< 14	< 14	< 14
	> 25	> 25	> 30	> 30	> 30	> 30
			Curl-ups (#)			
Good	≥20	≥25	≥30	≥35	≥35	≥35
Borderline	12	15	22	25	25	25
Needs work	≤5	≤10	≤13	≤15	≤15	≤15
			Sit-and-reach (in.)[a]			
Good	12	12	12	12	12	12
Borderline	8	8	8	8	8	8
Needs work	≤6	≤6	≤6	≤6	≤6	≤6
			Modified pull-ups (#)			
Good	≥10	≥12	≥15	≥15	≥15	≥15
Borderline	6	8	10	10	10	10
Needs work	≤2	≤4	≤5	≤5	≤5	≤5

Note. [a]The feet touch the base of the box at 9 in. A score of 9 indicates the person can touch his or her feet.
[b]Individuals over 70 years of age should be encouraged to do the walk test (chapter 11) and strive to monitor the other fitness components.
Adapted from *YMCA Youth Fitness Test Manual* (pp. 42-47) by B.D. Franks, 1989, Champaign, IL: Human Kinetics. Copyright 1989 by National Council of Young Men's Christian Associations of the United States of America. Adapted by permission.

3 **In Review:** **Test scores include the true score, constant error, and random error. The standard deviation from the mean can be used to describe variability. Fitness tests can provide good approximations of fitness levels; but rather than focusing on test scores it is more critical for individuals to be recognized and rewarded for healthy behaviors, improving in fitness status, achieving specific fitness goals, and maintaining a healthy fitness status in each component of physical fitness.**

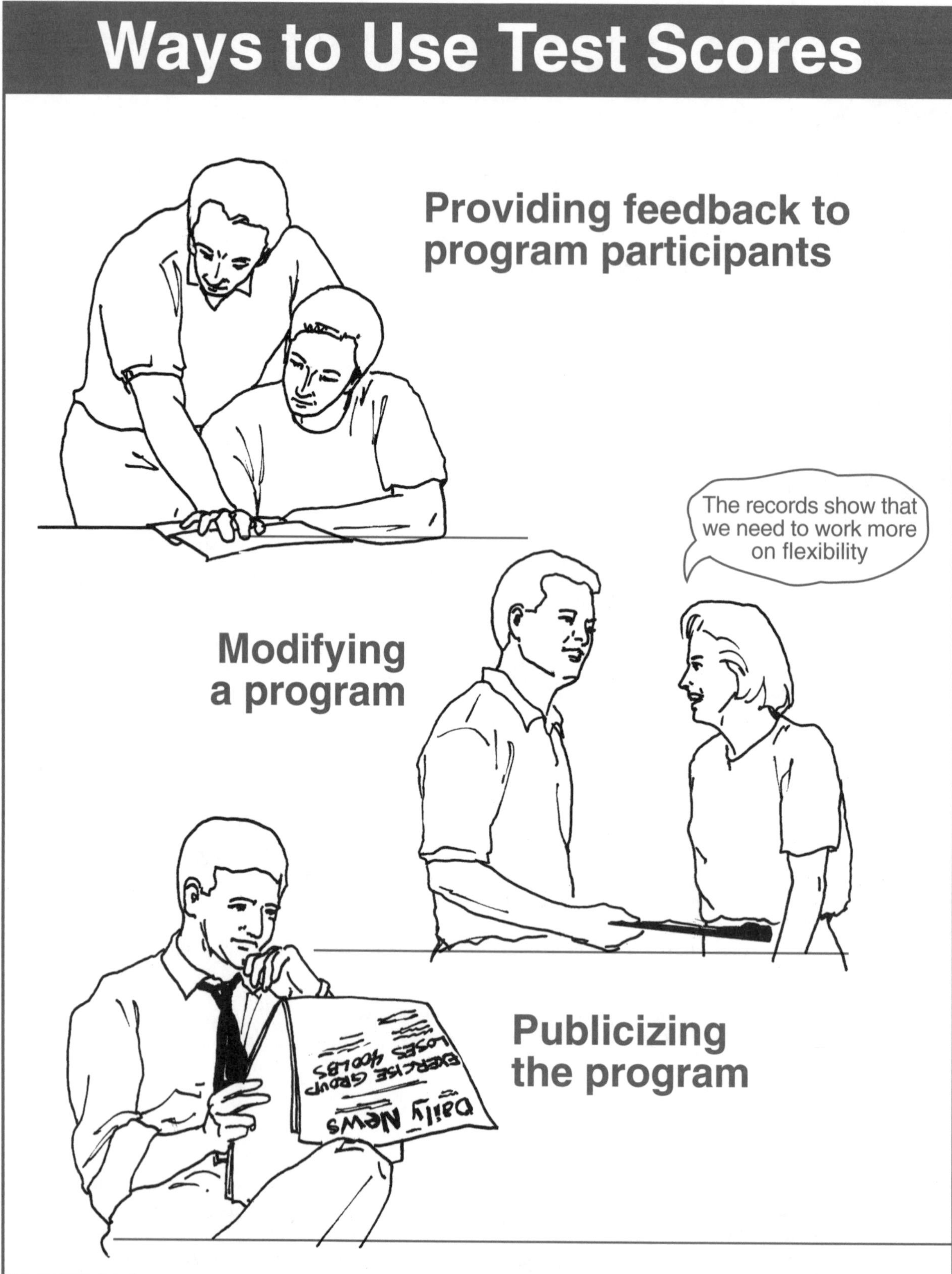
Ways to Use Test Scores
Providing feedback to program participants
The records show that we need to work more on flexibility
Modifying a program
Daily News
EXERCISE GROUP LOSES 400LBS
Publicizing the program

Fitness Testing for Individuals With Disabilities

Many individuals have one or more disabilities ranging from mild to severe limitations regarding physical activity and assessment. It is beyond the scope of this book to recommend specific activities and tests to deal with each possible condition (2). The following general principles, however, can be applied by the HFI:

- Almost all individuals with disabilities can benefit from regular physical activity.
- Most of these individuals can participate in a variety of activities with simple adaptations.
- Individuals with disabilities can gain motivation from periodic assessment.
- The same types of fitness tests can be used with simple adaptations.
- Adaptations in activity and assessment are often simply commonsense adjustments made by the HFI and the participant.
- Experts in adapted physical education and special education can provide additional assistance.

Providing Feedback Based on Test Results

The health standards and emphasis on improvement and healthy behaviors provide the basis for the feedback given to individual participants. Another factor to consider is the individual's own nature and likes and dislikes. The key to feedback is to provide the best recommendations concerning activities (type, total work, intensity, frequency) that would be healthy, helpful, and interesting to this individual (thus providing motivation to continue). Assistance is especially important early in the fitness program.

Using Testing to Guide Program Revision

Analysis of test scores from different fitness classes can assist in deciding what revisions need to be made in the overall fitness program. How many people drop out of various classes? What kinds of aerobic, body fatness, and low-back function changes are being made? How many injuries are related to the various classes? The answers to such questions help you to evaluate, revise, and improve your fitness programs. You might consider your programs to be improving steadily rather than having reached "perfection." This improvement can result from program evaluation.

Using Test Results to Promote Your Program

Another use of test scores is to help educate the public and to get positive attention for your program. What percentage of the participants stay with the program long enough to make important fitness gains? What is the total amount of fat lost by participants in 1 year? How many miles have the participants run during the year? Careful testing, record keeping, and analysis can provide helpful information about your program to the public.

4

In Review: Fitness scores, along with individuals' interests, can help HFIs to modify exercise recommendations for participants. The test results from all the participants can provide the basis for evaluating, modifying, and promoting your fitness center's program.

CALIBRATING EQUIPMENT

To **calibrate** is to check the accuracy of a measuring device by comparing it with a known standard and adjusting it to provide an accurate reading. This section explains how to calibrate the equipment used in exercise testing. These are suggestions only and should not be viewed as a replacement for the specific procedures recommended by the equipment manufacturer (9).

Treadmill Speed and Elevation Settings

The treadmill's speed and grade settings must be calibrated because they determine physiological

calibrate—To determine the accuracy of a measuring device by comparing it with a known standard and adjusting it to provide an accurate reading.

demand and are crucial in estimating cardiorespiratory fitness.

Calibrating Speed

An easy way to calibrate the speed on any treadmill is to measure the length of the belt and count the number of belt revolutions in a certain time period. To calibrate treadmill speed, follow these specific steps (9):

1. Measure the exact length of the belt in meters and record the value.
2. Place a small piece of tape near the edge of the belt surface.
3. Turn on the treadmill to a given speed using the speed control.
4. Count 20 revolutions of the belt while tracking time with a stopwatch. Start your watch as the tape first moves past the fixed point, beginning your counting with "zero."
5. Convert the number of revolutions to revolutions per minute (rev · min^{-1}). For example, if the belt made 20 complete revolutions in 35 s, then

$$35 \text{ s} / 60 \text{ s} \cdot \text{min}^{-1} = .583 \text{ min}$$

So,

$$20 \text{ rev} / .583 \text{ min} = 34.3 \text{ rev} \cdot \text{min}^{-1}$$

6. Multiply the calculated revolutions per minute (step 5) times the belt length (step 1). This will give you the belt speed in meters per minute (m · min^{-1}). For example, if the belt length is 5.025 m, then

$$34.3 \text{ rev} \cdot \text{min}^{-1} \cdot 5.025 \text{ m} \cdot \text{rev}^{-1} = 172.35 \text{ m} \cdot \text{min}^{-1}$$

7. To convert meters per minute to miles per hour (mi · hr^{-1}), divide the answer in step 6 by 26.8 (m · min^{-1}) · (mi · hr^{-1})$^{-1}$:

$$172.35 \text{ m} \cdot \text{min} / 26.8 ([\text{m} \cdot \text{min}^{-1}] \cdot [\text{mi} \cdot \text{hr}^{-1}]^{-1}) = 6.43 \text{ mi} \cdot \text{hr}^{-1}$$

8. The value obtained in step 7 is the actual treadmill speed in miles per hour. If the speed indicator does not agree with this value, adjust the dial to the proper reading. Check the instruction manual for the location of the speed adjustment.
9. Repeat for a number of different speeds to ensure accuracy across the speeds used in test protocols.

Calibrating Elevation

Treadmill manuals describe how to calibrate the grade using a simple carpenter's level and a square edge. This calibration procedure consists of three steps:

1. Use a carpenter's level to make sure that the treadmill is level, and check the zero setting on the grade meter under these conditions (with the treadmill electronics turned on). If the meter does not read zero, follow instructions to make the adjustment (usually by using the small screw on the face of the dial).
2. Elevate the treadmill so that the percentage-grade dial reads approximately 20%. Measure the exact incline of the treadmill as shown in figure 6.1. When the level's bubble is exactly in the center of the tube, the rise measurement is obtained.
3. Calculate the grade as the rise over the "run" (tangent), and adjust the treadmill meter to read that exact grade. For example, if the rise were 4.5 in. to the run's 22.5 in., the fractional grade would be

$$\text{Grade} = \text{tangent } ø = \text{rise} / \text{run} = 4.5 \text{ in.} / 22.5 \text{ in.} = 0.20 = 20\%$$

The rise-over-run method is a typical engineering method for calculating grade, giving the tangent of the angle (the opposite side divided by the horizontal distance, as shown in figure 6.1). Although the sine of the angle (opposite side divided by the hypotenuse) provides the most accurate setting of grade, table 6.2 shows that the tangent value is a good

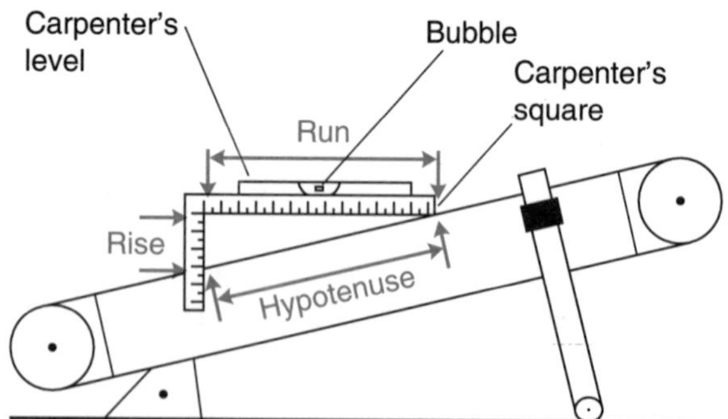

FIGURE 6.1 Calibrating grade by the tangent method (rise/run) with a carpenter's square and level.
Reprinted from Howley, 1988, The exercise testing laboratory. In *Resource manual for guidelines for exercise testing and prescription*. By permission of Lea & Febiger.

Table 6.2 Natural Sines and Tangents

Degrees	Sine	% Grade	Tangent	% Grade
0	0.0000	0.0	0.0000	0.0
1	0.0175	1.7	0.075	1.7
2	0.0349	3.5	0.0349	3.5
3	0.0523	5.2	0.0524	5.2
4	0.0698	7.0	0.0699	7.0
5	0.0872	8.7	0.0875	8.7
6	0.1045	10.4	0.1051	10.5
7	0.1219	12.2	0.1228	12.3
8	0.1392	13.9	0.1405	14.0
9	0.1564	15.6	0.1584	15.8
10	0.1736	17.4	0.1763	17.6
11	0.1908	19.1	0.1944	19.4
12	0.2079	20.8	0.2126	21.3
13	0.2250	22.5	0.2309	23.1
14	0.2419	24.2	0.2493	24.9
15	0.2588	25.9	0.2679	26.8
20	0.3420	34.2	0.3640	36.4
25	0.4067	40.7	0.4452	44.5

Reprinted from Howley, 1988, The exercise testing laboratory. In *Resource manual for guidelines for exercise testing and prescription*. By permission of Lea & Febiger.

approximation of the sine value for grades less than 20%, or 12° (see page 122). The rise-over-run method can also be used for calibrating steep grades: Obtain the tangent value as described above and simply look across table 6.2 to obtain the correct sine value to set on the treadmill dial. For example, if the rise-over-run method yielded 0.268, or 26.8% (tangent), the "correct" setting would be 25.9% (sine). The latter value is set on the grade dial of the treadmill.

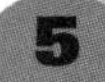

In Review: Calibrating the treadmill includes checking both the speed and elevation. Page 120 lists the steps for calibration.

Calibrating the Cycle Ergometer

The cycle ergometer must be calibrated on a routine basis to ensure that the work rate is accurate. The work rate on the mechanically braked cycle ergometer is varied by altering either the pedal rate or the load on the wheel. Work is equal to force times the distance through which the force acts: W = F × d. The kilopond (kp) is a common unit used to express force, not the kilogram, which is a unit of mass. The kilopond is defined as the force acting on a mass of 1 kg at the normal acceleration of gravity.

On a mechanically braked cycle ergometer, the force (kp) is moved through a distance (in meters, or m), so work is expressed in kpm. Because work is accomplished over some period of time (minutes, or min), the activity is referred to as a work rate or power output (kpm · min^{-1}), not a workload. On the Monark cycle ergometer, a point on the rim of the wheel travels 6 m per pedal revolution, so at 50 rev · min^{-1} the wheel travels 300 m · min^{-1}. If a force of 1 kp were hanging from that wheel, the work rate, or power output, would be 300 kpm · min^{-1}. From these simple calculations you can see the importance of maintaining a correct pedal rate during the test—if the subject were pedaling at 60 rev · min^{-1}, the work rate would actually be 20% higher (360 vs. 300 kpm · min^{-1}) than it appears to be. The force setting (resistance on the wheel) must also be carefully set and checked because it tends to drift as the test progresses. It is crucial that the force (resistance) values on the scale be correct. The following five steps outline the procedures for calibrating the Monark cycle ergometer scale (3) (refer to figure 6.2):

1. Using a carpenter's level, adjust a table to ensure that it is level, and put the ergometer on it.
2. Disconnect the "belt" at the spring.
3. Loosen the lock nut and use the adjusting screw on the front of the bike against which the force scale rests so that the vertical mark on the pendulum weight is matched with

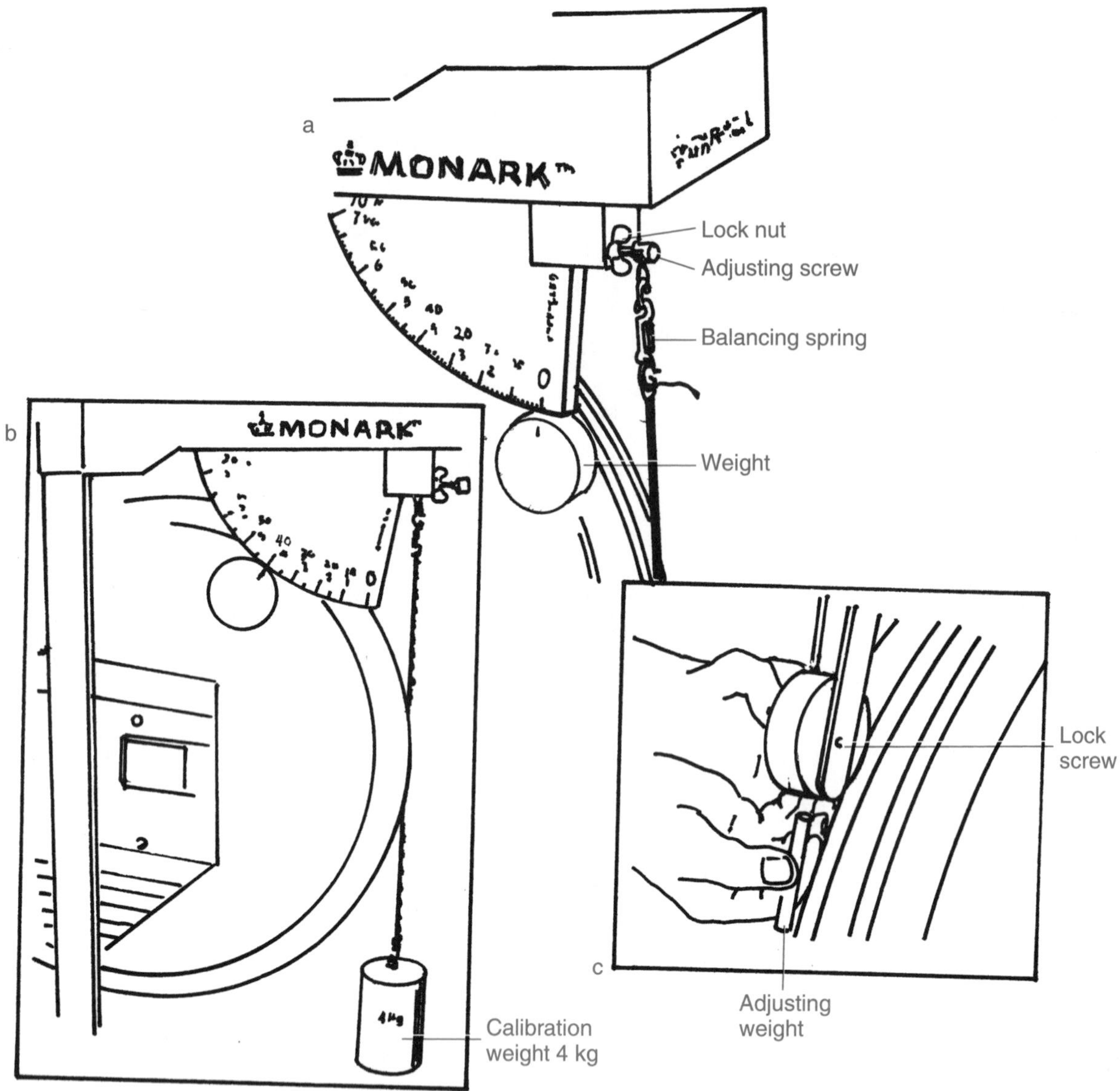

FIGURE 6.2 Calibrating the Monark cycle ergometer. Adjust the pendulum to align with 0 (a); suspend a 4.0 kg weight from the spring (b); and adjust the position or size of the weight in the pendulum (c).
Adapted from Monark Exercise AB.

"0" kp on the weight scale (see figure 6.2a). The pendulum must be free-swinging. Lock the adjustment screw with the lock nut.

4. Suspend a 4.0-kg weight from the spring so that no contact is made with the flywheel, and see if the pendulum moves to the 4.0-kp mark (see figure 6.2b). If it doesn't, alter the position or size of the adjusting weight in the pendulum (see figure 6.2c). When the lock screw on the back of the pendulum weight is loosened, the adjusting weight can be lowered or replaced. Check the force scale again and be sure to calibrate the ergometer through the range of values to be used in your tests.
5. Reassemble the cycle ergometer.

6 **In Review: Calibrating the cycle ergometer involves establishing a true zero, then hanging standard weights from the spring, and verifying that they line up with the readings on the scale. Specific steps are listed above.**

Calibrating the Sphygmomanometer

A **sphygmomanometer** is a blood-pressure measurement system composed of an inflatable rubber bladder, an instrument to indicate the applied pressure, an inflation bulb to create pressure, and an adjustable valve to deflate the system. The cuff and the measuring instrument are the most crucial in terms of measurement accuracy. The width of the cuff should be about 20% wider than the diameter of the limb to which it is applied, and when inflated, the bladder should not cause a bulging or displacement. If the bladder is too wide, blood pressure will be underestimated; if too narrow, pressure will be overestimated. Consequently, bladder size (length × width) varies with the type of cuff: child size (21.5 cm × 10 cm), adult size (24 cm × 12.5 cm), and large adult size (33 cm or 42 cm × 15 cm).

The pressure-measuring device, the manometer, can be a mercury or an aneroid type. The mercury type is the standard, and its calibration is easily maintained. The mercury column should rise and fall smoothly, form a clear meniscus, and read zero when the bladder is deflated. If the mercury sticks in the tube, remove the cap and swab out the inside. If it is very dirty, the tube should be removed and cleaned (with detergent, a water rinse, and alcohol for drying). If the mercury column falls below zero, add mercury to bring the meniscus exactly to the zero mark (4, 8, 9).

The aneroid gauge uses a metal bellows assembly that expands when pressure is applied, and the expansion moves the pointer on the indicator dial. A spring attached to the pointer moves the pointer downscale to zero when the bladder is deflated. This gauge should be calibrated at least once every 6 months at a variety of settings, using the mercury column just described. A simple Y tube is used to connect the two systems together (see figure 6.3). Readings should be taken with pressure falling to simulate the readings during an actual measurement (9).

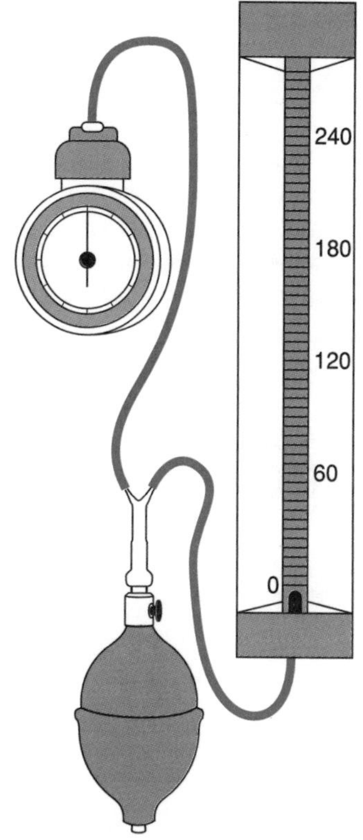

FIGURE 6.3 Calibrating an aneroid manometer with a mercury manometer.
Reproduced by permission. Human blood pressure determination by sphygmomanometer 1994. Copyright American Heart Association.

sphygmomanometer — A blood-pressure measurement system.

7 **In Review: It is important to have the correct size cuff when measuring blood pressure. The mercury sphygmomanometer is the standard, and the aneroid gauge should be calibrated against the mercury column every 6 months.**

Case Studies

You can check your answers by referring to appendix A.

6.1

You are contacted by an agency that wants you to recommend a running test to evaluate cardiorespiratory fitness. One part of your recommendations must provide a convincing argument that the test measures what you say it does. How would you do this?

6.2

A Monark cycle ergometer is calibrated with 0.5, 1.0, 1.5, and 2.0 kg weights, and each of the values are 0.25 kg too high on the scale. What could have caused this?

6.3

A male client who is beginning your fitness program completes a test to measure maximal aerobic power and wants to know how he compared to world-class runners. While you can obviously provide this information, how might you respond relative to (a) why the test is given and (b) the goals of the fitness program?

SOURCE LIST

1. American Alliance for Health, Physical Education, Recreation and Dance (1984)
2. American Association of Active Lifestyles (1995)
3. Åstrand (1979)
4. Baum (1961)
5. Canadian Association for Health, Physical Education, Recreation and Dance (1994)
6. Cooper's Institute for Aerobics Research (1992)
7. Franks (1989)
8. Frohlich et al. (1988)
9. Howley (1988)
10. Londeree & Moeschberger (1982)
11. President's Council on Physical Fitness and Sports (1996)
12. Safrit (1995)

CHAPTER

7

Energy Costs of Physical Activity

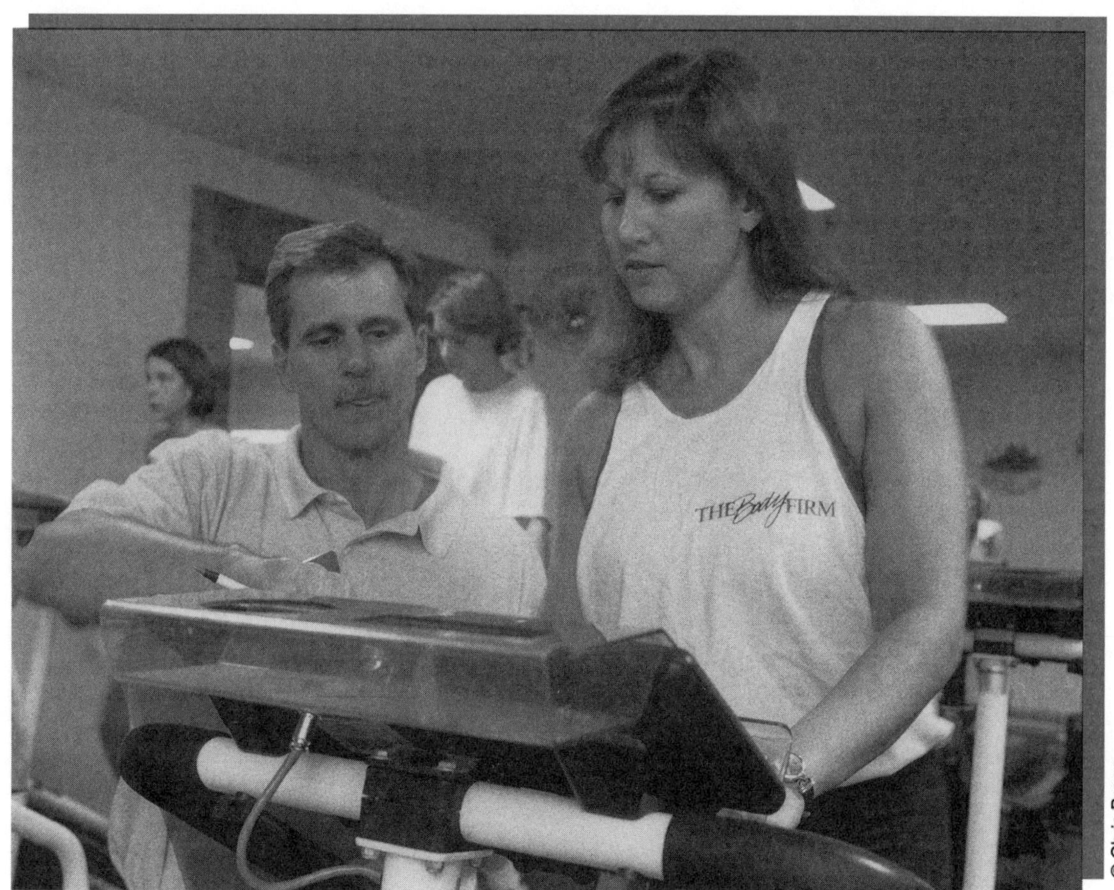

© Chris Brown

OBJECTIVES

The reader will be able to:

1. **Describe how oxygen consumption measurements can be used to estimate energy production, and list the number of calories derived per liter of oxygen and per gram of carbohydrate, fat, and protein.**
2. **Express energy expenditure as $L \cdot min^{-1}$, $kcal \cdot min^{-1}$, $ml \cdot kg^{-1} \cdot min^{-1}$, METs, and $kcal \cdot kg^{-1} \cdot hr^{-1}$.**
3. **Estimate the oxygen cost of walking, jogging, and running, including the cost of walking and running 1 mi.**
4. **Estimate the oxygen cost of cycle ergometry exercise for both arm and leg work.**
5. **Estimate the oxygen cost of bench stepping.**
6. **Identify the approximate energy cost of recreational, sport, and other activities; and describe the effect of environmental factors on the heart rate response to a fixed work rate.**

Health fitness instructors (HFIs) are usually concerned about the following two questions when they recommend specific physical activities to participants:

1. Are the activities appropriate, in terms of exercise intensity, to achieve the target heart rate (see chapter 14)?
2. Is the combination of intensity and duration appropriate for achieving an energy expenditure goal to balance or exceed caloric intake (see chapter 10)?

To answer these questions the HFI should become familiar with the energy costs of various activities. The purpose of this chapter is to offer some basic information about how to estimate the energy requirement of various physical activities and to summarize the values associated with common recreational activities.

WAYS TO MEASURE ENERGY EXPENDITURE

Energy expenditure can be measured by direct and indirect calorimetry. **Direct calorimetry** requires that the person perform an activity within a specially constructed chamber that is insulated and has water flowing through its walls. The water is warmed by the heat given off by the subject, and heat production can be calculated by knowing the volume of water flowing through the chamber per minute and the change in the temperature of the water from entry to exit. For example, a person does bench-stepping exercises in the chamber at the rate of 30 steps $\cdot$ min^{-1} using a 20-cm bench. The water flows through the walls of the chamber at 20 L $\cdot$ min^{-1}, and the increase in the temperature of the water from entry to exit is 0.5 °C. Because it takes approximately 1 kcal to raise the temperature of 1 L of water 1 °C, the following calculation yields the approximate energy expenditure.

$$\frac{20\ \text{L}}{\text{min}} \cdot \frac{1\ \text{kcal}}{°\text{C}} \cdot 0.5\ °\text{C} = \frac{10\ \text{kcal}}{\text{min}}$$

Additional heat is lost from the subject by evaporation of water from the skin and respiratory passages. This heat loss can be measured and added to that picked up by the water to yield the rate of energy produced by the individual for that task.

Indirect calorimetry estimates energy production by measuring oxygen consumption. This technique, already described in chapter 4, relies on certain constants to convert liters of oxygen consumption to kcal expended. The constants are derived from measurements made in a bomb calorimeter, a heavy metal chamber into which carbohydrate, fat, or protein can be placed with 100% oxygen under pressure. The chamber is immersed in a water bath, and the food stuff is oxidized to CO_2 and H_2O when an electric spark sets the process in motion. The heat given off by the combustion warms the water; and it has been determined that carbohydrates, fats, and proteins give off approximately 4, 9, and 5.6 kcal of heat per gram, respectively. Because the nitrogen in protein cannot be completely oxidized in the body and is excreted as urea, the physiological value for protein is actually 4.0 kcal $\cdot$ g^{-1}.

Knowing how much oxygen is required to oxidize 1 g of carbohydrate, fat, and protein allows one to calculate the number of kcal of energy produced when 1 L of oxygen is consumed. This is called the **caloric equivalent of oxygen**. Values for carbohydrate, fat, and protein are listed in table 7.1. The table shows that carbohydrates give about 6% more energy per liter of oxygen than fats (5.0 vs. 4.7 kcal $\cdot$ L^{-1}), whereas fats give more than twice as much energy per gram than carbohydrate (9 vs. 4 kcal $\cdot$ g^{-1}). If a person is deriving energy from a 50/50 mixture of carbohydrates and fats during exercise, the caloric equivalent is approximately 4.85 kcal $\cdot$ L^{-1}, halfway between the value of 4.7 for fat and 5.0 for carbohydrates (18). The ratio of carbon dioxide produced to oxygen consumed at the cell is called the respiratory quotient (RQ). The same ratio, when measured by conventional gas exchange procedures, is called the respiratory exchange ratio (R),

Table 7.1 Caloric Density, Caloric Equivalent, and Respiratory Quotient Associated With Oxidation of Carbohydrate, Fat, and Protein

Measurement	Carbohydrate	Fat	Protein[a]
Caloric density (kcal $\cdot$ g^{-1})	4.0	9.0	4.0
Caloric equivalent of 1 L of O_2 (kcal $\cdot$ L^{-1})	5.0	4.7	4.5
Respiratory quotient	1.0	0.7	0.8

Note. [a]Does not include the energy derived from the oxidation of nitrogen in the amino acids because the body excretes this as urea.

Adapted from "Energy Metabolism" by L.K. Knoebel. (18) In *Physiology* (5th edition) by E. Selkurt (Ed.), 1984, Boston: Little Brown & Co.

direct calorimetry — A method of measuring the metabolic rate using a closed chamber in which a subject's heat loss is picked up by water flowing through the wall of a chamber; the gain in temperature of the water, plus that lost in evaporation, determine the metabolic rate.

indirect calorimetry — The estimation of energy production on the basis of oxygen consumption.

caloric equivalent of oxygen — Approximately 5 kcal of energy are produced per liter of oxygen consumed (5 kcal $\cdot$ L^{-1})

and is used as an indicator of fuel use (carbohydrate vs. fat) during exercise (see chapter 4 for details).

Indirect calorimetry employs two techniques to measure oxygen consumption: **closed-circuit** and **open-circuit spirometry**. In the closed-circuit technique the subject usually breathes 100% oxygen from a spirometer, and the exhaled air passes through a chemical to absorb the carbon dioxide. Over time, the volume of oxygen contained in the spirometer decreases, giving us a measure of the oxygen consumption in ml $\cdot$ min^{-1}. Because the carbon dioxide is absorbed, one cannot calculate a respiratory exchange ratio, so a caloric equivalent of 4.82 kcal $\cdot$ L^{-1} is used to indicate that a mixture of carbohydrates, fats, and proteins is used. This closed-circuit technique has been used extensively to measure the basal metabolic rate (18).

The open-circuit technique for measuring oxygen consumption and carbon dioxide production is the most common indirect calorimetry technique. In this procedure, oxygen consumption is calculated by simply subtracting the volume of oxygen exhaled from the volume of oxygen inhaled. The difference is taken as the oxygen uptake or oxygen consumption (see chapter 4 for details). Carbon dioxide production is calculated in the same manner. This makes it possible to calculate the respiratory exchange ratio (R). One can then determine which substrate, fat or carbohydrate provided the most energy during work and also determine what value to use for the caloric equivalent of 1 L of oxygen in the calculation of energy expenditure (i.e., 5.0 kcal $\cdot$ L^{-1} for carbohydrates and 4.7 kcal $\cdot$ L^{-1} for fats).

1 **In Review: Oxygen consumption ($\dot{V}O_2$) is a measure of how much energy (kcal) is produced by the body. Knowing how many kcal are generated per gram of carbohydrate and fat and how much oxygen is used to do that, liters of oxygen used can be converted to kcal of energy produced. The following values are the number of kcal per gram of food when metabolized in the body: carbohydrates = 4 kcal $\cdot$ g^{-1}; fats = 9 kcal $\cdot$ g^{-1}; and protein = 4 kcal $\cdot$ g^{-1}. Knowing how much oxygen is used in the metabolism of a food, we know that we obtain 4.7 kcal $\cdot$ L^{-1} when fat is oxidized and 5.0 kcal $\cdot$ L^{-1} when carbohydrate is oxidized. When a 50/50 mixture of carbohydrates and fats are used for energy we obtain 4.85 kcal $\cdot$ L^{-1}.**

WAYS TO EXPRESS ENERGY EXPENDITURE

The energy requirement for an activity is calculated on the basis of a subject's steady-state oxygen uptake ($\dot{V}O_2$) measured during an activity. Once the steady-state (leveling off) oxygen uptake is reached, the energy (ATP) supplied to the muscles is derived from the aerobic metabolism of the various substrates. The measured oxygen uptake can then be used to express energy expenditure in different ways. The five most common expressions follow:

1. **$\dot{V}O_2$ (L $\cdot$ min^{-1})**. The calculation of oxygen uptake (see chapter 4) yields a value expressed in liters of oxygen used per minute. For example, the following data were collected during a submaximal run on a treadmill on an 80-kg man: ventilation (STPD) = 60 L $\cdot$ min^{-1}; inspired O_2 = 20.93%; expired O_2 = 16.93%.

$$\dot{V}O_2(\text{L}\cdot\text{min}^{-1}) = 60\ \text{L}\cdot\text{min}^{-1}\cdot\ (20.93\%\ O_2 - 16.93\%\ O_2)$$
$$= 2.4\ \text{L}\cdot\text{min}^{-1}$$

2. **kcal $\cdot$ min^{-1}**. Oxygen uptake can be expressed in kilocalories used per minute. The caloric equivalent of 1 L of O_2 ranges from 4.7 kcal $\cdot$ L^{-1} for fats to 5.0 kcal $\cdot$

L^{-1} for carbohydrates. For practical reasons, and with little loss in precision, 5 kcal per liter of O_2 is used to convert the oxygen uptake to kilocalories per minute. Energy expenditure is calculated by multiplying the kilocalories expended per minute ($kcal \cdot min^{-1}$) by the duration of the activity in minutes. For example, if the 80-kg man mentioned previously runs on the treadmill for 30 min at a $\dot{V}O_2 = 2.4\ L \cdot min^{-1}$, the total energy expenditure can be calculated as follows.

$$\frac{2.4\ L}{min} \cdot \frac{5\ kcal}{L\ O_2} = \frac{12\ kcal}{min}$$

$$\frac{12\ kcal}{min} \cdot 30\ min = 360\ kcal$$

3. **$\dot{V}O_2$ ($ml \cdot kg^{-1} \cdot min^{-1}$).** If the measured oxygen uptake, expressed in liters per minute, is multiplied by 1000 to yield milliliters per minute and then divided by the subject's body weight in kilograms, the value is expressed in ml O_2 per kilogram of body weight per minute, or $ml \cdot kg^{-1} \cdot min^{-1}$. This facilitates comparisons among people of different body sizes. For example, for the 80-kg man with a $\dot{V}O_2 = 2.4\ L \cdot min^{-1}$

$$\frac{2.4\ L}{min} \cdot \frac{1000\ ml}{L} \div 80\ kg = (30\ ml \cdot kg^{-1} \cdot min^{-1}).$$

4. **METs**. The resting metabolic rate (oxygen uptake) is approximately $3.5\ ml \cdot kg^{-1} \cdot min^{-1}$. This is called 1 MET. Activities are expressed in terms of multiples of the MET unit. For example, using the values presented above,

$$30\ ml \cdot kg^{-1} \cdot min^{-1} \div 3.5\ ml \cdot kg^{-1} \cdot min^{-1} = 8.6\ METs.$$

5. **$kcal \cdot kg^{-1} \cdot hr^{-1}$**. The MET expression of energy expenditure carries a special bonus; the value also indicates the number of kcal the subject uses per kg of body weight per hour. In the example mentioned above, the subject is working at 8.6 METs, or about $30\ ml \cdot kg^{-1} \cdot min^{-1}$. When this value is multiplied by $60\ min \cdot hr^{-1}$, it equals $1800\ ml \cdot kg^{-1} \cdot hr^{-1}$, or $1.8\ L \cdot kg^{-1} \cdot hr^{-1}$. If the person is using a mixture of carbohydrates and fats as the fuel, then this oxygen consumption is multiplied by 4.85 kcal per $L\ O_2^{-1}$ to give $8.7\ kcal \cdot hr^{-1}$. The following steps show the detail.

$$8.6\ METs \cdot \frac{3.5\ ml \cdot kg^{-1} \cdot min^{-1}}{MET} = 30\ ml \cdot kg^{-1} \cdot min^{-1}$$

$$30\ ml \cdot kg^{-1} \cdot min^{-1} \cdot 60\ min \cdot hr^{-1} = 1800\ ml \cdot kg^{-1} \cdot hr^{-1} = 1.8\ L \cdot kg^{-1} \cdot hr^{-1}$$

$$1.8\ L \cdot kg^{-1} \cdot hr^{-1} \cdot 4.85\ kcal \cdot L\ O_2^{-1} = 8.7\ kcal \cdot kg^{-1} \cdot hr^{-1}$$

2 **In Review: Energy expenditure can be expressed in $L \cdot min^{-1}$, $kcal \cdot min^{-1}$, $ml \cdot kg^{-1} \cdot min^{-1}$, METs, and $kcal \cdot kg^{-1} \cdot hr^{-1}$. To convert $L \cdot min^{-1}$ to $kcal \cdot min^{-1}$, multiply by $5.0\ kcal \cdot L^{-1}$. To convert $L \cdot min^{-1}$ to $ml \cdot kg^{-1} \cdot min^{-1}$, multiply by 1000 and divide by body weight in kilograms. To convert $ml \cdot kg^{-1} \cdot min^{-1}$ to METs or $kcal \cdot kg^{-1} \cdot hr^{-1}$, divide by $3.5\ ml \cdot kg^{-1} \cdot min^{-1}$.**

closed-circuit spirometry— The subject breathes 100% oxygen from a spirometer while carbon dioxide is absorbed; loss of volume of oxygen from the spirometer is proportional to the oxygen consumption.

open-circuit spirometry— The method of measuring oxygen consumption by breathing in room air while collecting and analyzing the expired air.

FORMULAS FOR ESTIMATING THE ENERGY COST OF ACTIVITIES

In the mid-1970s the American College of Sports Medicine (ACSM) identified some simple formulas to estimate the steady-state energy requirement associated with common modes of activities used in graded exercise stress tests (GXTs): walking, stepping, running, and cycle ergometry (3). The oxygen uptake calculated from these formulas is an *estimate*, and a typical standard deviation associated with the actual measured average value is about 9% of the value (10). This normal variation in the energy cost of activities is important to remember when using these equations in prescribing exercise.

The ACSM formulas have been applied to GXTs to estimate functional capacity, or maximal aerobic power. This application has been shown to give reasonable estimates when the subjects are healthy and the rate at which the GXT progresses is slow enough to allow a steady-state oxygen uptake to be achieved at each stage (20, 22). When the increments in the stages of the GXT are large or the individual being tested is somewhat unfit, his or her oxygen uptake will not keep pace with each stage of the test. In these cases the formulas overestimate the actual measured oxygen uptake (14). The fact that this overestimation is more likely to happen in diseased populations (e.g., cardiac) suggests that the GXTs used may be too aggressive. A test that progresses at a slower rate and allows the subject to reach the steady-state $\dot{V}O_2$ at each stage reduces the chance of an overestimation of functional capacity and still requires the subject to work at an appropriate metabolic rate to overload the system (see chapter 14). The previous information is presented to clarify the usefulness of the following equations. The formulas *estimate* the steady-state energy requirements for activities.

In developing the ACSM equations, an attempt was made to use a true physiological oxygen cost for each type of work. Each activity is broken down into the energy components. That is, in estimating the total oxygen cost of grade walking, add the net oxygen cost of the horizontal walk to the net oxygen cost of the vertical (grade) walk to the resting metabolic rate, which is taken to be 1 MET (3.5 ml · kg^{-1} · min^{-1}).

$$\text{Total } O_2 \text{ cost} = \text{net oxygen cost of activity} + 3.5 \text{ ml} \cdot \text{kg}^{-1} \cdot \text{min}^{-1}$$

Note that for the formulas to estimate the oxygen cost of the activity, the subject must follow instructions carefully (e.g., do not hold on to the treadmill railing; maintain the pedal cadence), and the work instruments (treadmill, cycle ergometer) must be calibrated so the settings are correct (see chapter 6).

ENERGY REQUIREMENTS OF WALKING, RUNNING, CYCLE ERGOMETRY, AND STEPPING

The following sections provide formulas to estimate the energy cost of walking, running, cycle ergometry, and stepping. These activities are common to cardiac rehabilitation and adult fitness programs. Examples are provided to show how the formulas are used in designing exercise programs.

Oxygen Cost of Walking

Formulas to determine the oxygen cost of walking differ depending on the walking speed and whether the walker is on a horizontal or a graded surface.

Walking on a Horizontal Surface

One of the most common activities used in an exercise program and in GXTs is walking. The following formula can be used to estimate the energy requirement between the walking speeds of 50 and 100 m · min^{-1}, or 1.9 to 3.7 mi · hr^{-1}. (Multiply miles per hour by 26.8 to obtain meters per minute. Divide meters per minute by 26.8 to obtain miles per hour.) The current edition of the ACSM Guidelines (3, p. 276) states that the formula can be used for speeds faster than 3.7 mi · hr^{-1} as long as the person is truly walking, not jogging or running. As you will see later in the chapter, such is not the case.

Dill (12) showed that the net cost of walking 1 m · min^{-1} on a horizontal surface is 0.100 to 0.106 ml · kg^{-1} · min^{-1}. A value of 0.1 ml · kg^{-1} · min^{-1} is used in the ACSM equations to simplify calculations without the loss of too much precision. The equation for calculating the oxygen cost (ml · kg^{-1} · min^{-1}) of walking on a flat surface is

$$\dot{V}O_2 = 0.1 \text{ ml} \cdot \text{kg}^{-1} \cdot \text{min}^{-1} \text{ (horizontal velocity)} + 3.5 \text{ ml} \cdot \text{kg}^{-1} \cdot \text{min}^{-1}.$$

QUESTION: What are the estimated steady-state $\dot{V}O_2$ and METs for a walking speed of 90 m · min^{-1} (3.4 mi · hr^{-1})?

Answer:

$$\dot{V}O_2 = 90 \text{ m} \cdot \text{min}^{-1} \cdot \frac{0.1 \text{ ml} \cdot \text{kg}^{-1} \cdot \text{min}^{-1}}{\text{m} \cdot \text{min}^{-1}} + 3.5 \text{ ml} \cdot \text{kg}^{-1} \cdot \text{min}^{-1}$$

$$\dot{V}O_2 = 9.0 \text{ ml} \cdot \text{kg}^{-1} \cdot \text{min}^{-1} + 3.5 \text{ ml} \cdot \text{kg}^{-1} \cdot \text{min}^{-1} = 12.5 \text{ ml} \cdot \text{kg}^{-1} \cdot \text{min}^{-1}$$

$$\text{METs} = 12.5 \text{ ml} \cdot \text{kg}^{-1} \cdot \text{min}^{-1} \div 3.5 \text{ ml} \cdot \text{kg}^{-1} \cdot \text{min}^{-1} = 3.6$$

The formulas can also be used to predict the level of activity required to elicit a specific energy expenditure.

QUESTION: An unfit participant is told to exercise at 11.5 ml · kg^{-1}·min^{-1} to achieve the proper exercise intensity. What walking speed would you recommend?

Answer:

$$11.5 \text{ ml} \cdot \text{kg}^{-1} \cdot \text{min}^{-1} = ? \text{ m} \cdot \text{min}^{-1} \cdot \frac{0.1 \text{ ml} \cdot \text{kg}^{-1} \cdot \text{min}^{-1}}{\text{m} \cdot \text{min}^{-1}} + 3.5 \text{ ml} \cdot \text{kg}^{-1} \cdot \text{min}^{-1}$$

Subtract the resting metabolic rate of 3.5 ml · kg^{-1} · min^{-1} from both sides of the equation. Subtracting 3.5 ml · kg^{-1} · min^{-1} from 11.5 ml · kg^{-1} · min^{-1} gives you the *net oxygen cost* of the activity (8.0 ml · kg^{-1} · min^{-1}).

$$8 \text{ ml} \cdot \text{kg}^{-1} \cdot \text{min}^{-1} = ? \text{ m} \cdot \text{min}^{-1} \cdot \frac{0.1 \text{ ml} \cdot \text{kg}^{-1} \cdot \text{min}^{-1}}{\text{m} \cdot \text{min}^{-1}}$$

The net cost is divided by 0.1 ml · kg^{-1} · min^{-1} per m · min^{-1} to yield 80 m · min^{-1} (3 mi · hr^{-1}). Divide both sides by 0.1 ml · kg^{-1} · min^{-1} / m · min^{-1}. Next, to obtain miles per hour, divide meters per minute by 26.8.

$$80 \text{ m} \cdot \text{min}^{-1} = 8 \text{ ml} \cdot \text{kg}^{-1} \cdot \text{min}^{-1} \div \frac{0.1 \text{ ml} \cdot \text{kg}^{-1} \cdot \text{min}^{-1}}{\text{m} \cdot \text{min}^{-1}}$$

$$3.0 \text{ mi} \cdot \text{hr}^{-1} = 80 \text{ m} \cdot \text{min}^{-1} \div \frac{26.8 \text{ m} \cdot \text{min}^{-1}}{\text{mi} \cdot \text{hr}^{-1}}$$

Walking Up a Grade

The oxygen cost of grade walking is the sum of the oxygen cost of horizontal walking, the oxygen cost of the vertical component, and the resting metabolic rate of 3.5 ml · kg^{-1} ·

min^{-1}. Studies have shown that the oxygen cost of moving (walking or stepping) 1 m · min^{-1} vertically is 1.8 ml · kg^{-1} · min^{-1} (7, 23). The vertical component (velocity) is calculated by multiplying the grade (expressed as a fraction) times the speed in meters per minute. A person walking at 80 m · min^{-1} on a 10% grade is walking 8 m·min^{-1} vertically (0.10 times 80 m · min^{-1}). The equation for calculating the oxygen cost (ml · kg^{-1} · min^{-1}) of walking on a grade is

$$\dot{V}O_2 = 0.1 \text{ ml} \cdot \text{kg}^{-1} \cdot \text{min}^{-1} \text{ (horizontal velocity)} + 1.8 \text{ ml} \cdot \text{kg}^{-1} \cdot \text{min}^{-1} \text{ (vertical velocity)} + 3.5 \text{ ml} \cdot \text{kg}^{-1} \cdot \text{min}^{-1}.$$

QUESTION: What is the total oxygen cost of walking 90 m · min^{-1} up a 12% grade?

Answer:

Horizontal component: Calculated as in preceding equation for walking on a horizontal surface and equals 9 ml · kg^{-1} · min^{-1}.

Vertical component:

$$\dot{V}O_2 = 0.12 \text{ (grade)} \cdot 90 \text{ m} \cdot \text{min}^{-1} \cdot \frac{1.8 \text{ ml} \cdot \text{kg}^{-1} \cdot \text{min}^{-1}}{\text{m} \cdot \text{min}^{-1}}$$
$$= 19.4 \text{ ml} \cdot \text{kg}^{-1} \cdot \text{min}^{-1}$$
$$\dot{V}O_2 \text{ (ml} \cdot \text{kg}^{-1} \cdot \text{min}^{-1}) = 9.0 \text{ (horizontal)} + 19.4 \text{ (vertical)} + 3.5 \text{ (rest)}$$
$$= 31.9 \text{ ml} \cdot \text{kg}^{-1} \cdot \text{min}^{-1}, \text{ or } 9.1 \text{ METs}$$

As indicated earlier, the formulas can be used to estimate the settings needed to elicit a specific oxygen uptake.

QUESTION: Set the treadmill grade to achieve an energy requirement of 6 METs (21.0 ml · kg^{-1} · min^{-1}) when walking at 60 m · min^{-1}.

Answer:

The net oxygen cost of the activity is equal to 21 minus 3.5 , or 17.5 ml · kg^{-1} · min^{-1}.

$$\text{Horizontal component} = 60 \text{ m} \cdot \text{min}^{-1} \cdot \frac{0.1 \text{ ml} \cdot \text{kg}^{-1} \cdot \text{min}^{-1}}{\text{m} \cdot \text{min}^{-1}}$$
$$= 6.0 \text{ ml} \cdot \text{kg}^{-1} \cdot \text{min}^{-1}$$
$$\text{Vertical component} = 17.5 - 6.0 = 11.5 \text{ ml} \cdot \text{kg}^{-1} \cdot \text{min}^{-1}$$
$$11.5 \text{ ml} \cdot \text{kg}^{-1} \cdot \text{min}^{-1} = \text{ fractional grade} \cdot 60 \text{ m} \cdot \text{min}^{-1} \cdot \frac{1.8 \text{ ml} \cdot \text{kg}^{-1} \cdot \text{min}^{-1}}{\text{m} \cdot \text{min}^{-1}}$$
$$11.5 \text{ ml} \cdot \text{kg}^{-1} \cdot \text{min}^{-1} = \text{ fractional grade} \cdot 108 \text{ ml} \cdot \text{kg}^{-1} \cdot \text{min}^{-1}$$
$$\text{Fractional grade} = 11.5 \div 108 = 0.106 \cdot 100\% = 10.6\% \text{ grade}$$

Walking at Different Speeds

The preceding formulas are useful within the range of walking speeds of 50 to 100 m · min^{-1} (1.9 to 3.7 mi · hr^{-1}); beyond that, the oxygen requirement for walking increases in a curvilinear manner (10). Because many people choose to walk at a fast speed rather than jog, knowledge of the energy requirements for walking at these higher speeds is useful in prescribing exercise. Values for the energy requirement for walking on the level and at various grades at these faster speeds (4.0 to 5.0 mi · hr^{-1}) are included in table 7.2.

One of the most common and useful ways the energy cost of walking can be expressed is in kilocalories per minute. In this way, the HFI can simply look up the speed of the walk in a table, identify the number of calories used per minute, and calculate the total energy

Table 7.2 Energy Requirement, in METs, for Walking at Various Speeds ($mi \cdot hr^{-1}$ or $m \cdot min^{-1}$) and Grades (%)

	Miles per hour/meters per minute						
% Grade	2.0/54	2.5/67	3.0/80	3.5/94	4.0/107	4.5/121	5.0/134
0	2.5	2.9	3.3	3.7	4.9	6.2	7.9
2	3.1	3.6	4.1	4.7	5.9	7.4	9.3
4	3.6	4.3	4.9	5.6	7.1	8.7	10.6
6	4.2	5.0	5.8	6.6	8.1	9.9	12.0
8	4.7	5.7	6.6	7.5	9.3	11.1	13.4
10	5.3	6.3	7.4	8.5	10.4	12.4	14.8
12	5.8	7.1	8.3	9.5	11.4	13.6	16.6
14	6.4	7.7	9.1	10.4	12.6	14.9	17.5
16	6.9	8.4	9.9	11.4	13.6	16.1	18.9
18	7.5	9.1	10.7	12.4	14.8	17.4	20.3
20	8.1	9.8	11.6	13.3	15.9	18.6	21.7
22	8.6	10.3	12.4	14.3	17.0	19.9	23.1
24	9.1	11.1	13.2	15.3	18.1	21.1	
26	9.7	11.9	14.0	16.2	19.2	22.3	
28	10.3	12.5	14.9	17.2	20.3	23.6	
30	10.8	13.2	15.7	18.2	21.4		

Note. Based on *ACSM's Guidelines for Exercise Testing and Prescription* (5th ed., 1995) (3) and W.J. Bubb, A.D. Martin, and E.T. Howley (1985) (10).

Table 7.3 Energy Costs of Walking ($kcal \cdot min^{-1}$)

Body weight		Miles per hour						
kg	lb	2.0	2.5	3.0	3.5	4.0	4.5	5.0
50.0	110	2.1	2.4	2.8	3.1	4.1	5.2	6.6
54.5	120	2.3	2.6	3.0	3.4	4.4	5.6	7.2
59.1	130	2.5	2.9	3.2	3.6	4.8	6.1	7.8
63.6	140	2.7	3.1	3.5	3.9	5.2	6.6	8.4
68.2	150	2.8	3.3	3.7	4.2	5.6	7.0	9.0
72.7	160	3.0	3.5	4.0	4.5	5.9	7.5	9.6
77.3	170	3.2	3.7	4.2	4.8	6.3	8.0	10.2
81.8	180	3.4	4.0	4.5	5.0	6.7	8.4	10.8
86.4	190	3.6	4.2	4.7	5.3	7.0	8.9	11.4
90.9	200	3.8	4.4	5.0	5.6	7.4	9.4	12.0
95.4	210	4.0	4.6	5.2	5.9	7.8	9.9	12.6
100.0	220	4.2	4.8	5.5	6.2	8.2	10.3	13.2

Note. Multiply value by the duration of the activity to obtain total calories expended.
Based on *ACSM's Guidelines for Exercise Testing and Prescription* (5th ed., 1995) (3) and W.J. Bubb, A.D. Martin, and E.T. Howley (1985) (10).

expenditure, depending on the duration of the walk. Table 7.3 presents the energy cost (in $kcal \cdot min^{-1}$) for walking at speeds of 2 to 5 $mi \cdot hr^{-1}$ and includes values for people of different body weights. It is no surprise that the energy cost of walking increases with the speed of the walk; however, the rate of increase is higher at the higher speeds. For example, when walking speed increases from 2 to 3 $mi \cdot hr^{-1}$ for a 170-lb participant, the energy cost increases from 3.2 to 4.2 $kcal \cdot min^{-1}$. But going from 4 to 5 $mi \cdot hr^{-1}$ requires an increase from 6.3 to 10.2 $kcal \cdot min^{-1}$. It is clear that the very sedentary individual can walk at slow speeds and achieve the desired exercise intensity, and the relatively fit individual can walk at high speeds at which the elevated energy requirement provides the necessary stimulus for a training effect. As a participant loses weight, the energy cost of walking at a certain speed decreases because the energy cost is dependent on body weight. One can compensate by walking for a longer period of time or for a greater distance.

Oxygen Cost of Jogging and Running

Jogging and running are common activities used in fitness programs for apparently healthy individuals. Using the ACSM equations it is possible to estimate the oxygen cost of these activities for a broad range of speeds, generally from 130 to 350 $m \cdot min^{-1}$. The equations are also useful at speeds below 130 $m \cdot min^{-1}$ as long as the person is really jogging. The fact that a person can walk or jog at speeds below 130 $m \cdot min^{-1}$ complicates the issue. The oxygen cost of walking is less than that of jogging at slow speeds; however, at approximately 135 to 140 $m \cdot min^{-1}$, the oxygen cost of jogging and walking are about the same. Above this speed the oxygen cost of walking exceeds that of jogging (5).

Jogging and Running on a Horizontal Surface

The net oxygen cost of jogging or running 1 $m \cdot min^{-1}$ on a horizontal surface is about twice that of walking, 0.2 $ml \cdot kg^{-1} \cdot min^{-1}$ per $m \cdot min^{-1}$ (6, 9, 19). Remember that the equation will, in general, yield a reasonable estimate of the oxygen cost of running for average individuals. However, it is well known that trained runners are more economical (in terms of energy expenditure) than the average person and also that running economy varies within any specific group, trained or untrained (9, 11, 21). The equation used to estimate the oxygen cost ($ml \cdot kg^{-1} \cdot min^{-1}$) of running is

$$\dot{V}O_2 = 0.2\ ml \cdot kg^{-1} \cdot min^{-1}\ (\text{horizontal velocity}) + 3.5\ ml \cdot kg^{-1} \cdot min^{-1}.$$

QUESTION: What is the oxygen requirement for running a 10K race on a track in 60 min?

Answer:

$$10\ 000\ m \div 60\ min = 167\ m \cdot min^{-1}$$

$$\dot{V}O_2 = 167\ m \cdot min^{-1} \cdot \frac{0.2\ ml \cdot kg^{-1} \cdot min^{-1}}{m \cdot min^{-1}} + 3.5\ ml \cdot kg^{-1} \cdot min^{-1}$$

$$\dot{V}O_2 = 36.9\ ml \cdot kg^{-1} \cdot min^{-1},\ \text{or } 10.5\ \text{METs}$$

QUESTION: A 20-year-old female distance runner with a $\dot{V}O_2max$ of 50 $ml \cdot kg^{-1} \cdot min^{-1}$ wants to run intervals at 90% of $\dot{V}O_2max$. At what speed should she run on a track given that one mile equals 1610m?

Answer:

90% of 50 = 45 $ml \cdot kg^{-1} \cdot min^{-1}$, and the net cost of the run is equal to 45 $ml \cdot kg^{-1} \cdot min^{-1}$ – 3.5 $ml \cdot kg^{-1} \cdot min^{-1}$, or 41.5 $ml \cdot kg^{-1} \cdot min^{-1}$.

$$41.5\ ml \cdot kg^{-1} \cdot min^{-1} \div \frac{0.2\ ml \cdot kg^{-1} \cdot min^{-1}}{m \cdot min^{-1}} = 207\ m \cdot min^{-1}$$

$$1610\ m \cdot min^{-1} \div 207\ m \cdot min^{-1} = 7.78\ min,\ \text{or 7:47 (min:s) mi pace}$$

Jogging and Running Up a Grade

There is not as much information about the oxygen cost of grade running as there is about the previous activities. But one thing is clear—the oxygen cost of running up a grade is about one half that of walking up a grade (8, 19). Some of the vertical lift associated with running on a flat surface is used to accomplish some grade work during inclined running, lowering the net oxygen requirement for the vertical work. The oxygen cost of running 1 m · min^{-1} vertically is about 0.9 ml · kg^{-1} · min^{-1}. As in grade walking, the vertical velocity is calculated by multiplying the fractional grade times the horizontal velocity. The following equation is used for calculating the oxygen cost of grade running.

$$\dot{V}O_2 = 0.2\ ml \cdot kg^{-1} \cdot min^{-1}\ (\text{horizontal velocity}) + 0.9\ ml \cdot kg^{-1} \cdot min^{-1}\ (\text{vertical velocity})\ +\ 3.5\ ml \cdot kg^{-1} \cdot min^{-1}$$

QUESTION: What is the oxygen cost of running 150 m · min^{-1} up a 10% grade?

Answer:

Horizontal component:

$$\dot{V}O_2 = 150\ m \cdot min^{-1} \cdot \frac{0.2\ ml \cdot kg^{-1} \cdot min^{-1}}{m \cdot min^{-1}} = 30\ ml \cdot kg^{-1} \cdot min^{-1}$$

Vertical component:

$$\dot{V}O_2 = 0.10\ (\text{fractional grade}) \cdot 150\ m \cdot min^{-1} \cdot \frac{0.9\ ml \cdot kg^{-1} \cdot min^{-1}}{m \cdot min^{-1}}$$

$$= 13.5\ ml \cdot kg^{-1} \cdot min^{-1}$$

$$\dot{V}O_2 = 30.0\ (\text{horizontal}) + 13.5\ (\text{vertical}) + 3.5\ (\text{rest}) = 47\ ml \cdot kg^{-1} \cdot min^{-1}$$

QUESTION: The oxygen cost of running 350 m · min^{-1} on a flat surface is about 73.5 ml · kg^{-1} · min^{-1}. What grade should be set on a treadmill for a speed of 300 m · min^{-1} to achieve the same $\dot{V}O_2$?

Answer:

Horizontal component:

$$\dot{V}O_2 = 300\ m \cdot min^{-1} \cdot \frac{0.2\ ml \cdot kg^{-1} \cdot min^{-1}}{m \cdot min^{-1}} = 60\ ml \cdot kg^{-1} \cdot min^{-1}$$

Vertical component:

$$\text{Net}\ \dot{V}O_2 = 73.5\ (\text{total}) - 60\ (\text{horizontal}) - 3.5\ (\text{rest}) = 10.0\ ml \cdot kg^{-1} \cdot min^{-1}$$

$$10\ ml \cdot kg^{-1} \cdot min^{-1} = \text{fractional grade} \cdot 300\ m \cdot min^{-1} \cdot \frac{0.9\ ml \cdot kg^{-1} \cdot min^{-1}}{m \cdot min^{-1}}$$

$$\text{Fractional grade} = 10\ ml \cdot kg^{-1} \cdot min^{-1} \div 270\ ml \cdot kg^{-1} \cdot min^{-1}$$

$$= .037\ \text{or}\ 3.7\%\ \text{grade}$$

Table 7.4 summarizes the values for oxygen cost of running on the level and up a grade.

Jogging and Running at Different Speeds

In contrast to walking, the energy cost of jogging and running increases in a linear and predictable manner with increasing speed. Table 7.5 shows the caloric cost of running, in kilocalories per minute, for participants of different body weights. If we consider the 170-lb participant, the energy cost increases from 7.2 to 11.2 kcal · min^{-1} when increasing speed from 3 to 5 mi · hr^{-1}; the increase is also 4 kcal · min^{-1} when increasing the speed from 7 to 9 mi · hr^{-1}. As with walking, the energy cost is higher for heavier individuals.

Table 7.4 Energy Requirement, in METs, for Jogging/Running at Various Speeds ($mi \cdot hr^{-1}$ or $m \cdot min^{-1}$) and Grades

	Miles per hour/meters per minute							
% Grade	3/80	4/107	5/134	6/161	7/188	8/215	9/241	10/268
0	5.6	7.1	8.7	10.2	11.7	13.3	14.8	16.3
1	5.8	7.4	9.0	10.6	12.2	13.8	15.4	17.0
2	6.0	7.7	9.3	11.0	12.7	14.4	16.0	17.7
3	6.2	7.9	9.7	11.4	13.2	14.9	16.6	18.4
4	6.4	8.2	10.0	11.9	13.7	15.5	17.3	19.1
5	6.6	8.5	10.4	12.3	14.2	16.1	17.9	19.8
6	6.8	8.8	10.7	12.7	14.6	16.6	18.5	20.4
7	7.0	9.0	11.0	13.1	15.1	17.1	19.1	21.1
8	7.2	9.3	11.4	13.5	15.6	17.7	19.7	21.8
9	7.4	9.6	11.7	13.9	16.1	18.3	20.3	22.5
10	7.6	9.9	12.1	14.3	16.6	18.8	21.0	23.2

Note. Based on equations published in *ACSM's Guidelines for Exercise Testing and Prescription* (5th ed.) 1995.

Table 7.5 Energy Costs of Jogging and Running ($kcal \cdot min^{-1}$)

Body weight		Miles per hour							
kg	lb	3.0	4.0	5.0	6.0	7.0	8.0	9.0	10.0
50.0	110	4.7	5.9	7.2	8.5	9.8	11.1	12.3	13.6
54.5	120	5.1	6.4	7.9	9.3	10.6	12.1	13.4	14.8
59.1	130	5.5	7.0	8.6	10.0	11.5	13.1	14.6	16.1
63.6	140	5.9	7.5	9.2	10.8	12.4	14.1	15.7	17.3
68.2	150	6.4	8.1	9.9	11.6	13.3	15.1	16.8	18.5
72.7	160	6.8	8.6	10.5	12.4	14.2	16.1	17.9	19.8
77.3	170	7.2	9.1	11.2	13.1	15.1	17.1	19.1	21.0
81.8	180	7.6	9.7	11.8	13.9	15.9	18.1	20.2	22.2
86.4	190	8.1	10.2	12.5	14.7	16.8	19.1	21.3	23.5
90.9	200	8.5	10.8	13.2	15.4	17.7	20.1	22.4	24.7
95.4	210	8.9	11.3	13.8	16.2	18.6	21.1	23.5	25.9
100.0	220	9.3	11.8	14.5	17.0	19.5	22.2	24.7	27.2

Note. Multipy value by the duration of the activity to obtain total calories expended.

Oxygen Cost of Walking and Running 1 Mile

In spite of the vast amount of information available regarding the costs of walking and running, a good deal of misunderstanding still exists. We hear claims that the energy cost of walking 1 mi is equal to that of running the same distance. In general, this is not the case (16). The formulas for estimating the energy cost of walking and running can be used to estimate the caloric cost of walking and running 1 mi, a piece of information that is useful in achieving energy expenditure goals.

If a person walks at 3 $mi \cdot hr^{-1}$ (80 $m \cdot min^{-1}$), 1 mi will be completed in 20 min. The caloric cost for walking 1 mi for a 70-kg person is

$$\dot{V}O_2 = 80\ m \cdot min^{-1} \cdot 0.1\ ml \cdot kg^{-1} \cdot min^{-1} + 3.5\ ml \cdot kg^{-1} \cdot min^{-1}$$

$$\dot{V}O_2 = 11.5\ ml \cdot kg^{-1} \cdot min^{-1}$$

$$\dot{V}O_2\ (ml \cdot mi^{-1}) = 11.5\ ml \cdot kg^{-1} \cdot min^{-1} \cdot 70\ kg \cdot 20\ min \cdot mi^{-1} = 16100\ ml \cdot mi^{-1}$$

$$\dot{V}O_2\ (L \cdot min^{-1}) = 16\ 100\ ml \cdot mi^{-1} \div 1000\ ml \cdot L^{-1} = 16.1\ L \cdot mi^{-1}.$$

At about 5.0 kcal per L O_2, the *gross caloric cost* per mi of walking is 80.5 kcal (5 kcal · 16.1 L · mi^{-1}). The *net caloric cost* for the mile walk can be calculated by subtracting the oxygen cost of 20 min of rest from the gross cost of the 3 mi · hr^{-1} walk. For example, 20 min of rest · 70 kg · (3.5 ml · kg^{-1} · min^{-1}) = 4900 ml, or 4.9 L. Using 5 kcal · L^{-1}, this equals 24.5 kcal for 20 min of rest. The net cost of the mile walk is 80.5 kcal – 24.5 kcal, or 56 kcal per mile.

If the same 70-kg individual ran the mile at 6 mi · hr^{-1} (161 m · min^{-1}), the oxygen cost could be calculated by the following method.

$$\dot{V}O_2 = 161\ \text{m} \cdot \text{min}^{-1} \cdot 0.2\ \text{ml} \cdot \text{kg}^{-1} \cdot \text{min}^{-1} + 3.5\ \text{ml} \cdot \text{kg}^{-1} \cdot \text{min}^{-1}$$

$$\dot{V}O_2 = 35.7\ \text{ml} \cdot \text{kg}^{-1} \cdot \text{min}^{-1}$$

$$\dot{V}O_2\ (\text{ml} \cdot \text{mi}^{-1}) = 35.7\ \text{ml} \cdot \text{kg}^{-1} \cdot \text{min}^{-1} \cdot 70\ \text{kg} \cdot 10\ \text{min} \cdot \text{mi}^{-1} = 25\ 000\ \text{ml} \cdot \text{mi}^{-1}$$

$$\dot{V}O_2\ (\text{L} \cdot \text{min}^{-1}) = 25\ 000\ \text{ml} \cdot \text{mi}^{-1} \div 1000\ \text{ml} \cdot \text{L}^{-1} = 25\ \text{L} \cdot \text{mi}^{-1}$$

At about 5 kcal per L O_2, 125 kcal are used to jog or run 1 mi (5 kcal · L^{-1} · 25 L · mi^{-1}). The gross caloric cost per mile is about 50% higher for jogging than for walking (125 vs. 80 kcal). The net caloric cost of jogging or running 1 mi (kcal used above resting), however, is relatively independent of speed and is about twice that of walking. For example, when we subtract the caloric cost for 10 min of rest (12 kcal) from the gross caloric cost of the run (125 kcal), the net cost is 113 kcal, or twice that for the walk (56 kcal). Table 7.6 lists values for the net and gross caloric costs of walking and running 1 mi for a variety of body weights, with the values expressed in kilocalories per mile.

For weight control it is important to use the net cost of the activity, as it measures the energy used over and above that of sitting around. When moving at slow to moderate speeds (2 to 3.5 mi · hr^{-1}), the net cost of walking a mile is about half that of jogging or running the mile. This means that a person who jogs a mile at 3 mi · hr^{-1} will be working at a higher metabolic rate than someone who walks at the same speed, and of course the heart rate response will be higher as well. Because many people walk at these slower speeds, it is important to remember that the net energy cost of the mile is half that of running. If we look at very high walking speeds (5 mi · hr^{-1}, or 1 mi in 12 min), however, we see that the net energy cost of walking 1 mi is only 10% less than that of running.

Table 7.6 shows that the net cost of running a mile is independent of speed. It does not matter whether participants jog at 3 mi · hr^{-1}—the net caloric cost is the same. At 6 mi · hr^{-1} the individual will be expending energy at about twice the rate measured at 3 mi · hr^{-1}; but because the mile is finished in half the time, the net energy expenditure is about the same. Heart rate will, of course, be higher in the 6 mi · hr^{-1} run in order to deliver the oxygen to the muscles at the higher rate.

In Review: The oxygen cost of walking increases linearly between the speeds of 50 and 100 m · min^{-1}; it increases faster at higher walking speeds. The oxygen cost of jogging or running increases linearly with speed from slow jogging (3 mi · hr^{-1}) to fast running. The net caloric cost of jogging or running a mile is twice that of walking a mile at a moderate pace.

Oxygen Cost of Cycle Ergometry

Cycle ergometry exercise is a popular exercise done at a sport club, at home, or as part of a rehabilitation program. Generally, energy expenditure is accomplished with less trauma to ankle, knee, and hip joints compared to jogging. Cycle ergometers are used for conventional leg-exercise programs, but they are also adapted for arm exercise (by placing the ergometer on a table). The following sections describe how to estimate the energy costs of doing leg and arm cycle ergometry.

Table 7.6 Gross and Net (Gross/Net) Cost in kcal · mi^{-1} for Walking and Running

Body weight		Walking						
		Miles per hour						
kg	lb	2.0	2.5	3.0	3.5	4.0	4.5	5.0
50.0	110	64/39	58/39	54/39	53/39	60/48	68/57	79/67
54.5	120	69/42	63/42	59/42	57/42	66/52	75/63	86/75
59.1	130	75/45	68/45	64/45	62/45	71/57	81/68	93/81
63.6	140	80/49	73/49	69/49	67/49	77/61	87/73	100/88
68.2	150	87/52	79/52	74/52	72/52	82/65	93/78	108/94
72.7	160	92/56	84/56	79/56	76/56	88/70	100/84	115/100
77.3	170	98/59	90/59	84/59	81/59	93/74	106/89	122/107
81.8	180	104/63	95/63	89/63	86/63	99/78	112/94	129/113
86.4	190	110/66	100/66	94/66	91/66	104/83	118/99	136/119
90.9	200	115/70	105/70	99/70	95/70	110/87	124/104	144/125
95.4	210	121/73	111/73	104/73	100/73	115/92	131/110	151/132
100.0	220	127/77	116/77	109/77	105/77	121/96	137/115	158/138

Body weight		Running							
		Miles per hour							
kg	lb	3.0	4.0	5.0	6.0	7.0	8.0	9.0	10.0
50.0	110	93/77	89/77	86/77	84/77	84/77	83/77	82/77	81/77
54.5	120	101/83	97/83	94/83	92/83	92/83	90/83	89/83	89/83
59.1	130	110/90	105/90	102/90	100/90	99/90	98/90	97/90	96/90
63.6	140	118/97	113/97	110/97	108/97	107/97	106/97	104/97	104/97
68.2	150	127/104	121/104	118/104	115/104	114/104	113/104	112/104	111/104
72.7	160	135/111	129/111	125/111	123/111	122/111	121/111	119/111	119/111
77.3	170	144/118	137/118	133/118	131/118	130/118	128/118	127/118	126/118
81.8	180	152/125	146/125	141/125	138/125	137/125	136/125	134/125	133/125
86.4	190	161/132	154/132	149/132	146/132	145/132	143/132	141/132	141/132
90.9	200	169/139	162/139	157/139	154/139	153/139	151/139	149/139	148/139
95.4	210	177/146	170/146	165/146	161/146	160/146	158/146	156/146	155/146
100.0	220	186/153	178/153	173/153	169/153	168/153	166/153	164/153	163/153

Note. Multiply value by the number of miles walked or run to obtain the total (gross/net) calories expended.

Leg Ergometry

In the previous activities the individual was carrying his or her body weight, and the oxygen requirement was therefore proportional to body weight (ml · kg^{-1} · min^{-1}). This is not the case in cycle ergometry, in which an individual's body weight is supported by the cycle seat and the work rate is determined *primarily* by the pedal rate and the resistance on the wheel. The oxygen requirement, in liters per minute, is *approximately* the same for people of different sizes for the same work rate. Thus, when a light person is doing the same work rate as a heavy person, the relative $\dot{V}O_2$ (ml · kg^{-1} · min^{-1}), or MET level, is higher for the lighter person.

The work rate is set on the simple, mechanically braked cycle ergometers by varying the force (weight, or load) on the wheel and the number of pedal revolutions per minute (rev · min^{-1}). On the Monark cycle ergometer the wheel travels 6 m per pedal revolution; on the Tunturi ergometer the wheel travels only 3 m per revolution. Using the Monark ergometer as an example, a pedal rate of 50 rev · min^{-1} causes the wheel to travel a distance of 300 m (6 m per pedal revolution times 50 rev · min^{-1}). If a 1-kp force (1-kg weight) were applied to the wheel, the work rate would be 300 kp meters per minute

(300 kpm · min^{-1}). Work rates are also expressed in watts (W), where 6.1 kpm · min^{-1} is equal to 1 W; the 300 kpm · min^{-1} work rate would be expressed as 50 W. The work rate can be doubled by changing the force from 1 kp to 2 kp or by changing the pedal rate from 50 to 100 rev · min^{-1}. In contrast, some cycle ergometers are electronically controlled to deliver a specific work rate somewhat independent of pedal rate; as the pedal rate falls, the load on the wheel is increased proportionally.

The oxygen cost of doing 1 kpm of work is approximately 1.8 ml. During cycle ergometer exercise, energy must also be expended to overcome the friction (unmeasured work) in the drive train of the cycle; this energy cost must be added to that required for the work rate that is set on the basis of pedal rate and force. This additional work requires about 10% of the oxygen required to do the measured work, so 0.2 ml · kpm^{-1} is added to the 1.8 ml · kpm^{-1} to get the net cost per kilopond meter of work on a cycle ergometer (2 ml · kpm^{-1}) (4). For the purposes of the ACSM formulas, the oxygen cost of sitting on the cycle ergometer is estimated to be 3.5 ml · kg^{-1} · min^{-1} (3). The estimates from the following equations are reasonable for work rates between approximately 150 and 1200 kpm · min^{-1} (see table 7.7).

$$\dot{V}O_2\ (\text{ml} \cdot \text{min}^{-1}) = \text{work rate (kpm} \cdot \text{min}^{-1})\ (2\ \text{ml}\ O_2 \cdot \text{kpm}^{-1}) + (3.5\ \text{ml} \cdot \text{kg}^{-1} \cdot \text{min}^{-1} \cdot \text{kg body weight})$$

$$\dot{V}O_2\ (\text{ml} \cdot \text{min}^{-1}) = \text{work rate (W)}\ (12\ \text{ml}\ O_2 \cdot \text{W}^{-1}) + (3.5\ \text{ml} \cdot \text{kg}^{-1} \cdot \text{min}^{-1} \cdot \text{kg body weight})$$

QUESTION: What is the oxygen cost of doing 600 kpm · min^{-1} (100 W) on a cycle ergometer for 50-kg and 100-kg subjects?

Answer:

$$\dot{V}O_2 = 600\ \text{kpm} \cdot \text{min}^{-1} \cdot 2\ \text{ml}\ O_2 \cdot \text{kpm}^{-1} + (3.5\ \text{ml} \cdot \text{kg}^{-1} \cdot \text{min}^{-1} \cdot \text{kg body weight})$$

For the 50-kg subject:

$$\dot{V}O_2 = 1200\ \text{ml} \cdot \text{min}^{-1} + (3.5\ \text{ml} \cdot \text{kg}^{-1} \cdot \text{min}^{-1} \cdot 50\ \text{kg})$$
$$= 1200\ \text{ml} \cdot \text{min}^{-1} + 175\ \text{ml} \cdot \text{min}^{-1} = 1375\ \text{ml} \cdot \text{min}^{-1}$$

Expressed per kilogram of body weight, the answer is 27.5 ml · kg^{-1} · min^{-1}, or 7.9 METs.

For the 100-kg subject:

$$\dot{V}O_2 = 1200\ \text{ml} \cdot \text{min}^{-1} + (3.5\ \text{ml} \cdot \text{kg}^{-1} \cdot \text{min}^{-1} \cdot 100\ \text{kg})$$
$$= 1200\ \text{ml} \cdot \text{min}^{-1} + 350\ \text{ml} \cdot \text{min}^{-1} = 1550\ \text{ml} \cdot \text{min}^{-1}$$

Expressed per kilogram of body weight, the answer is 15.5 ml · kg^{-1} · min^{-1}, or 4.4 METs.

Table 7.7 Energy Expenditure, in METs, for Cycle Ergometry for Legs and Arms

Body weight		Work rate (kpm · min^{-1}) and watts						
kg	lb	300/50	450/75	600/100	750/125	900/150	1050/175	1200/2000
50	110	4.4(6.1)	6.1(8.7)	7.9(11.3)	9.6(13.9)	11.3(–)	13.0(–)	14.7(–)
60	132	3.9(5.3)	5.3(7.4)	6.7(9.6)	8.1(11.7)	9.6(–)	11.0(–)	12.4(–)
70	154	3.4(4.7)	4.7(6.5)	5.9(8.3)	7.1(10.2)	8.3(12.0)	9.6(–)	10.8(–)
80	176	3.1(4.2)	4.2(5.8)	5.3(7.4)	6.4(9.0)	7.4(10.6)	8.5(12.3)	9.6(–)
90	198	2.9(3.9)	3.9(5.3)	4.8(6.7)	5.8(8.1)	6.7(9.6)	7.7(11.0)	8.6(12.4)
100	220	2.7(3.6)	3.6(4.9)	4.4(6.1)	5.3(7.4)	6.1(8.7)	7.0(10.0)	7.9(11.3)

Note. Values in ( ) are for arm work. Table is based on equations for estimating the oxygen cost of arm and leg work published in *ACSM's Guidelines for Exercise Testing and Prescription* (5th ed.) 1995.

As you can see, the oxygen cost of the work, expressed in $L \cdot min^{-1}$, is similar for people of different sizes (1.37 vs. 1.55 $L \cdot min^{-1}$), but relative cost is markedly different (7.9 vs. 4.4 METs).

In some exercise programs a participant might use a variety of pieces of exercise equipment to achieve a training effect and might like to be able to set about the same intensity on each. In this regard, the formula for the cycle ergometer can be used to set the load to achieve a particular MET value on the cycle ergometer and bring it in balance with what is done during walking or jogging.

QUESTION: A 70-kg participant must work at 6 METs to match the intensity of his walking program. What force (load) should be set on a Monark cycle ergometer at a pedal rate of 50 rev · min⁻¹?

Answer:

$$6 \text{ METs} = 6\ (3.5 \text{ ml} \cdot \text{kg}^{-1} \cdot \text{min}^{-1}) \cdot 70 \text{ kg} = 1470 \text{ ml} \cdot \text{min}^{-1}$$

$$1470 \text{ ml} \cdot \text{min}^{-1} = \text{kpm} \cdot \text{min}^{-1} \cdot 2 \text{ ml } O_2 \cdot \text{kpm}^{-1} + (3.5 \text{ ml} \cdot \text{kg}^{-1} \cdot \text{min}^{-1} \cdot 70 \text{ kg})$$

$$\text{Net cost of cycling} = 1470 - (70 \text{ kg} \cdot 3.5 \text{ ml} \cdot \text{kg}^{-1} \cdot \text{min}^{-1}) = 1225 \text{ ml} \cdot \text{min}^{-1}$$

$$1225 \text{ ml} \cdot \text{min}^{-1} = ?\ \text{kpm} \cdot \text{min}^{-1} \cdot 2 \text{ ml} \cdot \text{kpm}^{-1}$$

$$\text{Work rate } (\text{kpm} \cdot \text{min}^{-1}) = 1225 \div 2 = 612 \text{ kpm} \cdot \text{min}^{-1}$$

$$612 \text{ kpm} \cdot \text{min}^{-1} = (50 \text{ rev} \cdot \text{min}^{-1} \cdot 6 \text{ m} \cdot \text{rev}^{-1}) \cdot \text{force}$$

$$612 \text{ kpm} \cdot \text{min}^{-1} = 300 \text{ m} \cdot \text{min}^{-1} \cdot \text{force}$$

$$\text{Force} = 612 \text{ kpm} \cdot \text{min}^{-1} \div 300 \text{ m} \cdot \text{min}^{-1} = 2.04 \text{ or } 2.0 \text{ kp}$$

Arm Ergometry

A cycle ergometer can be used to exercise the arms and shoulder-girdle muscles by modifying the pedals and placing the cycle on a table. Arm ergometry is used on a limited basis as a GXT to evaluate cardiovascular function. It is used more generally as a routine exercise in rehabilitation programs (13).

There are a variety of factors to keep in mind when considering arm ergometry:

- Functional capacity ($\dot{V}O_2max$) for the arms is only 70% of that measured with the legs in a normal healthy population and less in an unfit, elderly, or diseased population.
- The natural endurance of the muscles used in this work is less than that of the legs.
- The heart rate (HR) and blood pressure (BP) responses are higher for arm work compared to leg work at the same $\dot{V}O_2$.
- The oxygen cost of doing 1 kpm of work is about 50% higher (3 ml $O_2 \cdot kpm^{-1}$) for arm work because of the action's inefficiency (3).

The formula for estimating the oxygen cost of arm work is

$$\dot{V}O_2 \ (\text{ml} \cdot \text{min}^{-1}) = \text{work rate } (\text{kpm} \cdot \text{min}^{-1}) \cdot 3 \text{ ml } O_2 \cdot \text{kpm}^{-1} + (3.5 \text{ ml} \cdot \text{kg}^{-1} \cdot \text{min}^{-1} \cdot \text{kg body weight}).$$

See table 7.7 for estimates of the oxygen cost of arm work on a cycle ergometer.

QUESTION: What is the oxygen requirement of doing 150 kpm · min⁻¹ on an arm ergometer for a 70-kg man?

Answer:

$$\dot{V}O_2 (\text{ml} \cdot \text{min}^{-1}) = 150 \text{ kpm} \cdot \text{min}^{-1} \cdot 3 \text{ ml } O_2 \cdot \text{kpm}^{-1} + (3.5 \text{ ml} \cdot \text{kg}^{-1} \cdot \text{min}^{-1} \cdot 70 \text{ kg})$$

$$= 695 \text{ ml} \cdot \text{min}^{-1}$$

In Review: The oxygen cost of cycle ergometry is primarily dependent on the work rate because body weight is supported. The net oxygen cost of leg ergometry is 2 ml · kpm^{-1} vs. 3 ml · kpm^{-1} for arm ergometry. Physiological responses (HR, BP) are exaggerated for arm work compared to leg work at the same work rate due to the fact that the oxygen cost is higher and represents a higher percentage of $\dot{V}O_2$max.

Oxygen Cost of Bench Stepping

One of the most useful and inexpensive forms of exercise is bench stepping. The activity is easily done at home and requires little or no equipment. The work rate is easily adjusted by simply increasing step height or cadence (number of lifts per minute).

The total oxygen cost of this exercise is the sum of the costs of (a) stepping up, (b) stepping down, and (c) moving back and forth on a level surface at the specified cadence. The oxygen cost of stepping up is 1.8 ml · kg^{-1} · min^{-1} per m · min^{-1}, as in walking (23). The oxygen cost of stepping down is a third of the cost of stepping up; therefore, the oxygen cost of stepping up and down is 1.33 times the cost of stepping up. The number of meters moved up or down per minute is calculated by multiplying the number of lifts per minute by the height of the step (e.g., if the step height is 0.2 m (20 cm) and the cadence is 27 steps · min^{-1}, then the total lift or descent per minute is 27 times 0.2 m, or 5.4 m · min^{-1}). To determine step height multiply inches by 2.54 to obtain centimeters, and divide centimeters by 100 to obtain meters.

The oxygen cost of stepping back and forth on a flat surface is proportional to the cadence (up, up, down, down). If the cadence is 15, the energy cost of moving back and forth at that rate is *about* 1.5 METs; if the cadence is 27, the energy requirement for moving back and forth on a flat surface is *about* 2.7 METs. In essence, the oxygen cost of stepping back and forth on a flat surface can be estimated in METs by dividing the step rate by 10. Because 1 MET is 3.5 ml · kg^{-1} · min^{-1}, the oxygen cost of stepping back and forth can be estimated as 0.35 times the step rate (step rate · 0.35 ml · kg^{-1} · min^{-1}). The formula for estimating the energy requirement for stepping is

$$\dot{V}O_2 = (\text{step height in meters})\ (\text{lifts} \cdot \text{min}^{-1})(1.33)(1.8\ \text{ml} \cdot \text{kg}^{-1} \cdot \text{min}^{-1}) + \text{step rate}\ (0.35\ \text{ml} \cdot \text{kg}^{-1} \cdot \text{min}^{-1}).$$

QUESTION: What is the oxygen requirement for stepping at a rate of 20 steps · min^{-1} on a 20-cm bench?

Answer:

$$\dot{V}O_2 = \frac{0.2\ \text{m}}{\text{lift}} \cdot \frac{20\ \text{lifts}}{\text{min}} \cdot 1.33 \cdot \frac{1.8\ \text{ml} \cdot \text{kg}^{-1} \cdot \text{min}^{-1}}{\text{m} \cdot \text{min}^{-1}} + 20\ (0.35\ \text{ml} \cdot \text{kg}^{-1} \cdot \text{min}^{-1})$$

$$= 9.6\ \text{ml} \cdot \text{kg}^{-1} \cdot \text{min}^{-1} + 7.0\ \text{ml} \cdot \text{kg}^{-1} \cdot \text{min}^{-1}$$

$$= 16.6\ \text{ml} \cdot \text{kg}^{-1} \cdot \text{min}^{-1}, \text{ or } 4.7\ \text{METs}$$

Table 7.8 presents a summary of the energy requirement of stepping at different rates.

In Review: The oxygen cost of bench stepping includes the cost of stepping up and down and moving horizontally back and forth. The oxygen cost of stepping up is the same as in walking. The oxygen cost of stepping down is 1.33 times the cost of stepping up. The oxygen cost of stepping back and forth is proportional to the cadence.

Table 7.8 Energy Expenditure in METs During Stepping at Different Rates on Steps of Different Heights

Step height		Steps per minute			
cm	in.	12	18	24	30
0	0	1.2	1.8	2.4	3.0
4	1.6	1.5	2.3	3.1	3.8
8	3.2	1.9	2.8	3.7	4.6
12	4.7	2.2	3.3	4.4	5.5
16	6.3	2.5	3.8	5.0	6.3
20	7.9	2.8	4.3	5.7	7.1
24	9.4	3.2	4.8	6.3	7.9
28	11.0	3.5	5.2	7.0	8.7
32	12.6	3.8	5.7	7.7	9.6
36	14.2	4.1	6.2	8.3	10.4
40	15.8	4.5	6.7	9.0	11.2

Reprinted from American College of Sports Medicine, 1980, *Guidelines for graded exercise testing and prescription*, 2nd ed. By permission of Lea & Febiger.

ENERGY REQUIREMENTS OF OTHER ACTIVITIES

Many activities are available to you when you are designing a fitness program (see chapter 17). These include exercising to music, rope skipping, swimming, and playing games. Not surprisingly, the energy expenditure associated with these activities is difficult to predict when compared to walking or running, in which the energy cost between people is similar because of the natural movements associated with those activities. In contrast, many activities have variable energy costs depending on the skill level of the participants and the motivation they bring to the activity. This will be clear in the following examples. Estimates of the energy requirements of some common aerobic activities are also presented.

Exercising to Music

Exercising to music is a fun alternative to walking and running. The energy requirement depends on whether the session is high or low impact; done at a low, medium, or high intensity; and done with or without hand weights (25). A person who is starting out might simply walk through the movements, whereas an experienced person might go through the full range of motion with each step. Thus the energy costs of this activity vary considerably. Values might range from as low as 4 METs for someone walking through the routine to 10 METs for the experienced participant working at a high intensity in either a low- or high-impact session (25). Remember that this activity often involves small-muscle groups and includes some static (stabilizing) muscle contractions; as a result, HR response is higher for the same oxygen uptake measured in walking and running. Table 7.9 summarizes the caloric expenditure associated with exercise to music when done at low, moderate, and high intensities.

Rope Skipping

In walking and running, the energy requirement is proportional to the rate at which the person moves. But the energy requirement for rope skipping at only 60 to 80 turns per

Table 7.9 Gross Energy Cost of Exercise to Music (kcal · min⁻¹)

Body weight kg	Body weight lb	Low intensity	Moderate intensity	High intensity
50.0	110	3.3	5.8	8.3
54.5	120	3.6	6.4	9.1
59.1	130	3.9	6.9	9.8
63.6	140	4.2	7.4	10.6
68.2	150	4.5	7.9	11.3
72.7	160	4.8	8.5	12.1
77.3	170	5.1	9.0	12.8
81.8	180	5.4	9.5	13.6
86.4	190	5.7	10.1	14.3
90.9	200	6.0	10.6	15.1
95.4	210	6.3	11.1	15.9
100.0	220	6.6	11.7	16.7

Note. Multiply value by the duration of the aerobic phase of the exercise-to-music class to obtain total calories expended.

Table 7.10 Gross Energy Cost of Rope Skipping (kcal · min⁻¹)

Body weight kg	Body weight lb	Slow skipping	Fast skipping
50.0	110	7.5	9.2
54.5	120	8.2	10.0
59.1	130	8.9	10.9
63.6	140	9.5	11.7
68.2	150	10.2	12.5
72.7	160	10.9	13.4
77.3	170	11.6	14.2
81.8	180	12.3	15.0
86.4	190	13.0	15.9
90.9	200	13.6	16.7
95.4	210	14.3	17.5
100.0	220	15.0	18.4

Note. Multiply value by the duration of the rope-skipping session to obtain total calories expended.

minute (about as slow as the rope can be turned) is about 9 METs. At 120 turns per minute the energy cost increases to only 11 METs (17). Consequently, rope skipping is not a graded activity as are walking and running. Secondly, the HR response is higher than expected from the oxygen cost of the activity. This, again, may be because a small-muscle mass (lower leg) is the primary muscle group involved in the activity. In spite of this, rope skipping can be included as an effective part of a fitness program when done intermittently using target heart rate (THR) as the guide (see chapter 14). Rope skipping should not be used, however, in the early part of a fitness program because the energy cost and loading on ankle, knee, and hip joints are relatively high. Table 7.10 presents a summary of the energy costs of skipping rope at two speeds.

Swimming

Swimming is a preferred activity for many people because of the dynamic, large-muscle nature of the task and because little joint trauma is associated with it. The limitation is in finding a convenient facility that allows lap swimming and, of course, having enough skill to do the activity. The energy requirement depends on the velocity of movement and the stroke being used, but it is also influenced by the skill of the swimmer. A skilled swimmer requires less energy to move through the water, so the skilled swimmer has to swim a greater distance than an unskilled person to achieve the same caloric expenditure.

The energy cost of simply treading water can be as high as 1.5 L · min^{-1} (7.5 kcal · min^{-1}). Elite swimmers use this same number of kilocalories per minute to swim at 36 m · min^{-1}, whereas an unskilled swimmer might require twice that to maintain the same velocity. For elite swimmers, the front and back crawl are the most efficient and the butterfly is the least efficient. The net caloric cost per mile of swimming has been estimated to be more than 400 kcal, or about 4 times that of running 1 mi and about 8 times that of walking 1 mi. However, the actual caloric cost per mile of swimming varies greatly, depending on skill and gender. Table 7.11 is a summary of the values presented by Holmer (15) for men and women.

Table 7.11 Caloric Cost Per Mile ($kcal \cdot mi^{-1}$) of Swimming the Front Crawl

Skill level	Women	Men
Competitive	180	280
Skilled	260	360
Average	300	440
Unskilled	360	560
Poor	440	720

Note. Adapted from "Physiology of Swimming Man" by I. Holmer. In *Exercise and Sport Sciences Review*, 7, by R.S. Hutton and D.I. Miller (Eds.), 1970. (15).

The HR response measured during swimming at a specific $\dot{V}O_2$ is lower than that measured during running at the same $\dot{V}O_2$. In fact, the maximal HR response is about 14 beats $\cdot$ min^{-1} lower for swimming (see chapter 17). With this in mind, the THR range should be decreased when prescribing swimming activities.

Estimation of Energy Expenditure Without Formulas

Appendix C contains a tabular summary of the energy requirements for a wide variety of physical activities, including exercises, sports, occupations, and home-related tasks (1). This is helpful in estimating the total daily energy expenditure of an individual. There is an easy way, however, to estimate the energy costs of an exercise session without using formulas.

The HFI selects activities that cause the fitness participant to exercise in the range of 60% to 80% of his or her $\dot{V}O_2max$, the intensity needed to improve or maintain cardiorespiratory fitness. It should therefore be possible to estimate the energy expenditure for each individual on the basis of the subject's $\dot{V}O_2max$ and the portion of the THR range at which the person is working. If a person has a $\dot{V}O_2max$ of 10 METs, energy expenditure can be estimated in the following way. Ten METs is equivalent to about 10 $kcal \cdot kg^{-1} \cdot hr^{-1}$. If a person is working at the bottom portion of the target heart rate range, at about 60% $\dot{V}O_2max$, then the energy expenditure should be about 6 METs (60% of 10 METs). If the person weighs 70 kg, then 420 kcal are expended per hour (70 kg $\cdot$ 6 $kcal \cdot kg^{-1} \cdot hr^{-1}$). A 30-min workout would require half this, or about 210 kcal. These simple calculations assume that the person is performing a large-muscle activity. Table 7.12 shows the estimated kcal expenditure for a 30-min workout at 70% $\dot{V}O_2max$ for a variety of fitness levels ($\dot{V}O_2max$ expressed as METs) and body weights (24).

Environmental Concerns

Although changes in temperature, relative humidity, pollution, and altitude do not change the energy requirements for submaximal exercise, they do change the participant's response to the exercise bout. Remember that a person's HR response is the best indicator of the relative stress being experienced due to the interaction of exercise intensity, duration, and environmental factors. The participant should be instructed to cut back on the intensity of the activity when environmental factors increase the HR response. The duration of the activity can be increased to accommodate any energy expenditure goal.

Table 7.12 Estimated Energy Expenditure for a 30-Min Workout at 70% Functional Capacity for People of Various Fitness Levels ($\dot{V}O_2$max) and Body Weights

$\dot{V}O_2$max (METs) ($kcal \cdot kg^{-1} \cdot hr^{-1}$)	70% max METs ($kcal \cdot kg^{-1} \cdot hr^{-1}$)	kcal/30 min		
		50 kg/110 lb	70 kg/154 lb	90 kg/198 lb
20	14.0	350	490	630
18	12.6	315	441	567
16	11.2	280	392	504
14	9.8	245	343	441
12	8.4	210	294	378
10	7.0	175	245	315
8	5.6	140	196	252
6	4.2	105	147	189

6 **In Review: The energy cost of exercise to music varies from 4 to 10 METs, depending on effort and whether the exercise is high or low impact. Rope skipping requires about 10 METs, while the oxygen cost of swimming is inversely related to skill. Energy expenditure can be estimated without formulas. If a person is working at 60% of $\dot{V}O_2$max and has a $\dot{V}O_2$max of 10 METs, the person is expending energy at 6 METs, or 6 $kcal \cdot kg^{-1} \cdot hr^{-1}$. If the person weighs 80 kg, 480 kcal are expended per hour. Environmental factors such as heat, humidity, altitude, and pollution can increase the heart rate response to work while not affecting the energy cost very much. Heart rate should be monitored more frequently in these settings to adjust the intensity of the activity downward to keep the person in the appropriate heart rate range.**

CASE STUDIES

You can check your answers by referring to appendix A.

7.1

A 75-kg man walks at 3.5 $mi \cdot hr^{-1}$ for 30 min. How many calories does he expend?

7.2

A 60-kg woman rides a cycle ergometer at a work rate of 100 W. What is her oxygen uptake?

7.3

A 70-kg college student runs 3 mi in 24 min. How many calories did he expend?

7.4

An 85-kg man with a functional capacity of 12 METs worked at 70% of his capacity for 30 min. How many calories did he expend?

7.5

A client has read that he can expend the same number of calories per mile, whether he walks it at 3 $mi \cdot hr^{-1}$ or jogs it at 6 $mi \cdot hr^{-1}$. How would you respond?

SOURCE LIST

1. Ainsworth et al. (1993)
2. American College of Sports Medicine (ACSM) (1980)
3. ACSM (1995)
4. Åstrand (n.d.)
5. Åstrand & Rodahl (1986)
6. Balke (1963)
7. Balke & Ware (1959)
8. Bassett, Giess, Nagle, Ward, Raab, and Balke (1985)
9. Bransford & Howley (1977)
10. Bubb, Martin, & Howley (1985)
11. Daniels (1985)
12. Dill (1965)
13. Franklin (1985)
14. Haskell, Savin, Oldridge, & DeBusk (1982)
15. Holmer (1979)
16. Howley & Glover (1974)
17. Howley & Martin (1978)
18. Knoebel (1984)
19. Margaria, Cerretelli, Aghemo, & Sassi (1963)
20. Montoye, Ayen, Nagle, & Howley (1986)
21. Morgan et al. (1995)
22. Nagle, Balke, Baptista, Alleyia, & Howley (1971)
23. Nagle, Balke, & Naughton (1965)
24. Sharkey (1990)
25. Williford, Scharff-Olson, & Blessing (1989)

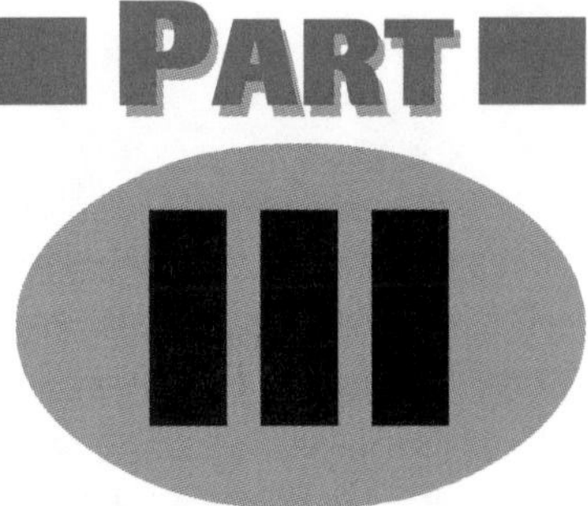

Part III

Nutrition, Body Composition, and Weight Management

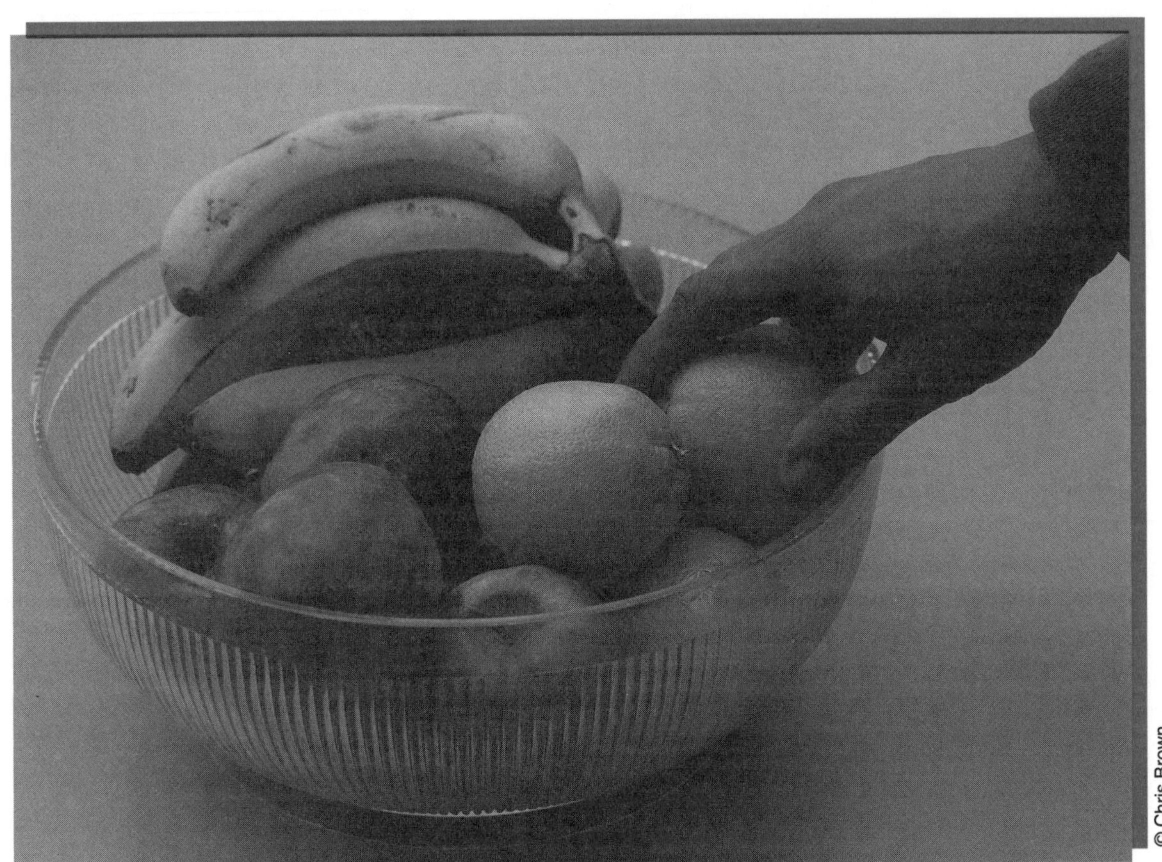

Part III summarizes the basic elements of nutrition, body composition, and weight management. Chapter 8 describes elements of nutrition related to health, blood lipids, and activity. Chapter 9 describes the methods available for assessing the different aspects of body composition. Chapter 10 discusses the importance of a healthy body weight and ways to utilize behavior in nutrition and exercise to achieve it.

CHAPTER

8

Nutrition

Dixie Thompson

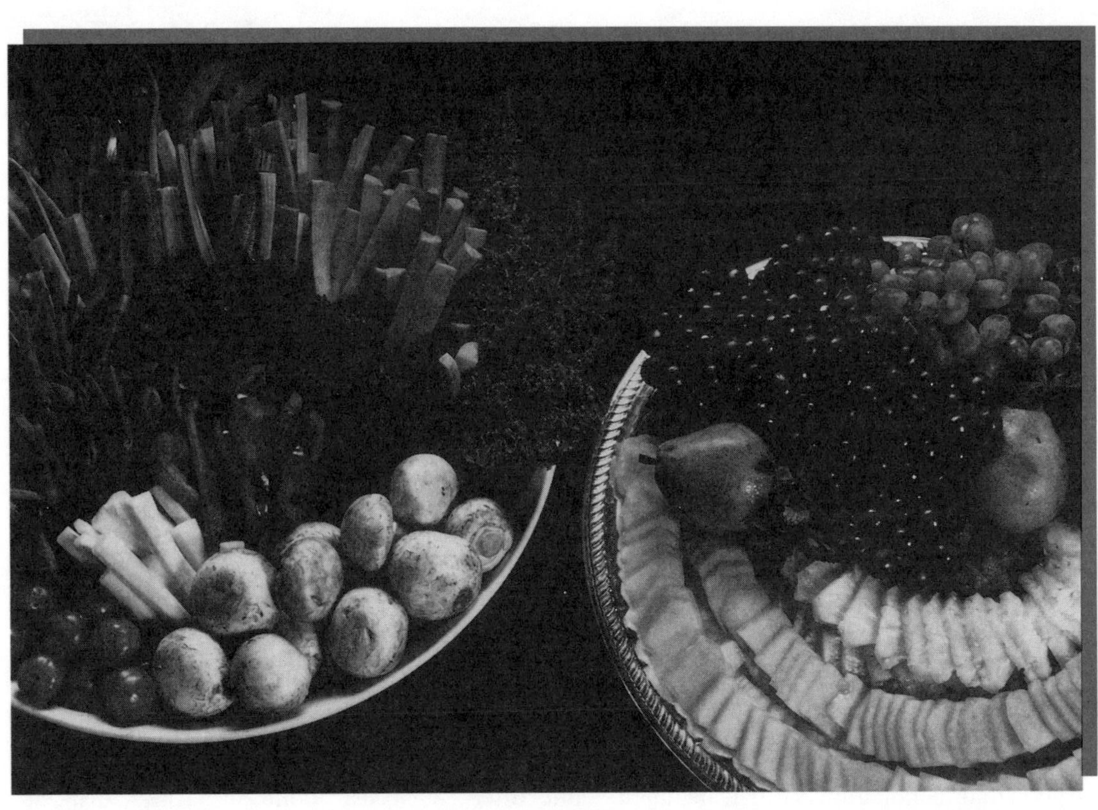

OBJECTIVES

The reader will be able to:

1. **List the six essential nutrients, describing their role in the proper functioning of the body, and list the recommended percentages of calories from fats, proteins, and carbohydrates.**
2. **Discuss appropriate assessment of dietary intake.**
3. **Describe the role of the USDA Food Guide Pyramid and the U.S. Dietary Guidelines in making healthy nutritional choices.**
4. **Explain the relationship between the blood lipid profile and cardiovascular disease and the role of diet and exercise in modifying blood lipids.**
5. **Describe appropriate methods for maintaining hydration during exercise.**
6. **Discuss the protein, vitamin, and mineral needs of a physically active person.**
7. **Describe an appropriate means for maximizing glycogen storage prior to competition.**
8. **List the three components of the female athlete triad.**

Good nutrition results from a diet in which foods are eaten in the proper quantities and with the needed distribution of nutrients to maintain good health in the present and in the future. **Malnutrition,** on the other hand, is the outcome of a diet in which there is an underconsumption, overconsumption, or unbalanced consumption of nutrients that leads to disease or an increased susceptibility to disease. Implicit in the above definitions is the fact that proper nutrition is essential to good health. A history of poor nutritional choices will eventually lead to health consequences. As will become apparent during this chapter, poor nutritional choices have been linked to chronic conditions including cardiovascular disease and cancer.

The public is bombarded with messages about nutrition, and it is often difficult for the layperson to distinguish good information from bad. The health fitness instructor (HFI) can play an important role in conveying basic nutritional information. It should be emphasized, however, that a registered dietitian is the appropriate health care professional to handle the nutritional counseling of individuals with special needs.

SIX CLASSES OF ESSENTIAL NUTRIENTS

There are many substances necessary for the proper functioning of the body. **Nutrients** are substances that the body requires for the maintenance of health, growth, and repair of tissues. Nutrients can be divided into six classes: carbohydrates, fats, proteins, vitamins, minerals, and water (17).

Carbohydrates

Carbohydrates are nutrients composed of carbon, hydrogen, and oxygen and are essential sources of energy in the body. Carbohydrates can be subdivided into three categories: monosaccharides, disaccharides, and polysaccharides (17). The monosaccharides and disaccharides are sometimes called simple sugars. Simple sugars provide a significant contribution to the caloric content of foods such as fruit juices, soft drinks, and candy. The most important simple sugar in the human body is **glucose**. The molecular formula for glucose is $C_6H_{12}O_6$. The polysaccharides are commonly referred to as complex carbohydrates or starches. These substances are formed by combining simple sugars. Rice, pasta, and whole grain breads are just a few examples of foods which are high in complex carbohydrates. When carbohydrates are stored in the human body, glucose molecules are joined together to form large molecules called **glycogen**. Glycogen is stored primarily in the liver and skeletal muscle.

Grains, vegetables, and fruits are excellent sources of carbohydrates. It is recommended that at least 55% to 60% of the total number of calories consumed come from carbohydrates (13) (figure 8.1). It is further recommended that 10% or less of the total calories consumed come from simple sugars. The reason for eating more complex rather than simple carbohydrates is the higher **nutrient density** in complex carbohydrates. Nutrient density refers to amount of essential nutrients in a food in comparison to the calories it contains. For example, a candy bar (simple sugars) has a low nutrient density whereas a slice of whole grain bread (complex sugars) contains a high nutrient density.

One of the benefits of consuming many foods that are high in complex carbohydrates is that they also typically contain **dietary fiber**. Dietary fiber is a term used when referring to substances found in plants that cannot be broken down by the human digestive system. Although fiber cannot be digested, it is important in helping to avoid cancers of the digestive system, hemorrhoids, constipation, and diverticular disease because it helps food move quickly and easily through the digestive system. It is recommended that people consume 20 to 35 g of fiber per day (13). Excellent sources of dietary fiber are grains, vegetables, legumes, and fruit.

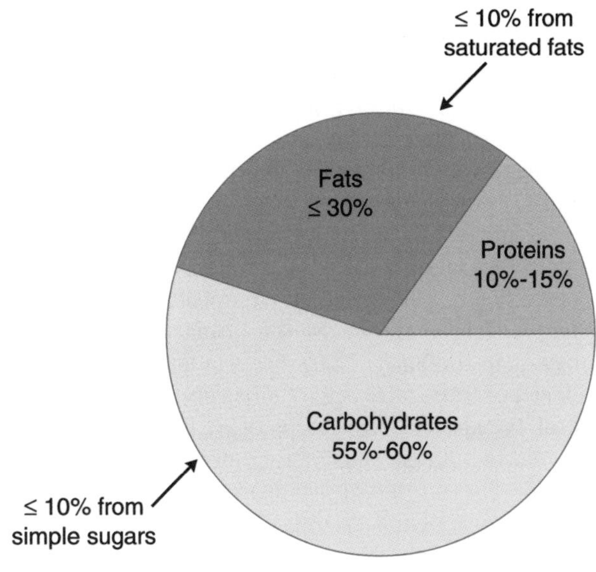

FIGURE 8.1 Recommended intake of carbohydrates, fats, and proteins.

As mentioned earlier, carbohydrates are a vital source of energy in the human body. During high-intensity exercise, carbohydrates are the primary fuel source for ATP production. When carbohydrates are broken down in the human body, they yield approximately 4 kcal of energy per gram. This relationship can also be viewed from the food intake perspective. For example, a person who eats 10 g of carbohydrate will have approximately 40 kcal of energy to use or store.

good nutrition — A diet in which foods are eaten in the proper quantities and with the needed distribution of nutrients to maintain good health in the present and in the future.

malnutrition — A diet in which there is an underconsumption, overconsumption, or unbalanced consumption of nutrients that leads to disease or an increased susceptibility to disease.

nutrient — A substance that the body requires for the maintenance of health, growth, and repair of tissues.

carbohydrate — An essential nutrient composed of carbon, hydrogen, and oxygen that is an essential energy source for the body.

glucose — A simple sugar that is a vital energy source in the human body.

glycogen — The storage form of carbohydrates in the human body.

nutrient density — The amount of essential nutrients in a food in comparison to the calories it contains.

dietary fiber — Substances found in plants that cannot be broken down by the human digestive system.

Fats

Fats are an essential part of a healthy diet and serve vital functions in the human body. Among the functions performed by fats are temperature regulation, protection of vital organs, distribution of some vitamins, energy production, and formation of component parts of cell membranes (17). Like carbohydrates, fats are composed of carbon, hydrogen, and oxygen; however, their chemical structure is different. **Triglycerides** are the primary storage form of fats in the body. These large molecules are composed of three fatty acid chains connected to a glycerol backbone. The majority of triglycerides are stored in adipose cells (sometimes referred to as fat cells). The aerobic metabolism of triglycerides provides most of the energy needed during rest and low-intensity exercise. When metabolized, 1 g of fat yields 9 kcal of energy. **Phospholipids** are another type of fat found in the body. As the name implies, these fats have phosphate groups attached to them. Phospholipids are important constituents of cell membranes. Cholesterol is a sterol (a fatty substance in which the carbon, hydrogen, and oxygen atoms are arranged in rings). In addition to the cholesterol we consume in our diet, the body constantly produces cholesterol, which is used in forming cell membranes and making steroidal hormones. Meat and eggs are the major sources of cholesterol in the typical American diet; however, it is recommended that people consume no more than 300 mg of cholesterol per day (19). **Lipoproteins** are large molecules that allow fats to travel through the bloodstream. The impact that these substances have on health is discussed later in the chapter.

Both animals and plants provide sources of fat. *Saturated fats* come primarily from animal sources and are typically solid at room temperature. Plant sources of saturated fats are palm oil, coconut oil, and cocoa butter. The chemical structure of saturated fats contains no double bonds between carbon atoms; in other words, the fat is "saturated" with hydrogen atoms. A high intake of saturated fat is directly related to increased cardiovascular disease. *Unsaturated fats* contain fewer hydrogen atoms because some double bonding between carbon atoms exists. These fats are typically liquid at room temperature. Corn, peanut, canola, and soybean oil are sources of unsaturated fats. It is recommended that no more than 30% of one's diet be composed of fats (figure 8.1). Ten percent or less of the total calories should come from saturated fats. One way to reduce saturated fat intake would be to substitute margarine for butter. Although both items have similar total fat content, over 60% of the butter's fat is saturated while approximately only 20% of margarine's fat is saturated.

Proteins

Proteins are substances composed of carbon, hydrogen, oxygen, and nitrogen. All proteins are made by combining **amino acids**. Amino acids are molecules composed of an amino group (NH_3), a carboxyl group (COO), a hydrogen atom, a central carbon atom, and a side chain. The body requires 20 amino acids; it is the difference in the side chains that gives unique characteristics to each amino acid (17). Amino acids can combine in innumerable ways to form proteins, and it is estimated that tens of thousands of different types of proteins exist in the body. It is the ordering of the amino acids that provides the unique structure and function of proteins. The unique chemical properties and structures of proteins allow them to serve many different functions in the body. Some of the most common functions are listed below:

- Carries oxygen (hemoglobin)
- Fights disease (antibodies)
- Catalyzes reactions (enzymes)
- Essential to movement (actin, myosin, and troponin)
- Acts as a connective tissue (collagen)
- Clots blood (prothrombin)
- Acts as a messenger (protein hormones such as growth hormone)

Of the 20 amino acids found in the body, most can be constructed from other substances in the body; however, there are eight **essential amino acids** that should be a part of one's regular diet. Eating a variety of protein-containing foods is typically adequate to meet this need. There are proteins in both meat products and plant products. Animal sources of protein such as meat, milk, and eggs contain the eight essential amino acids. Plant sources of protein such as beans, starchy vegetables, nuts, and grains do not always contain all eight essential amino acids. Because of this, vegetarians must consume a variety of protein-containing foods (17).

It is recommended that proteins make up 10% to 15% of one's daily calories (figure 8.1). This will ensure adequate protein for the growth, maintenance, and repair of cells. The protein requirement for adults is generally met by consuming 0.8 g of protein for each kilogram of body weight (14). As discussed later in this chapter, individuals who are training intensely may have higher protein requirements. In addition, children have higher protein needs in order to support their continually growing bodies. The recommended protein intake is approximately 2 g/kg for infants, 1.2 g/kg for 1- to 3-year-olds, 1.1 g/kg for 4- to 6-year-olds, 1 g/kg for 7- to 14-year-olds, and 0.9 g/kg for 15- to 18-year-old boys (14).

In addition to the functions of proteins listed above, these molecules can be metabolized for energy production. It is estimated that 5% to 15% of the energy needs during exercise come from the breakdown of proteins. The breakdown of 1 g of protein yields approximately 4 kcal of energy to be used by the body.

Vitamins

Vitamins are organic substances that are essential to the normal functioning of the human body. Although vitamins do not contain energy to be used by the body, these substances are essential in the metabolism of fats, carbohydrates, and proteins. The 13 vitamins are needed for numerous processes including blood clotting, protein synthesis, and bone formation. Because of the critical role vitamins play, it is necessary that they exist in proper quantities in the body. The major functions, important dietary sources, and the daily requirements of vitamins are listed in table 8.1. There are two major classifications of vitamins: fat-soluble and water-soluble (17).

The chemical structure of *fat-soluble vitamins* causes them to be transported and stored with lipids. The four fat-soluble vitamins are A, D, E, and K. Because these vitamins are stored in the body with fats, it is not necessary to continually ingest large amounts of them; however, a small intake of each is recommended on a daily basis.

The B vitamins and vitamin C are *water-soluble vitamins*. Water-soluble vitamins are not stored in large quantities and therefore must be consumed daily. Deficiencies related to water-soluble vitamins such as scurvy (vitamin C deficiency) and beriberi (thiamin deficiency) may appear in a rather short period of time. Overconsumption of either fat-soluble or water-soluble vitamins can lead to toxic effects; however, because fat-soluble vitamins are stored in the body, the potential for overdose with these substances is greater (17).

Antioxidant vitamins have received a great deal of media attention in the past few years. These substances are hypothesized to counteract the effects of aging and decrease the likelihood of developing cardiovascular disease and cancer. It is thought that antioxidants neutralize free radicals that are formed during metabolic processes. **Beta-carotene** (a precursor of vitamin A), vitamin C, and vitamin E are highly touted antioxidant substances. Several large epidemiological studies are currently underway that may help us understand more about the protective function of these substances. Because of the potential for toxic effects when an overdose of antioxidants occurs, it is wise to follow the recommended intake of these substances. Even though antioxidants may prove to be a factor in reducing chronic diseases, "antioxidant supplementation is not a substitute for tobacco cessation, a prudent diet, and regular exercise" (11, p. 245).

fats— Non-water-soluble substances composed of hydrogen, oxygen, and carbon that serve a variety of functions in the body including energy production.

triglycerides— The primary storage form of fat in the human body.

phospholipids— Fatty compounds that are essential constituents of cell membranes.

lipoproteins — Large molecules responsible for transporting fats in the blood.

proteins— Nutrients composed of amino acids that serve a variety of functions in the human body.

amino acids— Nitrogen-containing building blocks for proteins; can be used for energy.

essential amino acids — The eight amino acids that the body cannot synthesize and therefore must be ingested.

vitamins — Organic substances essential to the normal functioning of the human body. They may be subdivided into fat-soluble and water-soluble categories.

antioxidant vitamins— Substances that attach to harmful metabolic products (free radicals). Antioxidants are touted to be effective in decreasing the risk for developing cardiovascular disease and cancer.

beta-carotene— A precursor of vitamin A thought to be an important antioxidant vitamin.

Table 8.1 Vitamins and Their Functions

Vitamin	Function	Sources	Daily adult requirement[a] Men	Women
Thiamin (B-1)	Functions as part of a coenzyme to aid utilization of energy	Whole grains, nuts, lean pork	1.5 mg[b]	1.1 mg
Riboflavin (B-2)	Involved in energy metabolism as part of a coenzyme	Milk, yogurt, cheese	1.7 mg	1.3 mg
Niacin	Facilitates energy production in cells	Lean meat, fish, poultry, grains	19.0 mg	15.0 mg
Vitamin B-6	Absorbs and metabolizes protein; aids in red blood cell formation	Lean meat, vegetables, whole grains	2.0 mg	1.6 mg
Pantothenic acid	Aids in metabolism of carbohydrate, fat, and protein	Whole-grain cereals, bread, dark green vegetables	4-7 mg	4-7 mg
Folic acid	Functions as coenzyme in synthesis of nucleic acids and protein	Green vegetables, beans, whole-wheat products	200 μg	180 μg
Vitamin B-12	Involved in synthesis of nucleic acids, red blood cell formation	Only in animal foods, not plant foods	2 μg	2 μg
Biotin	Coenzyme in synthesis of fatty acids and glycogen formation	Egg yolk, dark green vegetables	30-100 μg	30-100 μg
C	Intracellular maintenance of bone, capillaries, and teeth	Citrus fruits, green peppers, tomatoes	60 mg	60 mg
A	Functions in visual processes; formation and maintenance of skin and mucous membranes	Carrots, sweet potatoes, margarine, butter, liver	1000 μg	800 μg[c]
D	Aids in growth and formation of bones and teeth; promotes calcium absorption	Eggs, tuna, liver, fortified milk	5 μg	5 μg
E	Protects polyunsaturated fats; prevents cell membrane damage	Vegetable oils, whole-grain cereal and bread, green leafy vegetables	10 mg	8 mg
K	Important in blood clotting	Green leafy vegetables, peas, potatoes	80 μg	65μg

Note. [a]Values are for adults 25 to 50 years of age. The requirements vary for children and pregnant or lactating women. See appendix D.
[b]mg = milligram, μg = microgram, IU = international unit.
[c]μg vitamin A requirements are expressed in microgram of Retinol equivalents.
Reprinted from Franks and Howley 1989.

Minerals

Minerals are inorganic molecules that serve a variety of functions in the human body. The minerals that appear in the largest quantities (calcium, phosphorus, potassium, sulfur, sodium, chloride, and magnesium) are often called macrominerals. Other minerals are also essential to normal functioning of the body, but because they exist in smaller quantities, they are called microminerals. The functions, dietary sources, and daily requirements of minerals are listed in table 8.2.

A mineral that is often consumed in inadequate amounts by Americans is calcium. Calcium is a mineral important in the mineralization of bone, muscle contraction, and transmission of nervous impulses. **Osteoporosis** is a disease characterized by a decrease in the total amount of bone mineral in the body and by a decrease in strength of the remaining bone. This condition is most common in the elderly but

Table 8.2 Minerals and Their Functions

Mineral	Function	Sources	Daily adult requirement[a] Men	Women
		Major minerals		
Calcium	Bones, teeth, blood clotting, nerve and muscle function	Milk, sardines, dark green vegetables, nuts	800 mg	800 mg
Chloride	Nerve and muscle function, water balance (with sodium)	Table salt	750 mg	750 mg[c]
Magnesium	Bone growth; nerve, muscle, and enzyme function	Nuts, seafood, whole grains, leafy green vegetables	350 mg	280 mg
Phosphorus	Bone, teeth, energy transfer	Meats, poultry, seafood, eggs, milk, beans	800 mg	800 mg
Potassium	Nerve and muscle function	Fresh vegetables, bananas, citrus fruits, milk, meats, fish	2000 mg	2000 mg[c]
Sodium	Nerve and muscle function, water balance	Table salt	500 mg	500 mg[c]
		Trace minerals		
Chromium	Glucose metabolism	Meats, liver, whole grains, dried beans	.05-.2 mg	.05-.2 mg
Copper	Enzyme function, energy production	Meats, seafood, nuts, grains	1.5-3 mg	1.5-3 mg
Fluoride	Bone and teeth growth	Drinking water, fish, milk	1.5-4 mg	1.5-4 mg
Iodine	Thyroid hormone formation	Iodized salt, seafood	150 μg	150 μg
Iron	O_2 transport in red blood cells; enzyme function	Red meat, liver, eggs, beans, leafy vegetables, shellfish	10 mg	15 mg
Manganese	Enzyme function	Whole grains, nuts, fruits, vegetables	2.5-5 mg	2.5-5 mg
Molybdenum	Energy metabolism in cells	Whole grains, organ meats, peas, beans	.075-.25 mg	.075-.25 mg
Selenium	Works with vitamin E	Meat, fish, whole grains, eggs	70 μg	55 μg
Zinc	Part of enzymes, growth	Meat, shellfish, yeast, whole grains	15 mg	12 mg

Note. [a]Values are for adults 25 to 50 years of age. Requirements vary for children and pregnant or lactating women. See appendix D.
[b]mg = milligram, μg = microgram
[c]Minimum requirements for healthy people. See appendix D.
Reprinted from Franks and Howley 1989.

may also exist in younger people who have diets inadequate in calcium or vitamin D, or both. It is estimated that in the United States osteoporosis results in 1.5 million fractures per year with resultant health care costs of more that $10 billion (12). Maximal bone density is achieved during the early adult years after which bone density declines in everyone. Those who achieve the highest bone density

minerals — Inorganic molecules that serve a variety of functions in the human body.

osteoporosis — A disease characterized by a decrease in the total amount of bone mineral and a decrease in the strength of the remaining bone.

Table 8.3 NIH Guidelines for Calcium Intake

Age	Recommended intake (mg/day)
0-6 months	400
6-12 months	600
1-5 years	800
6-10 years	800-1200
11-24 years	1200-1500
Women 25-50 years	1000
Pregnant or lactating women	1200-1500
Postmenopausal on estrogen	1000
Postmenopausal w/o estrogen	1500
Men 25-65 years	1000
All people > 65 years	1500
Up to 2000 mg/day appears safe in most individuals.	

Note. Data from *NIH Consensus Statement on Optimal Calcium Intake*, June 1994.

and maintain adequate intakes of calcium and vitamin D are most protected from the ravages of this disease. In 1994, the National Institutes of Health released recommendations for calcium intake for Americans of all ages (table 8.3). Milk, dark green vegetables, and nuts are excellent sources of calcium. For example, a 30-year-old male should consume 1000 mg of calcium daily. One cup (8 oz) of 1% milk has approximately 300 mg of calcium, which would be almost one third of this daily recommendation.

Iron is another mineral that is often underconsumed by Americans. This is especially true of women. The oxygen-carrying properties of hemoglobin depend on the presence of iron. **Anemia** is a condition characterized by a decreased capacity to transport oxygen in the blood. Red blood cells are produced continually. Although much of the iron needed for hemoglobin production comes from the breakdown of old red blood cells, it is recommended that iron be consumed daily. The recommended intake of iron for males and postmenopausal women is 10 mg per day (14). For females during the childbearing years, the recommended intake is 15 mg per day (14). Red meat and eggs are excellent sources of iron. Additionally, spinach, lima and navy beans, and prune juice are excellent vegetarian sources of iron. The consumption of vitamin C with meals increases the body's ability to absorb iron.

Sodium, on the other hand, is a mineral that many Americans *overconsume*. High sodium intake has been linked with hypertension. It is suggested that adults limit their sodium intake to no more than 2400 mg per day (13). People can substantially reduce their sodium intake by limiting consumption of processed foods and decreasing the amount of salt added to foods when cooking.

Water

Water is considered an essential nutrient because of its vital role in the normal functioning of the body. Water contributes approximately 60% of the total body weight and is essential in creating the environment in which all metabolic processes occur. Water is necessary to regulate temperature and transport substances throughout the body.

It is recommended that each day a person should ingest 1 to 1.5 ml of water for each kcal expended (14). For most adults, drinking approximately 2.5 L (10 glasses) of water each day will fulfill this requirement. As discussed later in this chapter, this need is higher for individuals exercising intensely. Water is consumed in both food and beverages. It is suggested that individuals limit their intake of caffeinated beverages because of the diuretic effects of these products.

1 **In Review: The six classes of nutrients are carbohydrates, fats, proteins, vitamins, minerals, and water. The metabolism of 1 g of carbohydrate yields 4 kcal of energy. Carbohydrates should contribute at least 55% to 60% of one's daily calories and no more than 10% of one's calories should come from simple sugars. Cholesterol intake should be limited to 300 mg per day. The breakdown of 1 g of fat yields 9 kcal of energy. Proteins are made of amino acids and serve numerous functions. To ensure that all needed amino acids are available in adequate amounts, people should eat a variety of protein-containing foods each day. The breakdown of 1 g of protein yields 4 kcal of energy. No more than 30% of one's daily calories should come from fats. No more than 10% of one's daily calories should come from saturated fats. Vitamins,**

minerals, and water do not provide energy, but they are essential in many other ways to the healthy functioning of the body. Ingesting more than the Recommended Dietary Allowance for antioxidants does not appear necessary. In general, Americans would benefit from limiting sodium consumption (to decrease blood pressure), increasing calcium intake (to improve bone strength), and increasing iron ingestion (to prevent anemia).

ASSESSING DIETARY INTAKE

Examining a person's dietary habits allows the HFI to make suggestions about how to better meet nutritional and weight loss/weight maintenance goals. This information is most often gathered through the use of a food log in which the client records everything that is consumed. These records are typically kept for 3 or 7 days. A 1-day food log may not provide enough information to develop a profile of a person's nutritional habits. Because of the time and effort required to record food intake, many people prefer 3-day rather than 7-day food logs. If a 3-day food record is kept, it is important that one of the days be a weekend day because many people eat differently on weekends than they do on weekdays (10). Once the records are compiled, there are a number of software packages that can provide an analysis of the diet. Although food logs provide important information, there are problems with this practice (20):

- People tend to underreport what they eat.
- People do not keep records specific enough to provide quality information.
- People often temporarily change how they eat when they are required to record their food intake.

There are steps that the HFI can take to minimize these problems. First, make sure that the client understands the importance of completely and honestly recording what is eaten. Emphasize to the client that the accuracy and usefulness of the feedback is dependent on the information he or she provides and that the client is not going to be criticized or judged for what he or she has eaten. The HFI should provide the client with models or descriptions of portion sizes. Examples can be found in the United States Department of Agriculture's (USDA) Information Bulletin, No. 364. Explicit instructions about how to complete the food record should be given to the client. Additionally, the food log should be user-friendly and include cues to elicit complete responses. A sample food log and instructions are provided on form 8.1.

As indicated earlier, the HFI can provide general nutrition information to the public. Clients with special metabolic needs such as diabetes mellitus should be referred to a registered dietitian. Explaining to a client how closely her or his nutritional profile matches the Recommended Dietary Allowances (see appendix D) is particularly informative. For the typical client, there are special areas of emphasis that should be provided with a nutritional profile:

- Total calories
- Percentage of calories from fats, carbohydrates, and protein
- Amount of saturated fat and cholesterol
- Sodium intake
- Iron intake
- Calcium intake
- Fiber

It is also important to examine the food log for emotional and/or social cues to eating behaviors. For example, some people eat when depressed or only eat when alone. This type of information can be quite helpful in making behavior changes needed for weight loss and weight maintenance.

2 **In Review: Food logs can be used to assess dietary practices. Detailed information must be provided by the client in order for the dietary assessment to be accurate.**

RECOMMENDATIONS FOR DIETARY INTAKE

Many different plans have been suggested to guide food intake. The USDA has suggested using the

anemia — A condition characterized by a decreased ability to transport oxygen in the blood.

FORM 8.1

Sample Food Log

Instructions

1. Record everything you eat. This should include foods and beverages eaten at meals and snacks.
2. Record carefully how the food was prepared. Be as descriptive as possible (e.g., fried in corn oil, broiled in 1 T of margarine).
3. Be sure to indicate the amount of food eaten. Use typical household measures when possible (t = teaspoon; T = tablespoon; c = cup; oz = ounce).
4. Provide brand names and labels for packaged foods.
5. For composite foods such as sandwiches, casseroles, and soups, indicate the ingredients contained in the food. For example, a turkey sandwich might be described as 2 slices of whole wheat bread, 1 oz of baked turkey breast without skin, 1 slice of tomato, 2 leaves of iceberg lettuce, 1 T light mayonnaise.
6. Indicate where and with whom you were when you ate. Also describe your feelings at the time—were you worried, content, lonely, stressed? (Be honest with yourself.)
7. Carry this form with you so that you can write down foods as they are eaten. Do not wait until the end of the day to record your food intake.

Food/drink	**Description** (e.g., amount, cooking method, brand name)	**Location** (e.g., place, people, alone)	**Feelings** (e.g., hunger, anger, joy)	**Time**

Food Guide Pyramid as a guide to eating (18). The Food Guide Pyramid is reproduced in figure 8.2, along with a quantification of serving sizes. This plan separates foods into six categories:

- Bread, cereal, rice, and pasta group (6 to 11 servings)
- Fruit group (2 to 4 servings)
- Vegetable group (3 to 5 servings)
- Milk, yogurt, and cheese group (2 to 3 servings)
- Meat, poultry, fish, dry beans, eggs, and nuts group (2 to 3 servings)
- Fats, oils, and sweets (use sparingly)

This helpful guide to eating provides a suggested number of servings for each group. It is important to note that there is a recommended range of servings for each group. The low end of the range should be used by a person who is smaller or less active, and a person who is very active or large should consume the higher number of servings. In addition to using the Food Guide Pyramid to guide nutritional choices, the USDA makes other general nutritional recommendations:

- Eat a variety of foods.
- Balance the food you eat with physical activity.
- Maintain or improve your weight.
- Choose a diet with plenty of grain products, vegetables, and fruits.
- Choose a diet low in fat, saturated fat, and cholesterol.
- Choose a diet moderate in sugars.
- Choose a diet moderate in salt and sodium.
- If you drink alcoholic beverages, do so in moderation.

The entire USDA Dietary Guidelines for Americans (19) can be accessed via the Internet at <http://www.usda.gov/fcs/cnpp.htm>.

The above guidelines can be used in an attempt to meet the **Recommended Dietary Allowances (RDAs)** (14). These guidelines, developed by the National Research Council of the National Academy of Sciences, suggest levels that appear to be adequate to meet the nutritional needs of practically all healthy people. The RDAs were determined by estimating the average need for the nutrient and then increasing the value. Ultimately, these recommendations are adequate for more than 97% of the population. The recommendations are divided into age and gender categories to allow more specificity. For nutrients about which less is known, an estimated safe and effective range of intakes is suggested. The RDAs for vitamins and minerals are given in appendix D. It can be assumed that, if a person regularly meets the RDAs, her or his intake of nutrients is adequate for good health.

The Food and Drug Administration publishes recommended **Daily Values (DV)** to be used in food labeling. The DVs were developed in an attempt to inform the public about the nutritional content of the foods they buy. All foods must have labeling containing information about the total calories, fat (including saturated fat), cholesterol, sodium, carbohydrates (including dietary fiber), protein, and various vitamins and minerals. The nutritional labels also contain the percentage of the recommended DVs provided by the food. For example, the suggested DV for cholesterol is 300 mg; therefore, if a food contains 15 mg of cholesterol, it will constitute 5% of the recommended daily intake of cholesterol. A more complete description of DVs can be found in nutrition textbooks such as Sizer and Whitney's *Nutrition: Concepts and Controversies* (17).

3 **In Review: The Food Guide Pyramid provides information about the amount and types of food that should be consumed daily. The RDAs provide specific information about needed nutrient intake. Daily Values allow consumers to evaluate the nutritional content of foods.**

DIET, EXERCISE, AND THE BLOOD LIPID PROFILE

Cardiovascular disease is the leading cause of death in the United States. One of the primary risk factors

Food Guide Pyramid — A system designed by the United States Department of Agriculture for making healthy food choices. It divides foods into six different categories and recommends daily servings from each.

Recommended Dietary Allowances (RDAs) — The recommended daily intake of nutrients. These values published by the National Research Council are thought to be adequate for good nutrition in the majority of healthy people.

Daily Values (DVs) — Amount of nutrients recommended by the Food and Drug Administration to be consumed each day. Daily Values are used in food labeling.

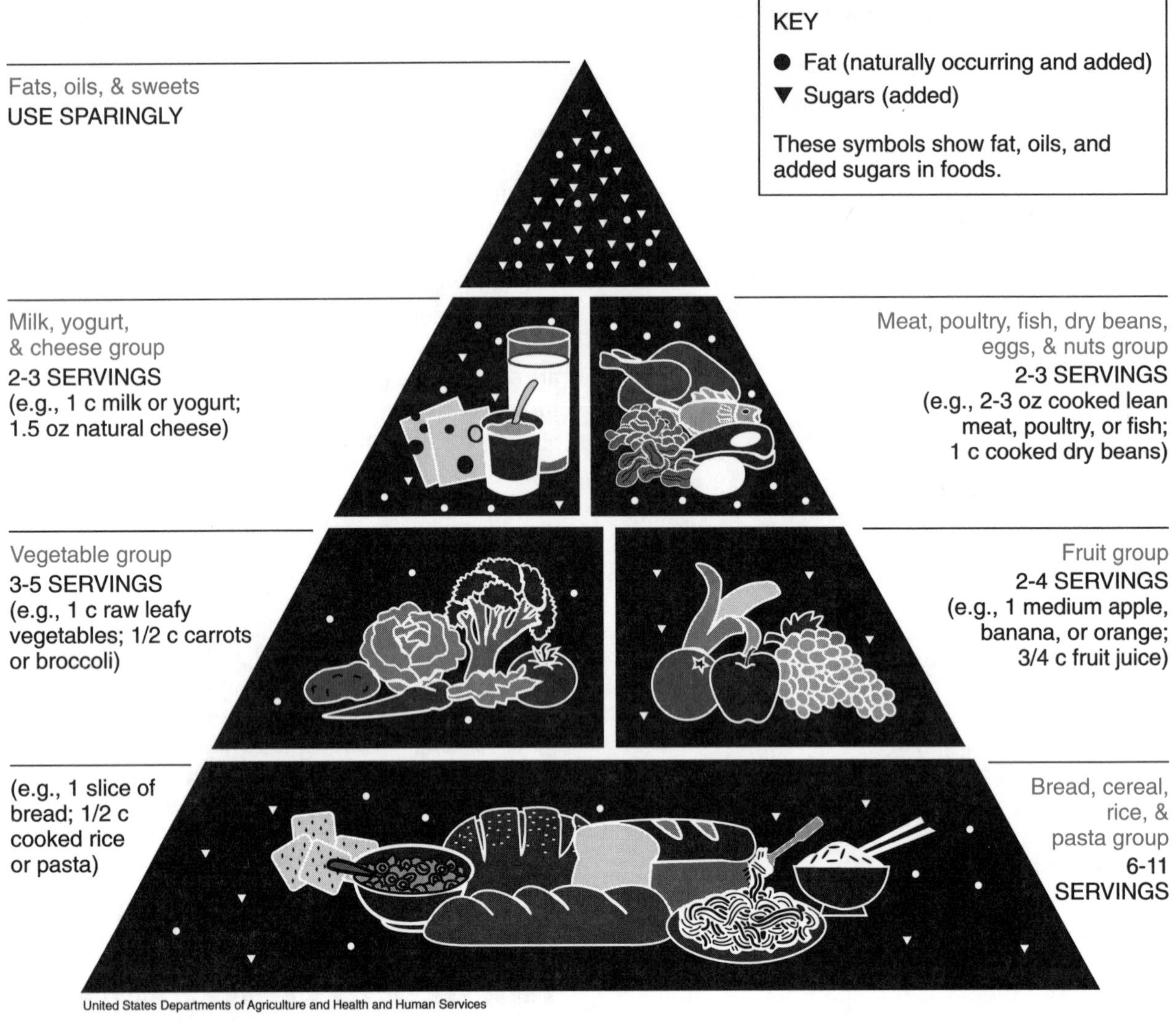

FIGURE 8.2 The Food Guide Pyramid.

for development of cardiovascular disease is a poor blood lipid profile. Both diet and exercise can have positive effects on this very important risk factor.

Lipoproteins and Risk of Cardiovascular Disease

Because lipids are hydrophobic (i.e., not water soluble) they need to bind with some other substance in order to be transported in the blood. Lipoproteins are macromolecules composed of cholesterol, triglycerides, protein, and phospholipids. Classifications for these molecules are based on their size and makeup. The two classes of lipoproteins most closely linked with cardiovascular disease are low-density lipoproteins (LDL) and high-density lipoproteins (HDL). LDL transports cholesterol and triglycerides from the liver to be used in various cellular processes. HDL retrieves cholesterol from the body's cells and returns it to the liver to be metabolized.

Elevated levels of total cholesterol (the sum of all forms of cholesterol) and low-density lipoprotein cholesterol (LDL-C) are linked with the development of atherosclerotic plaque in the arteries. Increased levels of high-density lipoprotein cholesterol (HDL-C) help prevent the atherosclerotic process. It is also apparent that the ratios of LDL-C to HDL-C and of total cholesterol to HDL-C are very important in assessing one's risk of developing cardiovascular disease. According to the National Cholesterol Education Program (NCEP) guidelines, total cholesterol levels below 200 mg/dl and LDL-C values below 130 mg/dl are desirable (8). Total cholesterol above 240 mg/dl and LDL-C above 160 mg/dl are considered high and are associated with greater risk of cardiovascular disease (8) (see table 8.4). In addition HDL-C below 35 mg/dl is considered too low and HDL-C 60 mg/dl or higher is considered ideal (8). A total cholesterol to HDL-C ratio less than 5 for men and 4.5 for women is preferred to keep risk of developing cardiovascular disease at low to moderate levels (4).

Table 8.4 Recommended Levels of Total Cholesterol (TC) and Low-Density Lipoprotein Cholesterol (LDL-C)

Category	TC	LDL-C
Desirable	< 200 mg/dl	< 130 mg/dl
Borderline high	200-239 mg/dl	130-159 mg/dl
High	≥ 240 mg/dl	≥ 160 mg/dl

Effects of Diet and Exercise on the Blood Lipid Profile

Consuming a diet low in saturated fat and cholesterol, losing weight, and participating in regular aerobic exercise have all been linked to positive changes in the blood lipid profile. The Step I Diet recommended by the NCEP (8) includes the following dietary practices to improve the blood lipid profile:

- Limiting total fat intake to no more than 30% of calories
- Limiting saturated fat intake to 8% to 10% of calories
- Limiting cholesterol intake to 300 mg/day

The Step II Diet recommended by the NCEP calls for an additional reduction in saturated fat intake (< 7% of total calories) and cholesterol (< 200 mg/day) if no success is seen with the Step I Diet (8).

People who engage in regular aerobic exercise typically have a better blood lipid profile than their sedentary counterparts. It is difficult to ascertain which of these changes are due to the exercise and which are related to a healthy body weight. It appears that the primary blood lipid changes due to aerobic exercise are increases in HDL-C and decreases in blood levels of triglycerides (7). Weight loss has been linked with lower total cholesterol, LDL-C, and triglycerides as well as higher HDL-C.

In Review: Elevated total cholesterol and LDL-C and depressed HDL-C are risk factors for development of cardiovascular disease. Aerobic exercise, weight loss, and low intake of saturated fat and cholesterol are effective means of improving the blood lipid profile.

NUTRITION FOR PHYSICALLY ACTIVE INDIVIDUALS

As discussed previously, nutrition plays an important role in health. Proper nutrition is also essential for optimal performance during physical activity. The American Dietetic Association (ADA) and the Canadian Dietetic Association (CDA) released a position statement in 1993 that addresses the needs of physically active adults (3). The HFI should be familiar with these guidelines in order to provide basic nutritional advice to clients who exercise on a regular basis.

Hydration Before, During, and After Exercise

Sweating is the body's primary mechanism for heat dissipation during exercise. The amount of sweat lost during exercise depends on the environmental heat and humidity, the type and intensity of exercise, and individual characteristics. Dehydration reduces the body's capacity for sweating and can impair performance by decreasing strength, endurance, and coordination. In addition, dehydration increases the risk of heat cramps, heat exhaustion, and heat stroke (see chapter 21).

The ADA (3) and ACSM (2) recommend that a person consume approximately 2 c (500 ml) of water 2 hr prior to beginning exercise and then drink an additional 2 c within 15 min of beginning an endurance exercise bout. Fluid replacement during exercise is essential in activities that last an hour or longer especially if they take place in hot, humid environments. During exercise, one should drink approximately 150 ml of water every 15 min. Water that is slightly chilled (5-10 °C) is absorbed most readily (3).

In activities where large amounts of sweat are lost, it is important that the fluid is fully replaced. Weighing prior to and after these types of activities is recommended. One should drink approximately 16 oz (475 ml) of water for each pound of weight lost. If on subsequent days the weight has not returned to normal, additional water should be consumed prior to beginning exercise (3).

> **5 In Review: Adequate hydration is essential to performance. Water should be consumed before, during, and after extended bouts of exercise.**

Protein Intake for Athletes

It has been reported that athletes who are training intensely may benefit from increasing their protein intake above the level recommended for a sedentary person. The ADA recommends that a person who is training intensely consume 1 to 1.5 g of protein per kilogram of body weight (3). This is slightly higher than the typical 0.8 g/kg recommended for adults (14). The additional protein requirements should be met through food choices, not supplements. The ADA states that "excessive protein intake, either through consumption of high-protein foods or protein/amino acid supplements, is unnecessary, does not contribute to athletic performance or increase muscle mass, and actually may be detrimental to health and athletic performance" (3). It should also be noted that because of a higher caloric intake, the normal diet of most athletes contains adequate amounts of protein so that additional increases in protein intake are rarely necessary (6).

Ergogenic Aids

The search for nutritional and/or pharmacological agents that improve performance has led to the marketing of numerous products touted as **ergogenic aids**. Some of these products (e.g., bee pollen, brewer's yeast) provide no physiological advantage. Other products such as caffeine may improve performance in some instances (1) and have been regulated by various sporting agencies such as the International Olympic Committee. Some "ergogenic aids" must be strictly avoided, such as anabolic-adrogenic steroids, due to severe and sometimes fatal side-effects (16).

Vitamins and minerals are often consumed by athletes in amounts higher than the RDA in an attempt to improve performance. There is no evidence that this costly practice enhances performance; however, if an athlete's diet provides inadequate amounts of any nutrient, health and performance could suffer. The two minerals that often need to be increased in the diet are iron and calcium (5). For athletes with anemia, increased iron consumption is advised. For female athletes with menstrual cycle irregularities, calcium supplementation is often prescribed.

> **6 In Review: The typical protein RDA for adults of 0.8 g/kg appears inadequate for athletes. People who are training intensely should consume 1 to 1.5 g of protein per kilogram of body weight. Ergogenic aids are pharmacological or nutritional agents thought to improve athletic performance. Although a few of these products may enhance performance, there are medical and ethical reasons for avoiding their use. Extra vitamins and minerals (i.e., above the RDAs) do not improve performance.**

Carbohydrate Loading and Intake During Exercise

Adequate intake of carbohydrates is necessary for optimal athletic performance. Glucose is the major source of energy during exercise; when blood glucose levels decline, the ability to continue exercise is limited. A physically active person should routinely consume a diet in which 60% to 65% of the calories are carbohydrates. For an athlete who trains heavily on consecutive days or who engages in frequent exhaustive exercise bouts, a diet in which 65% to 70% of the calories are carbohydrates is recommended (3).

Carbohydrate loading is a practice used to maximize glycogen storage prior to competition. This practice is most beneficial for athletes who compete in events lasting longer than an hour. The ADA recommends the following practices to enhance glycogen storage (3):

- Consume a diet in which 65% to 70% of the total calories are carbohydrates.
- Decrease the duration of exercise bouts during the week prior to competition.
- Rest completely on the day prior to competition.

During events that involve continuous vigorous activity for 60 min or more, it is beneficial to consume easily absorbed carbohydrates during the exercise. The ACSM recommends that solutions containing 4% to 8% carbohydrates (glucose, sucrose, or starch) are best to balance the need for blood glucose maintenance and fluid replacement. The solution should be consumed in small to moderate amounts (150 to 350 ml) every 15 to 20 min (2).

7 **In Review: Adequate glycogen is necessary for optimal performance. Carbohydrate loading is beneficial for extended exercise bouts. Glucose intake during exercise can be beneficial if vigorous exercise lasts 60 min or more.**

Female Athlete Triad

The **female athlete triad** is a condition characterized by the presence of disordered eating, amenorrhea, and osteoporosis (15). As discussed in chapter 10, disordered eating is more common in female athletes than in the general population. It is thought that the pressure to succeed and the drive to be thin leads many female athletes to begin unhealthy eating practices such as severe caloric restriction, purging of food after eating, and compulsive over-exercising. These unhealthy patterns interfere with normal hormone secretion and can eventually lead to irregular menses (**oligomenorrhea**) or a lack of menses altogether (**amenorrhea**). Because estrogen is essential in maintaining strong bones in women, the low estrogen levels observed in athletes with menstrual cycle irregularities can lead to a loss of bone. The weakening of the bones makes the athlete more susceptible to stress fractures and can lead to an early and severe onset of osteoporosis.

The HFI should encourage all physically active people to consume adequate calories and nutrients to support their energy expenditure. Active females who begin to miss menstrual periods should be referred to a physician to evaluate the need for hormonal therapy or calcium supplementation. Some signs of disordered eating are listed in chapter 10. Athletes who exhibit these signs should be referred to a nutritionist, a psychologist, or both, who is qualified to counsel a person with eating disorders.

8 **In Review: The female athlete triad (disordered eating, amenorrhea, and osteoporosis) can lead to serious health consequences. Athletes who exhibit signs of an eating disorder should be referred to a qualified nutritionist, psychologist, or both.**

Case Studies

You can check your answers by referring to appendix A.

8.1

Based on the dietary recommendations (expressed as a percent of total calories), how many grams of the following nutrients should be consumed by a 140-lb female with an average daily caloric intake of 2100 kcal?

Carbohydrate ______________

Saturated fat ______________

Unsaturated fat ______________

Protein ______________

8.2

You are asked to make a presentation to a fitness class regarding the use of the Food Guide Pyramid in meeting the recommended intake of carbohydrates, fats, and proteins. Develop an outline of your presentation.

Source List

1. American College of Sports Medicine (ACSM) (1987)

ergogenic aids — Substances taken in hopes of improving athletic performance.

carbohydrate loading — Practice of increasing carbohydrate intake and decreasing activity in the days preceding competition.

female athlete triad — A condition sometimes observed in female athletes that is characterized by disordered eating patterns, amenorrhea, and osteoporosis.

oligomenorrhea — Irregular menses.

amenorrhea — A cessation of menses.

2. ACSM (1996)
3. American Dietetic Association & Canadian Dietetic Association (1993)
4. Barrow (1992)
5. Berning (1995)
6. Brotherhood (1984)
7. Durstine & Haskell (1994)
8. Expert Panel on Detection, Evaluation, and Treatment of High Blood Cholesterol in Adults (1993)
9. Franks & Howley (1989a)
10. Gibson (1993)
11. Hoffman & Garewal (1995)
12. National Institutes of Health (1994b)
13. National Research Council, Committee on Diet and Health (1989)
14. National Research Council (1989)
15. Nattiv, Yeager, Drinkwater, & Agostini (1994)
16. Ruud & Wolinsky (1995)
17. Sizer & Whitney (1994)
18. United States Department of Agriculture (USDA) (1992)
19. USDA (1995)
20. Whitney & Hamilton (1987)

CHAPTER

9

Body Composition

Dixie Thompson

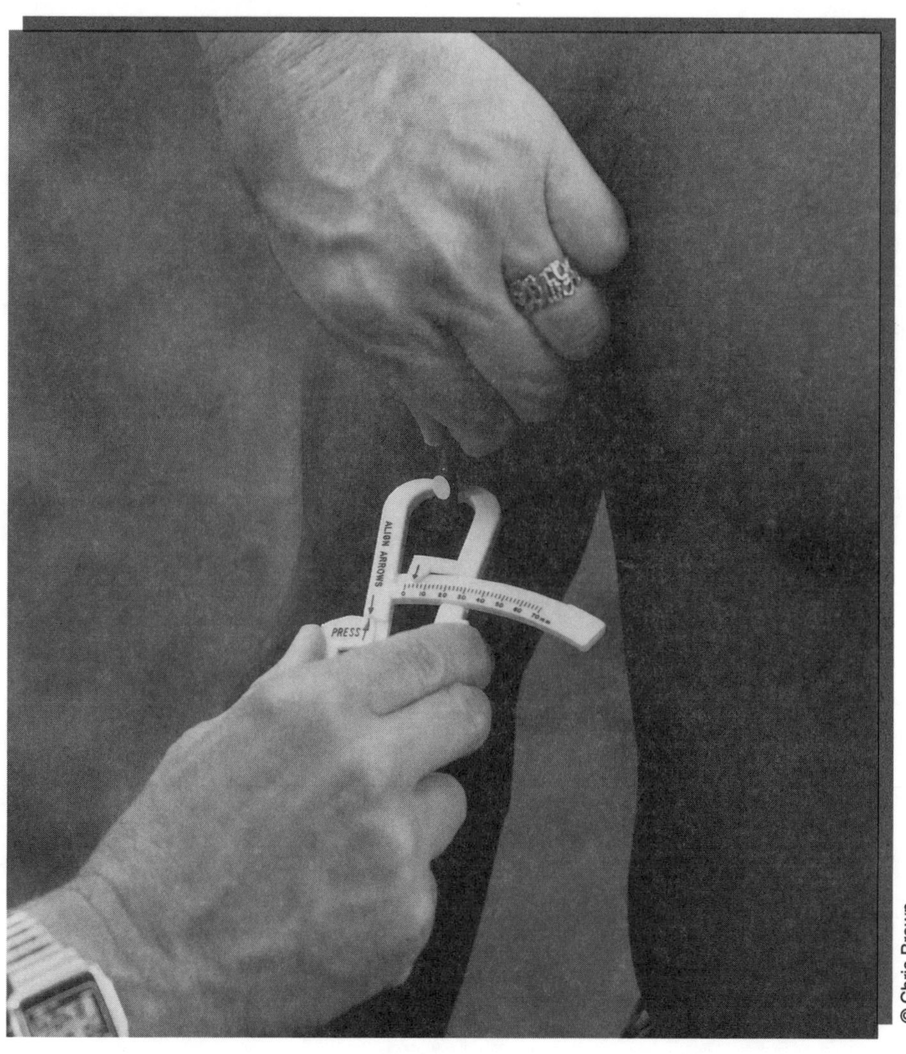

© Chris Brown

OBJECTIVES

The reader will be able to:

1. **Discuss the impact of weight and body composition on health and physical fitness and describe the health implications for different types of body fat distribution patterns.**
2. **Discuss the importance of body composition analysis in assessing physical fitness.**
3. **Describe the differences between two-compartment and multicompartment models of body composition and explain the purpose of the models.**
4. **Identify common measurement sites for skinfolds.**
5. **Identify common measurement sites for girths.**
6. **Assess body composition using a variety of techniques and describe the advantages and disadvantages of these techniques.**

American media is filled with advertisements for programs designed to help people "get in shape." One point of emphasis (many times the primary focus) in these programs is weight loss. An appropriate amount of body fat is an important part of a person's physical fitness. The HFI needs to understand the importance of appropriate amounts of body fat, become aware of the various means for assessing body fat, and become proficient at measuring body fat through skinfolds and girths. This chapter was written to assist the HFI in acquiring these skills.

HEALTH AND BODY COMPOSITION

It is estimated that approximately one third of American adults are obese (9). **Obesity** is a condition in which a person is **overfat** (i.e., has an excess of **adipose,** or fat, **tissue**) and is typically defined as a body fat percentage of greater than 32% for females and greater than 25% for males (11). Table 9.1 lists categories with which to interpret body fat percentage. Numerous negative health consequences of obesity have been documented including coronary artery disease, hypertension, stroke, non-insulin dependent diabetes mellitus, increased risk of various cancers, osteoarthritis, degenerative joint disease, abnormal blood lipid profile, and menstrual irregularities (14). In addition, obesity creates a severe psychological burden for many individuals. Because of the link between obesity and many diseases, it is essential that the health fitness instructor provide clients with an accurate assessment of this important fitness component.

Table 9.1 Body Fat Norms Based on Percentage of Body Weight That Is Fat

Classification	% Fat Women	 Men
Essential fat	11.0-14.0	3.0-5.0
Athletes	12.0-22.0	5.0-13.0
Fitness	16.0-25.0	12.0-18.0
Potential risk	26.0-31.0	19.0-24.0
Obese	32.0 and higher	25.0 and higher

Note. Females before puberty use male scale. There is no health reason for increased body fat with age, thus the same standards apply to all ages.
Adapted from Doxey et al. 1987.

When people gain excess fat, the adipose tissue tends to accumulate in certain areas of the body. Researchers are quite interested in learning how **body fat distribution,** or **fat patterning,** affects health. **Android-type obesity** (i.e., male-pattern obesity, apple shape) is the term used to describe the excessive storage of fat in the trunk and abdominal areas. Excessive fat in the hips and thighs is labeled **gynoid-type obesity** (i.e., female-pattern obesity, pear shape). In terms of negative health consequences, android-type obesity appears to be the most dangerous and is closely linked with cardiovascular disease. The use of waist-to-hip ratios is one of the most useful tools for differentiating gynoid-type and android-type obesity. A description of how to assess waist-to-hip ratio is presented later in this chapter.

Just as too much body fat can be unhealthy, too little body fat can also compromise one's wellness. Among the many important roles of fat are providing energy, helping with temperature regulation, and cushioning the joints. The minimal body fat level needed to maintain health varies among individuals and is dependent on gender and genetics. Infertility, depression, impaired temperature regulation, and even death are among the outcomes of excessive fat loss (18). Extreme fat loss is the result of starvation imposed by internal or external forces. Eating disorders that result in self-starvation are discussed in chapter 10. Because of the important link between health and body composition, an analysis of a client's body fat should be a part of physical fitness assessments.

1 **In Review: Significant health consequences (e.g., cardiovascular disease, non-insulin dependent diabetes mellitus) may result from obesity. Likewise, too little body fat can have negative physical outcomes. Cardiovascular disease risk is more closely linked with android-type obesity (apple shape) than with gynoid-type obesity (pear shape).**

INTRODUCTION TO BODY COMPOSITION ASSESSMENT

Body composition refers to the relative percentages of fat and nonfat tissues in the body. **Fat-free mass** and **percent body fat (%BF)** are typically the most frequently reported values from a body composition assessment. Percent body fat refers to the percentage of the total body weight that is composed of fat (%BF = fat weight/body weight). Fat-free mass refers to the weight of the nonfat tissues of the body and is often used synonymously with the term **lean body mass**. Technically, however, lean body mass refers to the combination of fat-free tissues and essential, life-sustaining lipids.

Various techniques are used to assess body composition, and the HFI should be skilled in their use. As with other aspects of fitness assessment, attention to detail and experience with the techniques employed are necessary in order to become proficient at estimating body composition.

2 **In Review: Because of the health implications of too much or too little body fat, body composition assessment (especially determination of percent body fat) is an essential component of a physical fitness profile.**

obesity — Condition of being **overfat**.

overfat — Condition in which one has excessive adipose tissue.

adipose tissue — Tissue composed of fat cells.

body fat distribution — Pattern of fat accumulation that is often inherited; also called **fat patterning**.

fat patterning — See **body fat distribution.**

android-type obesity — Obesity in which there is a disproportionate amount of fat in the trunk and abdomen.

gynoid-type obesity — Obesity in which there is a disproportionate amount of fat in the hips and thighs.

body composition — Relative percentages of fat and nonfat tissues in the body.

fat-free mass — Weight of the nonfat tissues of the body.

percent body fat (%BF) — Percentage of the total weight composed of fat tissue. Calculated by dividing fat mass by total weight.

lean body mass — Weight of fat-free tissues and essential, life-sustaining lipids.

METHODS FOR ASSESSING BODY COMPOSITION

Numerous techniques have been used successfully in estimating body composition. It is important for the HFI to understand that none of the methods currently used actually *measure* percentage of body fat. The techniques *estimate* body fat percentage based on the relationship between %BF and other factors that can be accurately measured such as skinfold thicknesses or underwater weight. The only way to truly measure the volume of fat in the body would be to dissect adipose tissue from other tissues in the body!

Each of the body composition techniques described in the following sections have inherent advantages and disadvantages. It is important that the HFI understand these so that wise decisions can be made when choosing the method for body composition assessment. In many situations encountered by the HFI, ease of measurement, relative accuracy, and cost will be the primary considerations when choosing a technique. In other situations (research or clinical conditions), the accuracy of the measurement may outweigh other considerations.

Hydrostatic Weighing

Hydrostatic (underwater) **weighing** is one of the most common means for estimating body composition in research settings and is often used as the **criterion method** for assessing body fat percentage. A criterion method provides the standard against which other methodologies are compared. In performing this procedure, a person gets into a tank of warm water, submerges him- or herself under the surface of the water, and then exhales fully while technicians record her or his weight (figure 9.1). The submerged weight is then compared with total body weight (taken on land) to calculate body

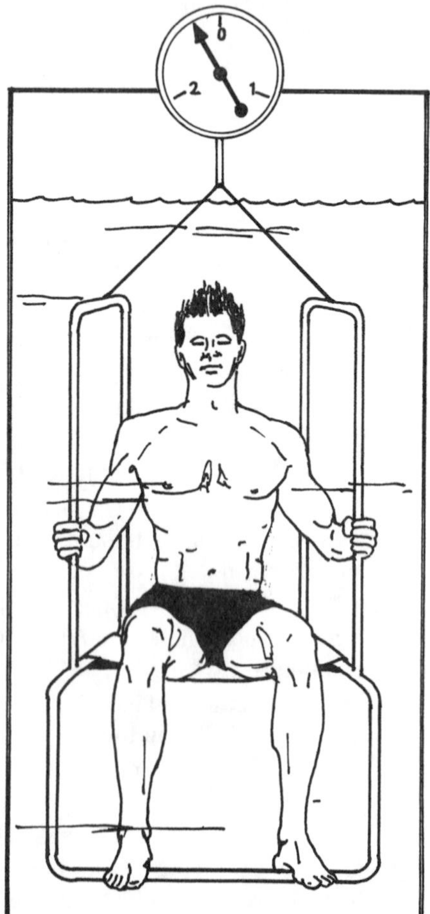

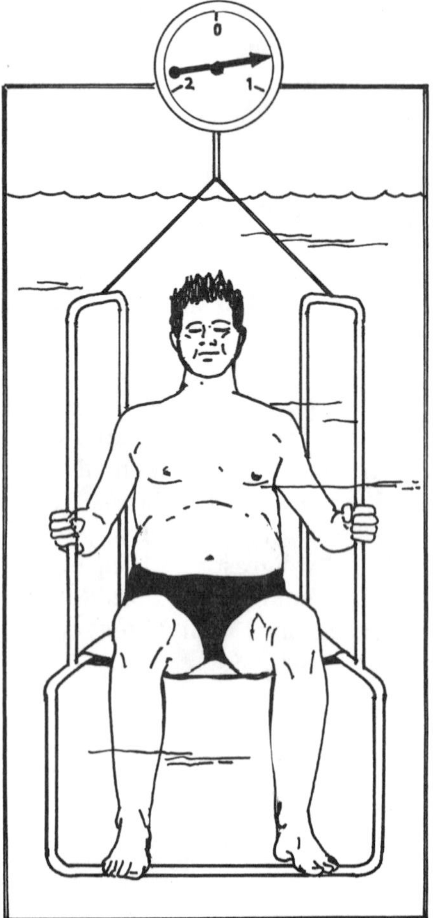

FIGURE 9.1 Hydrostatic weighing.
Adapted from Pollock and Wilmore 1990.

volume and subsequently body density and percentage of body fat.

Hydrostatic weighing utilizes a **two-compartment model** to assess body composition. This term is used because the assumptions upon which this methodology is based divide all body tissues into either a fat or a nonfat compartment. The fat-free portion of the body is composed of all tissues except lipids and is assumed to have a density of 1.1 g/cc. Fat is assumed to have a density of 0.9 g/cc. Density is the ratio of an object's weight to its volume. In other words, body density (D_b) is equal to body weight (BW) divided by body volume (BV).

$$D_b = \frac{BW}{BV}$$

Hydrostatic weighing is based on Archimedes' principle, which states that a submerged object is "buoyed up" by a force equal to the volume of the water it displaces. This buoyant force causes the object to weigh less under water than it does on land. The difference between land weight and underwater weight (UWW) is used to calculate body volume and subsequently body density.

$$D_b = \frac{BW}{\frac{(BW - UWW)}{D_{H_2O}} - RV}$$

You will note that in addition to body weight (BW) and underwater weight (UWW), one must measure the density of the water (D_{H_2O}) in the hydrostatic tank and the residual lung volume (RV). Water density is dependent on water temperature and is necessary to convert weight into volume; therefore, accurate measurement of the water temperature is essential. Also, one must correct for the residual lung volume of the person being weighed underwater because any air in the lungs will create an additional buoyant effect that will reduce underwater weight. The oxygen dilution technique described by Wilmore (22) is one of the most frequently used methods for assessing residual lung volume. If residual lung volume must be estimated, the accuracy of hydrostatic weighing is dramatically reduced. Since gender, age, and height are correlated with RV, an estimate of residual lung volume can be obtained using a formula that incorporates the client's age and height (3). The box on page 170 contains formulas for males and females.

Once the body density is calculated, this value must be converted into body fat percentage. One of the most commonly used equations for this procedure is the Siri (17) equation. This equation makes assumptions about the density and proportions of the component parts of the body. Estimation of %BF using the Siri equation works well for many in the population. It has been suggested that the inherent error (due to variations in hydration, bone density, etc.) of this method is 2% to 2.8% in young Caucasian adults (11). There are groups of people, however, for whom this equation may yield inaccurate results. The assumption that fat density is 0.9 g/cc appears to hold true for everyone; however, there are situations in which the density of the fat-free body is different from the assumed 1.1 g/cc. If a person's bone density is different from the standard used by Siri, the assumption that the density of fat-free body equals 1.1 g/cc becomes invalid. Because African-American adults typically have a higher bone density than their Caucasian counterparts, Schutte and colleagues (16) proposed that a different equation be used to calculate body fat percentage when African-Americans are being tested.

Controversy exists over the usefulness of a two-compartment model for assessing body composition in children and elderly individuals (11). Some equations have been proposed for use in specific populations. For example, there are equations to predict %BF from body density for boys ages 9 to 11 and girls ages 13 to 15 (10). It appears that, at the present, a multicompartment model that includes some measure of the body's water content and/or bone mineral content is more appropriate in these groups. Equations to predict body fat percentage for various individuals is presented on page 171.

As stated above, hydrostatic weighing provides an accurate estimation of body composition for most young, Caucasian adults, and this technique remains a standard of comparison for various other methods. Major disadvantages to this procedure are the time, expense, and technical expertise required. It should also be noted that many individuals are

hydrostatic weighing — Method of body composition assessment based on Archimedes' principle that is often used as the **criterion method**. Also called underwater weighing.

criterion method — Method used as the "gold standard" or the method against which other methods are compared.

two-compartment model — Refers to body composition assessment models that divide the body into fat and fat-free component parts.

Formulas to Calculate Residual Lung Volume From Height and Age (3)

Females:

$$(0.009 \times \text{age in yr}) + (0.08128 \times \text{ht in in.}) - 3.9 = \text{residual lung volume in L}$$

Males:

$$(0.017 \times \text{age in yr}) + (0.06858 \times \text{ht in in.}) - 3.447 = \text{residual lung volume in L}$$

unable to perform this procedure because of their discomfort in being underwater.

Following are guidelines that will help ensure accurate assessment of body composition using hydrostatic weighing techniques:

- Do not eat within 4 hr of testing.
- Urinate and defecate prior to testing.
- Wear as little clothing as possible. Remove any trapped air bubbles from clothing before weighing.
- Exhale completely while submerged. (This will take practice on the part of most individuals!)
- Remain as motionless as possible while submerged in order to increase accuracy.
- Perform several (5 to 10) trials to obtain consistent measurements.

Air Displacement Plethysmography

Another technique to determine body fat percentage that uses the concept of density as the ratio of body weight to body volume is **air displacement plethysmography**. In this method, a person sits in a sealed chamber and breathes through plastic tubing. By examining the pressure-volume relationship, body volume and therefore body density can be calculated (2, 13). The Siri equation (see equation 9.3) can then be used to estimate body fat percentage from body density.

The primary advantage of this method in comparison to hydrostatic weighing is that this technique is quicker and is less anxiety producing for many individuals. The major disadvantage to this method is the cost of the highly technical equipment needed to make the measurements. It remains to be seen if this promising methodology will be effective for assessing the body composition of people of different ages and from a variety of ethnic groups.

Total Body Water Measurement

Water is the most abundant substance in the body accounting for 67% to 74% of the body's weight. The amount of water contained in cells varies with different types of tissues. For example, adipose cells contain far less water than do muscle cells. If one assumes that the distribution of water in fat and fat-free tissues is fairly consistent among individuals, measuring the volume of water contained in the body (i.e., **total body water**) allows one to estimate body fat percentage. Like hydrostatic weighing, this methodology is considered a two-compartment model with the body being divided into fat and fat-free sections. Because of the variability in the water content of the lean compartment, Siri estimated that the error associated with this technique could be as high as 3.6% in the general population; however, in young, healthy adults, this error is probably closer to 2.6% (11).

In order to estimate total body water, one must ingest a substance that will be distributed equally throughout the water contained in the body. The substances most often used are deuterium and tritium. Deuterium is a rare, nonradioactive isotope of hydrogen. Tritium is a rare, radioactive isotope of hydrogen. Approximately 3 hr after ingestion of the isotope, a urine or blood sample is taken. Because the amount of isotope contained in the sample is inversely proportional to the amount of water in the body, total body water can be estimated.

Because of the expensive equipment and technical expertise required to measure deuterium or tritium in bodily fluids, this technique is rarely used outside of a research setting. As discussed next, the

Equations to Predict Body Fat Percentage From Body Density

Equation 9.3 — Siri Equation

$$\%BF = \frac{495}{D_b} - 450$$

EQUATION 9.4 — Schutte equation

$$\%BF = \frac{437}{D_b} - 393$$

Equation 9.5 — Prediction of %BF in 9- to 11-yr-old boys

$$\%BF = \frac{530}{D_b} - 489$$

Equation 9.6 — Prediction of %BF in 13- to 15-yr-old girls

$$\%BF = \frac{512}{D_b} - 469$$

assumptions from this methodology can be applied when total body water is estimated through other means.

Bioelectrical Impedance Analysis

The difficulty of measuring total body water by the method just described led researchers to search for other means for assessing this important variable. **Bioelectrical impedance analysis (BIA)** is a simple, quick, noninvasive method that can be used to estimate total body water. This technique is based on the assumption that tissues that are high in water content will conduct electrical currents with less resistance than those with little water (15). Because adipose tissue contains little water, fat will impede the flow of electrical current.

BIA requires that a small electrical current be sent through the body. This current (typically 800 μA at a frequency of 50 kHz) is undetectable to the person being tested (15). Typically four electrodes are placed on the individual (two on the hand and two on the foot). As the current passes through the body, the voltage difference between the electrodes is measured. This voltage drop (impedance) is then used to calculate body fat percentage. BIA has gained wide acceptance in the fitness industry because it is easy, inexpensive, and noninvasive. The accuracy of this technique is dependent on the type of equipment and equations used; however, a standard error of approximately ± 4% is commonly reported (11). A problem with the use of BIA is a lack of knowledge about its usefulness with non-Caucasian individuals and people of different age categories. Furthermore, BIA does not produce accurate results for

air displacement plethysmography— Method of body composition assessment that estimates body density from body volume and body weight.

total body water— Total amount of water in the body. This measure can be used to assess body composition.

bioelectrical impedance analysis (BIA) — Method of body composition assessment based on the electrical conductivity of various tissues in the body.

individuals with amputations, significant muscular atrophy, severe obesity, or diseases that alter the state of hydration. It has also been recommended that people with implanted defibrillators avoid BIA assessment until the safety of BIA with these individuals has been determined (15).

A person's state of hydration can greatly alter BIA results; therefore, it is essential that one standardize the methods used with this assessment technique (15). Below is a list of guidelines to follow when using BIA:

- Remove oil and lotions from the skin with alcohol before placing electrodes.
- Place electrodes precisely as directed by the manufacturer of the impedance device used. Incorrect electrode placement will greatly reduce the accuracy of the procedure.
- Many of the equations used with BIA require the measurement of height, weight, or both. Height should be measured to the nearest 0.5 cm and weight to the nearest 0.1 kg.
- Any substance that alters the body's hydration state such as alcohol or diuretics should be avoided for at least 48 hr prior to BIA.
- Individuals being assessed should limit eating and drinking 4 hr prior to assessment.
- Exercise should be avoided 12 hr preceding BIA. A state of euhydration should be restored after exercise and prior to BIA.
- Menstrual cycle phase should be noted because of its ability to alter hydration levels.

Multicompartment Models

A disadvantage to any two-compartment model of body composition is the number of assumptions that must be made about the density of various body tissues and the proportion of the total body weight accounted for by these various tissues. Researchers have proposed the use of several models in which multiple measurements are used in combination to estimate body composition. Although these techniques must still rely on some basic assumptions about the body's "makeup," fewer broad generalizations about the body's component parts are made. **Multicompartment models** provide, therefore, a potentially more accurate assessment of body composition.

Siri proposed a three-compartment model that divides the body into fat, water, and solids (protein and mineral) (17). This model requires the measurement of total body density and total body water. Because total body water accounts for the largest proportion of body weight and tends to be the most variable compartment, this model can be used effectively for many individuals. It is estimated that this technique will provide fat percentage values within 2% of the actual value (11).

Although Siri's equation is an advance over two-compartment models, it cannot accurately assess the body composition of individuals with significant alterations in bone density. Lohman's three-compartment model overcomes this difficulty by dividing the body into fat, mineral, and protein and water components (10). For this technique both total body density and bone mineral content must be measured; if these values are measured correctly, the error of this technique is estimated to be less than 2% (10).

Heymsfield and colleagues (4) and Lohman (10) developed four-compartment models that incorporate the advantages of both the Siri and Lohman three-compartment models. These four-compartment models assume that the body is divided into protein, mineral, fat, and water components. This technique requires the measurement of bone mineral content, total body water, and total body density. Theoretically, these methods provide a more accurate assessment of body composition than any of the two- or three-compartment models (11).

Although multicompartment models hold much promise as potential criterion measures of body composition, most are not easily used in a nonresearch setting. The cost of performing the multiple tests needed for using these models makes it impractical in screening settings. The one possible use of multicompartment methodology in the field setting is the Siri three-compartment model (17). This model, however, is dependent on the ability of BIA to precisely assess total body water and the ability to readily measure total body density through either hydrostatic weighing or air displacement plethysmography.

3 In Review: Two-compartment models assume that the body is divided into fat and fat-free components. Multicompartment models assume that the body is divided into a fat component and at least two other parts (protein, mineral, water). These models improve the accuracy with which body composition can be assessed and have both advantages and disadvantages in terms of expense, accuracy, and application.

Dual-Energy X-Ray Absorptiometry

Dual-energy X-ray absorptiometry (DEXA) was developed for measuring the density of bones. While this remains a primary use of this methodology, software has been developed that can estimate body fat percentage from DEXA scans. This procedure requires a total-body X ray using extremely low dosage energy beams. Assessment of body composition using DEXA requires the assumption that the body has three compartments (fat, bone mineral, and non-bone lean tissue) with each of the components having a different density (8). As the X-ray beams pass through the subject, the density of all parts of the body is determined. Because fat is less dense than bone or non-bone lean tissue, the percentage of the total body weight composed of fat can be calculated.

Although this technique requires a full-body X ray, the radiation exposure for the procedure is minimal and is roughly equivalent to one quarter of the radiation exposure of a dental X ray. Some claim DEXA as the new criterion method for body composition assessment; however, there are still technical aspects of the procedure that must be standardized. For example, differences in DEXA software packages may result in varied body fat outcomes. Also, variation in body segment thicknesses have a tendency to alter DEXA results (8). Studies investigating the error associated with this technique have reported errors ranging from 1.2% to 4.8% (11).

This procedure is relatively quick (5 to 20 min depending on the technique used) and has the potential for very accurate results no matter the age, gender, or race of the individual being tested. The major prohibitive factors to the HFI using this procedure are cost and access to the equipment. Because of the radiation exposure involved, DEXA equipment is housed in hospitals and/or clinically-oriented research centers. At present, DEXA methodology is most frequently used as a research tool and in the clinical assessment of body composition. In addition to the DEXA software assessment of body composition, bone mineral content measured by DEXA can be used as an integral part of various multicompartment models.

Skinfolds

The measurement of skinfolds is one of the most frequently performed tests to estimate body composition. This quick, noninvasive, inexpensive method can, in most cases, provide a fairly accurate assessment of body fat percentage. The fat percentage value obtained using skinfold equations is typically within 4% of the value measured using underwater weighing (11). This methodology is based on the assumption that, as one gains adipose tissue, the increase in skinfold thickness will be proportional to the additional fat weight. Because 50% to 70% of one's adipose tissue is stored subcutaneously, this assumption holds true in most cases.

Because of the widespread use of this type of assessment, the HFI should master the skills involved. Accurate measurement of skinfold thickness requires that several things be done correctly: locating the skinfold site, "pinching" the skinfold away from the underlying tissue, measuring with the caliper, and choosing the proper equation. The following sections address each of these important concerns.

Locating the Skinfold Site

It is critical that the site of the skinfold measurement be accurately determined. To increase the accuracy of the measurement, especially for the inexperienced technician, the site for measurement should be located and then marked with an erasable marker. This will help ensure that the calipers are placed in precisely the correct position each time the skinfold is measured. All skinfold measurements should be taken on the right side of the body unless otherwise specified. Refer to table 9.2 for some of the most commonly used measurement sites. For a more complete description of skinfold site determination refer to the *Anthropometric Standardization Reference Manual* (12). The HFI should also note that the measurement of skinfolds immediately after exercise may lead to inaccurate results because of fluid volume shifts.

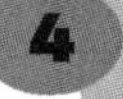

In Review: Common measurement sites for skinfolds are found in table 9.2.

"Pinching" the Skinfold

Once the correct location for the skinfold measurement is determined, the HFI must then gently but

multicompartment models — Theoretical models of body composition in which the body is assumed to consist of more than two compartments.

Table 9.2 Commonly Used Skinfold Site Locations

Skinfold site	Description
Abdominal	Measure vertical fold 2 cm to the right of and level with the umbilicus. Make sure the head of caliper is not in the umbilicus.
Triceps	Measure the vertical fold over the belly of the triceps muscle. The arm should be relaxed. The specific site is the posterior midline of the upper arm, half the distance between the acromion and olecranon processes.
Chest	The location for this site is half or a third the distance between the anterior axillary line and the nipple for men and women, respectively. The measurement should be a diagonal fold along the natural line of the skin.
Midaxillary	This vertical fold should be taken at the level of the ziphoid process on the midaxillary line.
Subscapular	This site is located 2 cm below the inferior angle of the scapula. The diagonal fold should be measured at a 45° angle.
Suprailiac	This diagonal fold should be measured in line with the natural angle of the iliac crest. The measurement should be taken along the anterior axillary line just above the iliac crest.
Thigh	Measure the vertical fold over the quadriceps muscle on the midline of the thigh. The measurement site is half the distance between the top of the patella and the inguinal crease.

firmly pinch and lift the skinfold away from the underlying muscle in order to measure it. The guidelines below describe proper methods for measuring skinfolds:

1. Place the fingers perpendicular to the skinfold approximately 1 cm from the site to be measured.
2. Gently yet firmly pinch the skinfold between the thumb and the first two fingers and lift away from the underlying tissues.
3. Place the jaws of the caliper at the measurement site perpendicular to the skinfold. The jaws of the caliper should be halfway between the bottom and top of the fold.
4. Read the measurement on the caliper approximately 2 s after the jaws come into contact with the skin.
5. Wait at least 15 s before taking a subsequent measurement. If the second measurement varies by more than 1 to 2 mm, repeat the measurement a third time.

Measuring the skinfolds of obese individuals can be difficult it not impossible. If the jaws of the caliper will not open wide enough to measure the skinfold, use an alternative method for assessing body composition. Girth measurements for predicting body fat percentage (20, 21), body mass index, and waist-to-hip ratio are methods that may be used for obese individuals. These methods are described later in the chapter.

Measuring With the Caliper

Skinfold thickness is measured with a skinfold caliper. There are a variety of commercially available calipers that vary in price and accuracy. The Lange and Harpenden calipers have traditionally been used most often in research settings because of their precision and reliability, however, other calipers may also be used effectively. Obviously if the calipers that are being used do not measure skinfolds accurately, the estimate of body fat will be compromised. It is wise to periodically test the accuracy of skinfold calipers using calibration blocks sold by various companies. It is also advisable to measure with calipers that closely match those utilized in the development of the equation you are using.

Choosing the Proper Equation

Most skinfold equations were developed using underwater weighing as the criterion method and are actually designed to estimate body density. To develop skinfold equations, the body density of a large number of people was measured (typically using hydrostatic weighing), and this value was compared to skinfold thickness through a statistical method called *regression analysis*. This statistical technique results in the development of an equation that reflects the relationship between skinfolds and body density. By inserting a client's skinfold measurements (and sometimes other information such as age) into these equations, the HFI obtains an estimate of the client's body density. Body density is then converted to percent body fat using the Siri equation (see equation 9.3).

Both generalized and population-specific skinfold equations have been developed (6, 11). Generalized equations are designed to estimate body composition in groups of people that vary greatly in age, body composition, and fitness. An advantage of these equations is that they can be used to estimate body composition in most people; however, these equations lose accuracy when testing individuals that are dissimilar from those used to develop the equation. Population-specific equations are designed to predict body composition in a particular subgroup of the population such as women runners. The advantage of using population-specific equations is that they tend to have higher accuracy when testing people that fit the physical profile of those in the subgroup of interest.

Because gender influences the areas in which fat is stored, separate skinfold equations for men and women have been developed. The Jackson and Pollock (5) equations for men and the Jackson, Pollock, and Ward (7) equations for women are generalized equations that are widely used. Note that the client's age is also used in these equations. This is because the relationship between total body fat and subcutaneous fat changes with age. Equations from these authors that require the measurement of 3 or 7 sites are listed in the box below. In addition, tables 9.3 and 9.4 provide quick references for estimating body fatness from skinfold thicknesses for men and women, respectively. To use these tables, total the

Equations to Estimate Body Density From Skinfold Thicknesses (5,6,7)

Women

3 sites

$$D_b = 1.099421 - 0.0009929(X1) + 0.0000023(X1)^2 - 0.0001392(X2)$$

3 sites

$$D_b = 1.089733 - 0.0009245(X3) + 0.0000025(X3)^2 - 0.0000979(X2)$$

7 sites

$$D_b = 1.097 - 0.00046971(X4) + 0.00000056(X4)^2 - 0.00012828(X2)$$

X1 = sum of triceps, suprailiac, and thigh skinfolds
X2 = age in yr
X3 = sum of triceps, suprailiac, and abdominal skinfolds
X4 = sum of triceps, abdominal, suprailiac, thigh, chest, subscapular, and midaxillary skinfolds

Men

3 sites

$$D_b = 1.10938 - 0.0008267(X1) + 0.0000016(X1)^2 - 0.0002574(X2)$$

3 sites

$$D_b = 1.1125025 - 0.0013125(X3) + 0.0000055(X3)^2 - 0.0002440(X2)$$

7 sites

$$D_b = 1.112 - 0.00043499(X4) + 0.00000055(X4)^2 - 0.00028826(X2)$$

X1 = sum of chest, abdomen, and thigh skinfolds
X2 = age in yr
X3 = sum of chest, triceps, and subscapular skinfolds
X4 = sum of triceps, abdominal, suprailiac, thigh, chest, subscapular, and midaxillary skinfolds

Table 9.3 Percentage Body Fat[a] Estimation for Men From Age and the Sum of Chest, Abdominal, and Thigh Skinfolds

Sum of skinfolds	Age to the last year								
(mm)	Under 22	23 to 27	28 to 32	33 to 37	38 to 42	43 to 47	48 to 52	53 to 57	Over 57
8-10	1.3	1.8	2.3	2.9	3.4	3.9	4.5	5.0	5.5
11-13	2.2	2.8	3.3	3.9	4.4	4.9	5.5	6.0	6.5
14-16	3.2	3.8	4.3	4.8	5.4	5.9	6.4	7.0	7.5
17-19	4.2	4.7	5.3	5.8	6.3	6.9	7.4	8.0	8.5
20-22	5.1	5.7	6.2	6.8	7.3	7.9	8.4	8.9	9.5
23-25	6.1	6.6	7.2	7.7	8.3	8.8	9.4	9.9	10.5
26-28	7.0	7.6	8.1	8.7	9.2	9.8	10.3	10.9	11.4
29-31	8.0	8.5	9.1	9.6	10.2	10.7	11.3	11.8	12.4
32-34	8.9	9.4	10.0	10.5	11.1	11.6	12.2	12.8	13.3
35-37	9.8	10.4	10.9	11.5	12.0	12.6	13.1	13.7	14.3
38-40	10.7	11.3	11.8	12.4	12.9	13.5	14.1	14.6	15.2
41-43	11.6	12.2	12.7	13.3	13.8	14.4	15.0	15.5	16.1
44-46	12.5	13.1	13.6	14.2	14.7	15.3	15.9	16.4	17.0
47-49	13.4	13.9	14.5	15.1	15.6	16.2	16.8	17.3	17.9
50-52	14.3	14.8	15.4	15.9	16.5	17.1	17.6	18.2	18.8
53-55	15.1	15.7	16.2	16.8	17.4	17.9	18.5	19.1	19.7
56-58	16.0	16.5	17.1	17.7	18.2	18.8	19.4	20.0	20.5
59-61	16.9	17.4	17.9	18.5	19.1	19.7	20.2	20.8	21.4
62-64	17.6	18.2	18.8	19.4	19.9	20.5	21.1	21.7	22.2
65-67	18.5	19.0	19.6	20.2	20.8	21.3	21.9	22.5	23.1
68-70	19.3	19.9	20.4	21.0	21.6	22.2	22.7	23.3	23.9
71-73	20.1	20.7	21.2	21.8	22.4	23.0	23.6	24.1	24.7
74-76	20.9	21.5	22.0	22.6	23.2	23.8	24.4	25.0	25.5
77-79	21.7	22.2	22.8	23.4	24.0	24.6	25.2	25.8	26.3
80-82	22.4	23.0	23.6	24.2	24.8	25.4	25.9	26.5	27.1
83-85	23.2	23.8	24.4	25.0	25.5	26.1	26.7	27.3	27.9
86-88	24.0	24.5	25.1	25.7	26.3	26.9	27.5	28.1	28.7
89-91	24.7	25.3	25.9	26.5	27.1	27.6	28.2	28.8	29.4
92-94	25.4	26.0	26.6	27.2	27.8	28.4	29.0	29.6	30.2
95-97	26.1	26.7	27.3	27.9	28.5	29.1	29.7	30.3	30.9
98-100	26.9	27.4	28.0	28.6	29.2	29.8	30.4	31.0	31.6
101-103	27.5	28.1	28.7	29.3	29.9	30.5	31.1	31.7	32.3
104-106	28.2	28.8	29.4	30.0	30.6	31.2	31.8	32.4	33.0
107-109	28.9	29.5	30.1	30.7	31.3	31.9	32.5	33.1	33.7
110-112	29.6	30.2	30.8	31.4	32.0	32.6	33.2	33.8	34.4
113-115	30.2	30.8	31.4	32.0	32.6	33.2	33.8	34.5	35.1
116-118	30.9	31.5	32.1	32.7	33.3	33.9	34.5	35.1	35.7
119-121	31.5	32.1	32.7	33.3	33.9	34.5	35.1	35.7	36.4
122-124	32.1	32.7	33.3	33.9	34.5	35.1	35.8	36.4	37.0
125-127	32.7	33.3	33.9	34.5	35.1	35.8	36.4	37.0	37.6

Note. [a]Percentage of fat is calculated by the formula of Siri: percent fat = $[(4.95/D_b) - 4.5] \times 100$, where D_b = body density.

Adapted from Pollock, Schmidt, and Jackson 1980.

sum of your client's skinfolds (chest, abdominal, and thigh for men; triceps, suprailium, and thigh for women) and locate the corresponding value in the far left column. Then, locate the client's age in the top row. The intersection of the row and column will be the client's estimated percent body fat.

Girth Measurements

Several girth measurements (body and limb circumferences) are used as ways to either estimate body composition or describe body proportions. Advantages of making girth measurements are

Table 9.4 Percentage Body Fat[a] Estimation for Women From Age and Triceps, Suprailium, and Thigh Skinfolds

Sum of skinfolds	Age to the last year								
(mm)	Under 22	23 to 27	28 to 32	33 to 37	38 to 42	43 to 47	48 to 52	53 to 57	Over 57
23-25	9.7	9.9	10.2	10.4	10.7	10.9	11.2	11.4	11.7
26-28	11.0	11.2	11.5	11.7	12.0	12.3	12.5	12.7	13.0
29-31	12.3	12.5	12.8	13.0	13.3	13.5	13.8	14.0	14.3
32-34	13.6	13.8	14.0	14.3	14.5	14.8	15.0	15.3	15.5
35-37	14.8	15.0	15.3	15.5	15.8	16.0	16.3	16.5	16.8
38-40	16.0	16.3	16.5	16.7	17.0	17.2	17.5	17.7	18.0
41-43	17.2	17.4	17.7	17.9	18.2	18.4	18.7	18.9	19.2
44-46	18.3	18.6	18.8	19.1	19.3	19.6	19.8	20.1	20.3
47-49	19.5	19.7	20.0	20.2	20.5	20.7	21.0	21.2	21.5
50-52	20.6	20.8	21.1	21.3	21.6	21.8	22.1	22.3	22.6
53-55	21.7	21.9	22.1	22.4	22.6	22.9	23.1	23.4	23.6
56-58	22.7	23.0	23.2	23.4	23.7	23.9	24.2	24.4	24.7
59-61	23.7	24.0	24.2	24.5	24.7	25.0	25.2	25.5	25.7
62-64	24.7	25.0	25.2	25.5	25.7	26.0	26.2	26.4	26.7
65-67	25.7	25.9	26.2	26.4	26.7	26.9	27.2	27.4	27.7
68-70	26.6	26.9	27.1	27.4	27.6	27.9	28.1	28.4	28.6
71-73	27.5	27.8	28.0	28.3	28.5	28.8	29.0	29.3	29.5
74-76	28.4	28.7	28.9	29.2	29.4	29.7	29.9	30.2	30.4
77-79	29.3	29.5	29.8	30.0	30.3	30.5	30.8	31.0	31.3
80-82	30.1	30.4	30.6	30.9	31.1	31.4	31.6	31.9	32.1
83-85	30.9	31.2	31.4	31.7	31.9	32.2	32.4	32.7	32.9
86-88	31.7	32.0	32.2	32.5	32.7	32.9	33.2	33.4	33.7
89-91	32.5	32.7	33.0	33.2	33.5	33.7	33.9	34.2	34.4
92-94	33.2	33.4	33.7	33.9	34.2	34.4	34.7	34.9	35.2
95-97	33.9	34.1	34.4	34.6	34.9	35.1	35.4	35.6	35.9
98-100	34.6	34.8	35.1	35.3	35.5	35.8	36.0	36.3	36.5
101-103	35.3	35.4	35.7	35.9	36.2	36.4	36.7	36.9	37.2
104-106	35.8	36.1	36.3	36.6	36.8	37.1	37.3	37.5	37.8
107-109	36.4	36.7	36.9	37.1	37.4	37.6	37.9	38.1	38.4
110-112	37.0	37.2	37.5	37.7	38.0	38.2	38.5	38.7	38.9
113-115	37.5	37.8	38.1	38.2	38.5	38.7	39.0	39.2	39.5
116-118	38.0	38.3	38.5	38.8	39.0	39.3	39.5	39.7	40.0
119-121	38.5	38.7	39.0	39.2	39.5	39.7	40.0	40.2	40.5
122-124	39.0	39.2	39.4	39.7	39.9	40.2	40.4	40.7	40.9
125-127	39.4	39.6	39.9	40.1	40.4	40.6	40.9	41.1	41.4
128-130	39.8	40.0	40.3	40.5	40.8	41.0	41.3	41.5	41.8

Note. [a]Percentage of fat is calculated by the formula of Siri: percent fat = $[(4.95/D_b) - 4.5] \times 100$, where D_b = body density.

Adapted from Pollock, Schmidt, and Jackson 1980.

that they provide quick and reliable information about the individual. These measurements are sometimes used in equations to predict body composition and may also be used to track changes in body shape and size during weight loss. The major disadvantage is that they provide little information about the fat and nonfat components of the body. For example, a body builder may have a thigh that has a larger circumference (yet less fat) than an obese individual. A description of several commonly measured girths follows (refer to the *Anthropometric Standardization Reference Manual* [12] or the *ACSM's Guidelines for Exercise Testing and Prescription* [1] for additional circumference sites):

- Waist—most narrow part of the torso between the ziphoid process and the umbilicus

- Abdomen—circumference of the torso at the level of the umbilicus
- Hips—maximal circumference of the buttocks above the gluteal fold
- Thigh—largest circumference of the right thigh below the gluteal fold

The **waist-to-hip ratio (WHR)** is one of the most used clinical applications of girth measurements. This value is often used to reflect the degree of abdominal, or android-type, obesity. A WHR greater than 0.95 for men or 0.86 for women is considered to place the individual at much greater risk for developing negative health consequences as a result of excess abdominal fat (1).

When assessing girths, use the following procedures to standardize the measurements.

- Make sure that the measuring tape is horizontal when making all trunk circumferences and is perpendicular to the long axis of the limb when measuring limbs. Using either a mirror or an assistant will help ensure the tape is placed properly.
- Apply constant pressure to the tape without pinching the skin. A tape measure fitted with a handle that indicates the amount of tension exerted is recommended.
- When measuring limbs, measure on the right side of the body.
- Ensure that the person is standing erect, relaxed, and with feet together.
- When measuring girths of the trunk, take the measurement after the person exhales and before beginning the next breath.

In Review:Common measurement sites for girths are the waist, abdomen, hips, and thigh.

Height-Weight Tables

One of the easiest ways to draw conclusions about the appropriateness of one's weight is to make a comparison between height and weight. Several different height-weight tables have been proposed as ways to determine appropriate weights based on height. The Metropolitan Life Insurance Company published a widely used height-weight table in 1959 (table 9.5). These data were based on the weights that were associated with the lowest mortality rates. In 1983, these values were revised to reflect an increase in acceptable weight for each height. Controversy exists over which of the values (1959 or 1983) have the most practical and meaningful applications. In 1995, the U.S. Department of Agriculture (19) released new healthy weight ranges for men and women (table 9.6). These new guidelines do not list separate weight ranges for men and women, but they do recommend that individuals who have a larger skeletal structure or more muscle mass should be at

Table 9.5 Metropolitan Life Height and Weight Tables (1959 version) for Men and Women Between the Ages of 25 and 59

Height[a]		Frame		
Feet	Inches	Small	Medium	Large
		Men		
5	2	112-120	118-129	126-141
5	3	115-123	121-133	129-144
5	4	118-126	124-136	132-148
5	5	121-129	127-139	135-152
5	6	124-133	130-143	138-156
5	7	128-137	134-147	142-161
5	8	132-141	138-152	147-166
5	9	136-145	142-156	151-170
5	10	140-150	145-160	155-174
5	11	144-154	150-165	159-179
6	0	148-158	154-170	164-184
6	1	152-162	158-175	168-189
6	2	156-167	162-180	173-194
6	3	160-171	167-185	178-199
6	4	164-175	172-190	182-204
		Women		
4	10	92-98	96-107	104-119
4	11	94-101	98-110	106-122
5	0	96-104	101-113	109-125
5	1	99-107	104-116	112-128
5	2	102-110	107-119	115-131
5	3	105-113	110-122	118-134
5	4	108-116	113-126	121-138
5	5	111-119	116-130	125-142
5	6	114-123	120-135	129-146
5	7	118-127	124-139	133-150
5	8	122-131	128-143	137-154
5	9	129-135	132-147	141-158
5	10	130-140	136-151	145-163
5	11	134-144	140-155	149-168
6	0	138-148	144-159	153-173

Note. [a]With shoes with 1-in. heels for men, 2-in. heels for women.

the higher end of each range while individuals with smaller frames and/or less muscle mass should expect their weight to be nearer the low end of the range.

It should be noted that height-weight tables do not directly reflect body fat percentage or body fat distribution. Also, much of the data collected in the development of the Metropolitan Life Tables came from upper- and middle-class Caucasians and therefore may not reflect appropriate weight for members of diverse ethnic and socioeconomic groups.

The 1959 Metropolitan Life Height-Weight Table is sometimes used to calculate **relative weight**. Relative weight is a reflection of the relationship of one's body weight to that recommended in height-weight tables. Relative weight is calculated by dividing body weight by the midpoint of the recommended weight range for a medium frame individual. A relative weight of 110% to 119% or higher is classified as **overweight** and a relative weight of 120% or higher is considered obese. See page 180 for an example of how to calculate relative weight.

Table 9.6 USDA Healthy Weight Ranges for Men and Women

Height	Weight
4' 10"	91-119
4' 11"	94-124
5' 0"	97-128
5' 1"	101-132
5' 2"	104-137
5' 3"	107-141
5' 4"	111-146
5' 5"	114-150
5' 6"	118-155
5' 7"	121-160
5' 8"	125-164
5' 9"	129-169
5' 10"	132-174
5' 11"	136-179
6' 0"	140-184
6' 1"	144-189
6' 2"	148-195
6' 3"	152-200
6' 4"	156-205
6' 5"	160-211
6' 6"	164-216

Note. The USDA recommends that individuals who have a larger skeletal frame or more muscle mass be at the higher end of each range; individuals with smaller frames and/or less muscle mass should expect their weight to be nearer the low end of the range.
From United States Department of Agriculture 1995.

Body Mass Index

A widely used clinical assessment of the appropriateness of a person's weight is the **body mass index (BMI)**, or Quetelet Index. This value is calculated by dividing the weight in kilograms by height in meters squared.

$$\text{BMI} = \frac{\text{kg}}{\text{m}^2}$$

BMI is a quick and easy method for providing a guide in determining if one's weight is appropriate for one's height. As is the case with girth measurements and height-weight tables, BMI does not provide a differentiation of fat and nonfat weight. For most adults, however, there is a clear correlation between elevated BMI and negative health consequences. When BMI climbs above 27 kg/m^2, the risk of developing cardiovascular disease rises dramatically. It is suggested that adults maintain a BMI below 25 kg/m^2. The USDA healthy weight guidelines (table 9.6) reflect a BMI ranging from 19 to 25 kg/m^2. When BMI is between 25 and 27 kg/m^2, one can be considered somewhat overweight with a slightly elevated risk of developing obesity-related conditions. When BMI rises above 27 kg/m^2, the risk for suffering negative health outcomes due to excess weight is significantly higher than a normal weight individual (18).

waist-to-hip ratio (WHR) — Waist circumference divided by hip circumference; often used as an indicator of android-type obesity.

relative weight — Reflection of the relationship of one's body weight to that recommended in height-weight tables. Calculated by dividing body weight by midpoint of recommended weight range.

overweight — Condition in which one weighs more than recommended by height-weight charts.

body mass index (BMI) — Measure of the relationship between height and weight; calculated by dividing the weight in kg by height in meters squared.

Calculating Relative Weight

Relative weight = (body weight/midpoint recommended range) × 100

Example: A 52-year-old man is 70 in. tall and weighs 185 lb. Using the 1959 Metropolitan Life Height-Weight Table calculate this individual's relative weight.

Relative weight = (185/153) × 100 = 117.6%

6 **In Review: The previous sections provide instructions for assessing body composition using hydrostatic weighing, air displacement plethysmography, total body water measurement, bioelectrical impedance analysis, dual-energy X-ray absorptiometry, skinfold measurements, girth measurements, height-weight tables, and body mass index. The following table summarizes the advantages and disadvantages of each.**

Body composition assessment method	Advantage	Disadvantage
Hydrostatic weighing	Accuracy	Expense, time, availability
Air displacement plethysmography	Accuracy	Expense, availability
Total body water measurement	Accuracy	Expense, time, availability
Bioelectrical impedance analysis	Easy	Accuracy if not done properly; accuracy in certain diseases
Dual-energy X-ray absorptiometry	Accuracy; also provides bone density	Expense, availability
Skinfold measurement	Easy, inexpensive	Accuracy can be problematic
Height-weight tables	Easy, inexpensive	Does not indicate amount of fat; inaccurate in very muscular people
Body mass index	Easy, inexpensive	Does not indicate amount of fat; inaccurate in very muscular people

CALCULATING TARGET BODY WEIGHT

As listed in table 9.1, healthy body fat percentage ranges for normally active adults are 16% to 25% and 12% to 18% for females and males, respectively. Once an estimate of body fat percentage has been obtained, the HFI can calculate an appropriate target weight. As discussed in chapter 10, setting reasonable goals for weight loss is a major factor in maintaining compliance. To calculate target body weight one must know body weight, body fat percentage (or fat-free mass), and the desired level of body fatness. See page 181 for an example on how to calculate target body weight.

CASE STUDY

You can check your answers by referring to appendix A.

9.1

Ms. Client requests a body composition assessment. Using the measurements below,

1. calculate her WHR,
2. calculate her %BF, and
3. calculate her relative weight.

Calculating Target Body Weight

Fat mass = current body weight × (%BF/100%)

Fat-free mass (FFM) = current body weight - fat mass

$$\text{Target body weight} \frac{\text{FFM}}{1 - \left(\frac{\text{Desired \%BF}}{100}\right)}$$

Example: A 40-year-old woman weighs 155 lb and has a body fat percentage of 28%. Her goal is to reach 23% body fat. What is her target weight?

Fat mass = 155 lb × 0.28 = 43.3 lb

FFM = 155 lb – 43.4 lb = 111.6 lb

$$\text{Target body weight} \frac{111.6}{1 - \left(\frac{23}{100}\right)} = 144.9 \text{ lb}$$

4. Based on your values, calculate her target weight assuming that her goal is to reach 25% body fat.

   age = 55 years
   height = 5′5″
   weight = 170 lb
   hip girth = 108 cm
   waist girth = 76 cm
   skinfolds
      triceps = 29 mm
      thigh = 50 mm
      suprailiac = 28 mm
      abdominal = 35 mm

SOURCE LIST

1. American College of Sports Medicine (1995)
2. Dempster & Aitkens (1995)
3. Goldman & Becklake (1959)
4. Heymsfield et al. (1990)
5. Jackson & Pollock (1978)
6. Jackson & Pollock (1985)
7. Jackson, Pollock, & Ward (1980)
8. Kohrt (1995)
9. Kuczmarski, Flegal, Campbell, & Johnson (1994)
10. Lohman (1986)
11. Lohman (1992)
12. Lohman, Roche, & Martorell (1988)
13. McCrory, Gomez, Bernauer, & Molé (1995)
14. National Institutes of Health (NIH) (1985)
15. NIH (1994a)
16. Schutte et al. (1984)
17. Siri (1961)
18. Sizer & Whitney (1994)
19. United States Department of Agriculture (1995)
20. Weltman, Levine, Seip, & Tran (1988)
21. Weltman, Seip, & Tran (1987)
22. Wilmore (1969)

Chapter 10

Weight Management

Dixie Thompson

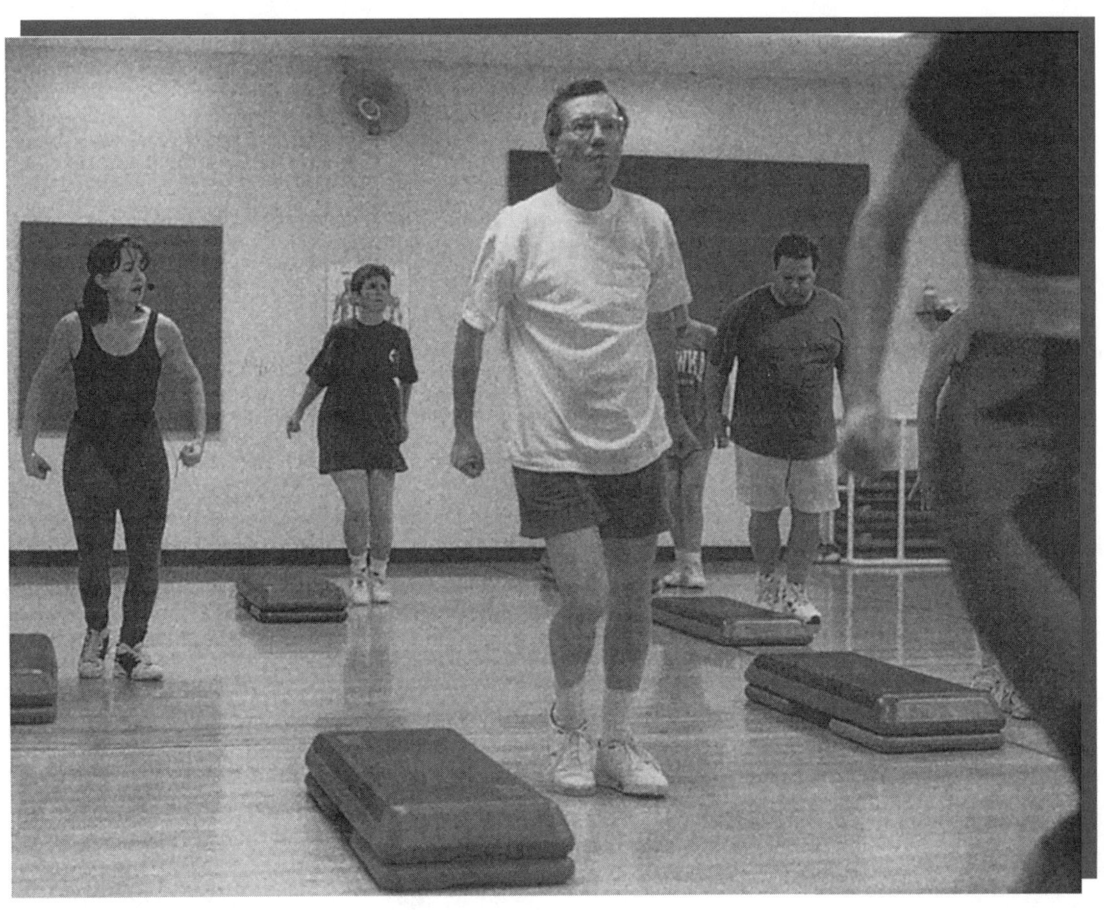

© Chris Brown

The reader will be able to: **OBJECTIVES**

1. Describe the typical changes in body composition that occur with aging.
2. Describe the role that energy balance plays in weight loss/weight maintenance.
3. Identify the factors that contribute to obesity.
4. Prescribe guidelines for caloric intake to facilitate weight loss or weight gain.
5. Describe appropriate and inappropriate weight loss goals, discuss the role of exercise in weight loss and weight maintenance, and prescribe safe and effective exercise programs for obese individuals.
6. Describe appropriate behavioral change strategies for modifying and/or maintaining body composition.
7. State the efficacy of quick-fix weight loss methods.
8. Discuss the link between body weight and self-esteem.
9. Recognize signs of eating disorders.
10. Prescribe healthy guidelines for gaining weight.

Take a look at the advertisements commonly appearing in the media, and you can see evidence of American's obsession with weight loss and "the body beautiful." It has been estimated that more than $30 billion is spent in the United States each year on weight loss efforts. This obsession with thinness is so prevalent that the National Institutes of Health (NIH) Consensus Panel on the health implications of obesity commented that the psychological burden of obesity was a major negative health consequence of being overweight (19). It has also been reported that people who are obese suffer both social and economic discrimination.

INCREASING PREVALENCE OF OBESITY IN THE UNITED STATES

In spite of the emphasis on being thin, Americans are getting fatter; and it is estimated that 58 million American adults are obese (14). Figure 10.1 demonstrates the trend for the increasing prevalence of obesity among American adults.

It is common for adults to accumulate additional adipose tissue as they age. This gradual accumulation of fat is sometimes called **creeping obesity**. Part of this change in body composition is due to a natural loss of muscle due to the aging process. A falling metabolic rate, a more sedentary lifestyle, and a lack of adjustment in eating patterns, however, appear to be the most important factors contributing to increased body fat (6). This additional increase in body fat should not be viewed as healthy, and the health fitness instructor (HFI) should encourage people of all ages to strive toward the standards for weight and body fat recommended in chapter 9.

1 **In Review: People tend to accumulate fat as they age, but creeping obesity is not healthy; a change in eating and exercise habits can often help to prevent it or mitigate its potential.**

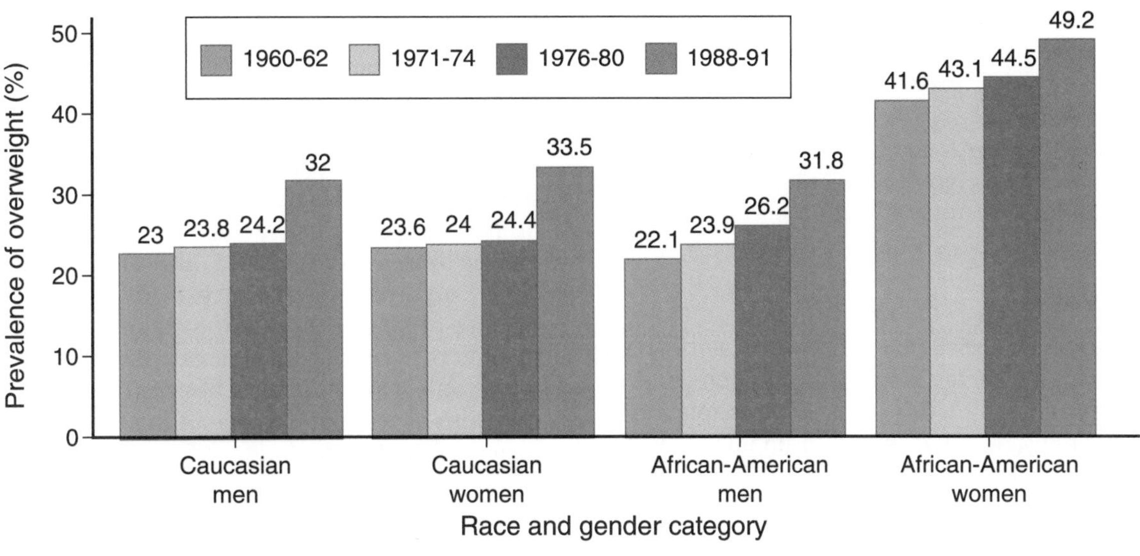

FIGURE 10.1 Changes in percentage of overweight American adults (1960-1991).
Adapted from Kuczmarski et al. 1994.

ETIOLOGY OF OBESITY

The cause of obesity cannot be simply defined because many factors contribute to the development of obesity. Ultimately, **positive caloric balance** (i.e., taking in more calories than are expended) leads to obesity. It is clear, however, that factors contributing to obesity can be discussed under two broad categories: genetics and lifestyle.

Genetics

Evidence exists that inheritance is a contributing factor in the development of obesity (3, 23). In evaluating the impact of genetics on the development of obesity, researchers have attempted to differentiate among factors that are truly genetic and sociocultural factors that are passed down through the generations. Bouchard and colleagues (3) estimated that approximately 25% of the variance in body fat percentage is due to genetics. Interestingly, these authors found that inheritance has a larger affect on total fat and deep deposits of adipose tissue than on subcutaneous fat. Lifestyle choices appear to have a greater impact on subcutaneous fat than do genetics. Additional evidence on the importance of genetics in the transmission of obesity comes from data demonstrating that the body mass index (BMI) (see chapter 9) of adopted children is more similar to their biological parents than to their adoptive parents (23). The recent discovery of a specific gene linked with obesity in mice provides additional evidence that genetics are important in determining the likelihood of obesity. The media attention on the inherited aspects of obesity may discourage those who are from families where many are overweight. Although genetics can be a major contributor to the development of obesity, the primary reason that an individual becomes obese is related to lifestyle. It is important that the HFI emphasize to clients that genetics may predispose one to obesity, but one still has the ability to make a significant impact on her or his body weight.

Lifestyle

The choices that one makes about caloric expenditure and caloric intake have a predominant impact on the development of obesity. The number of calories consumed, the types of foods eaten, and the amount of daily activity are essential contributing factors in assessing the influence of lifestyle on weight. If more calories are consumed than are expended, the positive caloric balance will result in weight (fat) gain. In order to lose fat weight, a

creeping obesity — Slow accumulation of adipose tissue with age.

positive caloric balance — A condition in which more calories are consumed than are expended, resulting in weight gain.

negative caloric balance must be established. This can be achieved through decreasing caloric intake and/or increasing caloric expenditure.

In Review: A positive caloric balance results in weight gain; a negative caloric balance results in weight loss.

Food Intake

When excess calories (particularly fat calories) are consumed, the energy is stored as fat. From an evolutionary standpoint, this is a positive adaptation to variations in food availability. In populations that have a relatively stable food supply, this mechanism results in excessive fat accumulation.

Health professionals argue about whether obese individuals typically consume more calories than their average weight counterparts. Dietary recall studies provide little clear information about this issue because people tend to underreport dietary intake and overestimate physical activity (16). Highly advanced research procedures in which people ingest isotopes of various molecules (doubly labeled water) indicate that overweight individuals expend and consume more calories than normal weight individuals (25). The higher energy expenditure is due to the metabolic cost of supporting the excess body weight. The reasons for consumption of extra calories are not well defined.

Types of Food Eaten and Obesity

When fat is consumed, it is more readily stored as fat than are either protein or carbohydrates. From a theoretical perspective, the low thermic effect of fat (i.e., the energy needed to digest, absorb, transport, and store fat), the ease with which fat is stored as adipose tissue, and the high-caloric density of high-fat foods make fat a likely culprit in the development of obesity.

Several studies indicate that obese and/or overweight individuals have a tendency to consume a higher percentage of calories from fat than normal weight individuals (8). It appears that the availability of foods high in fat and simple sugars puts individuals at higher risk for development of obesity. In cultures where the majority of calories consumed are complex carbohydrates, the rates of obesity are lower than in the United States. It is unclear whether palatability or sociocultural influences such as the frequent eating of fried foods in certain cultures, is more important in the food preferences and food choices of adults.

Daily Energy Expenditure

Data demonstrate that there is a relationship between low physical activity and the development of obesity (27). It is unclear, however, whether low physical activity leads to obesity or if obesity causes people to reduce their activity levels. The role of regular exercise in weight loss is complex and has been reviewed by several authors (11, 22, 26). Some studies have supported the role of exercise in the maintenance of fat-free mass and metabolic rate during periods of weight loss; whereas other researchers report little if any difference between caloric restriction with or without exercise. Although studies are equivocal in their findings of the short-term effects of exercise on weight loss, the long-term positive consequences of physical activity on weight maintenance are more clear. Exercise appears to be one of the strongest predictors of long-term weight maintenance (15, 27). Additionally, the positive physical and psychological benefits of regular physical activity, reviewed in chapter 1, make exercise a worthy investment regardless of its impact on weight.

In Review: Both genetics and lifestyle factors contribute to the development of obesity. Caloric intake, food choices, and daily physical activity are all aspects of lifestyle that have an impact on fat accumulation.

HEALTHY WAYS TO LOSE WEIGHT

There are numerous methods that can be used to lose weight. The HFI should encourage clients to choose weight loss techniques that are effective yet pose little threat to overall health. The following sections outline weight loss practices that can be implemented safely for the majority of adults.

Assessing Daily Caloric Need

Prior to designing an individualized weight loss program, it is often helpful to know the number of calories the client needs to sustain his or her current body weight. This can be done by estimating daily caloric need. **Daily caloric need** represents the number of calories a person needs to sustain current body weight and activity levels. The daily caloric need comprises the resting metabolic rate (RMR), the

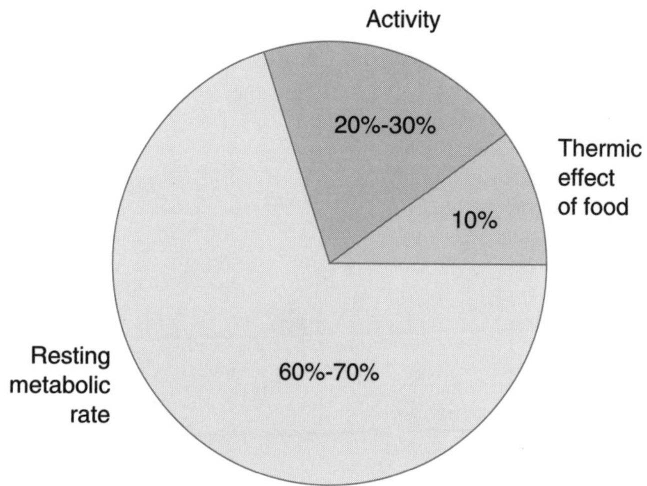

FIGURE 10.2 Contributors to daily caloric need.

thermic effect of food, and the calories used in daily activities (figure 10.2).

Resting metabolic rate (RMR) is the number of calories expended to maintain the body during resting conditions. For most individuals, RMR represents 60% to 70% of the daily caloric need. RMR is generally measured using indirect calorimetry. For reliable measurements of RMR, the assessment should occur when the client has not eaten for several hr; has not exercised vigorously for the past 12 hr; and has been in a resting, reclined position for 30 min (17). For these reasons, measuring RMR is not always practical; therefore, a number of equations have been developed to predict RMR. These RMR equations are based on the following principles:

- RMR is proportional to body size.
- RMR decreases with age.
- Muscle is more metabolically active than fat.

The larger the body size, the more calories it takes to sustain it. This relationship is reflected in all RMR equations. In addition to body size, age has a significant effect on RMR. As a person gets older, the RMR decreases, meaning that a person's daily caloric need will fall as he or she ages. Children typically have higher metabolic rates than adults of any age. RMR remains relatively stable during the early adult years; however, it begins to decline rather substantially after age 45. The effects of age and body size on RMR are reflected in the Revised Harris-Benedict equations (see page 188). Notice that these estimates of RMR use separate equations for males and females. This is because many males have more fat-free mass than females; and fat-free mass requires more energy to sustain it than does fat tissue.

If the HFI knows the fat-free mass of a client, the equation below can be used to predict RMR (7). There is no need for separate equations when fat-free mass is known because a gram of muscle has the same metabolic need whether it is housed in a male or a female body.

$$\text{RMR (kcal/day)} = 370 + (21.6 \times \text{fat-free mass in kg})$$

When attempting to determine daily caloric need, the HFI must also estimate the calories burned in physical activity. This assessment must contain information about work and leisure-time activity. Although there are numerous ways to gather information about daily activity, one method typically used is to have the client complete an activity log in which he or she records work and leisure activity. Once the activity pattern is established, the information in chapter 7 about the caloric cost of various activities

negative caloric balance — A condition in which less energy is consumed than is expended, resulting in a decrease in body weight.

daily caloric need — Number of calories needed to maintain current body weight. It is composed of **resting metabolic rate**, calories for activity, and the thermic effect of food.

resting metabolic rate (RMR) — Number of calories needed to sustain the body in a normal, resting condition.

Revised Harris-Benedict Equations for Estimating Resting Metabolic Rate (21)

Males:

RMR = 88.362 + (4.799 × ht) + (13.397 × wt) − (5.677 × age)

Females:

RMR = 447.593 + (3.098 × ht) + (9.247 × wt) − (4.33 × age)

RMR expressed in kilocalories per day
ht (height) expressed in centimeters
wt (weight) expressed in kilocalories
age expressed in years

can be used to estimate the energy burned in activity. Alternately, one can estimate daily caloric need using the methods outlined in the box on page 189.

The smallest part of the daily caloric need is the **thermic effect of food**. This is the energy needed to digest, absorb, transport, and store the food that is eaten. Although the types of food eaten may vary this value slightly, the thermic effect of food typically accounts for 10% of the daily caloric need (18).

Changing Lifestyle to Promote Weight Loss

Although each individual must assess which areas of her or his lifestyle most contribute to excessive weight accumulation, some common steps that would benefit the majority of people who are attempting to lose weight include the following:

- Reduce total calories.
- Reduce fat intake.
- Increase physical activity.
- Change eating behaviors.

As previously mentioned, a negative caloric balance must be established in order for weight loss to occur. The number of calories consumed while attempting to lose weight should be determined by the health of the client, the caloric need of the client, and the client's ultimate weight loss goals. The American College of Sports Medicine recommends that weekly weight loss goals should not exceed 1 kg (about 2.2 lb) per week (1). A general guideline is to establish a caloric deficit of 3500 to 7000 kcal per week (500 to 1000 kcal/day), which, theoretically, will result in a 1 to 2 lb loss of fat each week (1 lb of fat = 3500 kcal).

Most healthy adults can institute a daily caloric intake of 1000 to 1500 kcal/day without major adverse consequences; however, it is recommended that if a person is consuming 800 kcal per day or less a physician should supervise this severe caloric restriction (20). The ACSM recommends a daily caloric intake of no fewer than 1200 kcal/day (1). It should be noted that this is a general recommendation, and those with special needs (e.g., athletes, the elderly, people with metabolic disorders) may require a different caloric intake. With any caloric restriction, the potential negative side effects of decreases in RMR and fat-free mass can be expected. These negative side effects will be greater in those who establish large daily caloric deficits (20).

In Review: Assessing clients' daily caloric need provides guidelines for healthy weight loss. Daily caloric need is determined by the resting metabolic rate, the thermic effect of food, and activity levels. Some common steps from which many people who are attempting to lose weight could benefit are reducing total calories, decreasing fat intake, increasing physical activity, and changing eating behaviors.

Exercise Prescription for Weight Loss

From a theoretical perspective, the addition of exercise to one's everyday life can make a significant

Guidelines for Estimating Daily Caloric Need (9)

Once resting metabolic rate (RMR) has been assessed, use the following criteria for estimating daily caloric need. The calculated value will be a rough estimate of the calories needed to sustain current body weight.

- For a person who does little physical exertion during work (i.e., sitting most of the time) or recreation (i.e., no regular exercise routine), multiply RMR by 1.4.
- For those who are moderately active at work (i.e., walking and standing more than sitting) and/or who engage regularly (at least 3 days per week) in low to moderate exercise (e.g., walking or jogging), multiply RMR by 1.6.
- For individuals who are highly active at work (i.e., the job requires a large amount of physical exertion such as heavy lifting and carrying objects) and/or who engage regularly (4 or more days per week) in moderate to high activity (e.g., jogging or running), multiply RMR by 1.8.

Example:

Calculate the daily caloric need of a 50-year-old male office worker. He is 6'0" tall and weighs 215 lb. He walks 2 mi briskly 3 times per week but otherwise is rather inactive.

6 ft × 12 in./ft = 72 in.
72 in. × 2.54 cm/in. = 182.9 cm
215 lb divided by 2.2 lb/kg = 97.7 kg

1. Calculate RMR (see the box on page 188).
   RMR = 88.362 + (4.799 × ht) + (13.397 × wt) - (5.677 × age)
   RMR = 88.362 + (4.799 × 182.9) + (13.397 × 97.7) - (5.677 × 50)
   RMR = 1991 kcal per day
2. Add calories expended in activity

For a moderately active individual or one who engages in low to moderate activity 3 days per week, multiply RMR by 1.6.

Daily caloric need = RMR × 1.6
Daily caloric need = 1991 × 1.6 = 3186 kcal/day

alteration in one's weight. For example, if a person burns 100 kcal per day over his or her daily caloric need for a year, he or she will lose over 10 lb of fat. The ACSM recommends that a person attempting to lose weight combine exercise and moderate caloric restriction. Although debate continues over the precise contribution of exercise, this recommended combination appears to be the most effective in maintaining lean mass and avoiding excessive drops in

thermic effect of food — The energy needed to digest, absorb, transport, and store the food that is eaten.

RMR. A person who is attempting to lose weight should exercise at a low to moderate intensity for a length of time that will expend approximately 200 to 300 kcal.

According to ACSM guidelines (1), the initial exercise prescription for an obese person should be low-intensity aerobic exercise. The exercise session should be designed to expend approximately 200 to 300 kcal. As fitness improves, moderate-intensity exercise may become possible and the caloric expenditure may also be increased. Because of the excessive stress on the joints of obese individuals during weight-bearing exercise, low-impact activities (e.g., low-impact aerobics, walking, swimming) should be chosen to minimize the chance of orthopedic injury. The HFI should also be cognizant of the fact that obese individuals may feel self-conscious when exercising. Choosing an exercise setting that helps alleviate these feelings (such as specialized classes for weight loss) may improve exercise adherence.

It has also been suggested that some individuals who are restricting calories might benefit from resistance training. It should be understood that resistance training programs may help maintain (or even increase) lean body mass, but because of its relatively low caloric cost, it is not very effective in helping with weight loss. The HFI should encourage all participants to begin exercise, whether aerobic or resistance training, at low intensity and increase intensity slowly in order to decrease the chance of injury and encourage them to stick to the program (1).

In addition to the physical benefits of regular physical activity, psychological variables have also been reported to improve with exercise. Improvements in self-esteem and self-efficacy are commonly reported outcomes of engaging in regular exercise. The empowerment that comes from feeling oneself becoming more fit can add to the resolve to live a healthy lifestyle.

5 **In Review: Weight loss goals of 1 to 2 lb per week can be safely initiated by most healthy adults. The exercise prescription for weight loss should involve regular aerobic activity that burns 200 to 300 kcal per session. Resistance exercise may benefit weight loss efforts by maintaining or increasing lean mass. Keep joint stress and self-esteem issues in mind when choosing an exercise setting for people who are obese.**

BEHAVIOR MODIFICATION TECHNIQUES FOR WEIGHT LOSS AND MAINTENANCE

The majority of attempts to lose weight and maintain weight loss are unsuccessful. Behavior modification (changes in lifestyle habits and patterns) has been reported to be an important component of successful weight loss/weight maintenance programs (20). For additional information on behavior modification, see chapter 20 and refer to Randall Cottrell's book *Weight Control* (6).

Prior to beginning a weight loss program, it is important that individuals honestly assess their readiness for this task. Without a commitment to the time and effort involved in this endeavor, frustration is a likely outcome. This period of evaluation prior to beginning weight loss is called the "Preparation Stage" (see chapter 20). Brownell (4) suggested the use of "The Weight Loss Readiness Test" to help with this task. This questionnaire can be found in *The LEARN Program for Weight Control* published by the American Health Publishing Company (1-800-736-7323). The HFI should encourage all potential weight loss clients to examine their motivation for and commitment to weight loss.

If people are really committed to change, a number of strategies can be used to help improve the chances of long-term success. During the initial phase of weight loss (the "Action Stage"—see chapter 20), implementing these strategies requires a great deal of effort and there is a significant chance of failure (relapse). After 6 months or more of using these strategies (the "Maintenance Stage"—see chapter 20), changes in diet and lifestyle become a more natural part of one's routine. Some strategies shown to be effective for losing weight and maintaining weight loss are listed in the box on page 191. It should be remembered that not every client will respond well to the same techniques. Each situation should be considered separately, and an individualized weight loss/weight maintenance plan should be developed for each client.

Record Keeping

Prior to implementing a weight loss/weight maintenance program, it is wise to obtain information about the current eating patterns. This is most easily done through the use of an eating diary or food log. A sample food log and instructions are provided in

Strategies for Success in Weight Loss or Weight Maintenance

- Keeping records
- Planning meals and snacks
- Soliciting support
- Setting behavioral as well as outcome-oriented goals
- Developing a reward system
- Avoiding self-defeating behaviors
- Combining moderate caloric restriction with aerobic exercise
- Developing healthy eating patterns
- Committing to lifelong maintenance

chapter 8. Remember, it is important to gather information about the types and quantities of food eaten as well as the social and emotional circumstances surrounding eating.

Careful record keeping helps accomplish several objectives. First, food logs document the problem areas of food intake. Many individuals are unaware of the number of total calories or the amount of fat that they consume on a daily basis. Another important purpose of eating diaries is to document the social/emotional cues to eating. After a period of record keeping, individuals begin to recognize the factors, other than hunger, that lead to eating (e.g., socializing with friends, watching television, feeling stressed). In order to combat these cues to eating and, in many cases, overeating, the social and emotional situations one is in when one eats must be recognized and strategies developed to overcome them. A third major purpose of keeping eating records is to make eating a cognitive process. For many people eating is a habit, and the automatic choices that they make about how much and what to eat is done without conscious consideration. As discussed next, appropriate planning of meals and snacks is an important component in a successful weight loss plan.

Planning Meals and Snacks

Weight loss does not occur by accident; it takes a concentrated effort. Purchasing appropriate foods and planning meals is imperative in successful weight loss/weight maintenance. One of the most helpful practices in controlling food intake is avoiding the purchase of high-fat/high-caloric density food. If these foods are not in the home, the person will not be tempted to eat them. Substituting low-calorie and/or low-fat foods for high-calorie and/or high-fat foods can also have a substantial impact on weight loss. For example, substituting 1% milk for whole milk represents a decrease of approximately 50 kcal per cup. If a person drinks 2 c of milk per day, this will account for 36 500 kcal or 10.4 lb of fat intake in 1 year!

Meal planning is also essential. In households where the adults work outside of the home, there is little time for meal preparation. Buying breakfast foods that are quick to prepare, nutritious, and relatively low in calories (e.g., fresh fruit, bagels, low-fat yogurt, whole grain cereals) is helpful in providing a morning meal to offset hunger and provide important nutrients. Because many Americans are not at home for the noon meal, food choices are often dependent on the restaurants that are convenient, affordable, and quick. This leads many to visit fast-food restaurants. Although many of these restaurant chains have added lower fat items to their menus, the majority of fast-food items are high in both fat and calories. It has been shown that individuals who choose to eat fast foods are less successful at maintaining weight loss than those who avoid these food choices (12). Planning ahead might allow some individuals to carry their lunch to work and ensure that a variety of healthy, low-fat, low-calorie food choices are available for this important meal. The evening meal represents a significant percentage of the daily caloric intake of many Americans. It is not uncommon for individuals who may have limited their food intake during the day to overindulge at night. The effort to cook a meal often results in people choosing to eat at restaurants or purchase packaged meals that tend to be high in fat and calories. The effort necessary for cooking nutritious nightly meals can be reduced by the following:

- Cook and store meals ahead of time.
- Find a variety of quick and easy to prepare low-calorie meals.
- Purchase food items ahead of time to avoid unnecessary shopping.
- Keep a variety of fresh vegetables on hand to serve.

It is also important to consider what types of foods are available for snacks. Although avoiding food between meals may be ideal for many, there are times when food is needed between meals. Foods that provide nutrients and are also low calorie are the best choices (e.g, fresh fruit, raw vegetables, low-fat yogurt).

Establishing a Support System

A number of studies have shown the benefit that comes from having a support system when trying to lose weight (5). It is important to understand, however, that the source of the support will vary depending on the client. The support system may be a friend, spouse, significant other, parent, co-worker, therapist, or support group. No matter what the source of the support, the HFI should encourage clients in a weight loss/weight maintenance program to seek out individuals to encourage them in their efforts.

Many people are encouraged by the support of other people who are also attempting to lose weight. Many commercial weight loss centers provide support groups. These groups serve several functions: They provide a group to whom participants are accountable, a setting in which helpful hints and success stories can be shared, and a nonthreatening environment where all of the participants are ultimately chasing the same objective. For some people, the reasons for overeating are emotional and deeply rooted. In these cases, the guidance provided by a trained therapist may be needed.

Committing to Behavioral as Well as Outcome-Oriented Goals

It is important for clients to develop goals that encourage weight loss and healthy eating practices. Goal setting is important to help individuals remain focused on weight loss/weight maintenance. Goal setting should take place in a mutual exchange between the HFI and the client. The HFI's role is to provide information about healthy weight loss practices; the client is responsible for identifying the behavioral goals to which she or he is willing to commit.

Typically, weight loss is an outcome-oriented goal (i.e., the end result is the measure of success). In contrast to outcome goals, behavioral goals focus on the *process* of weight loss not the final outcome. Weight loss goals should be reasonable for the client involved and should follow the guidelines listed previously. Behavioral goals can be used to help make behavior/lifestyle changes that will have an impact on weight loss/weight maintenance. Among the areas that might be targeted by these goals are altering eating patterns, making wise food choices, and increasing daily energy expenditure. An example of a behavioral goal that might be implemented is "I will walk the stairs to my office daily rather than riding the elevator." More specific information on goal setting can be found in chapter 20.

Designing a Reward System

A part of human nature is the desire to be rewarded for accomplishing goals. When designing a weight loss program, it is wise to motivate the person losing weight by planning a way to reward success. As with goal setting, it is vital that the client be involved in developing the rewards that will be used. One rule that the HFI should encourage, however, is to avoid using food as a reward. It is important to establish a reward program that will recognize the achievement of both outcome-oriented and behavioral goals. This is important because the attainment of an outcome goal may take a substantial amount of time, longer than it may take to change certain behaviors. Also there will be times when a person's weight will plateau, and it is important that behavioral goals be rewarded during these times. Examples of rewards that might be suggested are

- purchasing new clothes,
- purchasing hobby items (e.g., books, compact discs, tools),
- taking a trip, and
- attending special events (movies, music and dance concerts, lectures).

Avoiding Self-Defeating Behaviors

For all of us, there are situations that increase the likelihood that overeating will occur. It is important when trying to lose weight to acknowledge these situations and institute measures to minimize the chance of falling victim to these self-defeating behaviors. For example, a person who has a tendency to snack on high-calorie foods late at night might avoid purchasing such foods and also implement a behavioral objective of not eating after 7:00 P.M. A person who loves pizza but tends to overindulge when going out to a restaurant might make pizza at home using low-fat ingredients and vegetables as toppings.

It is important to remember that we are all human. There are special times (birthdays, holiday dinners) when people will want to eat foods that are not a part of their weight loss plan. The HFI should explain to clients that there will be times when they will not meet all their behavioral objectives. A crucial factor for weight loss clients to keep in mind is that a lapse in eating (or activity) should not mean an end to the weight loss plan. The HFI should encourage individuals to immediately return to their healthy eating and exercise plan after the lapse. The HFI might help reduce some of the guilty feelings by helping the client view the lapse not as a failure but as an opportunity to renew his or her commitment to the weight loss/weight maintenance process.

Combining Moderate Caloric Restriction With Aerobic Exercise

Regular exercise has been shown to be an important facet of successful weight loss/weight maintenance programs. As mentioned previously, the ACSM and NIH support the use of exercise for weight loss and weight maintenance (1, 20). Regular aerobic activity expending 200 to 300 kcal each session is recommended for individuals attempting to lose weight.

Changing Unhealthy Eating Patterns

There are specific eating patterns that have been linked with excessive weight gain (6). Being aware of these behaviors and implementing plans to help avoid them increases the likelihood that weight loss techniques will be successful. These four changes in eating patterns are recommended:

- Slow down.
- Make wise substitutions.
- Keep variety in your diet.
- Eat smaller and fewer portions.

It is common for people to eat rapidly and then begin to feel uncomfortably full several minutes after they are finished eating. When food is eaten rapidly, inadequate time is allowed for the satiety mechanisms to help curb hunger. This results in people eating more than necessary before they realize that they are no longer hungry. Some ways that can help people slow their eating are to put down the eating utensil between bites, pause at least 30 s between bites, and chew food completely and swallow before taking another bite (6).

As mentioned previously, the substitution of foods that contain less fat and calories for foods that are high in fat and calories can make a significant contribution to reducing caloric intake. For example, if a person eats a roasted chicken breast without the skin instead of a fried chicken breast with the skin, approximately 160 kcal will be saved. It is important to remember that the wise consumer looks closely at both the total calories in a food as well as the calories that are contributed by fat. Not only will reducing fat intake help with weight control, it will also help improve the blood lipid profile.

One problem faced when trying to lose weight is "diet burnout." It is not uncommon to find people on "diets" who consume only certain foods. To help avoid becoming bored and frustrated with one's diet, it is important to consume a variety of healthy, low-calorie, and tasty foods. This objective is linked to the planning process that was described previously. Maintaining variety in the diet not only helps avoid boredom but also provides nutritional balance.

When one is attempting to lose weight, one of the most helpful changes is to decrease the portion size as well as the number of portions consumed. Many people are in the habit of completely filling their plates and eating everything that is on the plate. Additionally, one of the ways that Americans demonstrate to their host or hostess that the food is being enjoyed is by eating extra portions. Taking smaller portions of foods as well as avoiding "seconds" will make a significant contribution to caloric restriction.

Committing to Lifelong Maintenance

It is important to remember that weight loss is only a temporary condition unless a plan is in place to maintain the loss. In examining the variables that predict success in maintaining weight loss, Lavery and Loewy (15) concluded, "There are no quick-fix, easy solutions to obesity. The solution is the harsh realization of the need for permanent lifestyle changes to maintain a desired weight status." The HFI should help clients understand the need to commit to long-term lifestyle changes rather than focus solely on short-term weight loss goals.

6 **In Review: Some strategies leading to successful weight loss are keeping records, planning meals and snacks, developing a support system, designing a reward system, committing to both outcome-oriented and behavioral goals, avoiding self-defeating behaviors, combining moderate caloric restriction with aerobic exercise, changing unhealthy eating patterns, and committing to lifelong weight maintenance. People who are committed to long-term weight loss and lifestyle changes are more successful at maintaining their desired weight.**

GIMMICKS AND GADGETS FOR WEIGHT LOSS

Over the years numerous devices have been marketed for weight loss. The majority of these devices are ineffective, and, unfortunately, some are potentially harmful.

Saunas and sweat suits have, at times, been recommended to help weight loss by burning off or melting away fat. This is a false claim. These devices may induce short-term (i.e., a number of hours) loss of weight due to dehydration. These devices do not burn fat but can cause people to sweat profusely. Overuse of saunas and sweat suits can potentially lead to severe dehydration. Furthermore, the increase in core temperature that is caused by these devices could be potentially harmful to fetuses during the first trimester of pregnancy.

Other devices such as vibrating belts, body wraps, and electrical stimulators have been used in an attempt to lose weight. While these devices may not be harmful, they do not lead to weight loss. The money spent on these useless devices would be better spent on proven techniques. Additionally, if one puts faith and effort into these unproven techniques, one may delay making lifestyle changes that could lead to long-term weight changes.

A widely held myth is that exercise emphasizing a particular body part will cause that area to lose fat quicker than the rest of the body. This false theory is called **spot reduction**. Sit-ups are commonly used exercises that people perform in an attempt to decrease their waistlines. Sit-ups can be terrific exercises for increasing the muscular strength and endurance of the abdominal muscles, but they are not very effective for burning fat. As a person establishes a caloric deficit through regular aerobic exercise, fat loss will occur all over the body, not just the parts where he or she would like to see the decrease!

Programs that advertise rapid, large weight losses are typically deceptive. The rapid weight losses seen at the beginning of such a "diet" are primarily the result of reductions in water weight. It is also important to understand that dietary plans that establish extremely large caloric deficits will result in substantial reductions in RMR and lean body mass and do not establish healthy, lifelong eating habits. As stated earlier, anyone attempting to reduce daily caloric intake to 800 kcal or less should be under a physician's supervision (20).

In Review: A number of "quick fixes" for weight loss are marketed, but these products are at best ineffective and at worst potentially dangerous.

BODY WEIGHT AND PSYCHOLOGICAL FACTORS

It is crucial to understand that a single psychological profile does not apply to all individuals who are obese because a great deal of psychological heterogeneity exists in this population. It does not appear that depression, anxiety, or other pathopsychological conditions are more prevalent among obese individuals than among people with an average weight (10, 24). One condition that does appear to be more common in obese individuals than normal weight individuals is binge eating disorder (see following section), but it must be understood that not all people who are obese exhibit this eating behavior (10). Although overeating may be driven by emotional and/or psychological factors in some people, every situation must be examined on an individual basis.

The psychological consequences of dieting, weight loss, and weight gain have been recently reviewed (10, 24). In general, positive changes in psychological variables (e.g., mood, depression) that might result from weight loss typically disappear if the weight is regained. With successful weight loss and weight maintenance, generally positive changes in self-esteem and self-efficacy can be expected (10). It is important to note, however, that a formerly obese individual may find that his or her relationships with others will change. For example, some find the attention generated by their weight loss uncomfortable.

> **8** **In Review: People who are obese do not fit a single psychological profile. Typically, improvements in self-esteem and self-efficacy result when people make positive lifestyle changes.**

DISORDERED EATING PATTERNS

There are conditions in which the eating pattern of an individual has a negative impact on his or her health. **Eating disorders** are clinically diagnosed conditions in which the unhealthy eating patterns may lead to severe declines in health and even to death. **Anorexia nervosa, bulimia nervosa,** and **binge eating disorder** are three of the eating disorders recognized by the American Psychiatric Association (APA) (2). **Disordered eating** refers to subclinical, unhealthy eating patterns that are often the precursors of eating disorders.

In America, anorexia nervosa and bulimia nervosa occur at a rate of 0.5% to 1% and 2% to 4%, respectively (13). No single mechanism has been identified as the primary cause of disordered eating and/or eating disorders. It appears that genetic/biological, psychological, as well as sociocultural factors may predispose one for these conditions. The groups in the American population in which these conditions are most common are young women from middle- and high-socioeconomic environments and female athletes in sports that emphasize extreme leanness. It is hypothesized that the social pressure to be thin as well as discomfort with their developing sexuality contribute to unhealthy eating patterns in young women. For female athletes, the pressure to perform in some sports is, unfortunately, linked with extremely low body weights. For example, it is commonly reported that more than 60% of female gymnasts exhibit some type of disordered eating pattern (13).

Anorexia nervosa is an eating disorder in which a preoccupation with body weight leads to self-starvation. People with anorexia nervosa typically view themselves as overweight even when their weight is substantially below normal. The APA lists the following criteria for diagnosis of anorexia nervosa (2):

- Purposefully maintaining weight at less than 85% of expected weight for age and height
- Extreme fear of gaining weight and/or fat
- Unhealthy body image in which the person views her- or himself as overweight even when underweight; often associated with a severe intertwining of body image and self-esteem and/or a disregard for the seriousness of maintaining an extremely low body weight
- Absence of at least three consecutive menstrual cycles in postmenarchal women

Bulimia nervosa is characterized by consuming large amounts of food followed by periods of food purging (2). Misuse of laxatives, self-induced vomiting, and excessive exercise are among the methods that may be used to purge. To meet the diagnostic criteria established by the APA, one must engage in this behavior at least two times a week for a period of 3 months. Patients with bulimia nervosa, similar to those suffering from anorexia nervosa, have an impaired body image and a fear of losing control over their body weight. Both anorexia nervosa and bulimia nervosa should be considered life-threatening disorders.

Binge eating disorder is characterized by consuming large amounts of food in short periods of time (2). Unlike bulimia nervosa, binge eating is not associated with purging. Binge episodes are often initiated by emotional/psychological cues (e.g., loneliness, anxiety) rather than by physical hunger. These binges typically occur when alone and may be followed by feelings of shame, guilt, and depression.

spot reduction — The myth that exercise emphasizing a particular body part will cause that area to lose fat quicker than the rest of the body.

eating disorders — Clinical eating patterns that result in severe negative health consequences.

anorexia nervosa — An eating disorder in which a preoccupation with body weight leads to self-starvation.

bulimia nervosa — An eating disorder characterized by consuming large amounts of food followed by periods of food purging.

binge eating disorder — An eating disorder characterized by consuming large amounts of food in a short period of time.

disordered eating — Unhealthy eating pattern that can in some cases be a precursor to eating disorders.

To achieve a clinical diagnosis of binge eating disorder, a person must engage in at least two periods of bingeing per week for 6 months (2). The prevalence of binge eating disorder in the general population has been estimated at 2%. In contrast, 25% to 70% of obese individuals seeking treatment for weight loss may suffer from this disorder (24).

Recognition of the signs of disordered eating is necessary prior to successful intervention. The box below lists some of the common signs of disordered eating. If these signs are seen by the HFI, it is important that the individual be confronted; however, many people when approached about this issue will deny the existence of a problem. Gentle questions about the client's health (e.g., "How are you feeling?" or "You look a little tired.") is one way to attempt to break the ice on this very delicate subject. Successful intervention for eating disorders requires a multidisciplinary approach combining medical, nutritional, and psychological professionals. A knowledge of local support groups or professionals who work with patients suffering from eating disorders will allow the HFI to recommend places for clients to go for help.

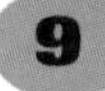

In Review: Eating disorders can significantly impair health and may even result in death. Anorexia nervosa, bulimia nervosa, and binge eating disorder are three eating disorders recognized by the American Psychiatric Association. HFIs should be aware of signs that may indicate a client has an eating disorder. Intervention for eating disorders should be multidisciplinary and should include psychological counseling.

STRATEGIES FOR GAINING WEIGHT

Before concluding this chapter it is important to mention that some individuals struggle to *increase*

Signs of Disordered Eating

- A preoccupation with food, calories, and weight
- Repeatedly expressed concerns about being or feeling fat, even when weight is average or below average
- Increasing self-criticism of one's body
- Secretly eating or stealing food
- Eating large meals, then disappearing or making trips to the bathroom
- Consumption of large amounts of food not consistent with the individual's weight
- Bloodshot eyes, especially after trips to the bathroom
- Swollen parotid glands at the angle of the jaw, giving a chipmunk-like appearance
- Vomitus, or odor of vomitus in the bathroom
- Wide fluctuations in weight over short periods of time
- Periods of severe caloric restriction
- Excessive laxative use
- Compulsive, excessive exercise that is not part of the individual's training regimen
- Unwillingness to eat in front of others
- Expression of self-deprecating thoughts following eating
- Wearing baggy or layered clothing
- Mood swings
- Appearing preoccupied with the eating behavior of others
- Continuous drinking of diet soda or water

Adapted from Johnson 1994.

Tips for Gaining Weight

- Increase caloric intake by 200 to 1000 kcal per day. This can be done by increasing meal size, number of meals, or number of between-meal snacks.
- Increase the number of healthy snacks consumed. Choose bread, fruit, granola, and other nutritious foods.
- The majority of additional calories consumed should be complex carbohydrates (e.g., pasta, bread, rice, potatoes).
- Add resistance training to the daily routine. Weight training is an effective means for increasing the body's fat-free mass.
- Increase consumption of milk and fruit juices. These excellent choices not only provide additional calories, but they also provide essential nutrients.

their body weight. The HFI should encourage these individuals to attempt to accumulate fat-free mass rather than all-fat weight. Above are some tips for increasing weight over time. It is important to note that when individuals continually lose weight or struggle to gain weight a physician should be consulted about the possibility of underlying conditions.

10 **In Review: The additional calories needed to increase weight should come from increasing the number of healthy snacks and/or the size of meals. The addition of resistance training to one's exercise routine may prove helpful in increasing muscle mass.**

Case Study

You can check your answers by referring to appendix A.

10.1

Mr. Jones is a healthy, sedentary 50-year-old male. At his last medical examination, his physician suggested that he lose weight and begin an exercise program. Mr. Jones weighs 215 lb, is 6′0″ tall, and has 29% body fat.

1. Assuming that Mr. Jones would like to reach 20% body fat, calculate his target weight.
2. Use the Revised Harris-Benedict equation for males to predict Mr. Jones' resting metabolic rate.
3. Assuming that Mr. Jones' RMR contributes 70% of his daily caloric need, calculate the number of calories Mr. Jones needs each day to maintain his current body weight.
4. Based on these calculations, recommend a daily caloric intake and an exercise plan that will help him safely reach his goal of 20% body fat.

SOURCE LIST

1. American College of Sports Medicine (1995)
2. American Psychiatric Association (1994)
3. Bouchard, Perusse, Leblanc, Tremblay, & Theriault (1988)
4. Brownell (1994)
5. Brownell & Kramer (1989)
6. Cottrell (1992)
7. Cunningham (1991)
8. Drewnowski (1994)
9. Food & Nutrition Board, National Research Council (1989)
10. Foster & Wadden (1994)
11. Grilo, Brownell, & Stunkard (1993)
12. Holden et al. (1992)
13. Johnson (1994)
14. Kuczmarski, Flegal, Campbell, & Johnson (1994)
15. Lavery & Loewy (1993)
16. Lichtman et al. (1992)
17. Molé (1990)
18. Montoye, Kemper, Saris, & Washburn (1996)
19. National Institutes of Health Consensus Development Panel (1985)

20. National Institutes of Health Technology Assessment Conference Panel (1993)
21. Roza & Shizgal (1984)
22. Saris (1993)
23. Stunkard et al. (1986)
24. Wadden & Stunkard (1993)
25. Welle, Forbes, Statt, Barnard, & Amatruda (1992)
26. Whatley & Poehlman (1994)
27. Williamson et al. (1993)

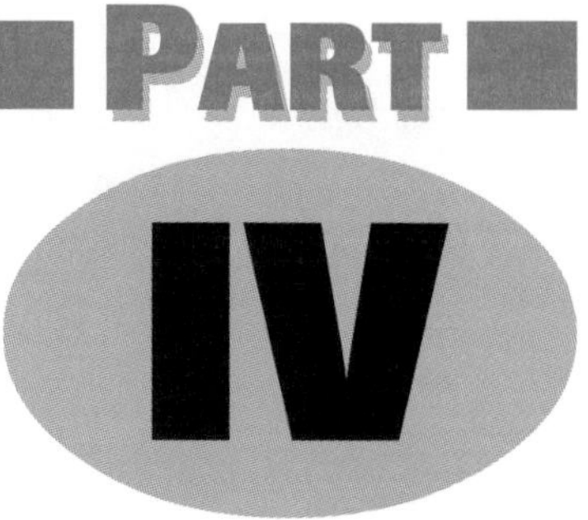

Part IV

Components of Fitness

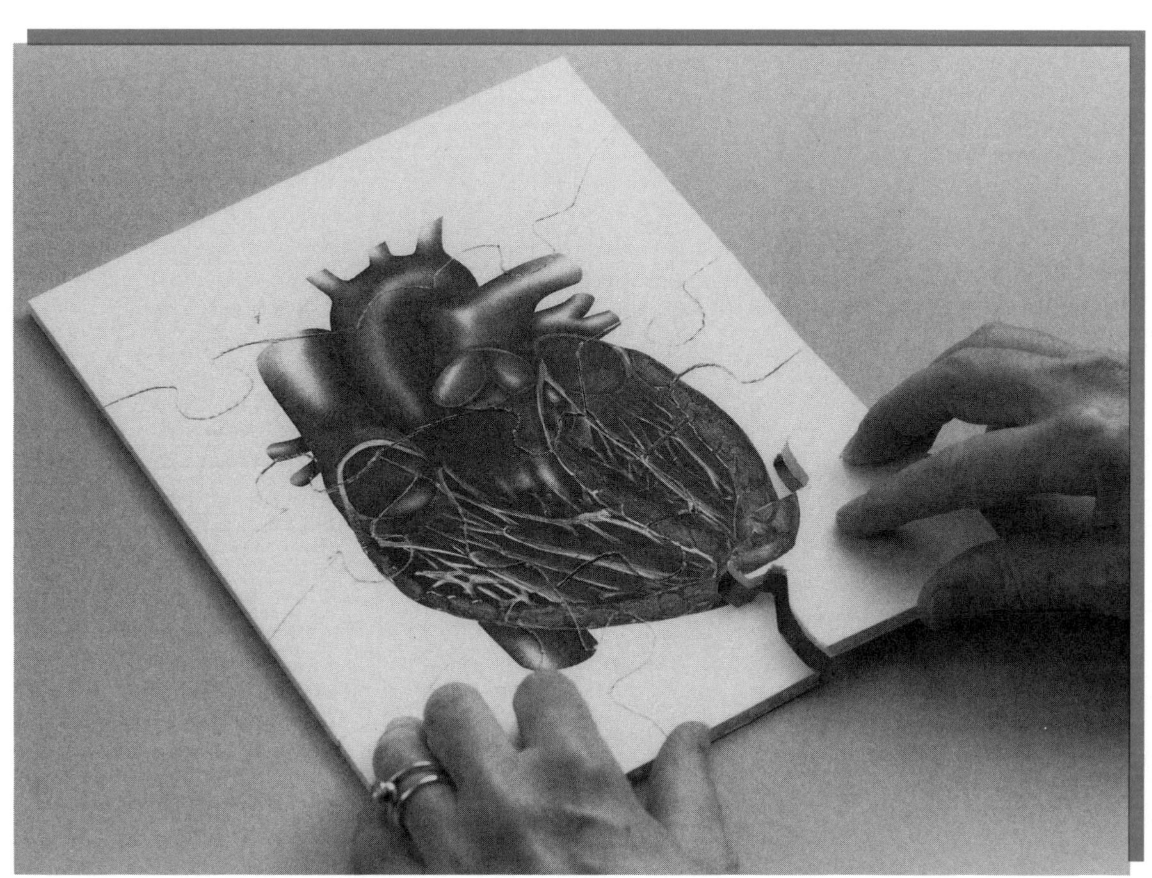

Part IV describes the components of physical fitness and assessment techniques for cardiorespiratory fitness (chapter 11), muscular strength and endurance (chapter 12), and flexibility and low-back function (chapter 13).

CHAPTER

11

Cardiorespiratory Fitness

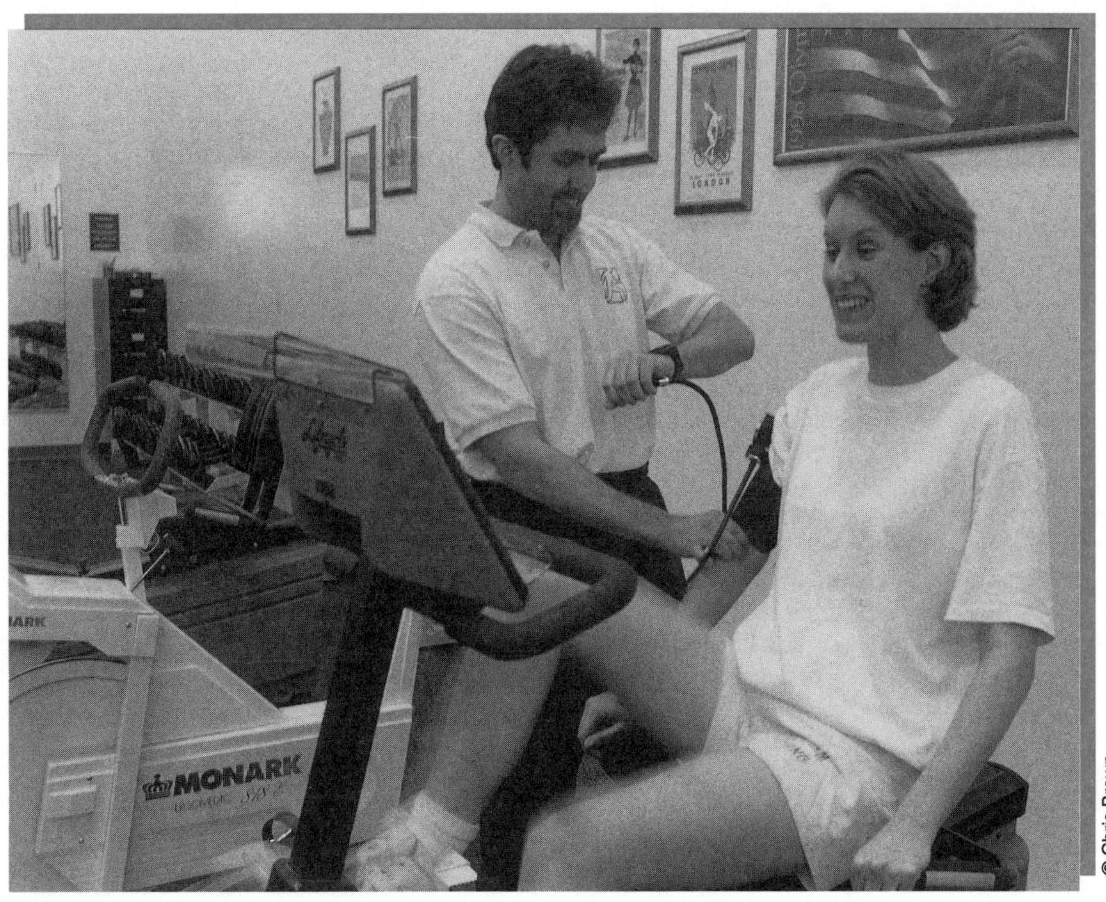

The reader will be able to: **OBJECTIVES**

1. **Describe the relationship of cardiorespiratory fitness (CRF) to health and list reasons for doing CRF testing as well as risks associated with CRF testing.**
2. **Present a logical sequence of testing.**
3. **Describe procedures for conducting walking and jogging/running field tests to estimate CRF.**
4. **Contrast the treadmill, cycle ergometer, and bench step as instruments to use in doing graded exercise tests (GXTs).**
5. **List variables measured during a GXT.**
6. **Describe procedures used prior to, during, and following testing.**
7. **Contrast submaximal and maximal GXTs.**
8. **Describe the heart rate extrapolation procedures to estimate $\dot{V}O_2$max using submaximal treadmill, cycle, and bench step GXTs.**

The usual introduction to cardiorespiratory fitness (CRF) delineates heart disease as the major cause of death and proceeds to describe the role of exercise in prevention and rehabilitation programs. It is also important, however, to focus attention on a high level of CRF as a normal, lifelong goal that makes life more enjoyable. That alone merits the inclusion of CRF in any discussion about positive health. Cardiorespiratory fitness, also called cardiovascular, or aerobic, fitness, is a good measure of the heart's ability to pump oxygen-rich blood to the muscles. Although the terms *cardio-* (heart), *vascular* (blood vessels), *respiratory* (lungs and ventilation), and *aerobic* (working with oxygen) differ technically, they all reflect different aspects of this component of fitness. The person with a healthy heart can pump great volumes of blood with each beat and will have a high level of CRF. CRF values are expressed in the following ways:

- Liters of oxygen used by the body per minute ($L \cdot min^{-1}$)
- Milliliters of oxygen used per kilogram of body weight per minute ($ml \cdot kg^{-1} \cdot min^{-1}$)
- METs, multiples of resting metabolic rate, where 1 MET = $3.5\ ml \cdot kg^{-1} \cdot min^{-1}$

A person with the ability to use $35\ ml \cdot kg^{-1} \cdot min^{-1}$ during maximal exercise is said to have a CRF equal to 10 METs ($35 \div 3.5 = 10$). Aerobic training programs increase the heart's ability to pump blood, so it is no surprise that CRF improves as a result of such programs.

Chapter 4 described how CRF variables respond to acute, or short-term exercise. Chapter 14 explains how to recommend activities to clients to improve their CRF. This chapter emphasizes the evaluation of CRF. The reader is referred to other resources for additional detail (2, 10, 19).

Historically, measurements of heart rate (HR), blood pressure (BP), and the electrocardiogram (ECG) taken at rest were used to evaluate CRF. In addition, some static pulmonary function tests (e.g., vital capacity) were used to characterize respiratory function. It became clear, however, that measurements made at rest told a physician little about the way a person's cardiorespiratory system responds to physical activity. We are now familiar with the use of a graded exercise test (GXT) to evaluate HR, ECG, BP, ventilation, and oxygen uptake responses during work.

WHY TEST CARDIORESPIRATORY FITNESS?

The results from cardiorespiratory fitness tests are used to write exercise recommendations and allow the HFI or physician to evaluate positive or negative changes in CRF as a result of physical conditioning, aging, illness, or inactivity. Given the recent increase in obesity and inactivity in children, it makes good sense to include an evaluation of CRF throughout life, from early childhood to old age. This information can serve as a marker of where the individual stands relative to health-criterion test scores, and it will alert the individual to subtle changes in lifestyle that may compromise positive health. The nature of the tests and the level of monitoring should vary across age groups to reflect the type of information that is needed.

CRF testing depends on the purpose(s) of the test, the type of person to be evaluated, and the work tasks available. Reasons for testing include

- determining physiological responses at rest and during **submaximal** and/or **maximal** work,
- providing a basis for exercise programming,
- screening for coronary heart disease (CHD), and
- determining one's ability to perform a specific work task.

The choice of an appropriate test depends on several factors. People differ in age, fitness levels, known health problems, and risks of CHD. Also, financial considerations determine the amount of time that can be devoted to each individual and the type of work tasks available.

RISKS OF CRF TESTING

As indicated in chapter 1, the risks associated with exercise testing are quite low, with the risk of a complication requiring hospitalization being 1 in 1000, and the risk of death being 1 in 10 000 (2). Health professionals should emphasize that the overall risk of a cardiovascular problem is greater for those who maintain sedentary habits than for those who take an exercise test and then embark on a regular exercise program (27, 39, 44). This is consistent with evidence showing that low levels of cardiorespiratory fitness are directly related to a higher risk of heart disease and death (11).

In Review: Cardiorespiratory fitness is an important aspect of quality of life for healthy individuals, as well as a risk factor for coronary heart disease. The ability to utilize oxygen during exercise is the basis for this fitness component and can be expressed in $L \cdot min^{-1}$, $ml \cdot kg^{-1} \cdot min^{-1}$, and METs. CRF testing is used for exercise programming, screening for heart disease, and determining one's ability to do a specific work task. The risk of death due to exercise testing is very low, 1 in 10 000.

TESTING SEQUENCE

A logical sequence for fitness testing (and activities) can be followed when people come to the same fitness center over a substantial period of time. This sequence progresses from the initial screening to fitness testing and programming, with opportunities for periodic retesting and revision of the program as fitness gains are made. The box on page 204 lists the sequence of testing and activity prescription. The rest of this section describes the process in detail. For people who come in for fitness testing but do not have continuing involvement with the fitness center, the submaximal and maximal tests are usually done on the same day and are a part of the same GXT protocol.

Informed Consent

Fitness participants should be informed volunteers. The fitness program should clearly describe all of its procedures and the potential risks and benefits of the fitness tests and activities. The participants

submaximal — Less than maximal (e.g., an exercise that can be performed with less than maximal effort).

maximal — The highest level possible, such as maximal heart rate or oxygen uptake.

Sequence of Testing and Activity Prescription

Step	Test or activity
1.	Informed consent
2.	Health history
3.	Screening
4.	Resting CRF, body composition, and psychological tests
5.	Submaximal CRF
6.	Tests for low-back function
7.	Begin light activity program here
8.	Tests for muscular strength and endurance
9.	Maximal CRF
10.	Revise activity program; include games and sports here
11.	Periodic retest (and activity revision)

should understand that their individual data will be confidential and that any test or activity can be terminated at any time should they feel uncomfortable. A written **informed consent** form should be signed by the participant after reading a description of the program and having all questions answered. A sample consent form is included in chapter 23.

Health History

Chapter 3 describes procedures for determining current health status. This information can be used to determine appropriate testing protocol and activity recommendations. In addition, follow-up testing should be advised for people with symptoms of health problems. Referrals to other professionals might be warranted based on the person's history.

Screening

We recommended in chapter 3 that individuals have regular medical examinations and health screening and engage in moderate-intensity exercise. Fitness programs need to determine whether the person needs medical permission to be in a fitness program involving vigorous-intensity activities. People with CHD or other known major health problems must have medical supervision or clearance before embarking on any fitness testing or program that goes beyond moderate-intensity exercise.

We've listed on page 205 the conditions (absolute contraindications) that the ACSM has identified in which the risk of testing outweighs the possible benefits. Other conditions (relative contraindications) may increase the risk of exercise testing; people with these conditions should only be tested if the medical judgment is that the need for the test outweighs the potential risk.

Apparently healthy people who have no known major health problems or symptoms can be tested or begin the type of fitness program recommended in this book with minimal risk. Chapter 3 identifies the people who need medical clearance, a carefully supervised program, and educational information about health problems and behaviors.

Resting Measurements

Typical resting tests may include CRF measures (e.g., 12-lead ECG, HR, BP, blood chemistry profile) as well as other fitness variables such as body composition and psychological traits. Evaluation of the ECG by a physician determines whether any abnormalities require further medical attention. People with extreme BP or blood chemistry values (see chapter 3) should also be referred to their personal physicians.

Submaximal Tests to Estimate CRF

If the resting tests reflect normal values, then a submaximal test is administered. The submaximal

Contraindications to Exercise Testing

Absolute contraindications:

1. A recent significant change in the resting ECG suggesting infarction or other acute cardiac event
2. Recent complicated myocardial infarction (unless patient is stable and pain-free)
3. Unstable angina
4. Uncontrolled ventricular arrhythmia
5. Uncontrolled atrial arrhythmia that compromises cardiac function
6. Third degree AV heart block without pacemaker
7. Acute congestive heart failure
8. Severe aortic stenosis
9. Suspected or known dissecting aneurysm
10. Active or suspected myocarditis or pericarditis
11. Thrombophlebitis or intracardiac thrombi
12. Recent systemic or pulmonary embolus
13. Acute infections
14. Significant emotional distress (psychosis)

Relative contraindications:

1. Resting diastolic blood pressure > 115 mmHg or resting systolic blood pressure > 200 mmHg
2. Moderate valvular heart disease
3. Known electrolyte abnormalities (hypokalemia, hypomagnesemia)
4. Fixed-rate pacemaker (rarely used)
5. Frequent or complex ventricular ectopy
6. Ventricular aneurysm
7. Uncontrolled metabolic disease (e.g., diabetes, thyrotoxicosis, or myxedema)
8. Chronic infectious disease (e.g., mononucleosis, hepatitis, AIDS)
9. Neuromuscular, musculoskeletal, or rheumatoid disorders that are exacerbated by exercise
10. Advanced or complicated pregnancy

Reprinted from American College of Sports Medicine 1995.

test usually provides the HR and BP responses to different intensities of work, from light intensity up to a predetermined point (usually 85% of predicted maximum HR). This test can use a bench step, cycle ergometer, or treadmill. Once again, if unusual responses to the submaximal test appear, then the person is referred for further medical tests. If the results appear normal, then an activity program is

informed consent — A procedure used to obtain a person's voluntary permission to participate in a program. Informed consent requires a description of the procedures to be used as well as the potential benefits and risks and written consent of the participant.

begun at intensities less than those reached on the test (e.g., a person goes to 85% of maximum HR on the test and starts the fitness program at 70%). After the person has become accustomed to regular exercise and appears to be adjusting to fitness activities, a maximal test can be administered.

Submaximal tests also can be used to estimate maximal functional capacity (maximal oxygen uptake) by extrapolating HR to a predicted maximum, then using the linear relationship between HR and oxygen uptake to estimate maximal oxygen uptake. Although this estimated maximum is useful for evaluating a person's current status and prescribing or revising exercise, there is considerable error involved in the estimation. In addition to measuring submaximal CRF, measurements of flexibility and muscular strength and endurance (especially related to low-back function) are often included at this stage (see chapters 12 and 13).

Maximal Tests to Estimate or Measure CRF

If no problems occur up to this point, a maximal test is administered. Two basic types of maximal tests are used to indicate CRF: laboratory tests involving the measurement of physiological responses (e.g., HR, BP) to increasing levels of work and all-out endurance performance tests (e.g., time on a 1-mi run). The results of the maximal test can be used to revise the activity program (i.e., the person's maximal functional capacity provides a new basis for selection of fitness activities). The person's measured maximal HR should now be used for determining target HR (instead of using the estimated maximal HR).

Program Modification and Periodic Retests

After a minimum level of fitness has been achieved, a wider variety of activities (e.g., games, sports) can be included in the fitness program. All of the tests should be retaken periodically to determine the progress being made and to revise the program in areas where the gains are not as great as desired.

2 **In Review: A logical sequence of steps to follow in fitness testing includes informed consent, health history, screening, resting CRF, submaximal CRF and other tests, light activity prescription, maximal CRF, program modification, and periodic retesting.** **(See the box on page 206.)**

FIELD TESTS

There are a variety of field tests that can be used to obtain an estimate of CRF. These are called "field tests" because they require very little equipment, can be done just about anywhere, and use the simple activities of walking and running. Because these tests involve running or walking as fast as possible over a set distance, they are *not recommended* at the start of an exercise program. Instead, we recommend that participants complete the graduated walking program before taking the walking test, and the graduated jogging program before taking the running test. The walk/jog programs are found in chapter 17. The graduated nature of the fitness program allows participants to start at a low and safe level of activity and gradually improve. It is then appropriate to administer an endurance run test to evaluate fitness status.

Field tests rely on the observation that for one to walk or run at high speeds over long distances, the heart must pump great volumes of oxygen to the muscles. It is in this way that the average speed maintained in these walk/run tests gives an estimate of CRF. The higher the CRF score, the greater the heart's capacity to transport oxygen. An endurance run of a set distance for a given time, or a set time for a given distance, provides information about a person's CR endurance as long as it is 1 mi or more. The advantages of an endurance run test include its moderately high correlation to maximum oxygen uptake, the use of a natural activity, and the large numbers of participants that can be tested in a short period of time. The disadvantages of endurance running are that it is difficult to monitor physiological responses, that other factors affect the outcome (e.g., motivation), and that it cannot be used for graded or submaximal testing.

1-Mi-Walk Test

A 1-mi-walk test to predict CRF has been developed to accommodate individuals of different ages and fitness levels. Follow the steps on page 209 to administer the mile-walk test.

Steps to Administer the Mile-Walk Test

Step **Activity**

Before test day

1. Arrange to have the following elements at the test site:
   - A person to start and read the time from a stopwatch
   - A partner with a watch (with a second hand) for each walker (perhaps with a sheet to mark off laps)
   - A stopwatch for the timer (with a spare ready)
   - A score sheet or scorecard
2. Explain the purpose of the test (i.e., to determine how fast they can walk a mile, which reflects the endurance of their cardiovascular system).
3. Select and mark off (if needed) a level area for the walk.
4. Explain to people being tested that they are to walk the mile in the fastest time possible. Only walking is allowed, and the goal is to cover the distance as fast as possible.

Test day

1. Participants warm up with stretching and slow walking.
2. Several people will walk at the same time.
3. The procedure is explained again.
4. The timer says, "Ready, go," and starts the stopwatch.
5. Each individual has a partner with a watch with a second hand.
6. The partner counts the laps and tells the individual at the end of each lap how many more lap(s) to walk.
7. The timer calls out the minutes and seconds as each person finishes the mile walk.
8. The partner listens for the time when his or her walker finishes the mile and records it (to the nearest second) immediately on a scorecard.
9. The walker takes a 10-s HR immediately after the end of the mile walk while the partner times.

In this test the individual walks as fast as possible on a measured track, and heart rate is measured at the end of the mile. The following equation is used to calculate $\dot{V}O_2max$ (ml · kg^{-1} · min^{-1}):

$$\dot{V}O_2max = 132.853 - 0.0769\ (\text{weight}) - 0.3877\ (\text{age}) + 6.315\ (\text{gender}) - 3.2649\ (\text{time}) - 0.1565\ (\text{HR})$$

where (weight) is body weight in pounds, (age) is in years, (gender) equals 0 for female and 1 for male, (time) is in minutes and hundredths of minutes, and (HR) is in beats · min^{-1}. The formula was developed and validated on men and women ages 30 to 69 years (32).

QUESTION: What is the CRF of a 25-year-old, 170-lb man who walks the mile in 20 min and has an immediate postexercise heart rate of 140 beats · min^{-1}?

Answer:

$\dot{V}O_2max = 132.853 - 0.0769 \text{ (weight)} - 0.3877 \text{ (age)} + 6.315 \text{ (gender)} - 3.2649 \text{ (time)} - 0.1565 \text{ (HR)}$

$\dot{V}O_2max = 132.853 - 0.0769\ (170) - 0.3877\ (25) + 6.315\ (1) - 3.2649\ (20.0) - 0.1565\ (140)$

$\dot{V}O_2max = 29.2 \text{ ml} \cdot \text{kg}^{-1} \cdot \text{min}^{-1}$

To simplify the steps in using this 1-mi-walk test, table 11.1 was generated on the basis of the above formula for men weighing 170 lb and women weighing 125 lb. For each 15 lb beyond these weights, subtract 1 ml · kg^{-1} · min^{-1}.

To use table 11.1, find the part of the table for the individual's gender and age, then go across the top until you find the time (to the nearest minute) it took to walk a mile, and then go down that column until it intersects with the person's postexercise HR (listed on the left side). The number at which the mile time and postexercise HR meet is the CRF value in terms of ml · kg^{-1} · min^{-1}. For example, a 25-year-old man who walked the mile in 20 min and had a postexercise HR of 140 would have an estimated maximal oxygen uptake of 29.2 ml · kg^{-1} · min^{-1}. You can evaluate cardiorespiratory fitness by using that number to compare with the standards presented in table 11.2. In the example of the 25-year-old man, his maximal oxygen uptake is less than 30, indicating a need for improvement. The standards in table 11.2 represent the levels of oxygen uptake for females and males with regard to health-related fitness. Those wishing to focus on performance should strive for higher values.

Jog/Run Test

One of the most common CRF field tests is the 12-min or 1.5-mi run popularized by Cooper (16). The idea in this test is very much like the walk test mentioned above: Jog or run as fast as possible for 12 min or for 1.5 mi. This test is based on original work by Balke (8), who showed that 10- to 20-min running tests could be used to estimate $\dot{V}O_2$max. Balke found the optimal duration to be 15 min. The test is based on the relationship between running velocity and the oxygen uptake required to run at that velocity (figure 11.1). The greater the running speed, the greater the oxygen uptake required. The reason for the duration of 12 to 15 min is that the running test has to be long enough to diminish the contribution of anaerobic sources of energy (immediate and short-term) to the average velocity. In essence, the average velocity that can be maintained in a 5- or 6-min run overestimates $\dot{V}O_2$max because the anaerobic energy sources contribute substantially to total energy production in a 5-min run compared to a 12 to 15 min run. If the run is too long, the person is not able to run close to 100% of $\dot{V}O_2$max, and the estimate is too low (figure 11.2).

The $\dot{V}O_2$ associated with a specific running speed can be calculated using the following formula (see chapter 7 for details):

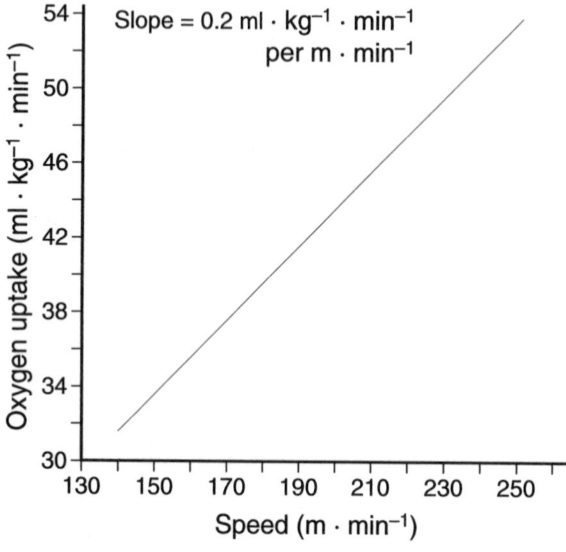

FIGURE 11.1 Relationship between steady-state oxygen uptake and running speed (14).

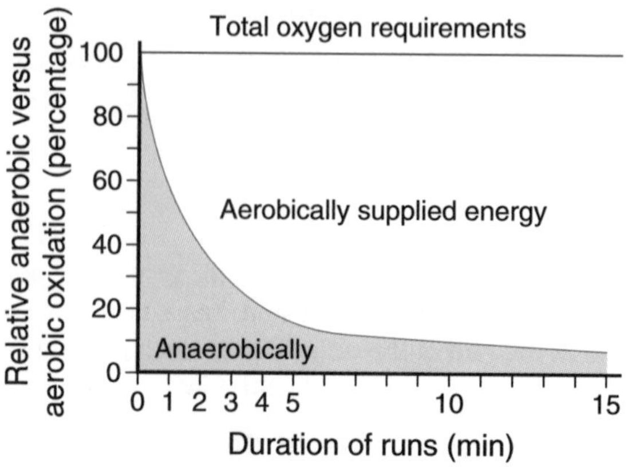

FIGURE 11.2 The relative role of aerobic and anaerobic energy sources in best-effort runs of various durations.

Reprinted from Balke 1963.

Table 11.1 Estimated Maximal Oxygen Uptake (ml · kg⁻¹ · min⁻¹) for Men and Women, 20-69 Years Old

	Min · mi^{-1}										
HR	10	11	12	13	14	15	16	17	18	19	20
					Men (20-29)						
120	65.0	61.7	58.4	55.2	51.9	48.6	45.4	42.1	38.9	35.6	32.3
130	63.4	60.1	56.9	53.6	50.3	47.1	43.8	40.6	37.3	34.0	30.8
140	61.8	58.6	55.3	52.0	48.8	45.5	42.2	39.0	35.7	32.5	29.2
150	60.3	57.0	53.7	50.5	47.2	43.9	40.7	37.4	34.2	30.9	27.6
160	58.7	55.4	52.2	48.9	45.6	42.4	39.1	35.9	32.6	29.3	26.1
170	57.1	53.9	50.6	57.3	44.1	40.8	37.6	34.3	31.0	27.8	24.5
180	55.6	52.3	49.0	45.8	42.5	39.3	36.0	32.7	29.5	26.2	22.9
190	54.0	50.7	47.5	44.2	41.0	37.7	34.4	31.2	27.9	24.6	21.4
200	52.4	49.2	45.9	42.7	39.4	36.1	32.9	29.6	26.3	23.1	19.8
					Women (20-29)						
120	62.1	58.9	55.6	52.3	49.1	45.8	42.5	39.3	36.0	32.7	29.5
130	60.6	57.3	54.0	50.8	47.5	44.2	41.0	37.7	34.4	31.2	27.9
140	59.0	55.7	52.5	49.2	45.9	42.7	39.4	36.1	32.9	29.6	26.3
150	57.4	54.2	50.9	47.6	44.4	41.1	37.8	34.6	31.3	28.0	24.8
160	55.9	52.6	49.3	46.7	42.8	39.5	36.3	33.0	29.7	26.5	23.2
170	54.3	51.0	47.8	44.5	41.2	38.0	34.7	31.4	28.2	24.9	21.6
180	52.7	49.5	46.2	42.9	39.7	36.4	33.1	29.9	26.6	23.3	20.1
190	51.2	47.9	44.6	41.4	38.1	34.8	31.6	28.3	25.0	21.8	18.5
200	49.6	46.3	43.1	39.8	36.5	33.3	30.0	26.7	23.5	20.2	16.9
					Men (30-39)						
120	61.1	57.8	54.6	51.3	48.0	44.8	41.5	38.2	35.0	31.7	28.4
130	59.5	56.3	53.0	49.7	46.5	43.2	39.9	36.7	33.4	30.1	26.9
140	58.0	54.7	51.4	48.2	44.9	41.6	38.4	35.1	31.8	28.6	25.3
150	56.4	53.1	49.9	46.6	43.3	40.1	36.8	33.5	30.3	27.0	23.8
160	54.8	51.6	48.3	45.0	41.8	38.5	35.2	32.0	28.7	25.5	22.2
170	53.3	50.0	46.7	43.5	40.2	36.9	33.7	30.4	27.1	23.9	20.6
180	51.7	48.4	45.2	41.9	38.6	35.4	32.1	28.8	25.6	22.3	19.1
190	50.1	46.9	43.6	40.3	37.1	33.8	30.5	27.3	24.0	20.8	17.5
					Women (30-39)						
120	58.2	55.0	51.7	48.4	45.2	41.9	38.7	35.4	32.1	28.9	25.6
130	56.7	53.4	50.1	46.9	43.6	40.4	37.1	33.8	30.6	27.3	24.0
140	55.1	51.8	48.6	45.3	42.1	38.8	35.5	32.3	29.0	24.7	22.5
150	53.5	50.3	47.0	43.8	40.5	37.2	34.0	30.7	27.4	24.2	20.9
160	52.0	48.7	45.4	42.2	38.9	35.7	32.4	29.1	25.9	22.6	19.3
170	50.4	47.1	43.9	40.6	37.4	34.1	30.8	27.6	24.3	21.0	17.8
180	48.8	45.6	42.3	39.1	35.8	32.5	29.3	26.0	22.7	19.5	16.2
190	47.3	44.0	40.8	37.5	34.2	31.0	27.7	24.4	21.2	17.9	14.6
					Men (40-49)						
120	57.2	54.0	50.7	47.4	44.2	40.9	37.6	34.4	31.1	27.8	24.6
130	55.7	52.4	49.1	45.9	42.6	39.3	36.1	32.8	29.5	26.3	23.0
140	54.1	50.8	47.6	44.3	41.0	37.8	34.5	31.2	28.0	24.7	21.4
150	52.5	49.3	46.0	42.7	39.5	36.2	32.9	29.7	26.4	23.1	19.9
160	51.0	47.7	44.4	41.2	37.9	34.6	31.4	28.1	24.8	21.6	18.3
170	49.4	46.1	42.9	39.6	36.3	33.1	29.8	26.5	23.3	20.0	16.7
180	47.8	44.6	41.3	38.0	34.8	31.5	28.2	25.0	21.7	18.4	15.2

(continued)

Table 11.1 *(continued)*

HR	10	11	12	13	14	15	16	17	18	19	20
						Min · mi^{-1}					
						Women (40-49)					
120	54.4	51.1	47.8	44.6	41.3	38.0	34.8	31.5	28.2	25.0	21.7
130	52.8	49.5	46.3	43.0	39.7	36.5	33.2	29.9	26.7	23.4	20.1
140	51.2	48.0	44.7	41.4	38.2	34.9	31.6	28.4	25.1	21.8	18.6
150	49.7	46.4	43.1	39.9	36.6	33.3	30.1	26.8	23.5	20.3	17.0
160	48.1	44.8	41.6	38.3	35.0	31.8	28.5	25.2	22.0	18.7	15.5
170	46.5	43.3	40.0	36.7	33.5	30.2	26.9	23.7	20.4	17.2	13.9
						Men (50-59)					
120	53.3	50.0	46.8	43.5	40.3	37.0	33.7	30.5	27.2	23.9	20.7
130	51.7	48.5	45.2	42.0	38.7	35.4	32.2	28.9	25.6	22.4	19.1
140	50.2	46.9	43.7	40.4	37.1	33.9	30.6	27.3	24.1	20.8	17.5
150	48.6	45.4	42.1	38.8	35.6	32.3	29.0	25.8	22.5	19.2	16.0
160	47.1	43.8	40.5	37.3	34.0	30.7	27.5	24.2	20.9	17.7	14.4
170	45.5	42.2	29.0	35.7	32.4	29.2	25.9	22.6	19.4	16.1	12.8
						Women (50-59)					
120	50.5	47.2	43.9	40.7	37.4	34.1	30.9	27.6	24.3	21.1	17.8
130	48.9	45.6	42.4	39.1	35.8	32.6	29.3	26.0	22.8	19.5	16.2
140	47.3	44.1	40.8	37.5	34.3	31.0	27.7	24.5	21.2	17.9	14.7
150	45.8	42.5	39.2	36.0	32.7	29.4	26.2	22.9	19.6	16.4	13.1
160	44.2	40.9	37.7	34.4	31.1	27.9	24.6	21.3	18.1	14.8	11.5
170	42.6	39.4	36.1	32.8	29.6	26.3	23.0	19.8	16.5	13.2	10.0
						Men (60-69)					
120	49.4	46.2	42.9	39.6	36.4	33.1	29.8	26.6	23.3	20.0	16.8
130	47.9	44.6	41.3	38.1	34.8	31.5	28.3	25.0	21.7	18.5	15.2
140	46.3	43.0	39.8	36.5	33.2	30.0	26.7	23.4	20.2	16.9	13.6
150	44.7	41.5	38.2	34.9	31.7	28.4	25.1	21.9	18.6	15.3	12.1
160	43.2	39.9	36.6	33.4	30.1	26.8	23.6	20.3	17.0	13.8	10.5
						Women (60-69)					
120	46.6	43.3	40.0	36.8	33.5	30.2	27.0	23.7	20.5	17.2	13.9
130	45.0	41.7	38.5	35.2	31.9	28.7	25.4	22.2	18.9	15.6	12.4
140	43.4	40.2	36.9	33.6	30.4	27.1	23.8	20.6	17.3	14.1	10.8
150	41.9	38.6	35.3	32.1	28.8	25.5	22.3	19.0	15.8	12.5	9.2
160	40.3	37.0	33.8	30.5	27.2	24.0	20.7	17.5	14.2	10.9	7.7

Note. Calculations assume 170 lb for men and 125 lb for women. For each 15 lb beyond these values, subtract 1 ml · kg^{-1} · min^{-1}.
Adapted from Kline et al. 1987.

$$\dot{V}O_2 = \text{horizontal velocity } (\text{m} \cdot \text{min}^{-1}) \cdot \frac{0.2\,\text{ml} \cdot \text{kg}^{-1} \cdot \text{min}^{-1}}{\text{m} \cdot \text{min}^{-1}} + 3.5\ \text{ml} \cdot \text{kg}^{-1} \cdot \text{min}^{-1}$$

These estimates are reasonable for adults who jog/run the entire 12 min or 1.5 mi. The formula will underestimate $\dot{V}O_2$max in children because of the higher oxygen cost of running in children (18). In contrast, the formula will overestimate $\dot{V}O_2$max in trained runners due to their better running economy (17) and in those who walk through the test because the net oxygen cost of walking is half that of running (see chapter 7).

QUESTION: A 20-year-old woman takes the Cooper 12-min-run test following a 15-week walk/jog program and completes 6 laps on a 440-yd (402.3-m) track. What is her $\dot{V}O_2$max?

Table 11.2 Standards for Maximal Oxygen Uptake and Endurance Runs

Age[a]	$\dot{V}O_2max$ (ml · kg^{-1} · min^{-1}) Female[b]	$\dot{V}O_2max$ Male	1.5-mi run (min:s) Female	1.5-mi run Male	12-min run (mi) Female	12-min run Male
			Good			
15-30	>40	>45	<12	<10	>1.5	>1.7
35-50	>35	>40	<13:30	<11:30	>1.4	>1.5
55-70	>30	>35	<16	<14	>1.2	>1.3
			Adequate for most activities			
15-30	35	40	13:30	11:50	1.4	1.5
35-50	30	35	15	13	1.3	1.4
55-70	25	30	17:30	15:30	1.1	1.3
			Borderline			
15-30	30	35	15	13	1.3	1.4
35-50	25	30	16:30	14:30	1.2	1.3
55-70	20	25	19	17	1.0	1.2
			Needs extra work on CRF			
15-30	<25	<30	>17	>15	<1.2	<1.3
35-50	<20	<25	>18:30	>16:30	<1.1	<1.2
55-70	<15	<20	>21	>19	<0.9	<1.0

Note. These standards are for fitness programs. People wanting to do well in endurance performance need higher levels. For those at the *Good* level, the emphasis is on maintaining this level the rest of their lives. For those in the lower levels, emphasis is on setting and reaching realistic goals.
[a]CRF declines with age.
[b]Women have lower standards because they have a larger amount of essential fat.
Reprinted from Howley and Franks 1986.

Answer:

$$402.3 \text{ m} \cdot \text{lap}^{-1} \cdot 6 \text{ laps} = 2414 \text{ m}$$

$$2414 \text{ m} \div 12 \text{ min} = 201 \text{ m} \cdot \text{min}^{-1}$$

$$\dot{V}O_2 = 201 \text{ m} \cdot \text{min}^{-1} \cdot \frac{0.2 \text{ ml} \cdot \text{kg}^{-1} \cdot \text{min}^{-1}}{\text{m} \cdot \text{min}^{-1}} + 3.5 \text{ ml} \cdot \text{kg}^{-1} \cdot \text{min}^{-1}$$

$$\dot{V}O_2 = 43.7 \text{ ml} \cdot \text{kg}^{-1} \cdot \text{min}^{-1}$$

Applying the 12-Min Run Test

The advantage of the 12-min run is that it can be used on a regular basis to evaluate current CRF without expensive equipment. It is easily adapted to cyclists and swimmers, who can evaluate their progress by determining how far they can ride or swim in 12 min. Although no equations exist that can relate cyclists' and swimmers' respective performances to $\dot{V}O_2max$, each participant is able to make a personal judgment about her or his current state of CRF and improvement due to training.

As Cooper (16) and others agree, an endurance run should *not* be used for testing at the beginning of an exercise program. A person new to exercise should progress through the jogging program at low intensities to make some fitness improvements before using an endurance-run field test.

Table 11.2 lists values for CRF as *good, adequate, borderline,* and *needs extra work*. The table takes age and gender into consideration. For example, a 40-year-old woman who runs 1.5 mi in 14 min and 15 s (14:15) would rate between adequate and good. Her time of 14:15 corresponds to a CRF value of about 35 to 40 ml · kg^{-1} · min^{-1}. We recommend that you encourage participants to try to achieve and maintain the "good" value for age and gender. If people are not at that level, help them to plan on making small and systematic progress toward that goal using the walking and jogging programs in chapter 17.

Administrating an Endurance-Run Test

The 1-mi run is used in many youth fitness programs (1). The steps to administering the 1-mi run are listed on page 213. They can be used for other endurance runs (e.g., 1.5-mi or 12-min run). The mile run is used as an example.

3 **In Review: A 1-mi walking test can be used to estimate CRF. The time for the mile as well as the heart rate measured at the end of the walk are used in a formula to calculate $\dot{V}O_2max$. A 1.5-mi run test can also be used to estimate CRF. The time for the 1.5 mi is used to determine average velocity and a formula (see chapter 7) is used to calculate $\dot{V}O_2max$.**

GRADED EXERCISE TESTS (GXTs)

Many fitness programs use a **graded exercise test (GXT)** to evaluate CRF. These multilevel tests can be administered using a bench, cycle ergometer, or treadmill.

Bench Step

Bench stepping is very economical. It can be used for both submaximal and maximal testing. The disadvantages include the limited number of stages that can be feasibly included for any one bench height and individual fitness level and the difficulty of taking certain measurements during the test (e.g., BP). The oxygen cost for stepping at different rates on steps of different heights was presented in chapter 7.

Cycle Ergometer

Cycle ergometers are portable, moderately priced work instruments that allow measurements to be made easily because the upper body is essentially stationary. Among their disadvantages, however, are that the exercise load is self-paced and that leg-muscle fatigue may be a limiting factor (43). On mechanically braked cycle ergometers such as the Monark models, the work rate can be changed by altering the pedal rate or the resistance on the flywheel. Generally, the pedal rate is maintained constant during a GXT at a rate appropriate to the individuals being tested: 50 to 60 rev · min^{-1} for the low to average fit, 70 to 100 rev · min^{-1} for the highly fit and competitive cyclists (26). The pedal rate is maintained by having the individual attend to a metronome or by providing some other source of feedback such as a speedometer. The resistance (load) on the wheel is increased sequentially to systematically overload the cardiovascular system. The starting work rate and the increment from one stage to the next depend on the fitness of the person being tested and the purpose of the test. $\dot{V}O_2$ can be estimated from a formula that gives reasonable estimates of $\dot{V}O_2$ up to work rates of about 1200 kpm · min^{-1} (see chapter 7 for details):

$$\dot{V}O_2\,(ml \cdot min^{-1}) = \text{work rate}\,(kpm \cdot min^{-1}) \cdot 2\,ml\,O_2 \cdot kpm^{-1} + (3.5\,ml \cdot kg^{-1} \cdot min^{-1} \cdot \text{kg body weight})$$

The cycle ergometer differs from the treadmill in that the body weight is supported by the seat and the work rate depends primarily on pedal rate and the load on the wheel. This means that the relative $\dot{V}O_2$ at any work rate is higher for a small person than for a big person.

QUESTION: What is the relative difficulty of a work rate of 900 kpm · min^{-1} for two individuals, one weighing 60 kg and the other 90 kg?

Answer:

$$\dot{V}O_2 = \text{work rate}\,(kpm \cdot min^{-1}) \cdot 2\,ml\,O_2 \cdot kpm^{-1} + (3.5\,ml \cdot kg^{-1} \cdot min^{-1} \cdot \text{kg body weight})$$

For the 60-kg subject,

$$\dot{V}O_2 = 900\,kpm \cdot min^{-1} \cdot 2\,ml\,O_2 \cdot kpm^{-1} + (3.5\,ml \cdot kg^{-1} \cdot min^{-1} \cdot 60\,kg)$$
$$= 1800\,ml \cdot min^{-1} + 210\,ml \cdot min^{-1}$$
$$= 2010\,ml \cdot min^{-1}, \text{ or } 2.0\,L \cdot min^{-1}$$

Expressed per kilogram of body weight, the answer is 33.5 ml · kg^{-1} · min^{-1}, or 9.6 METs.

For the 90-kg subject,

$$\dot{V}O_2 = 900\,kpm \cdot min^{-1} \cdot 2\,ml\,O_2 \cdot kpm^{-1} + (3.5\,ml \cdot kg^{-1} \cdot min^{-1} \cdot 90\,kg)$$
$$= 1800\,ml \cdot min^{-1} + 315\,ml \cdot min^{-1}$$
$$= 2115\,ml \cdot min^{-1}, \text{ or } 2.1\,L \cdot min^{-1}$$

Expressed per kilogram of body weight, the answer is 23.5 ml · kg^{-1} · min^{-1}, or 6.7 METs.

In addition, the increments in the work rate, by demanding a fixed increase in the $\dot{V}O_2$ (e.g., an increment of 150 kpm · min^{-1} is equal to a $\dot{V}O_2$ change of 300 ml · min^{-1}), force the small or unfit subject to make larger cardiovascular adjustments than a large or highly fit subject. As we will see, these factors are considered in the selection of the work rates when a cycle ergometer test is used to evaluate CRF. Table 11.3 summarizes the effects that differences in body weight have on the metabolic responses to

Steps to Administer the 1-Mile Run

Step **Activity**

Before test day

1. Arrange to have the following elements at the test site:
   - A person to start and read the time from a stopwatch
   - A partner for each runner (perhaps with a sheet to mark off laps)
   - A stopwatch for the tester (with a spare ready)
   - A score sheet or scorecard
2. Explain the purpose of the test (i.e., to determine how fast participants can run a mile, which reflects the endurance of their cardiovascular system).
3. Do *not* administer the test until participants have had several fitness sessions, including some with running.
4. Have participants practice running at a set submaximal pace for one lap, then two, and so on, several times prior to test day.
5. Select and mark off (if needed) a level area for the run.
6. Explain to people being tested that they are to run the mile in the fastest time possible. Walking is allowed, but the goal is to cover the distance as fast as possible.

Test day

1. Participants warm up with stretching, walking, and slow jogging.
2. Several people will run at the same time.
3. The procedure is explained again.
4. The timer says, "Ready, go," and starts the stopwatch.
5. Each individual has a partner with a watch with a second hand.
6. The partner counts the laps and tells the individual at the end of each lap how many more lap(s) to run.
7. The timer calls out the minutes and seconds as the runner finishes the mile run.
8. The partner listens for the time when the runner finishes the mile and records it (to the nearest second) immediately on a scorecard.
9. The runners continue to walk one lap after finishing the run.

graded exercise test (GXT) — A multistage test that determines a person's physiological responses to different intensities of exercise and/or the person's peak aerobic capacity.

bench stepping — Can be used for both submaximal and maximal testing to evaluate cardiorespiratory function. The height of the bench and the number of steps per minute determine the intensity of the effort. Also a very popular conditioning exercise.

cycle ergometer — A one-wheeled stationary cycle with adjustable resistance used as a work task for exercise testing or conditioning.

Table 11.3 Work Differences Based on Body Weight in Work Tasks

Work task	$\dot{V}O_2max$ $L \cdot min^{-1}$	$\dot{V}O_2max$ $ml \cdot kg^{-1} \cdot min^{-1}$	Total work (kcal)	METs
A heavier person will respond with the following differences compared with a lighter person when doing the task at the same rate:				
Carry body weight				
Bench	↑	=	↑	=
Walk	↑	=	↑	=
Job	↑	=	↑	=
Body weight supported				
Cycle	=	↓	=	↓

weight-supported (e.g., cycle ergometry) and weight-carrying (e.g., bench stepping, jogging) work tasks. Thus a larger person does more total work and has the same MET level for tasks in which the body weight provides the resistance (weight-carrying tasks). In cycling (a weight-supported task), the same total work is done, but the larger person has a lower MET level.

Treadmill

Treadmill protocols are very reproducible because they set the appropriate pace for the subject, whereas the subject may go too slow or too fast on either the bench step or the cycle ergometer. Treadmill tests can accommodate the least to the most fit and use the natural activities of walking and running, with the running tests placing the greatest potential load on the cardiovascular system. Treadmills, however, are expensive, not portable, and make some measurements (BP and blood sampling) difficult (43). The type of treadmill test influences the measured $\dot{V}O_2max$, with the graded running test giving the highest value, a running test at 0% grade the next highest, and the walking test protocols the lowest value (7, 34).

For estimates of $\dot{V}O_2$ to be obtained from grade and speed considerations, the grade and speed settings must be calibrated correctly (29) (see chapter 6 for details on how to calibrate a treadmill and other equipment). Furthermore, the subject must carefully follow the directions of not holding onto the treadmill railing during the test if the estimated $\dot{V}O_2$ values are going to be reasonable (5, 40). For example, it has been observed that HR decreased 17 beats $\cdot$ min^{-1} when a subject who was walking on a treadmill at 3.4 mi $\cdot$ hr^{-1} and a 14% grade held onto the treadmill railing (5). This would result in an overestimation of the $\dot{V}O_2max$ because the HR would be lower at any stage of the test and test duration would be extended. Lastly, there is no need to make adjustments to the $\dot{V}O_2$ calculation due to differences in body weight because treadmill tests require the person being tested to carry his or her own weight; therefore, the $\dot{V}O_2$ ($ml \cdot kg^{-1} \cdot min^{-1}$) is proportional to the body weight (35).

4 **In Review: CRF responses to different levels of exercise can be determined using a bench-stepping, cycle ergometer, or treadmill protocol. The oxygen uptake values (expressed in $ml \cdot kg^{-1} \cdot min^{-1}$) are similar for most adults at specific stages of a treadmill or step test because the energy cost is proportional to the body weight, which is carried along. In contrast, the oxygen uptake (expressed in $L \cdot min^{-1}$) is similar for most adults at each stage of a cycle ergometer test; however, the relative cost ($ml \cdot kg^{-1} \cdot min^{-1}$) is higher for the lighter participant.**

COMMON VARIABLES MEASURED DURING A GXT

The variables that are commonly measured for resting and submaximal tests include HR, BP, and rating of perceived exertion (RPE). For maximal testing, $\dot{V}O_2max$ and the final stage achieved on a GXT are often measured.

Heart Rate

Heart rate (HR) is often used as a fitness indicator at rest and during a standard submaximal work task.

Table 11.4 Effects of Conditioning on HR

Condition	Effects of fitness on HR
Rest	↓
Standard submaximal work (same external work rate)	↓
Maximal work	no change
Set % of maximal	no change

Maximal HR is useful for determining the target heart rate (THR) for fitness workouts (see chapter 14), but it is not a good fitness indicator because it changes very little with training. Table 11.4 summarizes the effects of aerobic exercise or conditioning on HR in different situations.

When an ECG is being recorded, the HR can be taken from the ECG strip (see chapter 22). When no ECG is being recorded, HR can be taken by a heart rate watch, a stethoscope, or manual palpation of an artery at the wrist or neck. Heart rate watches (getting signals similar to an ECG from a strap around the chest) have been found to be accurate and are the easiest way to measure HR. Fingers (not the thumb) should be used to take HR, preferably at the wrist (radial artery). If a person takes HR at the neck (carotid artery), caution should be used not to apply too much pressure because it could trigger a reflex that causes the HR to slow down. Reliable measures are obtained, however, when people are trained in this procedure (38, 41). The HR *at rest* or *during a steady-state exercise* should be taken for 30 s for higher reliability. However, when taking HRs *after exercise*, the measurement should begin soon after termination of exercise (e.g., 5 s) and be taken for 10 or 15 s because the heart rate changes so rapidly. The 10-s or 15-s rate is multiplied by 6 or 4, respectively, to calculate beats per minute. For example, if a 10-s postexercise HR is 20 beats · min^{-1}, the HR is 120 beats · min^{-1} (6×20).

Blood Pressure

Systolic blood pressure (SBP) and diastolic blood pressure (DBP) are often determined at rest, during work, and after work. The proper size of the cuff (in which the bladder overlaps two thirds of the arm) and a sensitive stethoscope are required to get accurate values at rest and during work (see figure 6.3 for an illustration of blood pressure measuring equipment). At rest, the person should have both feet flat on the floor and be in a relaxed position with the arm supported. The cuff should be wrapped securely around the arm at heart level, usually with the tube on the inside of the arm. The stethoscope should be below (not under) the cuff—the placement will depend on where the sound can be most easily heard, often toward the inside of the arm (24, 31). The first and fourth Korotkoff sounds (the first sound heard and the sound when the tone changes or becomes muffled) should be used for SBP and DBP, respectively, during exercise. If SBP fails to increase or the DBP increases excessively (> 115 mmHg) with increased work, the test should be stopped.

Rating of Perceived Exertion

Borg introduced the **rating of perceived exertion (RPE)**, that is, how hard the participant perceives his or her workout to be, using a scale from 6 to 20 (roughly based on resting to maximal HR, i.e., 60 to 200 beats · min^{-1}). Table 11.5 presents this scale as well as Borg's revised 10-point RPE scale (12). Either can be used with a GXT to provide useful information during the test as the person approaches exhaustion and to be a reference point for exercise prescription. The following instructions are recommended when administering the RPE scale (2):

> During the exercise test we want you to pay close attention to how hard you feel the exercise work rate is. This feeling should reflect your total amount of exertion and fatigue, combining all sensations and feelings of physical stress, effort, and fatigue. Don't concern yourself with any one factor such as leg pain, shortness of breath, or exercise intensity,

treadmill — A machine with a moving belt that can be adjusted for speed and grade, allowing a person to walk or run in place. Treadmills are widely used for exercise-tolerance testing.

heart rate (HR) — The number of beats of the heart per minute.

rating of perceived exertion (RPE) — A scale, by Borg, used to quantify the subjective feeling of physical effort. The original scale was from 6 to 20; the revised scale is from 0 to 10.

Table 11.5 Rating of Perceived Exertion Scales

Original rating scale	Revised rating scale
6	0 Nothing at all
7 Very, very light	0.5 Very, very light (just noticeable)
8	
9 Very light	1 Very light
10	
11 Fairly light	2 Light (weak)
12	3 Moderate
13 Somewhat hard	4 Somewhat hard
14	
15 Hard	5 Heavy (strong)
16	6
17 Very hard	7 Very heavy
18	8
	9
19 Very, very hard	10 Very, very heavy (maximal)
20	

Reprinted from Borg 1985.

but try to concentrate on your total, inner feeling of exertion. Try not to underestimate or overestimate your feeling of exertion; be as accurate as you can.

Estimating Versus Measuring Functional Capacity

Functional capacity is defined as the highest work rate (oxygen uptake) reached in a GXT during which time HR, BP, and ECG responses are within the normal range for heavy work. For cardiac patients, the highest work rate does not normally reflect a measure of the maximal capacity of the CR systems because the GXT might be stopped for ECG changes, angina, claudication pain, and so on. For the apparently healthy person, functional capacity can be called maximal aerobic power or maximal oxygen uptake ($\dot{V}O_2$max). (See chapter 4 for procedures to be used in measuring oxygen uptake.)

Oxygen uptake increases with each stage of the GXT until the upper limit of CRF is reached. At that point, $\dot{V}O_2$ does not increase further when the test moves to the next stage; the person's $\dot{V}O_2$max has been reached. Given the complexity and cost of these procedures, $\dot{V}O_2$max is usually estimated with equations relating the stage of the GXT to a specific oxygen uptake.

As discussed in chapter 7, a variety of formulas may be used to estimate oxygen uptake on the basis of the stage reached in a GXT. In general, these formulas give reasonable estimates of the $\dot{V}O_2$ achieved in a GXT if the test has been suited to the individual. However, if the increments in the stages of the GXT are too large relative to the person's CRF, or if the time for each stage is too short, then the person might not be able to reach the steady-state oxygen requirement associated with that stage (21, 28, 36). Failure to achieve the oxygen requirement for a GXT stage results in an overestimation of the $\dot{V}O_2$ at each stage of the test, with the overestimation growing larger with each stage. Inability to reach the oxygen requirement is a common problem with less fit individuals (e.g., cardiac patients). This inability suggests that more conservative (i.e., smaller increments between stages) GXT protocols should be used to allow the less fit individual to reach the oxygen demand at each stage. A more complete explanation of this problem is found in chapter 4.

In contrast, shorter stages and larger increments between stages in a GXT can be used if the purpose of the test is to screen for ECG abnormalities (rather than to estimate $\dot{V}O_2$max). In addition, changes in CRF over time can be determined by periodically using the same GXT on an individual.

5 **In Review: Common variables measured during a resting or submaximal GXT include heart rate, blood pressure, and rating of perceived exertion (RPE). Oxygen uptake can be measured at each stage of a test and at maximal exertion; however, $\dot{V}O_2$max is usually estimated from the final stage achieved using the formulas described in chapter 7.**

EXERCISE TESTING EQUIPMENT AND CALIBRATION

Fitness testing requires the purchase of high-quality equipment that can be calibrated (see chapter 6) and hold that calibration from one test to the next. This section provides an overview of the equipment used in testing centers that conduct submaximal fitness tests. Submaximal tests are used to evaluate a person's HR, BP, and RPE responses either to a single work rate or to a series of progressive work rates. The test is usually stopped at 70% to 85% of estimated maximal HR. The HR data are then used to estimate $\dot{V}O_2max$ by an extrapolation procedure or with specific formulas. The equipment and supplies used for such tests include

- the cycle ergometer, bench step (and metronome), or treadmill;
- a sphygmomanometer (blood pressure measuring device) and stethoscope;
- a clock or stopwatch;
- an RPE chart; and
- recording forms.

PROCEDURES FOR GRADED EXERCISE TESTING

This section provides information about how to administer a GXT and uses examples of different testing protocols. Before administering any GXT, the tester should

- calibrate the equipment;
- check supplies and data forms;
- select the appropriate test protocol for the participant;
- obtain informed consent;
- provide instruction in the task, including the cool-down procedure;
- have the participant practice the task, if needed; and
- check to see that pretest instructions were followed.

Because HR, BP, and RPE responses to submaximal work are influenced by a variety of factors, care must be taken to minimize the variation in each from one testing period to the next. These factors include, but are not limited to,

- temperature and relative humidity of the room;
- number of hours of sleep prior to testing;
- emotional state;
- hydration state;
- medication;
- time of day;
- time since last meal, cigarette smoking, caffeine intake, and exercise; and
- psychological environment for the test (i.e., the participant's comfort level with his or her surroundings during testing).

Attention to these factors increases the likelihood that changes in HR, BP, or RPE from one test to the next are actually caused by changes in physical fitness and physical activity habits. A form such as the Pretest Instructions for a Fitness Test (see form 11.1) is helpful in ensuring that the client will be ready for testing.

Typical procedures to follow in doing GXTs are shown on page 219, Steps to Administering a GXT.

A series of end points should be used to stop a GXT (see General Indications for Stopping a GXT in Apparently Healthy Adults on page 220 (2). These guidelines are for nondiagnostic testing performed without direct physician involvement or electrocardiographic monitoring.

6 **In Review: Equipment to measure and record CRF variables should be checked for availability and calibration prior to testing. Careful attention to procedures before and during a test will enhance the safety and accuracy of the test (see page 219). The tester should know when to stop a test, based on signs, symptoms, or CRF measurements (see page 220).**

WHEN TO USE SUBMAXIMAL AND MAXIMAL TESTS

GXTs have been used to evaluate CRF in fitness programs for healthy populations and in the clinical assessment of ischemic heart disease—a condition in which an inadequate blood flow to the heart muscle can cause changes in the ECG. Exercise is used to place a load on the heart to determine the cardiovascular response and to see if changes occur in the ECG (20). Some controversy has arisen concerning whether to use submaximal or maximal tests. On the basis of thousands of exercise stress tests conducted since the mid-1950s, it is generally recommended that a maximal exercise test be used to determine the presence of ischemic heart disease in asymptomatic individuals (2). Although

functional capacity — Maximal oxygen uptake, expressed in milliliters of oxygen per kilogram of body weight per minute, or in METs.

FORM 11.1

Pretest Instructions for a Fitness Test

Name ______________________________ Test date __________ Time __________

Report to ____

Instructions. Please observe the following:

1. Wear running shoes, shorts, and a loose-fitting shirt.
2. No food, drink (except water), tobacco, or medication for 3 hours prior to test.
3. Minimal physical activity on day of test.

Cancellation

If you cannot keep this appointment, please call _________ or _________.

submaximal exercise tests are not as effective in identifying disease conditions, they are appropriate for evaluating cardiorespiratory fitness prior to and following exercise programs.

When a fitness center is responsible for both fitness testing and the fitness program, the sequence of testing and activity recommended earlier provides the advantages of each while minimizing the disadvantages. The main objection to maximal tests is the stress they put on a person who has been inactive. Although the risk of a maximal GXT is very small with adequate screening and qualified testing personnel, the discomfort of going to one's maximum without prior conditioning may discourage some people from participating in a fitness program. Objections to the submaximal test include finding fewer abnormal responses to exercise and inaccurately estimating $\dot{V}O_2$max from submaximal data. In a fitness program for apparently healthy people, the objections against either maximal or submaximal tests given alone are overcome by administering the submaximal test early in the fitness program and waiting until the participant has been involved in a regular exercise program to administer the maximal test. Any of the GXT protocols can be used for submaximal or maximal testing—the only difference is the criteria for stopping the test. Either test is stopped if any of the abnormal responses listed on page 220 occur. In the absence of abnormal responses, the submaximal test is usually terminated when the person reaches a certain HR (often 85% of maximum HR), and the maximal test is stopped when the person reaches a state of voluntary exhaustion.

Maximal Exercise Test Protocols

No one GXT protocol is appropriate for all types of people. The duration, starting points, and increments between stages should vary with the type of person. Young active, normal sedentary, and people with questionable health status should start at 6, 4, and 2 METs, respectively. The same three groups should increase 2 to 3, 1 to 2, and 0.5 to 1 METs, respectively, for progressive stages of the test. If the test is being used to compare CRF at different times, then 1 or 2 min per stage can be used. If trying to predict $\dot{V}O_2$max, however, the time per stage should be 2 to 3 min. Table 11.6 illustrates how these criteria might be used for a bench, cycle, or treadmill test for different fitness levels.

The following testing protocols are examples of tests that could be used for different populations. The first protocol, shown in table 11.7, could be used with deconditioned subjects by starting at a very low MET level, walking slowly, and increasing 1 MET per 3-min stage (37). The Balke Standard (9) protocol could be used for typical inactive adults by progressing at 1 MET per 2-min stage and starting at a higher MET level. More active or younger people could be tested on the Bruce (15) protocol, which starts at a moderate MET level and goes up 2 or 3 METs per 3-min stage. Unfortunately, some testing centers attempt to use the same testing protocol for all people, with the result that the initial stage is often too high or too low and the work increments for each stage are either too small or too large for the individual being tested.

Steps to Administering a GXT

Step **Activity**

1. Greet patient/client.
2. Obtain consent (oral and written).
3. Record age and measure height and weight. Calculate and record estimated HRmax and 70% to 85% HRmax.
4. Obtain resting HR and BP.
5. Instruct participant in how to do a step test.
   - Step all the way up and all the way down.
   - Keep pace with the metronome.

   OR

   Instruct participant on how to use the cycle ergometer.
   - Adjust seat height so the knee is slightly flexed when the foot is at the bottom of the pedal swing and parallel to the floor.
   - Keep pace with the metronome.
   - Do not hold tightly onto the handlebars; release hold when blood pressure is taken.

   OR

   Instruct participant on how to walk on the treadmill.
   - Hold onto railing; get "feel" of belt speed by putting one foot on the belt, keeping up with belt speed.
   - Step on, keeping eyes ahead and back straight; walk relaxed with arms swinging.
   - Initially, person can hold on for balance, then use just finger or back of hand to touch railing lightly.
6. Follow test protocol.
   - Advise person to talk during the test about how he or she feels.
   - Follow criteria for termination of the test.

Note. For fitness evaluations HR, BP, and RPE are the usual variables measured.
Adapted from Howley 1988.

Submaximal Exercise Test Protocols

Any GXT protocol can be used for submaximal or maximal testing. The HFI typically uses a submaximal GXT to estimate a person's $\dot{V}O_2max$ or to simply show before-and-after changes in selected variables due to the exercise program. It needs to be emphasized that predicting maximal oxygen uptake from any submaximal test involves substantial error. However, it can provide useful information in a fitness program to estimate a person's functional capacity and to determine in what fitness category the person belongs and what exercise programming would therefore be most appropriate. The only way to determine an individual's true functional capacity is to measure it during a maximal test (13). Changes in HR, BP, and RPE as a result of an exercise conditioning program make a submaximal test a good mechanism for showing improvements in CRF.

General Indications for Stopping a GXT in Apparently Healthy Adults*

1. Onset of angina or angina-like symptoms
2. Significant drop (20 mmHg) in systolic blood pressure or a failure of the systolic blood pressure to rise with an increase in exercise intensity
3. Excessive rise in blood pressure: systolic pressure > 260 mmHg or diastolic pressure > 115 mmHg
4. Signs of poor perfusion: light-headedness, confusion, ataxia, pallor, cyanosis, nausea, or cold and clammy skin
5. Failure of heart rate to increase with increased exercise intensity
6. Noticeable change in heart rhythm
7. Subject requests to stop
8. Physical or verbal manifestations of severe fatigue
9. Failure of the testing equipment

*Assumes that testing is nondiagnostic and is being performed without direct physician involvement or electrocardiographic monitoring.

Reprinted from American College of Sports Medicine 1995.

Table 11.6 Testing Protocol for Different Groups

		Bench		Cycle		Treadmill	
Stage	METs	Height (cm)	Steps · min^{-1}	Work rate (kpm · min^{-1})	RPM	Speed (km · hr^{-1})	Grade (%)
			Individuals with questionable health				
1	2	0	24	0	50	3.2	0
2	3	16	12	150	50	4.8	0
3	4	16	18	300	50	4.8	2.5
4	5	16	24	450	50	4.8	5.0
5	6	16	30	600	50	4.8	7.5
			"Normal" sedentary individuals				
1	4	16	18	360	60	4.8	2.5
2	6	16	30	540	60	4.8	7.5
3	7-8	36	18-24	720-900	60	4.8-5.5	10.0
4	9	36	27	1010-1080	60	5.5	12.0
5	10-11	36	30-33	1080-1260	60	9.7	0-1.75
			Young active individuals				
1	6	16	30	630	70	4.8	7.5
2	9	36	27	1060	70	5.5	12.0
3	12	36	36	1270	70	9.7	3.5
4	15	50	33	1900	70	11.3	7.0
5	17	50	39	2110	70	11.3	11.0

Reprinted from Franks 1979.

Table 11.7 Treadmill Protocols for Various Categories

Stage	METs	Speed (km · hr^{-1})	Grade (%)	Time (min)
For deconditioned people[a]				
1	2.5	3.2	0	3
2	3.5	3.2	3.5	3
3	4.5	3.2	7	3
4	5.4	3.2	10.5	3
5	6.4	3.2	14	3
6	7.3	3.2	17.5	3
7	8.5	4.8	12.5	3
8	9.5	4.8	15	3
9	10.5	4.8	17.5	3
For normal inactive people[b]				
1	4.3	4.8	2.5	2
2	5.4	4.8	5	2
3	6.4	4.8	7.5	2
4	7.4	4.8	10	2
5	8.5	4.8	12.5	2
6	9.5	4.8	15	2
7	10.5	4.8	17.5	2
8	11.6	4.8	20	2
9	12.6	4.8	22.5	2
10	13.6	4.8	25	2
For young active people[c]				
1	5	2.7	10	3
2	7	4	12	3
3	9.5	5.4	14	3
4	13	6.7	16	3
5	16	8	18	3

[a]From "Methods of Exercise Testing" by J.P. Naughton and R. Haider. In *Exercise Testing and Exercise Training in Coronary Heart Disease*, by J.P. Naughton, H.R. Hellerstein, and L.C. Mohler (Eds.), 1973, New York: Academic Press.
[b]From "Advanced Exercise Procedures for Evaluation of the Cardiovascular System," *Monograph*, by B. Balke, 1970, Milton, WI: The Burdick Corporation.
[c]From "Multi-Stage Treadmill Test of Maximal and Submaximal Exercise" by R.A. Bruce. In American Heart Association, *Exercise Testing and Training of Apparently Healthy Individuals: A Handbook for Physicians* (pp. 32-34), 1972, New York: American Heart Association.

7 In Review: GXT protocols can be used for submaximal tests (early in the testing sequence) or maximal tests (for active persons who have reached minimal fitness levels). Submaximal and maximal tests can use the same GXT protocol; however, the criteria for test termination differ. Maximal tests are more effective in determining the presence of ischemic heart disease. Submaximal tests are useful in assessing fitness and are relatively inexpensive to administer. Although the $\dot{V}O_2$max value estimated from a submaximal test is not as accurate as that obtained from a maximal test, the information is useful in evaluating CRF prior to and following an exercise program.

Submaximal Treadmill Test Protocol

The initial stage and rate of progression of the GXT should be selected on the basis of the criteria mentioned earlier. In the following example, a Balke Standard protocol (3 mi · hr^{-1}, 2.5% grade increase every 2 min) was used; HR was monitored in the last 30 s of each stage. The test was terminated at 85% of age-adjusted maximal HR. Maximal aerobic power was estimated by extrapolating the HR response to the person's estimated maximal HR. Figure 11.3 presents the results of this test with a graph showing the HR response at each work rate. Note that the HR response is rather flat between the 0% and 5% grades. This is not an uncommon finding (see the discussion that follows of the YMCA test); perhaps the subject is too excited, or perhaps the stroke volume changes are accounting for the changes in cardiac output at these low work rates. The HR response is usually quite linear between 110 beats · min^{-1} and the subject's 85% of maximal HR cutoff.

To estimate $\dot{V}O_2$max, the procedures of Maritz et al. (33) are followed. A line is drawn through the HR points from 7.5% grade to the final work rate. The line is extended (extrapolated) to the person's estimated maximal HR (183 beats · min^{-1}). A vertical line is dropped from the last point to the baseline to estimate the subject's maximal aerobic power, which is 11.8 METs, or 41.3 ml · kg^{-1} · min^{-1}. Remember that the estimated maximal HR may be inaccurate and that the estimate of maximal oxygen uptake will be influenced by this possible inaccuracy. If this person's true (measured) maximal HR were 173 or 193 beats · min^{-1}, the estimated maximal MET level would have been 11.0 METs and 12.6 METs, respectively.

Submaximal Cycle Ergometer Test Protocol

The steps in the administration of submaximal cycle ergometer tests are on page 223. One of the most

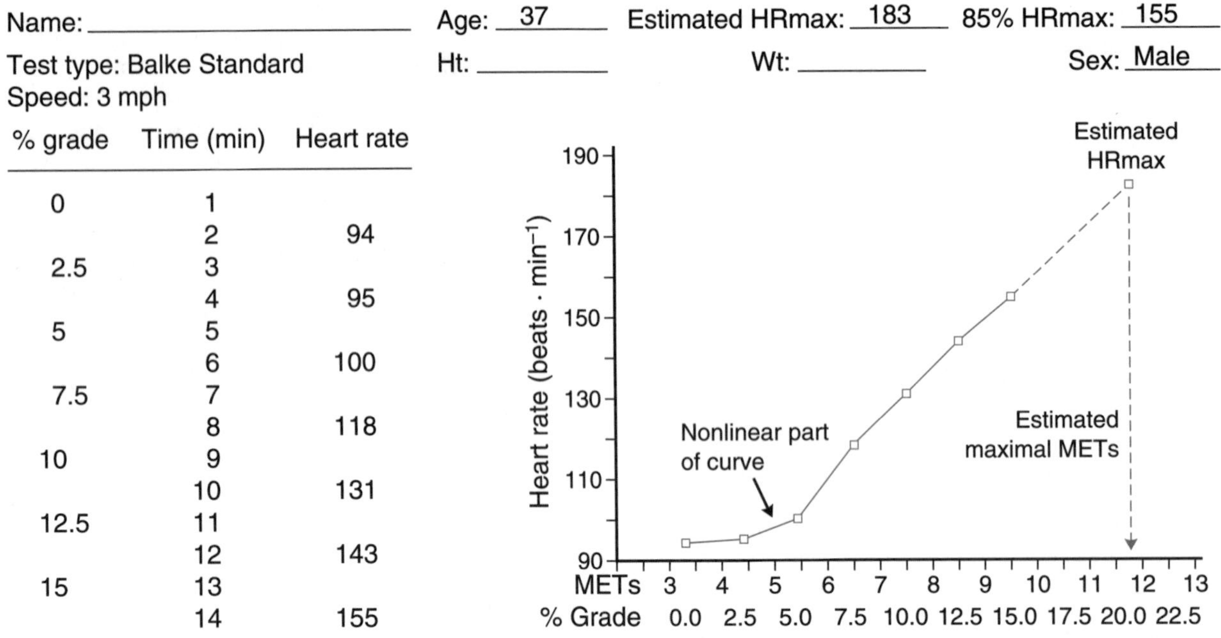

FIGURE 11.3 Maximal aerobic power estimated by measuring the heart rate response to a submaximal graded exercise test on a treadmill.

common submaximal cycle ergometer protocols (figure 11.4) is taken from the *Y's Way to Physical Fitness* (25). This protocol relies on the observation that there is a linear relationship between HR and work rate ($\dot{V}O_2$) once a HR of approximately 110 beats · min^{-1} is reached. The test requires the person to complete one more stage past the one causing a HR of 110 beats · min^{-1}. The intent of the test is to extrapolate the line describing the HR-work rate relationship out to the person's age-adjusted maximal HR (as was done for the treadmill protocol) to estimate the person's $\dot{V}O_2$max. Each stage of the test lasts 3 min, unless a person's HR has not yet reached a steady state (greater than 5 beats · min^{-1} difference between 2nd- and 3rd-min HR). In that case, an extra minute is added to that stage. The pedal rate is maintained at 50 rev · min^{-1}, so that, on a Monark cycle ergometer, a 0.5-kp increase in load is equal to 150 kpm · min^{-1} (25 W). Seat height is adjusted so that the knee is slightly bent (5°) when the pedal is at the bottom of the swing through 1 revolution. The seat height is recorded for future reference. HR is monitored during the later half of the 2nd and 3rd min of each stage.

Proper selection of the initial work rate and the rate of progression of the work rate on the cycle ergometer should take into consideration body weight, sex, age, and level of fitness. In general, absolute $\dot{V}O_2$max (L · min^{-1}) is lower in smaller people; women have lower absolute $\dot{V}O_2$max values than men; $\dot{V}O_2$max decreases with age; and inactivity is associated with low $\dot{V}O_2$max. The YMCA test addresses the concerns of body weight, fitness, and so on by starting everyone at 150 kpm · min^{-1} and using the HR response to that specified work task to set subsequent stages in the test (see figure 11.4). Large or fit individuals would have a low HR response to this work rate and would use the most strenuous sequence of work rates (far left boxes in the figure). A small or unfit individual would have a high HR response to the 150 kpm · min^{-1} work rate and would follow a sequence of work rates with small increments in the power output. People being tested should complete only one additional work rate beyond the one demanding a HR of 110 beats · min^{-1}.

The HR values for the 2nd and 3rd min of each work rate are recorded, and directions are followed to estimate $\dot{V}O_2$max in liters per minute. The YMCA protocol directions and an example are presented in figure 11.5 for a 50-year-old woman. The stages followed the pattern dictated by the HR response to the initial work rate of 150 kpm · min^{-1}. A line was drawn through the last two HR values and extrapolated to the estimated maximal HR. The $\dot{V}O_2$max was estimated to be 1.77 L · min^{-1}; this value was multiplied by 1000 to give 1770 ml · min^{-1} and divided by the 59-kg body weight to give an estimated $\dot{V}O_2$max of 30 ml · kg^{-1} · min^{-1}.

Steps to Administering a Submaximal Cycle Ergometer Test

Step	Activity
1.	Complete pretest items.
2.	Select the test protocol.
3.	Estimate the participant's HRmax (220 – age = beats · min^{-1}).
4.	Determine 85% of participant's HRmax (HRmax × .85 = 85% HRmax).
5.	Review the procedure with participant.
6.	Set and record the seat height (leg should be slightly bent at the knee when foot is at the bottom of the pedaling stroke).
7.	Start the metronome (set at 100 beats · min^{-1} so that one foot is at the bottom of the pedaling stroke on each beat, resulting in 50 complete rev · min^{-1}).
8.	Have the participant begin pedaling in rhythm with the metronome.
9.	As soon as the correct pace is achieved, set the resistance according to the protocol chosen.
10.	Start the timer for the beginning of the 3-min stage.
11.	Check the resistance setting (it may drift) and observe the participant for signs or symptoms that require terminating the test.
12.	At 1:30 into the stage, take and record BP.
13.	At 2:30, take and record HR either from ECG or manually from 2:30 to 2:45.
14.	At 2:50, get and record the participant's RPE.
15.	At 2:55, ask the participant, "How are you doing?"
16.	At 3:00, if HR is less than 85% of HRmax, blood pressure is responding normally, and participant is all right, increase resistance to the next stage.
17.	Repeat steps 10 through 16 until the participant reaches 85% of HRmax or there is another reason to stop the test. Go back to stage 1 (for cooldown) and repeat steps 10 through 15, stopping at 3:00 in the cool-down stage.
18.	Talk with the participant and check out any problems.

Reprinted from Franks and Howley 1989.

In contrast to the YMCA test, the Åstrand and Ryhming cycle ergometer test (6) requires the subject to complete only one 6-min work rate demanding a HR between 125 and 170 beats · min^{-1}. These investigators observed that for young (18 to 30 years) subjects, the average HR was 128 beats · min^{-1} for males and 138 beats · min^{-1} for females at 50% $\dot{V}O_2max$, and at 70% $\dot{V}O_2max$ the average HRs were 154 and 164 beats · min^{-1}, respectively. Based on these observations, if you know from a HR response that a person is at 50% $\dot{V}O_2max$ at a work rate equal to 1.5 L · min^{-1}, then the estimated $\dot{V}O_2max$ would be twice that, or 3.0 L · min^{-1}. Table 11.8 is used to estimate $\dot{V}O_2max$ based on the subject's HR response to one 6-min work rate (4).

Using the data collected for the YMCA test displayed earlier, we can see how $\dot{V}O_2max$ is estimated in the Åstrand and Ryhming protocol. The 50-year-old woman had a HR of 140 beats · min^{-1} at a work rate of 450 kpm · min^{-1}. Using table 11.8, for women, look down the leftmost column to a HR of 140, and look across to the second column (450 kpm · min^{-1}). The estimated $\dot{V}O_2max$ is 2.4 L · min^{-1}. Because maximal HR decreases with increasing age,

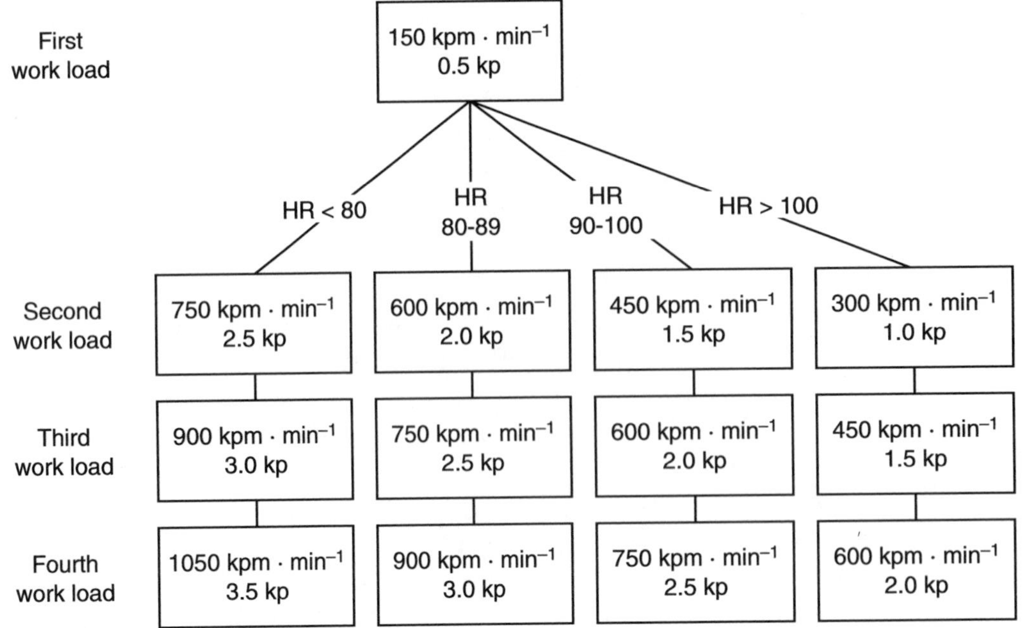

Directions:

1. Set the first work load at 150 kpm · min^{-1} (0.5 kp).
2. If the HR in the 3rd minute is
   - less than (<) 80, set the second load at 750 kpm · min^{-1} (2.5 kp);
   - 80 to 89, set the second load at 600 kpm · min^{-1} (2.0 kp);
   - 90 to 100, set the second load at 450 kpm · min^{-1} (1.5 kp);
   - greater than (>) 100, set the second load at 300 kpm · min^{-1} (1.0 kp).
3. Set the third and fourth (if required) loads according to the loads in the boxes below the second loads.

FIGURE 11.4 Guide for setting power outputs (work loads) for men and women on YMCA submaximal cycle ergometer test.

Reprinted from *Y's way to physical fitness: The complete guide to fitness testing and instruction*, 3rd ed., with permission of the YMCA of the USA, 101 N. Wacker Dr., Chicago, IL 60606.

however, and the data in table 11.8 were collected on young subjects, Åstrand (3,4) established the following correction factors with which one could multiply the estimated $\dot{V}O_2$max to correct for the lower maximal HR:

Age	*Factor*
15	*1.10*
25	*1.00*
35	*0.87*
40	*0.83*
45	*0.78*
50	*0.75*
55	*0.71*
60	*0.68*
65	*0.65*

One of the correction factors is multiplied by the estimated $\dot{V}O_2$max to calculate the corrected $\dot{V}O_2$max. For our 50-year-old subject, the correction factor is 0.75, and the corrected $\dot{V}O_2$max is 0.75 · 2.4 L · min^{-1} = 1.8 L · min^{-1}. This value compares well with that estimated by the YMCA protocol. The Åstrand and Ryhming calculations can be simplified using formulas developed by Shephard (42).

Submaximal Step Test Protocol

A multistage step test can be used to estimate $\dot{V}O_2$max and to show changes in CRF with training or detraining. As always, attention must be given to the initial stage and rate of progression of the stages so that the test is suited to the individual. Table 11.6 presented three examples of step

Name: ______________________

Sex: Female Age: 50

Estimated HRmax: 170 Ht: ______ in. Wt: ______ lb

85% HRmax: 145 ______ cm ______ kg

Work rate kpm · min^{-1}	Heart rate 2nd min	Heart rate 3rd min
150	95	96
300		
450	138	140
600	153	156

YMCA Protocol

1. Plot 3rd min HR for each work rate.
2. Draw line though points starting at HR > 110.
3. Extrapolate line to subject's estimated HRmax.
4. Drop vertical line from HRmax to baseline.
5. Record estimated $\dot{V}O_2$ max in L · min^{-1}.

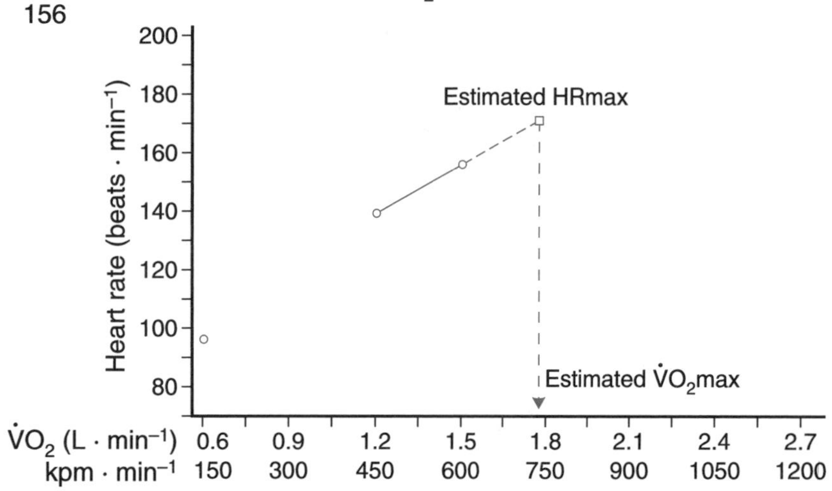

Heart rate (beats · min^{-1})

Estimated HRmax

Estimated $\dot{V}O_2$max

$\dot{V}O_2$ (L · min^{-1}) 0.6 0.9 1.2 1.5 1.8 2.1 2.4 2.7

kpm · min^{-1} 150 300 450 600 750 900 1050 1200

FIGURE 11.5 Maximal aerobic power estimated by measuring the heart rate response to a submaximal graded exercise test on a cycle ergometer, using the *Y's Way to Physical Fitness* protocol.

Reprinted from *Y's way to physical fitness: The complete guide to fitness testing and instruction*, 3rd ed., with permission of the YMCA of the USA, 101 N. Wacker Dr., Chicago, IL 60606.

test protocols. The subject must be instructed to follow the metronome (4 counts per cycle, i.e., up-up-down-down) and step all the way up and all the way down. Each stage should last at least 2 min, with HR monitored in the last 30 s of each 2-min period.

HR is more difficult to monitor during a step test protocol if the palpation technique is used. The heart rate watch simplifies the process, but when one is not available, a BP cuff can be used. When a HR measure is needed, pump the cuff up just above diastolic pressure (around 100 mmHg). With the stethoscope, the pulse rate can be counted for 15 to 30 s. The pressure is released after each measurement. An alternative is to stop stepping after each stage, taking the HR for a 10-s count 5 s after the stage is completed.

As in most submaximal test protocols, HR is plotted against $\dot{V}O_2$ for each stage, and a line is drawn through the points to the age-adjusted maximal HR. A line is drawn to the baseline to obtain an estimate of $\dot{V}O_2$max. Figure 11.6 shows the results of a step test for a sedentary 55-year-old man prior to a training program. His estimated $\dot{V}O_2$max was about 29 ml · kg^{-1} · min^{-1}, or 8.3 METs.

8 **In Review: A graphical plot of heart rate responses (> 110 beats · min^{-1}) to a graded exercise test on a treadmil, cycle ergometer, or bench step can be used to estimate $\dot{V}O_2$max. A line is drawn through the heart rate values and is extrapolated to the subject's age-adjusted estimate of maximal heart rate. A vertical line is drawn to the x-axis to estimate the work rate and $\dot{V}O_2$max the person would have achieved if the test had been a maximal test.**

Posttest Procedures

When the test is over, the tester should conduct a cool-down phase, monitor test variables, and give posttest instructions. The tester should also organize the test data (see Posttest Protocol on page 227).

Table 11.8 Predicting Maximal Oxygen Uptake From Heart Rate and Work Load During a 6-Min Cycle Ergometer Test

	Values for women $\dot{V}O_2max$ (L · min^{-1})						Values for men $\dot{V}O_2max$ (L · min^{-1})				
Heart rate	300 kpm/min	450 kpm/min	600 kpm/min	750 kpm/min	900 kpm/min	Heart rate	300 kpm/min	600 kpm/min	900 kpm/min	1200 kpm/min	1500 kpm/min
120	2.6	3.4	4.1	4.8		120	2.2	3.5	4.8		
121	2.5	3.3	4.0	4.8		121	2.2	3.4	4.7		
122	2.5	3.2	3.9	4.7		122	2.2	3.4	4.6		
123	2.4	3.1	3.9	4.6		123	2.1	3.4	4.6		
124	2.4	3.1	3.8	4.5		124	2.1	3.3	4.5	6.0	
125	2.3	3.0	3.7	4.4		125	2.0	3.2	4.4	5.9	
126	2.3	3.0	3.6	4.3		126	2.0	3.2	4.4	5.8	
127	2.2	2.9	3.5	4.2		127	2.0	3.1	4.3	5.7	
128	2.2	2.8	3.5	4.2	4.8	128	2.0	3.1	4.2	5.6	
129	2.2	2.8	3.4	4.1	4.8	129	1.9	3.0	4.2	5.6	
130	2.1	2.7	3.4	4.0	4.7	130	1.9	3.0	4.1	5.5	
131	2.1	2.7	3.4	4.0	4.6	131	1.9	2.9	4.0	5.4	
132	2.0	2.7	3.3	3.9	4.5	132	1.8	2.9	4.0	5.3	
133	2.0	2.6	3.2	3.8	4.4	133	1.8	2.8	3.9	5.3	
134	2.0	2.6	3.2	3.8	4.4	134	1.8	2.8	3.9	5.2	
135	2.0	2.6	3.1	3.7	4.3	135	1.7	2.8	3.8	5.1	
136	1.9	2.5	3.1	3.6	4.2	136	1.7	2.7	3.8	5.0	
137	1.9	2.5	3.0	3.6	4.2	137	1.7	2.7	3.7	5.0	
138	1.8	2.4	3.0	3.5	4.1	138	1.6	2.7	3.7	4.9	
139	1.8	2.4	2.9	3.5	4.0	139	1.6	2.6	3.6	4.8	
140	1.8	2.4	2.8	3.4	4.0	140	1.6	2.6	3.6	4.8	6.0
141	1.8	2.3	2.8	3.4	3.9	141		2.6	3.5	4.7	5.9
142	1.7	2.3	2.8	3.3	3.9	142		2.5	3.5	4.6	5.8
143	1.7	2.2	2.7	3.3	3.8	143		2.5	3.4	4.6	5.7
144	1.7	2.2	2.7	3.2	3.8	144		2.5	3.4	4.5	5.7
145	1.6	2.2	2.7	3.2	3.7	145		2.4	3.4	4.5	5.6
146	1.6	2.2	2.6	3.2	3.7	146		2.4	3.3	4.4	5.6
147	1.6	2.1	2.6	3.1	3.6	147		2.4	3.3	4.4	5.5
148	1.6	2.1	2.6	3.1	3.6	148		2.4	3.2	4.3	5.4
149		2.1	2.6	3.0	3.5	149		2.3	3.2	4.3	5.4
150		2.0	2.5	3.0	3.5	150		2.3	3.2	4.2	5.3
151		2.0	2.5	3.0	3.4	151		2.3	3.1	4.2	5.2
152		2.0	2.5	2.9	3.4	152		2.3	3.1	4.1	5.2
153		2.0	2.4	2.9	3.3	153		2.2	3.0	4.1	5.1
154		2.0	2.4	2.8	3.3	154		2.2	3.0	4.0	5.1
155		1.9	2.4	2.8	3.2	155		2.2	3.0	4.0	5.0
156		1.9	2.3	2.8	3.2	156		2.2	2.9	4.0	5.0
157		1.9	2.3	2.7	3.2	157		2.1	2.9	3.9	4.9
158		1.8	2.3	2.7	3.1	158		2.1	2.9	3.9	4.9
159		1.8	2.2	2.7	3.1	159		2.1	2.8	3.8	4.8
160		1.8	2.2	2.6	3.0	160		2.1	2.8	3.8	4.8
161		1.8	2.2	2.6	3.0	161		2.0	2.8	3.7	4.7
162		1.8	2.2	2.6	3.0	162		2.0	2.8	3.7	4.6
163		1.7	2.2	2.6	2.9	163		2.0	2.8	3.7	4.6
164		1.7	2.1	2.5	2.9	164		2.0	2.7	3.6	4.5
165		1.7	2.1	2.5	2.9	165		2.0	2.7	3.6	4.5
166		1.7	2.1	2.5	2.8	166		1.9	2.7	3.6	4.5
167		1.6	2.1	2.4	2.8	167		1.9	2.6	3.5	4.4
168		1.6	2.0	2.4	2.8	168		1.9	2.6	3.5	4.4
169		1.6	2.0	2.4	2.8	169		1.9	2.6	3.5	4.3
170		1.6	2.0	2.4	2.7	170		1.8	2.6	3.4	4.3

Reprinted from Åstrand 1979.

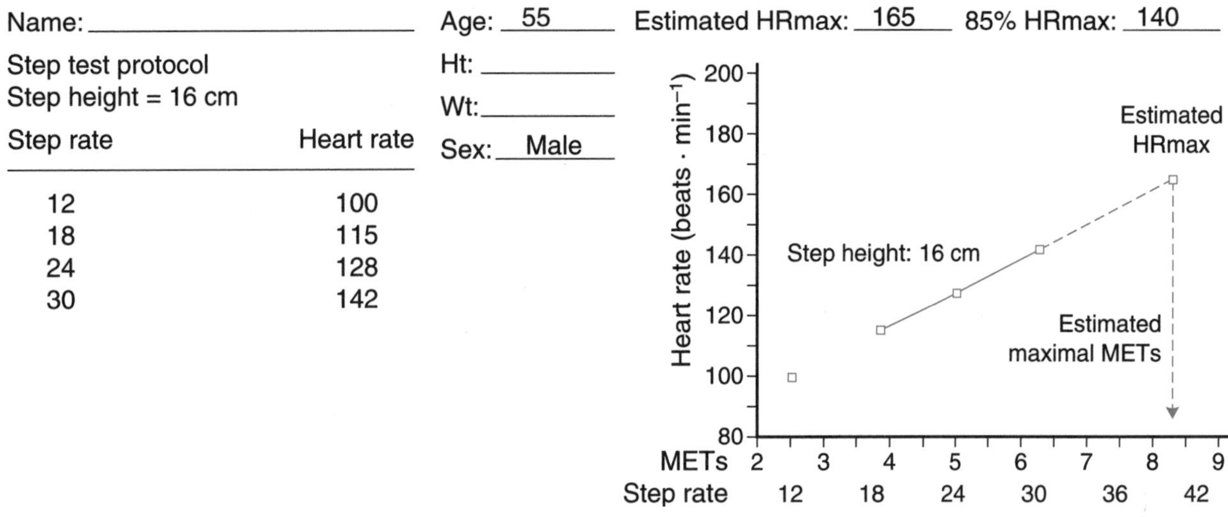

FIGURE 11.6 Maximal aerobic power estimated by measuring the heart rate response to a submaximal graded exercise step test.

Posttest Protocol

Use a cool-down as programmed per physician and other posttreadmill tests.

Have the individual sit down or lie down depending on posttests (nuclear).

Monitor HR, BP, and ECG immediately and after 1, 2, 4, and 6 min.

Remove cuff and electrodes when double product (HR × systolic BP) is close to pretest value.

Provide instructions for showering:

- Ask subject to wait for about 30 min before showering.
- Ask subject to move around in the shower and use warm (not hot) water.
- Check for return of person from the shower.

Organize test data and discuss test results with the participant.

Adapted from Howley 1988.

CASE STUDIES

You can check your answers by referring to appendix A.

11.1

You are contacted by a fitness club to review the test they have used to evaluate cardiorespiratory fitness on middle-age participants. The club requires the participants to perform the 1.5-mi-run test during their first exercise session. The club director says he uses this test because so much data exists for it—the test has been used for more than 10 years. What is your reaction?

11.2

You conduct the 1-mi-walk test with a 45-yr-old male client and record the following information: time = 15 min; heart rate = 140 beats · min^{-1}; weight = 170 lb. Calculate and evaluate his estimated $\dot{V}O_2max$.

11.3

A 50-year-old male, weighing 180 lb, completes a submaximal GXT on a cycle ergometer and the following data are obtained:

$kpm \cdot min^{-1}$	Heart rate
300	100
450	110
600	125
750	140

Estimate the subject's $\dot{V}O_2max$ by the extrapolation procedure. Express the value in METs.

11.4

A 30-year-old woman, weighing 120 lb, completes four stages of a submaximal Balke treadmill test ($3\ mi \cdot hr^{-1}$), and the following data are obtained:

% Grade	Heart rate
2.5	96
5	120
7.5	135
10	150

Estimate the subject's $\dot{V}O_2max$ by the extrapolation method, and express it in $ml \cdot kg^{-1} \cdot min^{-1}$, $L \cdot min^{-1}$, and METs.

SOURCE LIST

1. American Alliance for Health, Physical Education, Recreation and Dance (1988)
2. American College of Sports Medicine (1995)
3. Åstrand (1960)
4. Åstrand (1979)
5. Åstrand (1984)
6. Åstrand & Ryhming (1954)
7. Åstrand & Saltin (1961)
8. Balke (1963)
9. Balke (1970)
10. Blair, Painter, Pate, Smith, & Taylor (1988)
11. Blair et al. (1989)
12. Borg (1982)
13. Bouchard, Shephard, Stephens, Sutton, & McPherson (1990b)
14. Bransford & Howley (1977)
15. Bruce (1972)
16. Cooper (1977)
17. Daniels (1985)
18. Daniels, Oldridge, Nagle, & White (1978)
19. Durstine, King, Painter, Roitman, Zwiren, & Kenney (1993)
20. Ellestad (1994)
21. Foster et al. (1984)
22. Franks (1979)
23. Franks & Howley (1989)
24. Frohlich et al. (1988)
25. Golding, Myers, & Sinning (1989)
26. Hagberg, Mullin, Giese, & Spitznagel (1981)
27. Hanson (1988)
28. Haskell, Savin, Oldridge, & DeBusk (1982)
29. Howley (1988)
30. Howley & Franks (1986)
31. Kirkendall, Feinlieb, Freis, & Mark (1980)
32. Kline et al. (1987)
33. Maritz, Morrison, Peter, Strydom, & Wyndham (1961)
34. McArdle, Katch, & Pechar (1973)
35. Montoye & Ayen (1986)
36. Montoye, Ayen, Nagle, & Howley (1986)
37. Naughton & Haider (1973)
38. Oldridge, Haskell, & Single (1981)
39. Paffenbarger, Hyde, & Wing (1990)
40. Ragg, Murray, Karbonit, & Jump (1980)
41. Sedlock, Knowlton, Fitzgerald, Tahamont, & Schneider (1983)
42. Shephard (1970)
43. Shephard (1984)
44. Thompson (1988)

CHAPTER

12

Muscular Strength and Endurance

Vernon Bond

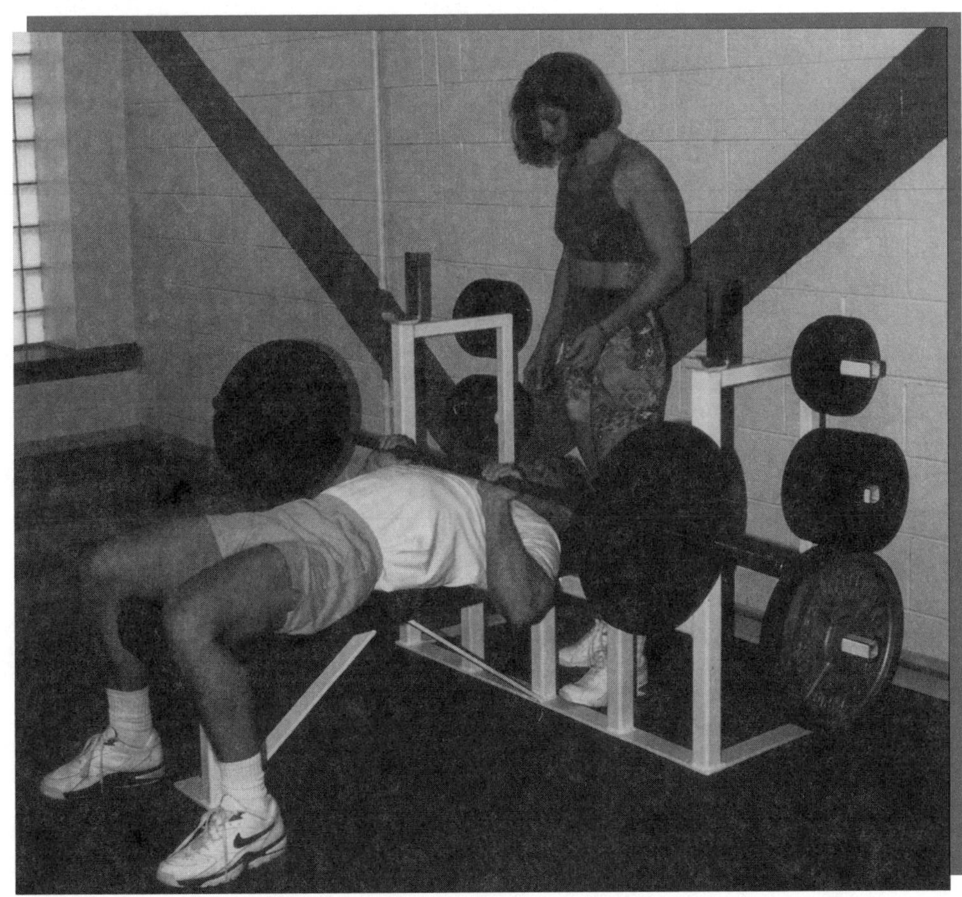

The reader will be able to: **OBJECTIVES**

1. Define muscular strength and endurance and list the factors related to muscle strength.
2. List the physiological adaptations associated with strength training in males and females and describe maturational changes in bone and muscle as people age.
3. Describe the common theories related to the cause of delayed-onset muscle soreness (DOMS).
4. List the factors related to muscle fatigue and contrast fast-twitch with slow-twitch muscle fibers in terms of fatigue.
5. Describe isometric, dynamic (isotonic), and isokinetic tests to assess muscular strength.
6. Describe field tests to evaluate muscular endurance.

Muscular strength and endurance are important components contributing to health and physical fitness. Four out of five Americans experience low-back discomfort, and 80 percent of low-back problems are muscular in nature (45) and can be corrected with strengthening exercises for the lower back and abdominal areas. Studies have shown that strength training reduces the risk of joint and/or muscle injuries that may occur during physical activity (20, 42). Also, strength training can attenuate the loss in muscle strength and bone density associated with the universal process of aging (22, 39). Osteoarthritis is the most common form of arthritis and is associated with a progressive loss of articular cartilage around the involved joint. Strength training is thought to reduce functional instability and pain in osteoarthritic patients by improving the strength and function of the surrounding connective tissue, which is often damaged by the disease (32). Not only does strength training help with health problems, but it also can increase muscle tone and improve one's personal appearance and self-esteem. Unless regular strength training exercises are performed, up to one-half pound of muscle may be lost every year after age 25 (45). Under most conditions, an annual increase in body fatness would not be desired as an ego boost to increase self-esteem.

Skeletal muscle is more metabolically active than fat, and one of the primary results of strength training is an increase in muscle mass. This causes a corresponding increase in resting energy expenditure (called resting metabolic rate), which is important in the prevention and management of obesity. From the standpoint of daily living, increased levels of muscular strength due to strength training can enhance the efficiency with which we carry out the usual routines (e.g., carrying loads such as groceries, boxes, children).

In this chapter we describe the factors influencing muscle strength, physiological adaptations to resistance training, muscle soreness, muscle fatigue, and methods for measuring muscular strength and endurance.

MUSCULAR STRENGTH AND ENDURANCE

Muscular strength is defined as the capacity of a muscle to exert maximum contractile force against a load. Muscular endurance is defined as the ability of a muscle to perform repetitive contractions, generating force for an extended period of time. If the resistance (load) during muscle contraction is equal to the contractile force of the muscle, the muscle contraction is isometric or static. If the resistance during muscle contraction is less than the contractile force of the muscle, the muscle contraction is isotonic or dynamic. Return to chapters 4 and 5 to review your understanding of the mechanism of skeletal muscle contraction (sliding-filament theory) and the types of muscle contractions (isometric, isotonic, eccentric, concentric).

Factors Influencing Muscle Strength

During muscle contraction the force generated can vary due to the following factors:

- The number of motor units activated
- The type of motor unit activated
- The size of the muscle
- The muscle's initial length when activated
- The muscle's speed of action

The motor unit is composed of a single motor neuron and all the muscle fibers innervated by that neuron. Greater muscle force is generated as the number of activated motor nerves increases. Fast-twitch motor units generate more force than slow-twitch motor units (see chapters 4 and 5). When a single stimulus is applied to a motor unit, a muscle twitch results (see figure 12.1). When the muscle receives repeated stimuli at a frequency such that the muscle cannot completely relax from the previous stimulus, the force produced increases to a value greater than after a single stimulus is received (summation). High-frequency stimulation results in a tetanus contraction and greater force production. Large muscles can generate greater force than small muscles due to the greater number of contractile filaments in the larger muscles. Muscles have the property of elasticity (ability to lengthen passively), and greater force can be generated when the muscle is stretched prior to contraction. The amount of force generated during muscle contraction is a function of the contraction speed. Muscles contracting at slow speeds produce greater force than muscles contracting at very rapid speeds.

> 1 **In Review: Muscle function can be classified in terms of strength or endurance. Muscle strength is the capacity of the muscle to generate force. Muscle endurance is the ability of the muscle to sustain continuous work. Muscular strength is influenced by the number and types of motor units recruited, muscle size, initial length, and velocity of contraction.**

GENERAL ADAPTATIONS TO RESISTANCE TRAINING

The muscular and skeletal systems are two of the ultimate targets of most resistance training programs. The following musculoskeletal adaptations are usually observed with resistance training:

- Increased muscle strength
- Increased muscle size
- Increased bone density

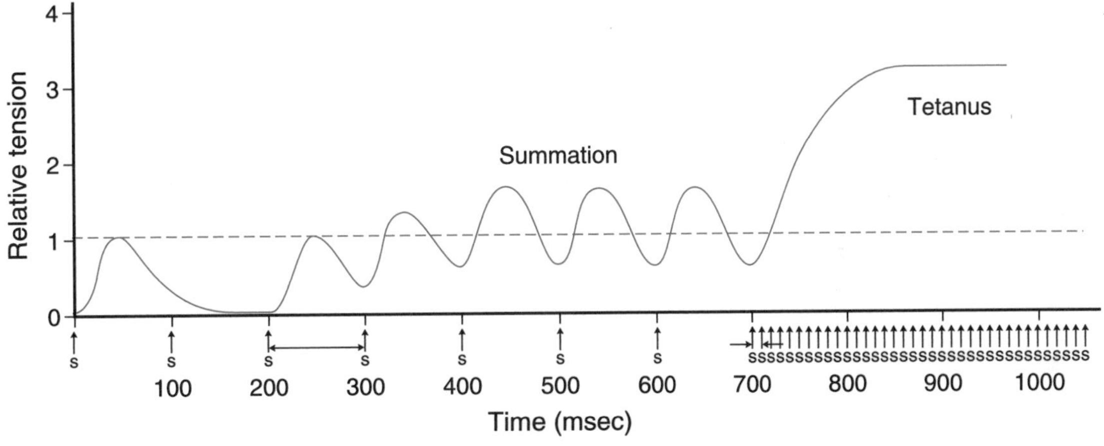

FIGURE 12.1 Repeated stimuli (S), each of a given strength, can produce a tension that adds up to be greater than the twitch tension. Continual stimulation results in a tetanic contraction (tetanus) three to five times stronger than the twitch tension.

Reprinted, by permission of McGraw-Hill, from Luciano, Vander, and Sherman 1978, *Human function and structure.*

Muscle Strength

Resistance training can produce significant strength gains (25% to 100% improvement) within 3 to 6 months. The nervous system and the increased muscle mass are the primary factors accounting for the increase in strength. Initial gains in muscle strength during the first few weeks of resistance training occur without an increase in the size of the muscle. Figure 12.2 shows that in the early phase of resistance training, the increases in muscle strength are associated primarily with that of neural adaptations. The neural adaptations can be explained by factors such as improved coordination and increased activation of the skeletal muscle prime movers. Figure 12.2 also illustrates that after 8 to 10 weeks of training, strength gains are associated with the combined effect of neural adaptation and increases in muscle mass (hypertrophy). It is noteworthy that after 3 to 4 months of training, further increases in muscle strength are attributed primarily to increases in muscle mass.

An increase in the level of physical fitness in the general population is an objective of the *Healthy People 2000* national fitness goals. Until about 15 years ago, most of what we knew about strength training was based on studies using young, healthy male subjects. Fortunately, that has changed. The following paragraphs examine what is known about the adaptations to resistance training in adolescents, the elderly, and females.

Research studies (29, 36, 37) have shown that resistance training done 3 times per week for 8 to 24 weeks will produce significant gains in strength among girls and boys 11 to 12 years of age. Testosterone is believed to be necessary for increases in muscle mass, but serum testosterone levels do not rise after exercise in prepubescent males as they do in adults. Because of the immature nature of the hormonal system in children, strength gains may be primarily a function of neural adaptations rather than an increase in muscle size.

It is well established that muscle strength decreases after the age of 30. In fact, loss of muscle mass is a primary factor responsible for the age-associated loss of strength. Loss of muscle mass can be alleviated, however. In a research study (16) it was shown that males, 60 to 72 years of age, who resistance trained the knee extension and flexion muscle groups for 12 weeks at 80% of their **one repetition maximum (1-RM)** (the greatest amount of weight a person can lift one time in good form), experienced gains of 107% and 227% in extension and flexion strength, respectively. A further significant finding was that the strength gains were associated with increased muscle size. Until the 1980s, it was assumed that increases in strength following resistance training in the elderly were primarily attributed to neural adaptations, rather than increases in muscle mass. Regardless of these findings, in strength training programs for older adults, exercises requiring maximal effort to exhaustion should be avoided to minimize adverse blood pressure responses and muscle injury.

Differences in measures of absolute muscle strength between males and females have been ob-

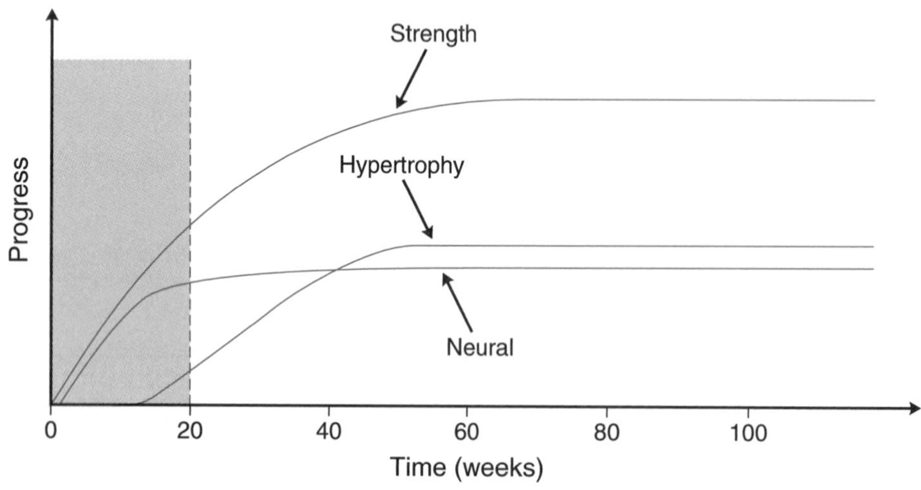

FIGURE 12.2 Neural and muscular adaptations during training. Most training studies span only 8 to 20 weeks. However, long-term studies reveal that neural adaptations dominate early in training, whereas most changes that occur during later training phases are associated with muscle hypertrophy.
Adapted from Sale, 1988, "Neural adaptation to resistance training." *Medicine and Science in Sports and Exercise*, 20: S142.

served for some time. Generally, a female's total body strength is 63.5% of a male's total body strength (23). However, this difference in muscle strength between genders appears to be a function of the specific body part. Laubach (23) reported that the upper extremity strength of females averaged 55.8% that of males', whereas lower extremity strength in women averaged 71.9% of the males' value.

The question has often been asked, "Does resistance training produce the same training effects in women as in men?" The answer is yes, but there is a difference in the magnitude of the training effects. The muscle's ability to exert force is the same for men and women (about 6 kg/cm^2) (14). However, there are variations both within and between genders in the adaptations to resistance training programs. Women will show increases in muscular strength and endurance as a result of a resistance training program, but the magnitude of the increase in absolute upper and lower body strength is less than that of men. This can be explained in part by the fact that females experience less of an increase in muscle mass with training than males. While some women might not choose to participate in resistance training programs because they are afraid their muscles will increase in size to such a degree that it will make them appear less feminine, in general, this will not happen. For example, it has been observed that following 10 weeks of resistance training, females exhibited a 0.6 cm increase in various body circumferences, an increase that would not be that noticeable (46).

Muscle Size

An increase in muscle size is one of the effects of a resistance training program but, as we just mentioned, there is great variation in this effect both within and between genders, and the effect occurs later rather than earlier in a training program. In untrained individuals a training period of 4 weeks or more is necessary before a measurable change in muscle size can be observed (44). Although it is well established that increases in muscle size occur with resistance training, there is some debate about *how* the muscles increase in size. One factor contributing to muscle enlargement is muscle fiber **hypertrophy**, an increase in the cross-sectional area of the existing muscle fibers. An opposing view suggests that muscle enlargement is attributed to **hyperplasia**, an increase in the total number of muscle fibers. Most physiologists agree, however, that the increase in muscle size in humans is due primarily to an enlargement of the muscle fibers (fiber hypertrophy).

Muscle hypertrophy can be attributed to transient and chronic effects of training. Transient hypertrophy is that "pumping up" of the muscle during a workout. This is due to fluid accumulation in the interstitial and intracellular spaces of the muscle. Approximately 1 hr after exercise the accumulated fluid returns to the blood and muscle size will decrease. Chronic hypertrophy refers to increases in muscle size over long-term resistance training with structural changes in the muscle (increased fiber size). The hormone **testosterone,** which is dominant in males, is important in stimulating muscle growth. Males experience greater muscle hypertrophy in comparison to females in response to resistance training, and this is attributed to differences in testosterone levels between the sexes.

Just as a muscle increases in size and strength with weight training, when the muscle is immobilized or training is stopped, the muscle also adapts to these conditions. When the muscle is immobilized there is a decrease in the size of the muscle (**atrophy**) because of muscle protein loss. Muscle strength decreases about 3% to 4% per day during the first week of immobilization (2). This decrease is associated with muscle atrophy and decreased neuromuscular activity of the immobilized muscle. When a muscle atrophies it appears that the slow-twitch muscle fibers are affected more than fast-twitch fibers. When the immobilized muscles become physically active, the atrophy effects can be reversed. The period of time needed for recovery of muscle size and strength, however, is longer than the period of immobilization.

one repetition maximum (1-RM) — The greatest amount of weight a person can lift one time in good form.

hypertrophy — An increase in the size of a muscle, organ, or other body part caused by an enlargement of its constituent cells.

hyperplasia — An increase in the size of the muscle due to an increase in the number of muscle fibers.

testosterone — Primary male hormone responsible for skeletal muscle development.

atrophy — A decrease in the size of skeletal muscle or other tissue because of disuse associated with muscle injury or sedentary lifestyle.

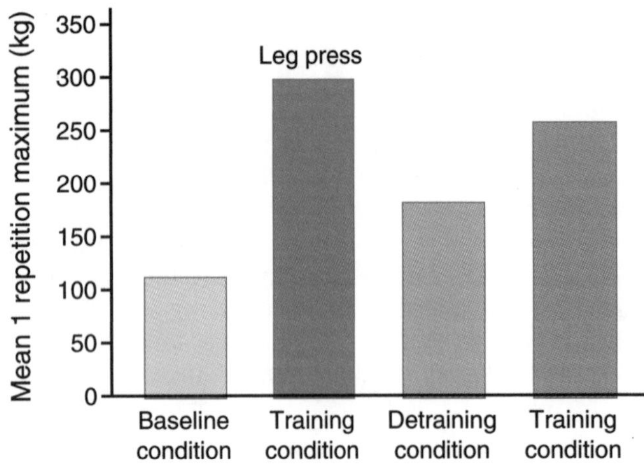

FIGURE 12.3 Changes in muscle strength, assessed by the leg press, with resistance training and detraining in women. Reproduced from Staron et al. 1991.

When individuals become inactive following an exercise program, their training adaptations are lost; that is, they experience a detraining effect. Endurance adaptations are most sensitive to periods of inactivity because the mitochondrial enzymes, the basis of endurance adaptations, change quickly during detraining. In contrast, strength changes appear more resistant to short periods of inactivity and decay over time at a much slower rate (21). Figure 12.3 shows the results of a study in which the lower extremities of females were resistance trained for 20 weeks; the training was then stopped for 30 to 32 weeks and was resumed for 6 weeks only (41). The study showed that detraining causes a loss of some of the strength gains associated with training. However, this loss was reversed once strength training was resumed.

Bone Density

The skeletal system consists of bones to which muscles are attached. Does weight training cause a change in the actual skeletal structure due to the increase in strength associated with weight training? Cross-sectional studies examining the bone mineral content in athletes who train with weights found a greater bone mineral content than that measured in sedentary individuals (30). Recent longitudinal studies have employed whole-body strength training and have shown a 2.8% increase in femoral neck bone mineral density (34) and a 1.2% increase in lumbar spine bone mineral density (40). Bone loss (osteoporosis) is a major health issue experienced by sedentary and older individuals; strength training can contribute to the prevention of osteoporosis.

A concern has often been expressed that resistance training might harm the skeletal system of young children. The long bones of the body grow in length from the epiphyseal plates located at each end of the bone (see chapter 5). Because of hormonal changes the epiphyseal plates do not ossify until after puberty. In children the most common risk of acute injury due to weight training is a fracture at the epiphyseal plate. This area is prone to injury in children because the epiphyseal plate is not ossified and does not have the structural strength of mature adult bone. Because of the concern for injury to growth cartilage in children due to resistance training, their training program should not focus on lifting maximal or near-maximal loads. The number of repetitions per set of exercise should be approximately 10, with a resistance of no greater than 10 repetition maximum.

2 **In Review: Early gains in muscle strength appear to be attributed to neural adaptations to strength training, but long-term gains are due to increased muscle size. Muscle enlargement associated with strength training is due primarily to an increase in the size of the individual muscle fibers (hypertrophy). Transient muscle hypertrophy associated with a workout results from fluid accumulating in the muscle and is short-lived. Chronic**

muscle hypertrophy results from prolonged periods of training that alters the structure of the muscle. The muscles of females hypertrophy with strength training but to a lesser degree than those of males because women have less testosterone. A muscle will atrophy (decrease in size and strength) when the muscle becomes immobilized or when training is discontinued. Bone loss (osteoporosis) associated with aging can be prevented or minimized by strength training. Due to risk of injury to epiphyseal (growth) plates in the long bones of children, resistance training should emphasize muscular endurance exercises.

MUSCLE SORENESS

Often with training a certain degree of muscle soreness or pain may be experienced. Muscle soreness might be present during the exercise period or during recovery immediately following exercise (**acute muscle soreness**). Also muscle soreness or discomfort may appear 12 to 48 hr after exercise (**delayed-onset muscle soreness**, or **DOMS**). Acute muscle soreness may persist for up to 1 hr following exercise and then disappear. This acute soreness or pain may be due to a reduction in blood flow to the muscle (ischemia) and the accumulation of metabolic products (hydrogen ions from lactic acid) in the muscle. DOMS appears to be related to the type of muscle contraction. Eccentric-type muscle contractions generate greater DOMS than concentric and isometric types of muscle contractions, and isokinetic exercises produce minimum DOMS (5). The physiological mechanism causing DOMS is not completely understood but several hypotheses have been offered that are discussed next.

Spasm Hypothesis

The muscular spasm hypothesis proposes that DOMS is due to ischemia during exercise, which results in an accumulation of a pain-causing substance in the muscle. This pain stimulates reflex muscular contractions or spasms that produce more ischemia that contributes to the pain occurring 12 to 48 hr after exercise (12).

Connective Tissue Damage Hypothesis

The connective tissue damage hypothesis suggests that DOMS is due to disruption in the connective tissue of the muscle and tendinous attachments. To support this theory Abraham (1) demonstrated that the excretion of hydroxyproline, a metabolic product of connective tissue damage, was higher in the urine of individuals who experienced muscle soreness than in those who did not.

Skeletal Muscle Damage Hypothesis

This hypothesis proposes that tears or ruptures of individual muscle fibers cause DOMS. Friden et al. (15), using muscle samples taken after intense eccentric exercise, showed structural damage to the myofibril Z lines of the sarcomere. Cellular enzymes representative of tissue damage (e.g., creatine kinase) have also been used as indicators of muscle damage. Clarkson et al. (10) found that after concentric, eccentric, and isometric types of muscle contraction the serum creatine kinase concentration was elevated. Interestingly, the subjects perceived greater muscle soreness associated with the eccentric muscle contractions.

Preventing Muscular Soreness

During the initial phase of exercise training some degree of muscle soreness or pain will most likely be experienced. To minimize or prevent muscular soreness, use of eccentric-type muscle contractions should be minimized. Warm-up exercise should always be done prior to resistance training, and the initial training program should begin with low-intensity exercises and progressively increase with time. To prevent muscle soreness during weight training McArdle et al. (27) suggest using 12 to

acute muscle soreness — Muscle soreness present during exercise or in recovery immediately following exercise.

delayed-onset muscle soreness (DOMS) — Muscle soreness that occurs 12 to 48 hr after the exercise bout.

15 repetition maximum (RM) at the onset of training, and after 2 weeks increase the intensity to between 6- to 8-RM.

> 3 **In Review: Acute muscle soreness can occur during an exercise bout and during the immediate recovery period lasting about 1 hr. Delayed-onset muscle soreness (DOMS) occurs 12 to 48 hr after the exercise bout. Eccentric-type muscle contractions are more strongly associated with DOMS than either isometric or isotonic contractions. Accumulation of metabolic products and ischemia are proposed causes for acute muscle soreness. DOMS may be caused by accumulation of waste products and/or structural damage to muscle cells and connective tissue. Muscle soreness can be prevented or minimized by limiting eccentric-type muscle contractions, beginning the training with low-intensity exercises with a gradual increase in progression, and warming up prior to each exercise session.**

MUSCLE FATIGUE

During repetitive muscle contractions fatigue is experienced and the total work produced is decreased. Fatigue experienced during physical exertion is associated with the intensity of the work involved. High-intensity work is primarily anaerobic (energy yielded without oxygen utilization) and the muscles fatigue relatively fast. Low-intensity work relies primarily on aerobic metabolism (energy yielded with oxygen utilization), and work can be sustained for a long period of time. The absolute ability of the muscle to generate power or resist fatigue is related to the muscle fiber type (see chapter 4 for a review). Fast-twitch fibers are characterized by anaerobic metabolism and can produce a large power output, but fatigue quickly. Slow-twitch fibers are characterized by aerobic metabolism and generate a low power output, but are fatigue resistant. The phosphagen system provides ATP primarily for anaerobic short-term, high-intensity work. This energy system relies on ATP and creatine phosphate, which are stored in limited amounts in the muscle and cannot supply energy for more than a few seconds. Activity such as high-intensity weight training relies primarily on the phosphagen system. Depletion of ATP and CP stores contribute to the fatigue experienced during high-intensity resistance training.

Also associated with short-term, high-intensity exercise is the production of lactic acid. At a physiological pH, lactic acid, a strong organic acid, releases a proton (H^+ ion). It is the H^+ rather than the lactate ion that causes pH to decrease. The H^+ accumulation resulting from glycolysis may interfere with Ca^{++} (calcium) binding to troponin, thereby interfering with muscle contraction and causing fatigue (4) (see also chapter 4).

Glucose stored in the muscle (muscle glycogen) is available for the production of energy during work. However, stores of glycogen in the muscle for exercise are limited (300 to 400 g of glycogen are stored in the body's total muscle mass) (4); and once muscle glycogen is depleted, the muscle begins to fatigue. The rate of glycogen depletion is related to the exercise intensity (38). Very high-intensity, intermittent exercise, such as weight training, can cause substantial depletion of muscle glycogen (20% to 50%) with relatively few sets of exercise (low total work) (33). Although phosphagens may be the primary limiting factor for resistance training with few repetitions or few sets (26), muscle glycogen may become the limiting factor for resistance training with many total sets and larger total amounts of work (33, 43).

> **In Review: Factors leading to muscle fatigue during short-term, high-intensity exercise include H^+ accumulation due to lactic acid production and decreases in ATP and CP. Muscle fatigue during prolonged low-intensity work can be explained by a decrease in muscle glycogen. Fast-twitch muscle fibers used during high-intensity exercise fatigue quickly, whereas the slow-twitch fibers utilized during low-intensity exercise can work for long periods of time without fatiguing.**

ASSESSING MUSCULAR STRENGTH

Muscle strength is generally assessed by the methods of cable tensiometry; dynamometry; the 1-RM method; and computerized, electromechanical, isokinetic dynamometers. It is very important that before any phase of muscle testing or exercise training, participants should do a complete warm-up (see chapter 15). See the appendix to this chapter that begins on page 240 for illustrations, protocols, and norms for each assessment method.

Cable Tensiometry

Cable tensiometry assesses muscular strength generated during a static or isometric contraction (28). Standardized testing procedures have been described in detail and should be followed to ensure the validity and reliability of the test results (8). The instrumentation includes a tensiometer, steel cables, testing table, wall hooks, straps, and a goniometer. The cable is attached to the wall or table hooks and the other end is attached with a strap to the body part to be tested. The cable is always positioned at right angles to the pulling bony lever. The goniometer is used to measure the appropriate joint angle. The tensiometer is placed on the cable and the individual exerts a maximal effort, pulling on the cable. As force is exerted on the cable, the riser of the tensiometer is depressed and the needle on the tensiometer indicates the peak force produced (19). See page 240 for instructions on how to administer this test. Although tensiometers vary in size and measure between 0 and 182 kg of force, a tensiometer that measures between 0 and 45 kg of force gives the highest degree of accuracy. Because this test can isolate the muscle groups at varying joint positions, it can be used as an objective diagnostic test to evaluate skeletal muscle function during rehabilitative treatment.

Dynamometers

Dynamometers are used to measure the strength of the forearm grip-squeezing muscles and leg and back muscles. When assessing grip strength the dynamometer is adjusted to a position that is comfortable to fit a particular hand size. The individual stands erect with the arm extended at the side and squeezes the dynamometer with maximal effort without moving the arm. Usually several trials are administered for each hand with a 1-min rest between trials. See page 241 for instructions on how to administer this test.

When assessing static leg strength using the back and leg dynamometer, the subject stands with the trunk erect and the knees flexed to an angle of 130° to 140°. The handbar is held using a pronated grip; and, without using the back, the subject slowly extends the legs with a maximal muscle contraction. The indicator needle remains at the peak force achieved. Two to three trials are conducted with a 1-min rest interval between trials (8). See page 241 for instructions on how to administer this test.

In assessing static back strength using the dynamometer, the individual stands with the knees fully extended and the head and trunk erect. The handbar is positioned across the thigh and grasped using a pronated (right hand) and supinated (left hand) grip. Without leaning backward, the subject pulls the handbar straight upward using only the back muscles. The shoulders are rolled backward during the pull. Individuals should be instructed to flex the trunk minimally and to keep the head and trunk erect during the lift (19). See page 242 for instructions on how to administer this test.

1-RM Method

Maximum strength during dynamic (isotonic) muscle contractions is often determined by the 1-RM method. To test 1-RM for any particular muscle group(s) such as the forearm flexors, leg extensors, or shoulders, a suitable starting weight is selected close to but below the subject's maximum lifting capacity (28). After each successful trial the individual should rest for 2 to 3 min, and the weight should be increased by 5, 2, or 1 kg (28). Gettman (17) recommends the bench press and leg press for assessing maximal strength in the upper and lower body, respectively. See pages 243-245 for instructions on how to administer these tests.

Computerized, Isokinetic Dynamometers

An isokinetic dynamometer is an electromechanical device containing a speed-controlling mechanism that is used to measure strength. With the limb speed of movement kept at a constant preselected velocity, the isokinetic dynamometer accommodates automatically to provide a counter force once the preselected velocity is reached. Thus, maximum

> **cable tensiometry** — An instrument that measures muscular strength during a static or isometric contraction.
>
> **dynamometer** — A device used to measure static strength of the forearm grip-squeezing muscles and the leg and back muscles.

force can be applied throughout the joint's complete range of motion. It is this characteristic of a dynamic isokinetic exercise that is different from a dynamic isotonic muscle contraction. The dynamometer is often interfaced with a computer or recorder that displays the force-velocity curve during each contraction cycle. The highest point on the force-velocity curve is defined as **peak torque** and represents the maximal strength achieved. Figure 12.4 illustrates the measurement of muscle strength in the lower extremity using a commercially available isokinetic dynamometer. While isokinetic testing applies the most advanced technology in muscle testing, its use is restricted to clinical or research applications due to its high cost.

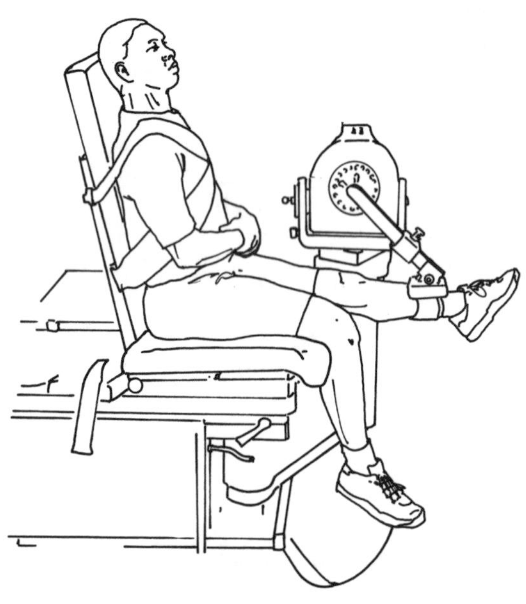

FIGURE 12.4 Measuring muscle strength in the lower extremity using a commercially available isokinetic dynamometer.

5 **In Review: Muscular strength testing can be done with static or dynamic contractions. Static muscle strength can be assessed through methods of cable tensiometry and dynamometry. Dynamic muscle strength can be assessed through the 1-RM method, which uses a specific load for resistance, and isokinetically at fixed joint velocities. When selecting different strength tests it is best to use those for which norms have been established.**

ASSESSING MUSCULAR ENDURANCE

Dynamic muscular endurance is measured by the maximum number of repetitions that can be executed during a given exercise. Two of the most common ways to measure muscular endurance are the curl-up test and the push-up test. See the appendix to this chapter that begins on page 240 for illustrations, protocols, and norms for each endurance assessment method.

Curl-Up Endurance Test

The curl-up test is used to determine the endurance capacity of the abdominal muscle group. For the partial curl-up test, the individual being tested assumes a supine position with the knees flexed and the feet about 12 in. from the buttocks. The arms are extended with the fingers positioned palm-down on the thighs and pointing toward the knees. The tester kneels behind the head of the individual with her or his hands cupped under the individual's head. The individual curls up slowly sliding the fingers up the legs until the fingertips touch the knee caps (patellas); this is followed by a slow return to the starting position with the back of the head touching the tester's hands. No assistance is provided to anchor or support the feet of the individual during the test. The movement is always slow, continuous, and well controlled, at a rate of 20 curl-ups per minute (i.e., 3 s per curl-up, with the metronome set at 40 beats $\cdot$ min^{-1}). Subjects perform as many curl-ups as they can without pausing, up to a maximum of 75 (24). See page 245 for instructions on how to administer this test.

Push-Up Endurance Test

The push-up test is used to determine the endurance capacity in the upper body. Following is a description of the protocol used in conducting the full-body and modified push-up. In the full-body push-up the individual assumes a position that is essentially a straight line from the head to the ankles. The hands are placed where they are most comfortable (approximately shoulder-width apart). In a rigid erect position with the arms extended, the individual lowers the body down until the elbows reach an angle of 90° flexion; then the individual pushes upward until the arms are once again fully extended. The push-ups should be done in a continuous motion with the score being the total number of push-ups to exhaustion. In the modified push-up the protocol is the same as described for the full-body push-up, except the individual assumes the bent-knee position with the hips and buttocks pressing downward, in line with the neck and shoulders. The individual's hands should be slightly ahead of the shoulders in the up position and directly under the shoulders in the down position. See page 246 for instructions on how to administer this test.

6 **In Review: Local muscle endurance of the abdominal and upper-body muscles is commonly assessed using the curl-up and push-up tests, respectively. Individuals with less upper-body strength should use the bent-knee position for the push-up test.**

CASE STUDIES

You can check your answers by referring to appendix A.

12.1

You are invited to make a presentation to a weight-training class at a local college. The teacher would like you to discuss the changes in muscle size and strength that might result from participation in a 7-week resistance training program, and indicate how the results might differ for male and female students. Prepare an outline for your presentation.

12.2

When you visit the class to make your presentation, one of the students asks you if lactic acid build up causes the muscle soreness he experienced a day or two after his first workout. Another wants to know if there is anything that can be done to prevent muscle soreness. How would you respond to these questions?

SOURCE LIST

1. Abraham (1977)
2. Appell (1990)
3. Baechle (1994)
4. Brooks, Fahey, & White (1996)
5. Byrnes, Clarkson, & Katch (1985)
6. D. Clarke (1966)
7. D. Clarke & H.H. Clarke (1984)
8. H.H. Clarke (1973)
9. H.H. Clarke, Bailey, & Shay (1952)
10. Clarkson, Byrnes, McCormick, Turcotte, & White (1986)
11. Corbin, Dowell, Lindsey, & Tolson (1978)
12. deVries (1980)
13. Faulkner, Springs, McQuarrie, & Bell (1988)
14. Fleck & Kraemer (1987)
15. Friden, Sjostrom, & Ekblom (1983)
16. Frontera, Meredith, O'Reilly, Knuttgen, & Evans (1988)
17. Gettman (1988)
18. Gettman (1993)
19. Heyward (1991)
20. Kibler, Chandler, & Stracener (1992)
21. Kramer (1994)
22. Larsson (1982)
23. Laubach (1976)
24. Liemohn & Sharpe (1992)
25. Luciano, Vander, & Sherman (1978)
26. MacDougall et al. (1988)
27. McArdle, Katch, & Katch (1981)
28. McArdle, Katch, & Katch (1991)
29. Micheli (1983)
30. Nilsson & Westlin (1977)
31. Pollock, Wilmore, & Fox (1978)
32. Pothier & Allen (1991)
33. Robergs et al. (1991)
34. Ryan et al. (1994)
35. Sale (1988)
36. Servedio et al. (1985)
37. Sewall & Micheli (1984)
38. Sherman & Wimer (1991)
39. Snow-Harter, Bousxein, Lewis, Carter, & Marcus (1992)
40. Snow-Harter & Marcus (1991)
41. Staron et al. (1991)
42. Stone (1990)
43. Stone & O'Bryant (1987)
44. Tesch (1988)
45. Westcott (1991)
46. Wilmore (1974)

peak torque — Highest point on the force-velocity curve measured during testing on an isokinetic dynamometer.

APPENDIX

Assessing Muscular Strength and Endurance

Muscular Strength Tests

Cable Tensiometry. While this figure illustrates only the cable tensiometer assessing muscular strength of the knee extensors, a variety of cable strength tests have been developed for most of the major muscle groups (6, 7, 9).

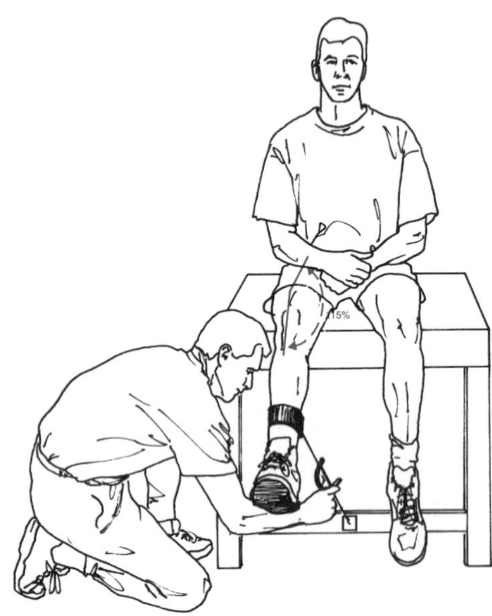

1. Attach one end of the cable to the wall or table hooks and the other end to the body part to be tested. Always position the cable at right angles to the pulling bony lever.
2. Use a goniometer to measure the appropriate joint angle.
3. Place the tensiometer on the cable.
4. Instruct the individual to exert a maximal effort, pulling on the cable.

Dynamometer Grip Test

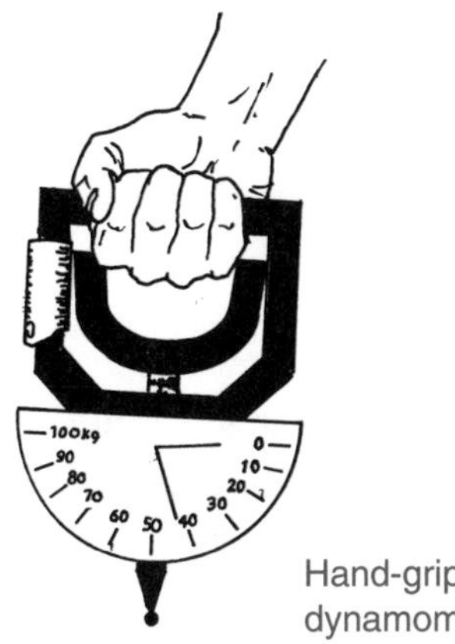

Hand-grip dynamometer

1. Adjust the dynamometer to a position that is comfortable to fit the subject's hand size.
2. Have the individual stand erect with the arms extended at the side and squeeze the dynamometer with maximal effort without moving the arm.
3. Administer several trials for each hand, with a 1-min rest between trials.

Static Leg Strength Dynamometer Test

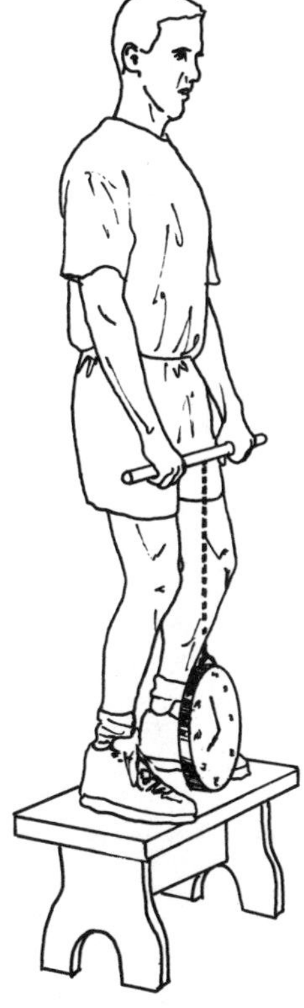

1. Have the subject stand with the trunk erect and the knees flexed to an angle of 130 to 140°.
2. Make sure the subject holds the handbar using a pronated grip.
3. Without using the back, the subject slowly extends the legs with a maximal muscle contraction.
4. Complete 2 to 3 trials with a 1-min rest interval between trials (8).

Static Back Strength Dynamometer Test

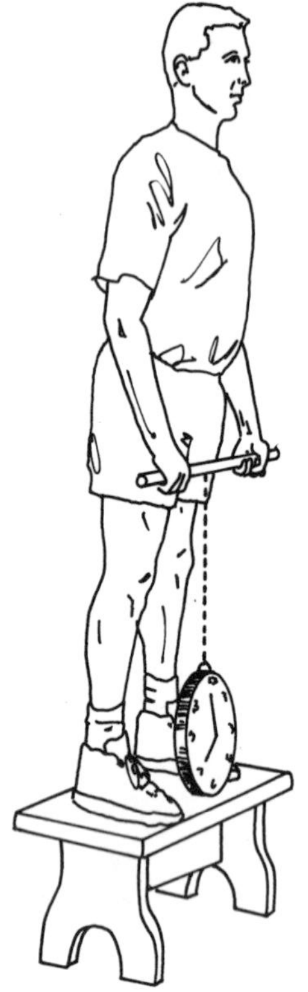

1. Have the subject stand with the knees fully extended and the head and trunk erect.
2. Make sure the subject holds the handbar across the thighs using a pronated (right hand) and supinated (left hand) grip.
3. Without leaning backward, the subject pulls the handbar straight up using only the back muscles. The shoulders are rolled backward during the pull.
4. Instruct individuals to flex the trunk minimally, and to keep the head and trunk erect during the lift (19).

Static Strength Norms

Classification	Left grip (kg)	Right grip (kg)	Back strength (kg)	Leg strength (kg)	Total strength[a] (kg)	Relative strength[b]
Men						
Excellent	> 68	> 70	> 209	> 241	> 587	> 7.50
Good	56-67	62-69	177-208	214-240	508-586	7.10-7.49
Average	43-45	48-61	126-176	160-213	375-507	5.21-7.09
Poor	39-42	41-47	91-125	137-159	307-374	4.81-5.20
Very poor	< 39	< 41	< 91	< 137	< 307	< 4.81
Women						
Excellent	> 37	> 41	> 111	> 136	> 324	> 5.50
Good	34-36	38-40	98-110	114-135	282-323	4.80-5.49
Average	22-33	25-37	52-97	66-113	164-281	2.90-4.79
Poor	18-21	22-24	39-51	49-65	112-163	2.10-2.89
Very poor	< 18	< 22	< 39	< 49	< 117	< 2.10

Note. For persons over age 50, reduce scores by 10% to adjust for muscle tissue loss due to aging.
[a]Total strength = left and right grip strength plus back strength plus leg strength.
[b]Relative strength is determined by dividing total strength score by body weight (in kg).
Data adapted with permission from C.B. Cobin et al.

1-RM Bench Press Test (Modified from Baechle [3])

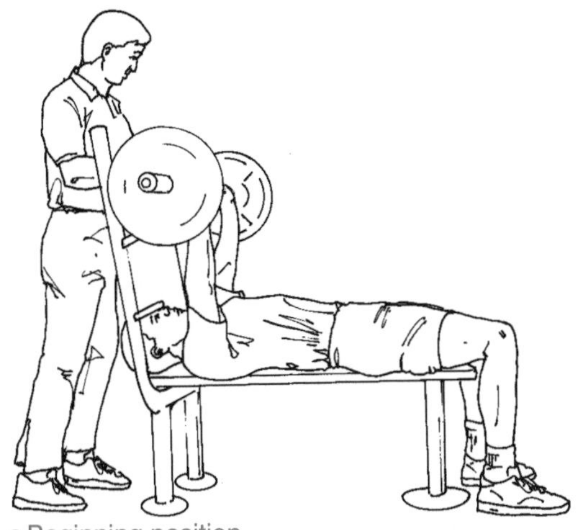

a Beginning position

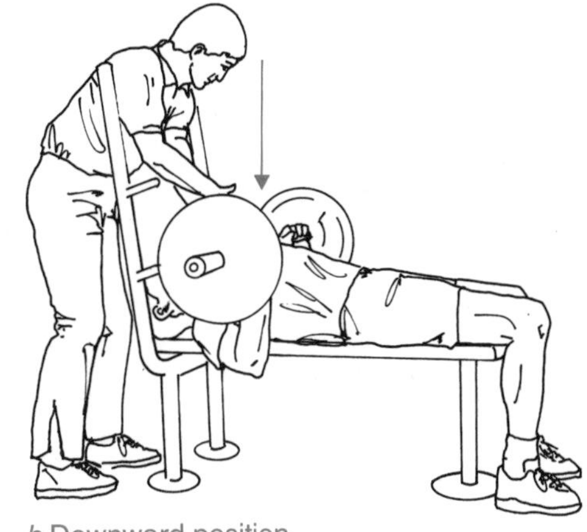

b Downward position

1. Have the individual lie face up on the bench in the beginning position (*a*). Feet are flat on the floor. The individual signals the spotter, then positions the bar over the chest with elbows fully extended.
2. In the downward movement phase (*b*), the subject lowers the bar to touch the chest as the body position is maintained and the wrists are kept straight.
3. In the upward movement phase (*c*), the subject pushes the bar up to full elbow extension while maintaining body position without arching the back.

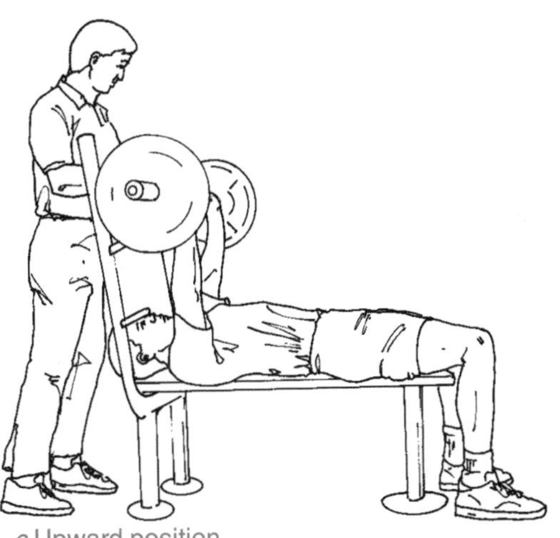

c Upward position

Standard Values for Bench Press Strength in 1-RM lb/lb Body Weight

Rating	Age (yr) 20-29	30-39	40-49	50-59	60 +
Men					
Excellent	> 1.25	> 1.07	> 0.96	> 0.85	> 0.77
Good	1.117-1.25	1.01-1.07	0.91-0.96	0.81-0.85	0.74-0.77
Average	0.97-1.16	0.86-1.00	0.78-0.90	0.70-0.80	0.64-0.73
Fair	0.88-0.96	0.79-0.85	0.72-0.77	0.65-0.69	0.60-0.63
Poor	< 0.88	< 0.79	< 0.72	< 0.65	< 0.60
Women					
Excellent	> 0.77	> 0.65	> 0.60	> 0.53	> 0.55
Good	0.72-0.77	0.62-0.65	0.57-0.60	0.51-0.53	0.51-0.54
Average	0.59-0.71	0.53-0.61	0.48-0.56	0.43-0.50	0.41-0.50
Fair	0.53-0.58	0.49-0.52	0.44-0.47	0.40-0.42	0.37-0.40
Poor	< 0.53	< 0.49	< 0.44	< 0.40	< 0.37

Note. Adapted from the Cooper Institute for Aerobics Research 1997.

1-RM Leg Press Test (Modified from Baechle [3])

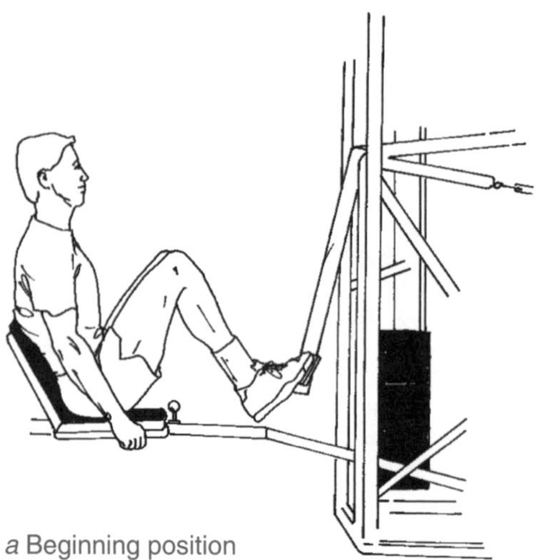

a Beginning position

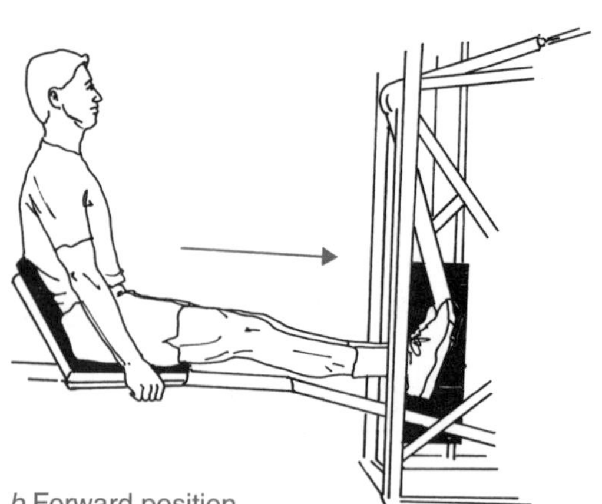

b Forward position

1. Have the individual sit on the machine in the beginning position (*a*) with the legs parallel to each other and the feet on the pedals.
2. In the forward movement phase (*b*), the subject pushes the foot pedals forward while avoiding forcefully locking out the knees on the extension.
3. In the backward movement phase (*c*), the subject moves the foot pedals backward to the beginning position slowly and under control.

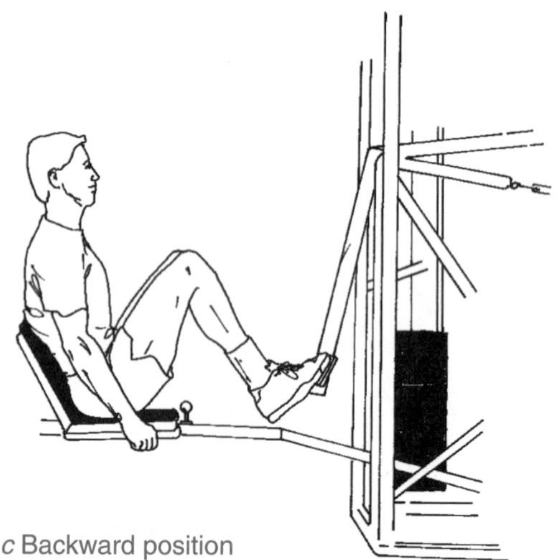

c Backward position

Standard Values for Leg Press Strength in 1-RM lb/lb Body Weight

	Age (yr)				
Rating	20-29	30-39	40-49	50-59	60 +
Men					
Excellent	> 2.07	> 1.87	> 1.75	> 1.65	> 1.55
Good	2.00-2.07	1.80-1.87	1.70-1.75	1.60-1.65	1.50--1.55
Average	1.83-1.99	1.63-1.79	1.56-1.69	1.46-1.59	1.37-1.49
Fair	1.65-1.82	1.55-1.62	1.50-1.55	1.40-1.45	1.31-1.36
Poor	< 1.64	< 1.54	< 1.49	< 1.39	< 1.30
Women					
Excellent	> 1.62	> 1.41	> 1.31	> 1.25	> 1.14
Good	1.54-1.62	1.35-1.41	1.26-1.31	1.13-1.25	1.08-1.14
Average	1.35-1.53	1.20-1.34	1.12-1.25	0.99-1.12	0.92-1.07
Fair	1.26-1.34	1.13-1.19	1.06-1.11	0.86-0.98	0.85-0.91
Poor	< 1.25	< 1.12	< 1.05	< 0.85	< 0.84

Note. Adapted from the Cooper Institute for Aerobics Research 1997.

Curl-Ups Test

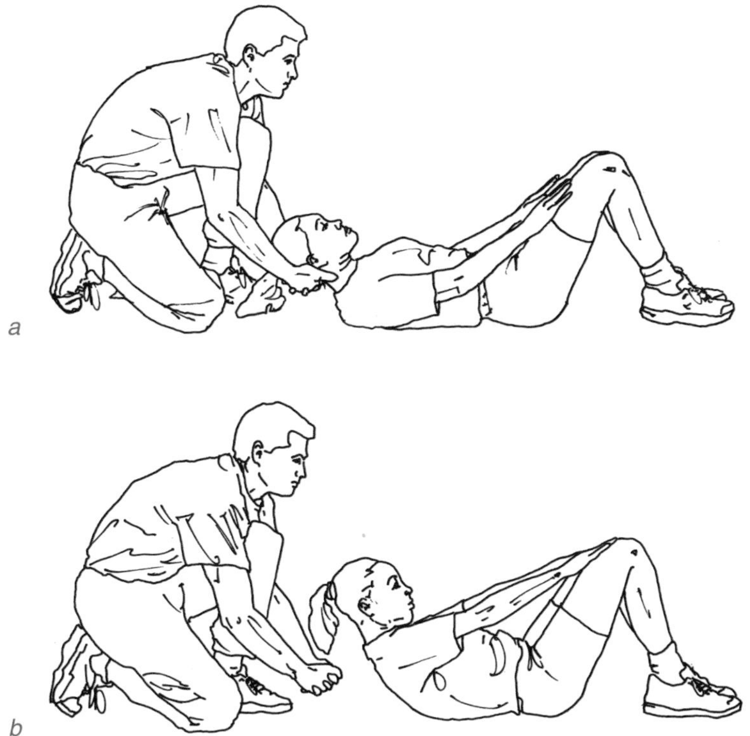

1. Have the subject start in a supine position with the knees flexed at 90° and the fingers resting on the upper legs (*a*).
2. The individual curls up slowly and touches the knees (*b*).
3. The individual returns to the starting position until the head touches the tester's hands (*a*).

Standards for Partial Curl-Up Test

	Number completed					
	Men/age			Women/age		
Rating	<35	35-44	>45	<35	35-44	>45
Excellent	60	50	40	50	40	30
Good	45	40	25	40	25	15
Marginal	30	25	15	25	15	10
Needs work	15	10	5	10	6	4

Note. Adapted from Liemohn and Sharpe 1992. Adaptation based on research by Faulkner et al. 1988.

Push-Ups Test

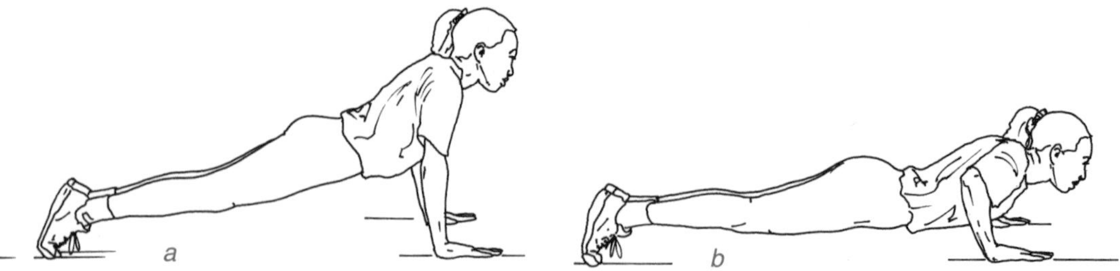

1. Have the individual assume a position that is essentially a straight line from the shoulders to the ankles. The hands are placed where they are most comfortable (approximately shoulder-width apart).
2. In a rigid erect position with the arms extended (*a*), the individual lowers the body down until the elbows reach an angle of 90° flexion (*b*).
3. The subject then pushes upward until full extension of the arms is reached (*a*).

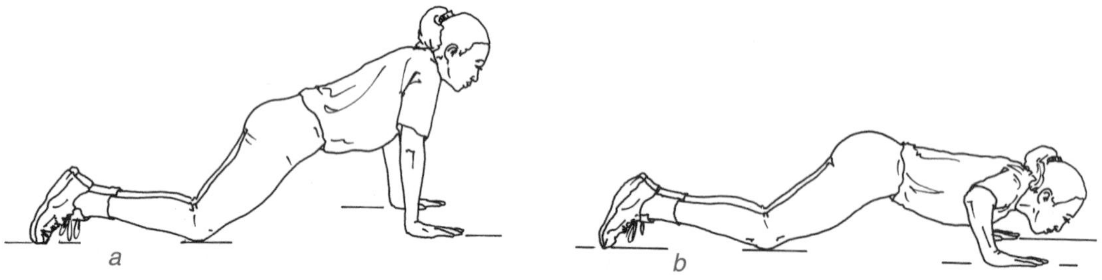

In the modified body push-up, the protocol is the same, except the individual assumes the bent-knee position with the buttocks down. The individual's hands should be slightly ahead of the shoulders in the up position (*a*), and directly under the shoulders in the down position (*b*).

Standard Values for Push-Up Test

Rating	Age (yr)				
	20-29	30-39	40-49	50-59	60 +
Full-body push-up					
Excellent	> 54	> 44	> 39	> 34	> 29
Good	45-54	35-44	30-39	25-34	20-29
Average	35-44	24-34	20-29	15-24	10-19
Fair	20-34	15-24	12-19	8-14	5-9
Poor	< 20	< 15	< 12	< 8	< 5
Modified-body push-up					
Excellent	> 48	> 39	> 34	> 29	> 19
Good	34-48	25-39	20-34	15-29	5-19
Average	17-33	12-24	8-19	6-14	3-4
Fair	6-16	4-11	3-7	2-5	1-2
Poor	< 6	< 4	< 3	< 2	< 1

Note. Modified from M.L. Pollock et al. 1978.

CHAPTER 13

Flexibility and Low-Back Function

Wendell Liemohn

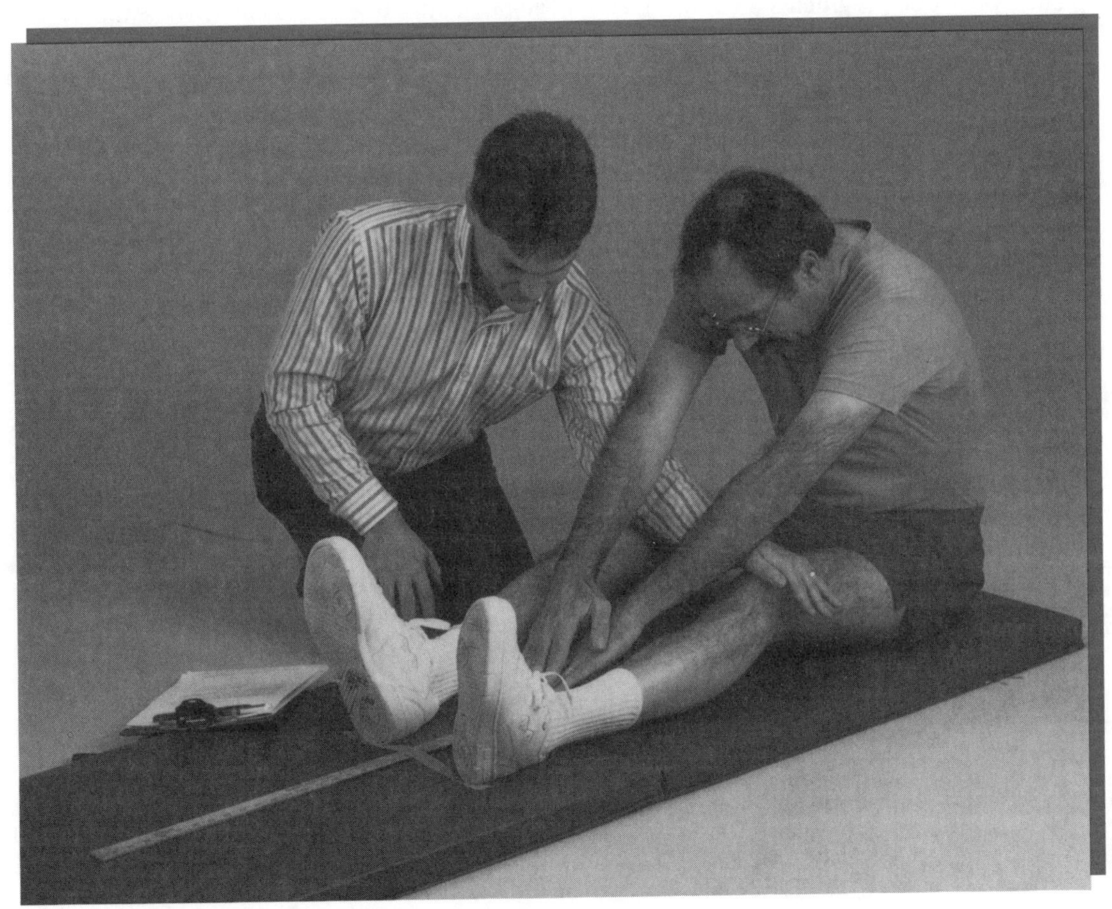

© Chris Brown

The reader will be able to: **OBJECTIVES**

1. Describe the relationship between flexibility/range of motion (ROM) and low-back function.
2. List five factors that can affect the degree of an individual's flexibility/ROM.
3. Describe the amount of flexion that can occur between the rib cage and the sacrum and state a rule of thumb to follow in performing lumbar extension exercises.
4. Explain why having good ROM at the hip joint is important to having a healthy back.
5. Describe the pluses and minuses of the sit-and-reach test.

Flexibility relates to the ability to bend without breaking; the related word *flexion* is the act of bending or being bent. In applied anatomy the term flexion is used to denote a bending movement in the sagittal plane as two body segments are moved in approximation to each other (see chapter 5). If you were to bend over and touch your toes from the standing position, you would be demonstrating flexion at both iliofemoral (hip) joints and limited flexion in the lower intervertebral joints of the spine.[1] To return to the standing position, the movement would be called extension; further movement of the trunk backwards beyond your normal standing posture would be called hyperextension (see chapter 5). What is somewhat ironic is that individuals may be called flexible if they can show an extreme amount of mobility in either forward bending (i.e., flexion) or backward bending (i.e., hyper*extension*) because the movements meet the criteria for the definition of flexion. In part because there is potential confusion in describing an individual's ability to hyperextend as being indicative of flexibility, *range of motion* (ROM) is frequently used in place of flexibility. The terms flexibility and ROM, however, are often interchanged.

Having functional ROM at all joints of the musculoskeletal system is desirable to ensure efficient body movement; this is one reason why flexibility is a key component of physical fitness. Although some individuals might be considered to have very good ROM at all their joints, flexibility is considered a joint-specific characteristic. In other words, having good trunk flexion ROM does not guarantee having good trunk extension ROM. Moreover, sometimes ROM might be related to one's genotype (i.e., heredity related). In other cases ROM might be related more to the activities in which one participates. For example, many years of ballet or gymnastics training would be expected to make an individual more flexible than someone with no such training.

When low-back function is considered, good ROM is of increased importance because it can decrease the probability of having a back problem. Furthermore, once a low-back problem occurs, increasing ROM can be a factor in reducing both the severity of the problem and the amount of time it takes to recover and return to work.

1 **In Review: Flexibility/ROM are joint specific. Having good ROM can decrease chances of having a low-back problem. Once a low-back problem has occurred, increasing ROM is a goal in most therapeutic exercise programs.**

[1]The greatest amount of intervertebral movement occurs between the fifth lumbar vertebra (L5) and the fused sacrum (which begins with S1); this is referred to as the lumbosacral joint. The intervertebral joint between L4–L5 also permits a substantial portion of the movement in the lower portion of the spine; however, the amount of movement permitted between L1–L4 is nominal.

FACTORS AFFECTING RANGE OF MOTION (ROM)

There are many different factors that affect ROM. Although age, gender, and genotype may be good predictors, there are always exceptions.

Effect of Age and Gender on ROM

The amount of ROM one has is dependent upon several demographic variables. For example, ROM typically decreases in adulthood; however, what is uncertain is how much of this diminution in ROM is due to aging per se or to the activity reduction related to aging. The gender factor is another consideration; although females are generally considered the more flexible gender, these differences are sometimes joint specific. For example, although females are generally considered to be more flexible than males, the opposite has been found to be true in flexion/extension movements of the spine.

Nature/Nurture Considerations

The statement has been made that if one wants to live to a ripe old age with a minimum amount of disease, simply "pick your parents." Similarly one could say that if one wants to have extremely good flexibility, pick your parents. Although marked increases in ROM can be achieved by participating in good flexibility training programs, one's genotype imposes limitations. Some people have relatively poor flexibility; no matter how hard they trained, their flexibility would improve nominally. Although an individual with great flexibility may devote a considerable amount of time to stretching exercises, one's genotype is most important.

Postural Considerations

If individuals did not use their full ROM at any joint, tendinous tissue would compensate by shortening. It would then become very difficult to make some of the movements used by many in activities of daily living. For example, a person sitting at a computer terminal for many hours each day without adequate postural support might develop a greater thoracic curve (e.g., a dorsal kyphosis) and round shoulders (see figure 13.1). If habitual postures such as this are maintained excessively, tendinous tissue that used to permit a wide degree of movement would shorten and impede movement.

Effects of Disease Processes on ROM

The process of disease can have a significant negative impact on a person's ROM. The disease processes of arthritis and osteoporosis and their effect on ROM are discussed next.

Arthritis

Arthritis can have debilitating effects on ROM; two of the more common types are **rheumatoid arthritis** and **osteoarthritis**. Rheumatoid arthritis is polyarticular in nature, affecting many joints; it is seen more in females than in males and it can affect any age. Conversely, the much more prevalent osteoarthritis (accounting for 90% to 95% of all arthritis cases) is seen more in joints in which damage or injury has occurred to the articular cartilage. Articular cartilage, also called hyaline cartilage, is **avascular** (i.e., it does not have a blood supply); because of this its healing capability is not good. Thus, if there is an injury to complex joints such as the knee or shoulder, or even to the simple hinge joints of the fingers, the body's compensatory adaptations may work for a while but often become deficient as the individual ages. After articular cartilage is damaged, fibrocartilage and/or bony spicules are often the replacement tissues and joint movement tends to diminish further.

Lack of mobility due to arthritis is often seen in joints such as the fingers or the knee; however, arthritis can also decrease mobility in the spine. Because it is avascular, articular cartilage depends on the diffusion of nutrients from tissue fluid; further deterioration can result from lack of movement. Thus, in as much as it is possible, it is desirable for the individual with arthritis to maintain movement.

arthritis — Inflammation of a joint.

rheumatoid arthritis — Debilitating form of arthritis involving many joints (polyarticular).

osteoarthritis — Most common form of arthritis (90% to 95% of all cases); affects joints whose articular cartilage is damaged or injured.

avascular — Without a blood supply.

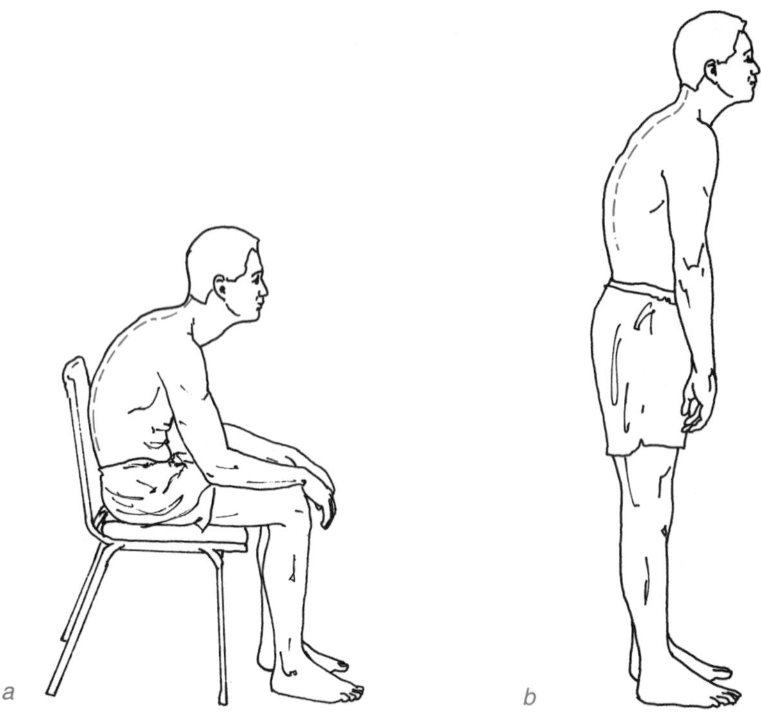

FIGURE 13.1 Connective tissue structures (e.g., ligaments and tendons) adapt to habitual poor sitting posture by lengthening in response to stress and shortening in the absence of stress (*a*). Eventually, if no attempt is made to remove these stresses and/or develop counterbalancing ones, poor sitting postures transfer to poor standing postures (*b*).

Osteoporosis

Osteoporosis is characterized by a loss in bone mineral density or bone mass. Although it is particularly a problem seen in women after menopause, it can also affect males and is genetically influenced. Common osteoporotic sites include the hip, wrist, and vertebrae; a common characteristic of these sites is that cancellous bone predominates (see chapter 5). In the spine osteoporosis can cause an actual buckling or compression of vertebrae; a person afflicted with this condition may show extreme curves in the spine as well as loss of ROM. The individual depicted in figure 13.2 shows the result of sustained buckling or crushing of vertebrae in the thoracic area; this condition is sometimes called *dowagers' hump*. Fortunately cancellous bone can, however, become more dense through activities such as weight training.

2 **In Review: Factors that relate to the degree of one's ROM are age, gender, heredity, posture, and disease. If joint ROM is not used it will be lost; although declines in ROM relate to increased age, some declines in ROM are related to a decline in physical activity. ROM relates to both nature and nurture; in other words it is affected by one's genotype as well as the type of activities in which one participates. Habitual poor posture also causes a decrease in ROM. Arthritis is a disease of joints and thus tends to reduce joint ROM. Osteoporosis can reduce spine ROM by damaging vertebrae.**

RANGE OF MOTION AND LOW-BACK FUNCTION

Spinal carriage is functionally integrated to all movements because all movements emanate from the spine. A strong argument has also been made that the spine and its associated tissues are the primary engine of locomotion in our species (5); any acceptance of this view demands an appreciation of the importance of maintaining good spinal mobility. Gracovetsky supported this contention with a graphic presentation in the book entitled *The Spinal Engine*.

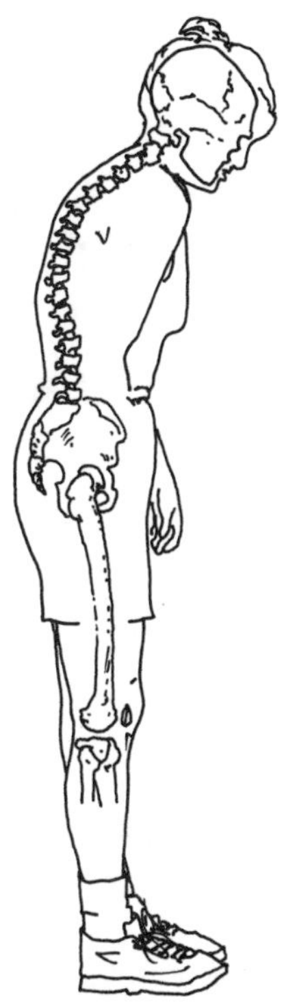

FIGURE 13.2 The condition of osteoporosis can result in a crushing or buckling of cancellous bone; here the cancellous vertebrae bones have been crushed. Osteoporosis is related to aging and is most prevalent in women after menopause; however, weight-bearing exercise and weight training can be a factor in reducing the seriousness of the condition.

Spine ROM

ROM deficiencies in the spine and its supporting structures have been viewed as prognostic indicators of low-back pain (1, 14). ROM by itself, however, is not that good a predictor of impending low-back problems (2). In other words ROM can be a major factor in some cases of low-back pain, but more often two or more variables are jointly responsible for the problem. It should be noted, however, that individuals with chronic low-back pain can establish therapeutic stretching regimens to improve trunk and hip-joint ROM (see chapter 16).

A very important concept to understand is that the flexion movement between the rib cage and the sacrum is in essence a straightening of one's "normal" **lordotic curve**; this concept is also mentioned in chapter 16 in conjunction with trunk strengthening exercises. Although there may be a progressive decline in spinal mobility in all planes with aging, McKenzie (12) contends that there is a greater decline in extension movement because this movement is used less as a person ages. Unfortunately extension of the spine is an issue often ignored or misinterpreted in exercise programs (see chapter 16). Although ballistic extension movements of the spine (and ballistic rotation movements) are totally inappropriate, "slow and controlled" extension movements to strengthen the erector spinae are appropriate for inclusion in exercise programs *if* active back extension does not exceed the upper limit of normal lumbar lordosis as seen in standing (15). (See figure 13.3.)

An extreme lateral curvature is called a **scoliosis**; the Adam's test can be used if an exercise leader wishes to get a better perception of the presence or absence of a scoliosis in a client (figure 13.4). Although many causes have been identified for scoliosis, usually the cause is unknown. It is not surprising that leg-length discrepancy leading to a lateral tilt of the pelvis is associated with scoliosis and low-back pain; however, the evidence of scoliosis causing low-back pain is not conclusive.

Iliofemoral-Joint ROM

The muscles crossing the hip joint can be viewed as guy wires bracing the pelvis (see figure 13.5); if any of these "guy wires" are too tight, the trunk musculature, regardless of how well it is developed, may have difficulty controlling pelvic position. Because the sacral portion of the pelvis is the foundation for the 24 vertebrae stacked on it, pelvic positioning plays an important role in the integrity of the spine. For example, tightness in the hip flexors such as the iliopsoas will produce an anterior or forward pelvic tilt; tightness in the hip extensors such as the hamstrings will produce a backward or posterior pelvic tilt (see figure 5.10). Thus if either of these muscle groups are tight, the ability of the abdominal muscles to control pelvic positioning will be adversely affected. Individuals who cannot control their pelvic positioning with their abdominal muscles are vulnerable to having the low-back pain malady; this is one of the reasons why good ROM at the iliofemoral joint is most important.

lordotic curve — Describes the condition of lordosis, a forward, concave curve of the lumbar spine when viewed from the side.
scoliosis — An abnormal lateral curvature of the spine.

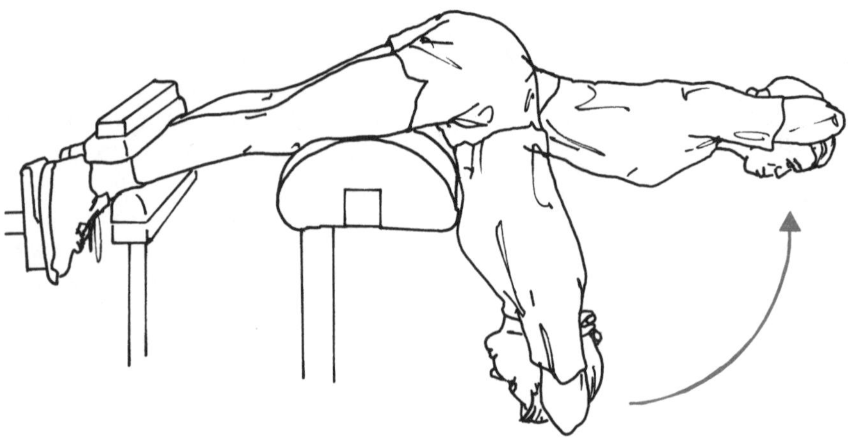

FIGURE 13.3 This exercise can be used to strengthen the erector spinae musculature. To be on the safe side, however, active extension movements should not exceed one's normal lordotic curve.

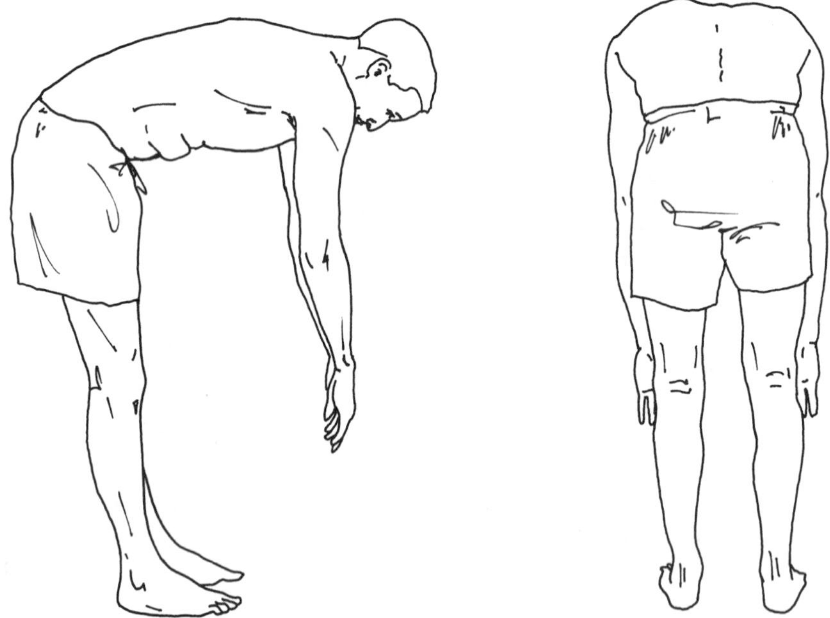

FIGURE 13.4 Adam's test. Viewing the spinous processes as the subject is standing does not always reveal scoliotic curves even if present. However, it is much easier to see a scoliotic curve after the subject bends forward at the waist.

3 **In Review:** Spine flexion between the rib cage and the sacrum is limited to the straightening of one's normal lordotic curve. Although maintenance of spine extension ROM is important, ballistic back extension movements should be avoided and back extension should not exceed the exerciser's normal lumbar lordosis.

MEASURING SPINE AND HIP-JOINT RANGE OF MOTION

Some of the techniques used to measure ROM as it relates to low-back function are specific to the spine or to the hip joint; other techniques purport to measure spine and hip-joint ROM concurrently. This discussion first reviews techniques that are specific to

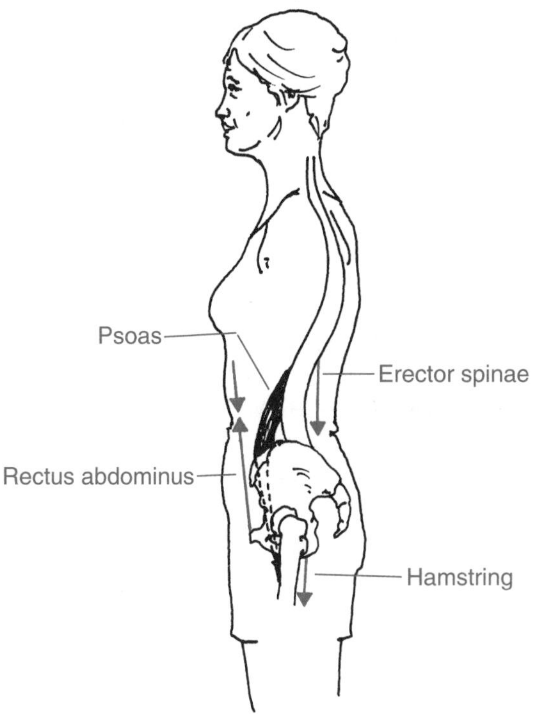

FIGURE 13.5 The muscles crossing the hip joint can be viewed as guy wires. If, for example, the hamstring guy wires are too tight, the rectus abdominis will have difficulty in controlling pelvic positioning. Inability to control pelvic positioning with the abdominal musculature makes one vulnerable to low-back problems.

either the measurement of spine or hip-joint ROM; then techniques that purport to measure both hip and spine ROM are reviewed. All techniques are illustrated in this chapter's appendix.

Trunk-Extension ROM

In Imrie and Barbuto's (8) test for back extension, the back musculature is not actively used; it is considered a *passive* test of back ROM because the extension movement in the spine is the result of arm and shoulder movement. Table 13.1 shows a scoring protocol for this test. An *active* test of spine-extension ROM was developed by the Cooper Institute for Aerobics Research (4). It is an active test because muscles of the spine contract actively to perform movement. It should be noted, however, that because both trunk-extensor muscle strength *and* trunk-extension ROM contribute to performance on this test, it is difficult if not impossible to pinpoint the basis for poor performance (and, consequently, the basis for therapeutic exercise prescription) should it exist in a given individual.

Table 13.1 Standards for Back Extension Test

Rating	Back extension (cm)
Excellent	> 30
Good	20-29
Marginal	10-19
Needs work	< 9

Note. Adapted from Imrie & Barbuto 1988.

Hip-Joint Flexion ROM

The Thomas test is typically used to measure tightness in the hip flexors. It is important that individuals using this test are familiar with its nuances. For example, if the contralateral leg is brought too close to the chest, a false positive might result (i.e., the extra posterior rotation of the pelvis may cause the tested limb to rise suggesting tightness at its hip joint). Although hip-flexor tightness is not seen as much as hip-extensor tightness, if there is tightness in the former and it is not realized, subsequent measurement of hip-extensor ROM is apt to be invalid.

Hip-Joint Extension ROM

Two of the more popular tests used to measure tightness in the hip extensors include the Passive Straight-Leg Raise and the Active Knee-Extension Tests. In either test a goniometer or an inclinometer may be used to make the measurement. If large groups are going to be tested, a protractor-type instrument can be used to expedite the procedure.

In Review: Good ROM at the hip joint is important to having good biomechanics of the spine. Although hip-flexor tightness is not seen as often as hip-extensor tightness, it too can be an important factor in the maintenance of a healthy spine. If any of the muscles crossing the hip joint are too tight, one is susceptible to low-back problems.

Combined Tests of Trunk- and Hip-Joint Flexion ROM

The fingertips-to-floor and the sit-and-reach tests have often been used under the pretense that they measure flexibility in the low-back area as well as at the hip joint. It has been shown conclusively, however, that although both can be used as measures of hip-joint flexibility (e.g., hamstring length), in their conventional use neither test is an effective measure of low-back ROM. Because the sit-and-reach is used more as a field test than the fingertips-to-floor test, it is examined here in greater detail; however, most of the following comments apply to its use either as an exercise or as a test.

The sit-and-reach test as an exercise has been questioned clinically. For example, if the hamstrings are tight and one performs the sitting stretch ballistically, the structures of the spine are obligated to absorb these stresses; over time these repetitive motions may have a serious consequence on low-back function. Moreover, it has also been shown that even if the sit-and-reach is done slowly, the static postures resulting during the stretching phase can place high compressive forces on the intervertebral discs (13). Cailliet (3) cautioned that this exercise might damage ligaments of the spine, particularly if the sit-and-reach performer's hamstrings are tight.

To reduce the stress on the spine incumbent in the sit-and-reach, Cailliet (3) recommended as an exercise what he called a "protective hamstring stretch" (see the appendix to this chapter). In this exercise the hamstrings of each leg are stretched alternately while the nonstretched limb is bent at the knee joint with its foot flat on the floor next to the contralateral knee. Cailliet contends that lumbosacral stress is less in his hamstring stretch than in the more typical sit-and-reach with both legs extended; if this is true, the same reasoning would warrant administering the sit-and-reach test with only one leg extended. However, we examined lumbosacral movement in university students tested with both legs extended as well as with just one leg extended and found that less flexion movement (which would imply less stress) was not seen in Cailliet's version of the sit-and-reach (11). Nevertheless, Cailliet's protective hamstring stretch has other factors in its favor (e.g., permits checking for symmetry) and is deemed to be a safer activity for the spine than the sit-and-reach with both legs extended.

The sit-and-reach test was originally used under the pretense that it measured both low-back and hamstring flexibility; however, research has shown conclusively that although it can be used as a measurement of hamstring length, it is not a valid measurement of low-back ROM when centimeters reached is the criterion. The sit-and-reach has also been questioned because it does not make allowance for proportional differences between arm, trunk, and leg length. In response to the latter, Hopkins and Hoeger (7) developed a protocol that controls for some of this variance by first determining how far the subject can reach (i.e., with the back positioned against the wall); from this position the subject then bends forward and the reach determination is again made. The second score minus the first one is net reach.

More recently we noted that performance on the sit-and-reach was significantly better with the ankles in passive plantar flexion as opposed to the fixed dorsiflexion posture usually required when the test is administered (10). Our research suggests that factors such as tightness in the connective tissue structures located behind the knee and/or tension on the **sciatic nerve** can affect performance on the sit-and-reach.

Even though the sit-and-reach activity has medical contraindications and a host of factors that can affect its performance, it can still be of value as a field test *provided* that test users are aware of these shortcomings. Following are suggestions that can make the sit-and-reach a better test:

- It is argued that the number of centimeters reached is not the most valid indicator of performance. The test administrator is better advised to examine the quality of the movement of the individual being tested. Quality points to look for include the angle of the sacrum (see figure 13.6) and the "smoothness" of the spinal curve. These relatively simple determinations can be used to make the sit-and-reach a measure of low-back mobility as well as a measurement of hamstring length. These and other quality points are delineated in figure 13.6.
- It is recommended that the sit-and-reach be administered with only one leg extended. Although this technique doubles the number of measurements required, the tester will also be able to evaluate symmetry.
- If a sit-and-reach box is used to make measurements, it is recommended that it be altered to permit passive plantar flexion at the ankle joint. This may be done by converting the standard box: The vertical surface under the cantilever extension can be replaced by a 4-cm rod, which permits plantar flexion into the box but restrains the heel.

If you are interested in other tests that are specifically designed to measure spine ROM, two suggestions are offered; however, both require a good knowledge of anatomy (e.g., ability to locate bony landmarks on the pelvis and spine). Keeley et al. (9) described a test protocol for a double inclinometer

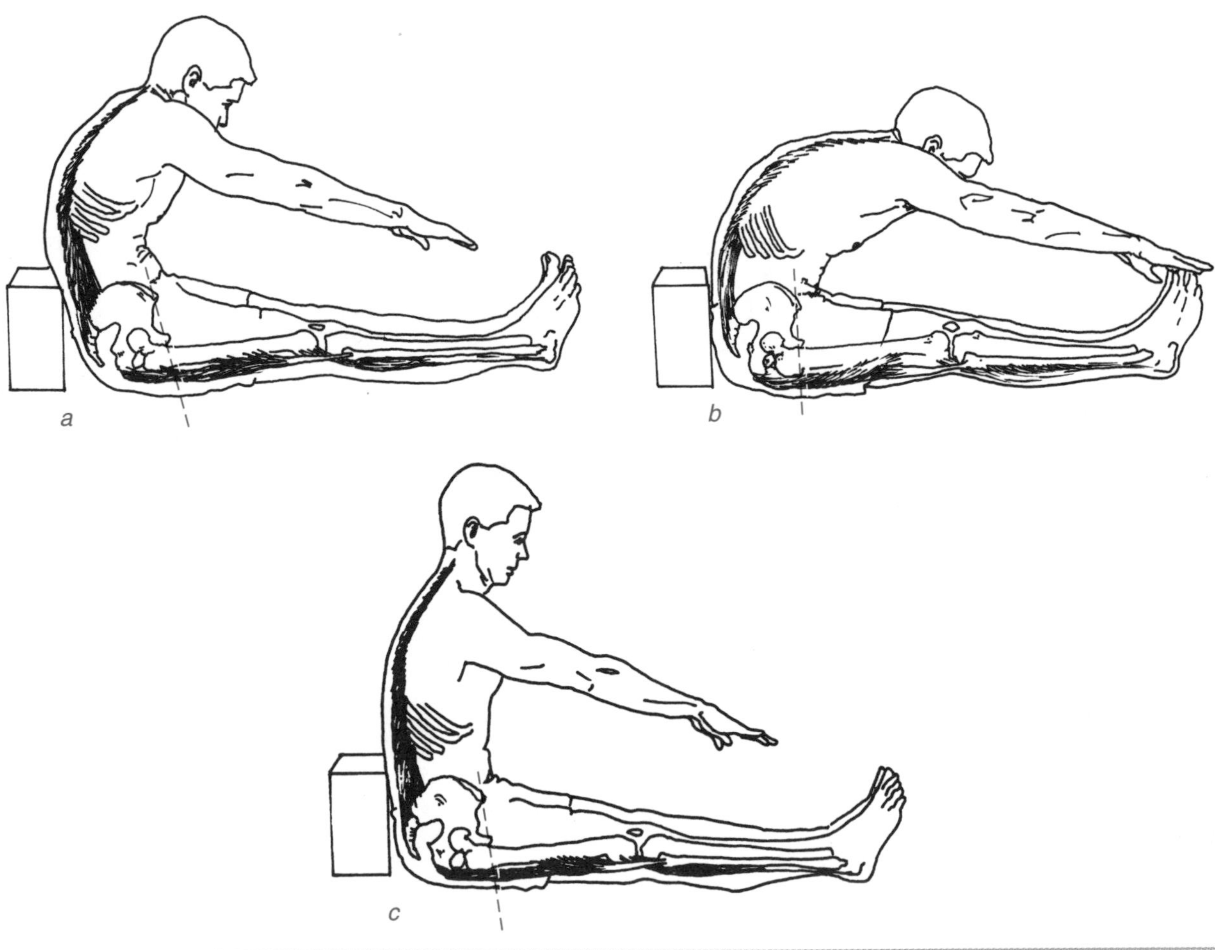

FIGURE 13.6 Sit-and-reach test. Quality points to look for: Tight hamstrings (note tilt of pelvis), tight low back and stretched upper back (*a*); normal length of hamstrings and low back (*b*); tight hamstrings (note tilt of pelvis), tight low back (*c*).

technique that is used in clinical settings; although inclinometers are expensive (approximately $100 each), they are more versatile than the less expensive goniometer. Williams et al. (16) described a modification of the Schober technique that is used to measure spine ROM; although a tape measure is the only equipment required, this test is primarily used in clinical settings in part because the location of bony landmarks requires the removal of clothing.

5 **In Review: If a person with tight hamstrings practices the sit-and-reach maneuver with both legs extended, damage to the soft tissue structures of the spine can occur. In administering the sit-and-reach test, the quality of the movement should be considered; it can be more important than the number of centimeters reached.**

Case Studies

You can check your answers by referring to appendix A.

13.1

After learning that one of the individuals participating in your physical fitness program was told that his hamstrings were tight, you administer the sit-and-reach test in order to get some baseline data on his tightness. Somewhat to your surprise you find that he can reach beyond the plane of his toes. What

sciatic nerve — Nerve originating at area of the hip; involved in low-back problems that can result in loss of feeling and control in the legs.

quality factors (i.e., something other than cm reached) in his sit-and-reach performance might you further examine to explain this disparity? What other hamstring length test might you administer?

13.2

Assume that this individual's record indicates that she has very tight hip flexors based on an administration of the Thomas test. However, when you administer the Thomas test, you do not find evidence of hip-flexor tightness. Assume that this individual has done nothing to increase her ROM and that you are confident that you administered the Thomas test correctly. Explain how the prior administrator of the test might have erred.

SOURCE LIST

1. Biering-Sorensen (1984)
2. Cady, Bischoff, & O'Connell, et al. (1979)
3. Cailliet (1988)
4. Cooper Institute for Aerobics Research (1992)
5. Gracovetsky (1988)
6. Gracovetsky & Farfan (1986)
7. Hopkins & Hoeger (1992)
8. Imrie & Barbuto (1988)
9. Keeley, Mayer, Cox, Gatchel, & Mooney (1986)
10. Liemohn, Martin, Sharpe, & Thompson (1996)
11. Liemohn, Sharpe, & Wasserman (1994)
12. McKenzie (1981)
13. Nachemson (1975)
14. Pope, Bevins, & Wilder, et al. (1985)
15. Saal, J.S., & Saal, J.A. (1991)
16. Williams, Binkley, Bloch, Goldsmith, & Minuk (1993)

APPENDIX

Tests for Measuring ROM as It Relates to Low-Back Function

Spine ROM

Passive-Back ROM Test

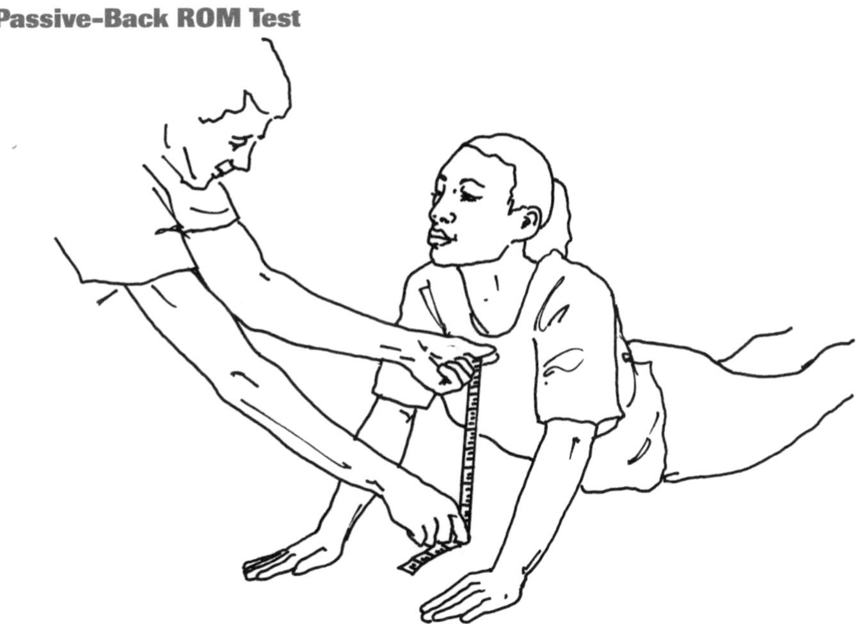

While keeping the anterior part of the pelvis (i.e., anterior superior iliac spines) in contact with the floor, the subject elevates the torso with arm action; the muscles of the back are *not* used in this movement. The score is the perpendicular distance from the suprasternal notch to the floor; from a geometric perspective it should be easy for individuals with longer trunks to have better scores.

Active-Back ROM/Strength Test

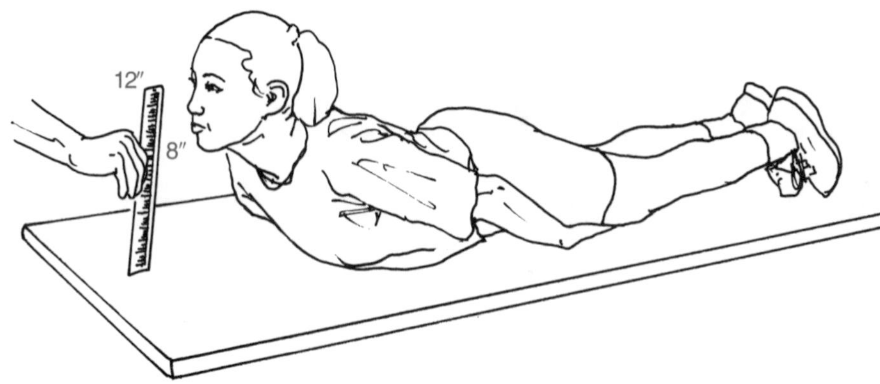

In this test the individual slowly lifts up the torso by contracting the erector spinae muscle group until the chin is a maximum of 12 in. (i.e., 12 in. is the top score). A drawback to this test is that performance is dependent upon both strength and ROM; if performance is poor, it can be difficult to determine if the cause is lack of strength or a lack of ROM.

Hip-Joint ROM

Thomas Test

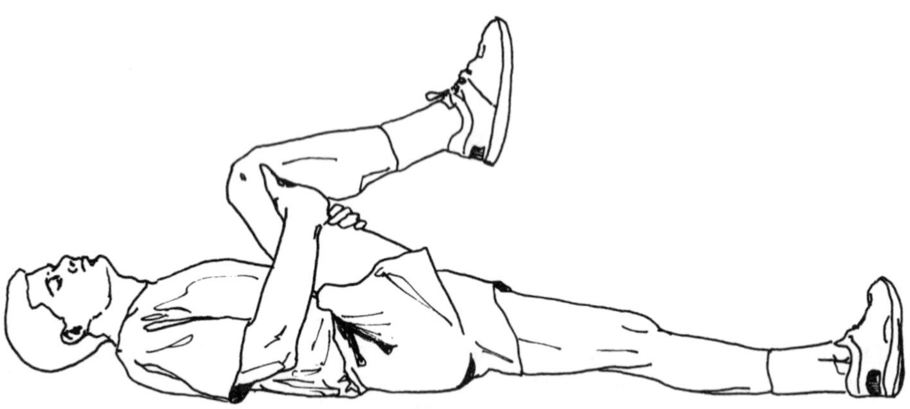

It is important that the contralateral leg be brought in the direction of the chest *only* to the point where the lumbar spine is snug against the floor or table. If the tested leg remains in contact with the testing surface during this maneuver, the hip flexors of that leg are of adequate length; however, if the tested leg raises, its hip flexors are more than likely short.

Passive Straight-Leg-Raise (PSLR) Test

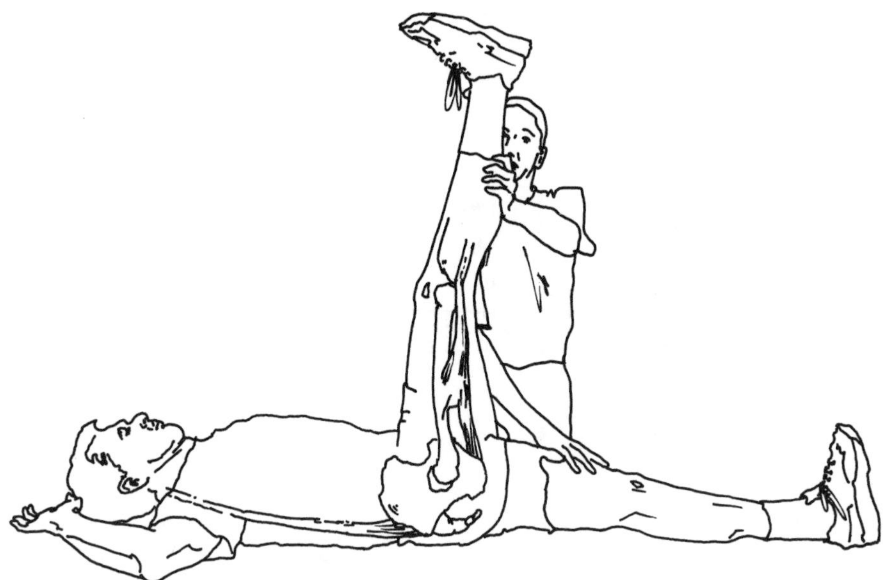

In the straight-leg-raise test recommended, the pelvis is first posteriorly rotated until the low back is snug against the table; one leg is then raised by the tester while ensuring that the other one remains extended and flat on the testing surface. ROM in flexion can be determined with (a) a goniometer by placing its axis on the greater trochanter or (b) an inclinometer placed just below the tibial tubercle. A minimum of 80° is desirable on the passive straight-leg-raise; however, most therapists would like to see 90°. If large numbers of subjects are being tested, a protractor-type device can be contrived to speed up the testing process; however, the measurement will not be as precise.

Active Knee-Extension (AKE) Test (Also Called the 90/90 Test)

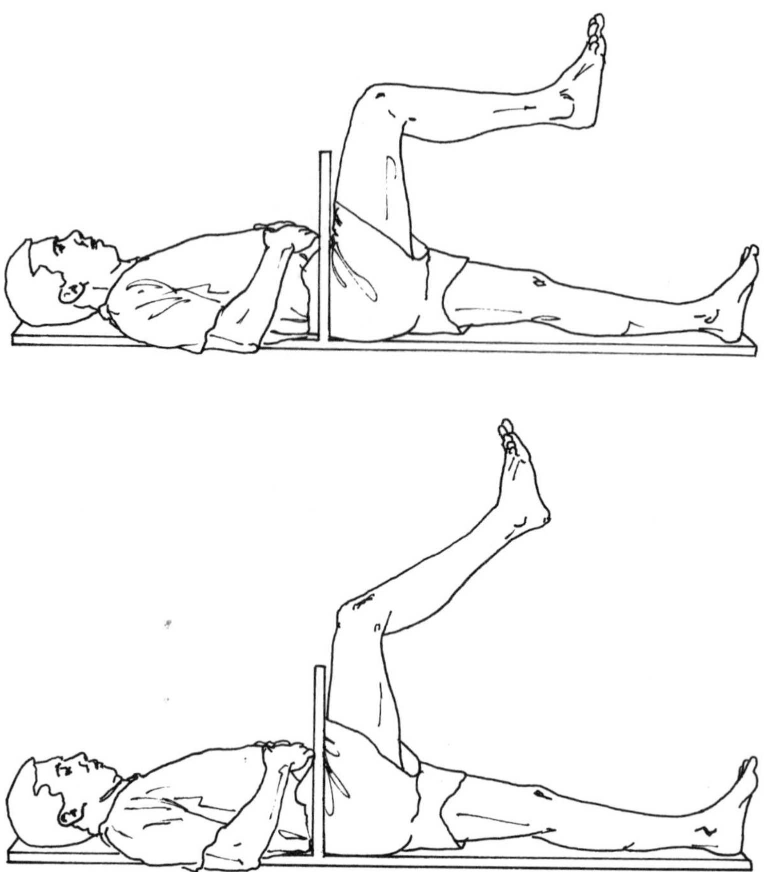

In this test the thigh of one leg is raised to the perpendicular with the lower 90 ° to the thigh (the tester will have to hold it in this position). The subject then actively extends the lower leg. A zero score would indicate that the leg was moved 90° (i.e., perpendicular to the table and in line with the thigh); a score of 10 would indicate that the leg was moved 80°.

Combined Tests of Trunk and Hip-Joint Flexion

Calliet Protective Hamstring Stretch

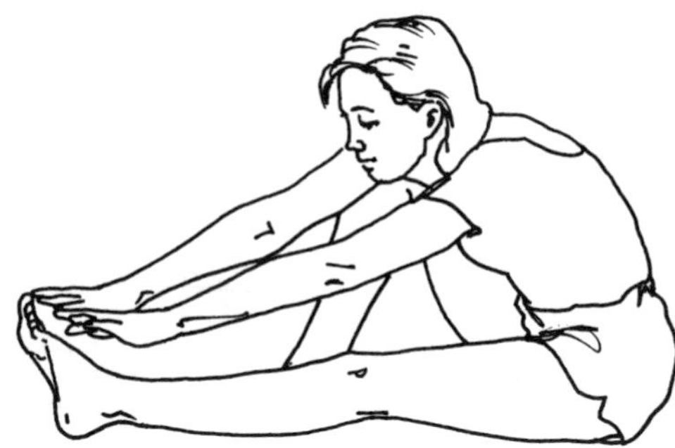

By flexing the hip and knee of the contralateral leg, the attendant posterior rotation of the pelvis decreases the turning moment of inertia of the torso; this is one reason why it is believed that this exercise/test is safer than the bilateral sit-and-reach activity (11).

Hopkins and Hoeger Sit-and-Reach (7)

A reach score is first determined with the back against the wall; this score is then subtracted from the maximum reach score.

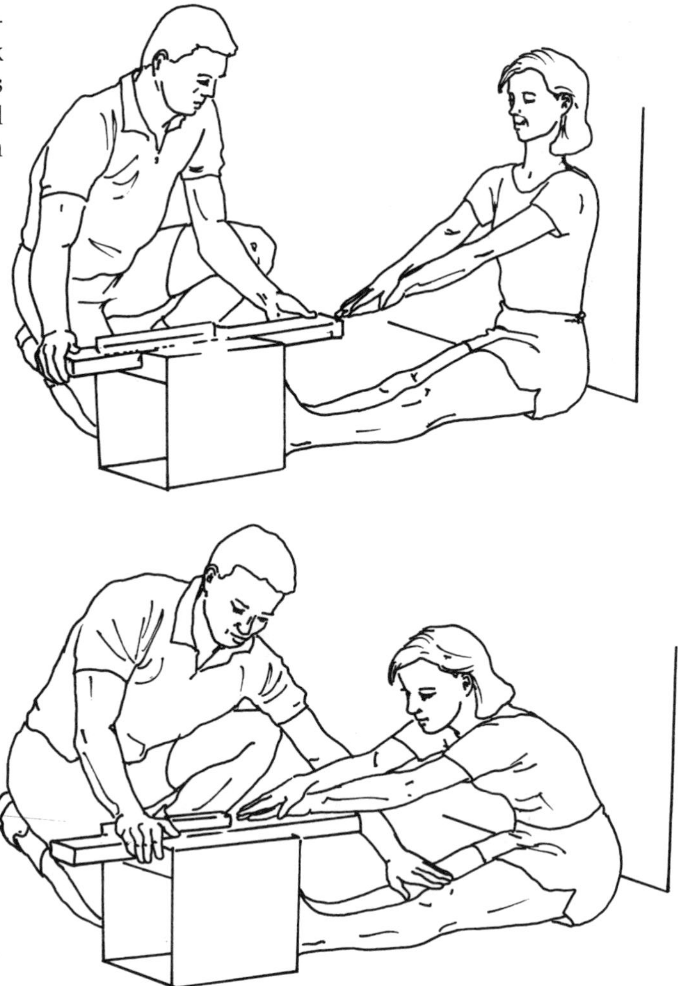

Modified Sit-and-Reach

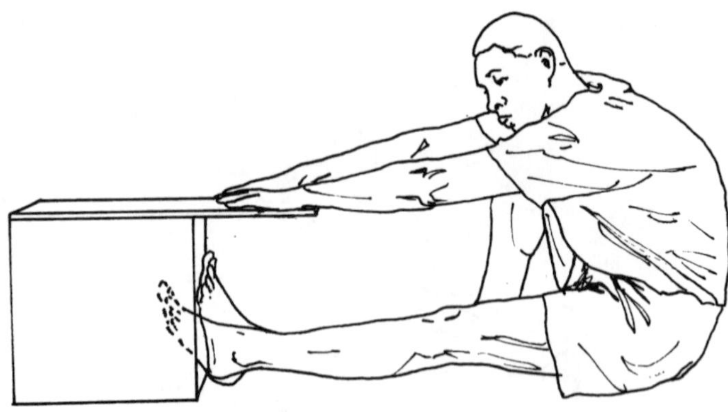

In the sit-and-reach depicted, passive plantar flexion of the ankle is permitted; this limits the role that connective tissue tightness behind the knee (as well as other factors such as nerve tension) has on performance.

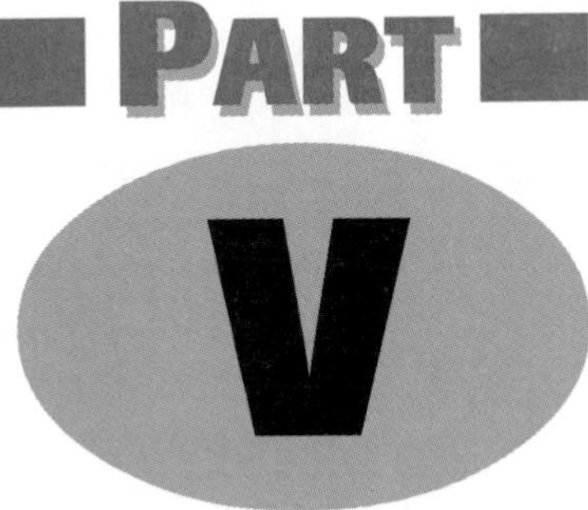

Part V

Exercise Prescription for Health and Fitness

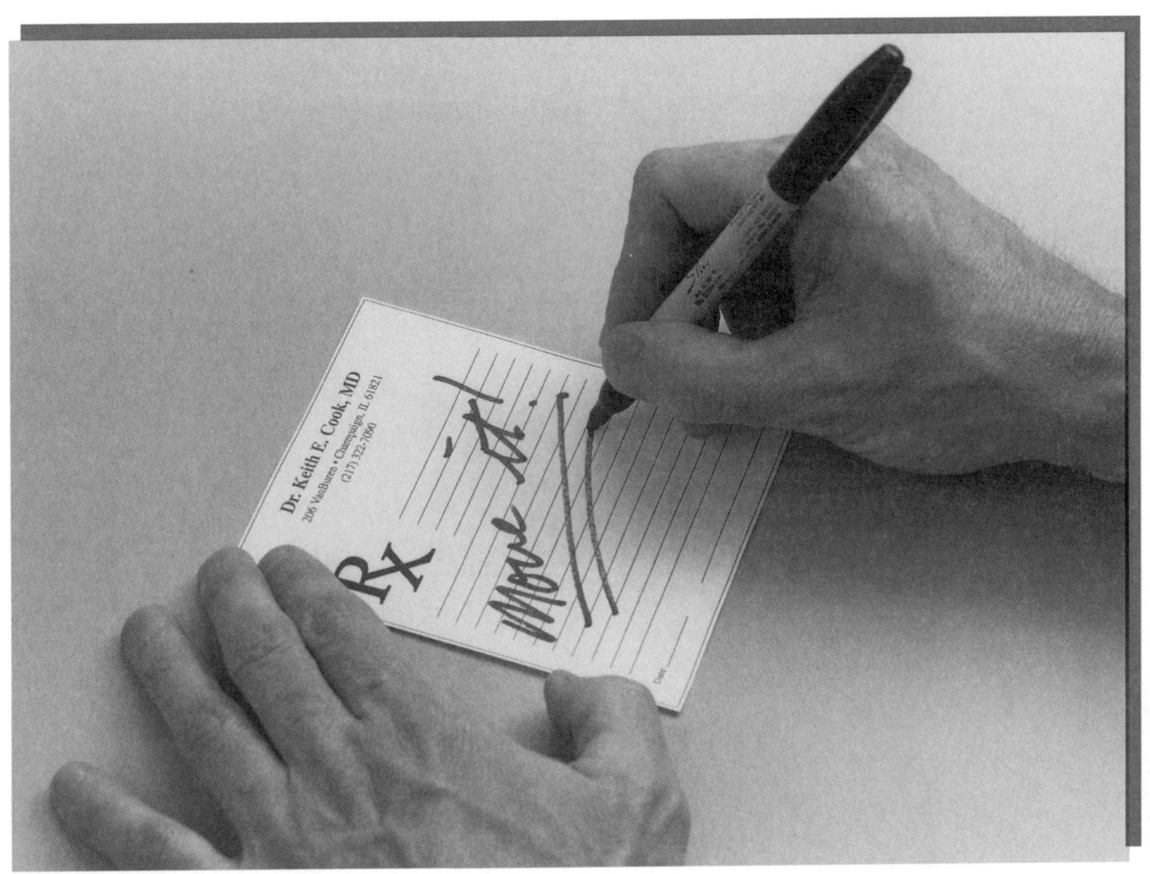

© Chris Brown

Part V provides guidelines and recommendations for exercise programming for each of the fitness components: cardiorespiratory fitness (chapter 14), muscular strength, endurance, and bone density (chapter 15), and flexibility and low-back function (chapter 16). Chapter 17 describes the importance of exercise leadership with examples of a variety of activities. Chapter 18 includes modifications recommended for individuals with special characteristics or conditions.

CHAPTER

14

Exercise Prescription for Cardiorespiratory Fitness

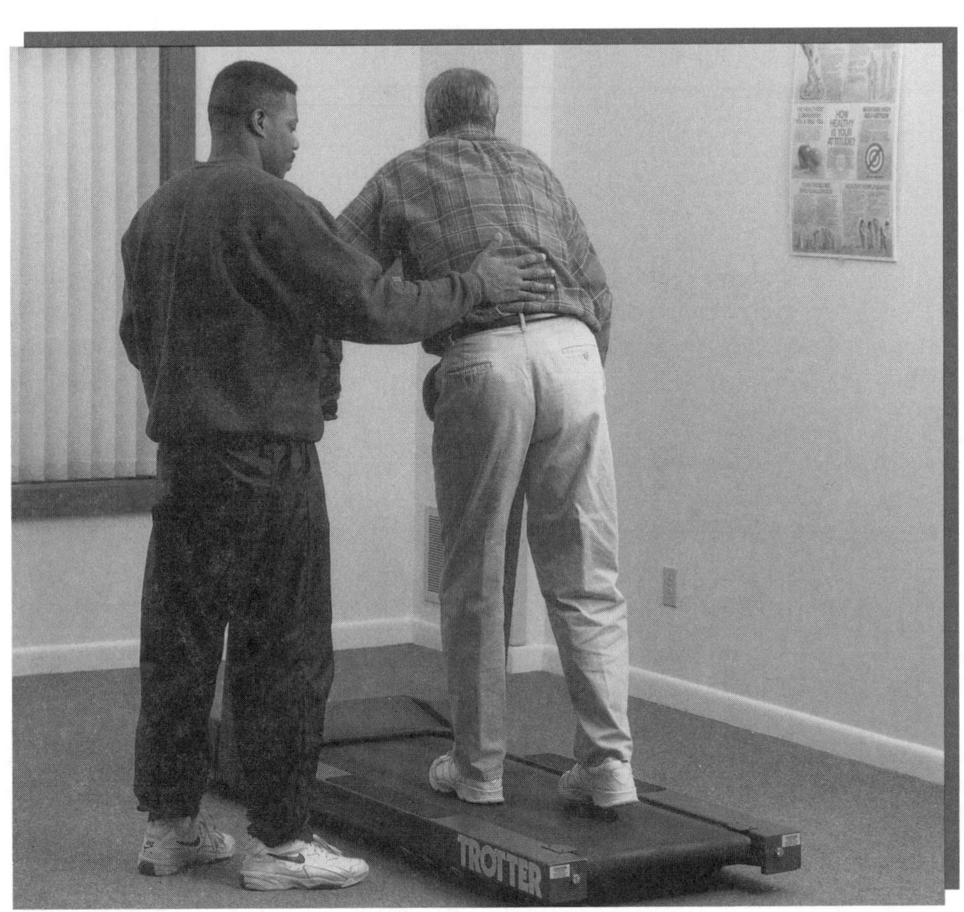

OBJECTIVES

The reader will be able to:

1. **Characterize the "dose" of exercise in an exercise prescription and identify means by which a health-related effect might occur.**
2. **Describe the "Exercise Lite" exercise prescription.**
3. **Explain the concepts of overload and specificity as they relate to training programs.**
4. **Describe general guidelines related to cardiorespiratory fitness programs, including those related to warm-up and cool-down.**
5. **Develop an exercise prescription for correct exercise intensity, duration, and frequency to achieve and maintain cardiorespiratory fitness goals.**
6. **Express exercise intensity in terms of energy production, heart rate, and rating of perceived exertion.**
7. **Contrast the approaches used for developing exercise prescriptions for the general public, the fit population, and for people whose complete GXT results are available; and describe the differences between a supervised and an unsupervised program.**
8. **Describe the effects of temperature and humidity, altitude, and pollution on the exercise prescription.**

In the introductory chapters to this text we indicated that physical inactivity had long been considered only a secondary risk factor in the development of coronary heart disease (CHD); that is, an inactive lifestyle would increase a person's risk for CHD only if other primary risk factors were present. This, of course, is no longer the case. Physical inactivity is now recognized as a primary risk factor for CHD, similar to smoking, hypertension, and high serum cholesterol (6, 44, 45, 51, 61). Studies also show that regular vigorous physical activity is instrumental in reducing the risk of CHD in those who smoke or are hypertensive (46). Furthermore, epidemiological studies show that increases in physical activity (47) and fitness (8) are associated with a reduced death rate from all causes as well as from CHD. Consequently, there is considerable agreement about the importance of physical activity in prevention as well as a therapeutic intervention in cardiovascular, respiratory, and metabolic diseases. The important question is how much activity is needed to bring about the desired effect.

PRESCRIBING EXERCISE

There is a close parallel between the HFI wishing to know the proper **dose** of exercise needed to bring about a desired **effect** (response) and the physician's need to know the type and quantity of a drug needed to cure a disease. We recognize that there is a difference between what is needed to cure a headache and what is needed to cure tuberculosis. In concert with that, there is no question that the dose of physical activity necessary to achieve a high-level of *performance* is different from that required to improve a *health-related outcome* (e.g., lowered blood pressure, reduced risk of coronary heart disease). Similarities can be drawn between the dose-response relationship for medications and that for exercise in figure 14.1.

- Potency: The potency of a drug is a relatively unimportant characteristic in that it makes little difference whether the effective dose is 1 μg or 100 mg as long as it can be administered in an appropriate dosage (20). Applied to exercise prescriptions, walking 4 mi is as effective in expending calories as running 2 mi.
- Slope: The slope of the curve describes how much of an effect is obtained from a change in dose (20). Some physiological measures such as heart rate and lactate responses to a fixed exercise task change quickly (in days) for a given dose of exercise, while some health-related effects (e.g., changes in serum cholesterol) are realized only after many months of exercise.
- Maximal effect: The maximal effect (efficacy) of a drug varies with the type of drug. For example, morphine can relieve pain of all intensities while aspirin is effective against only mild to moderate pain (20). Similarly, strenuous exercise can cause an increase in $\dot{V}O_2$max as well as modify risk factors, while light to moderate exercise can change risk factors with only a minimal impact on $\dot{V}O_2$max.
- Variability: The effect of a drug varies between individuals, and within individuals depending on the circumstances. The intersecting brackets in figure 14.1 indicate the variability in the dose required to bring about a particular effect and the variability in the effect associated with a given dose (20). For example, gains in $\dot{V}O_2$max due to endurance training show considerable variation, even when the initial $\dot{V}O_2$max value is controlled for (14).
- Side effect: A last point worth mentioning is that no drug produces a single effect (20). The effects might include adverse (side) effects that limit the usefulness of the drug. For exercise, the side effects might include an increased risk of injury.

In contrast to most drugs that individuals stop taking when a disease is cured, there is a need to engage in some form of physical activity throughout life to experience the health-related and fitness effects.

The exercise dose is usually characterized by the intensity, frequency, duration, and type of activity; and we discuss each of these in detail later in this chapter. It should be pointed out, however, that in contrast to what we know about the role of each of these variables in improving $\dot{V}O_2$max, little is known about the minimum or optimal quantities of each variable related to achieving health outcomes (27).

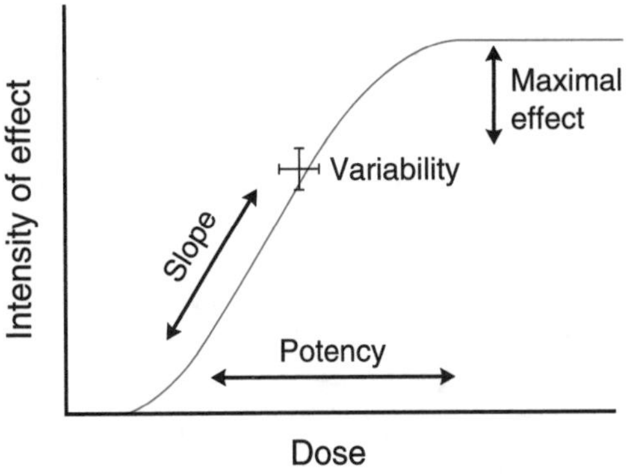

FIGURE 14.1 Representative log dose-effect curve, illustrating its four characterizing parameters.
Reprinted from Goodman and Gilman 1975.

Cause and Effect

The response (effect) generated by a particular dose of exercise can include changes in $\dot{V}O_2$max, resting blood pressure, insulin sensitivity, body weight (percentage body fat), and depression. However, as Haskell (26, 27) pointed out, we may have to reexamine our understanding of *cause and effect* when we study how a dose of physical activity is related to the responses of physical fitness and health. Physical activity could bring about favorable changes by

- improving fitness (especially cardiovascular fitness) and thereby improving health,
- improving fitness and health simultaneously and separately,
- improving fitness but not a specific health outcome, or
- improving some specific health outcome but not fitness.

dose — The quantity (intensity, frequency, and duration) of exercise needed to bring about a response (e.g., lower resting blood pressure).

effect — The desired response resulting from exercise training (e.g., lower resting blood pressure).

It has become clear that improvements in a variety of health-related concerns are not dependent on an increase in $\dot{V}O_2max$; this distinction is important to mention at the beginning of this chapter that concerns itself with appropriate ways to improve $\dot{V}O_2max$.

In Review: An exercise dose reflects the interaction of the intensity, frequency, duration, and type of exercise. The cause of the health-related response may be related to an improvement in $\dot{V}O_2max$ or may act through some other mechanism, making health-related outcomes and gains in $\dot{V}O_2max$ independent of each other.

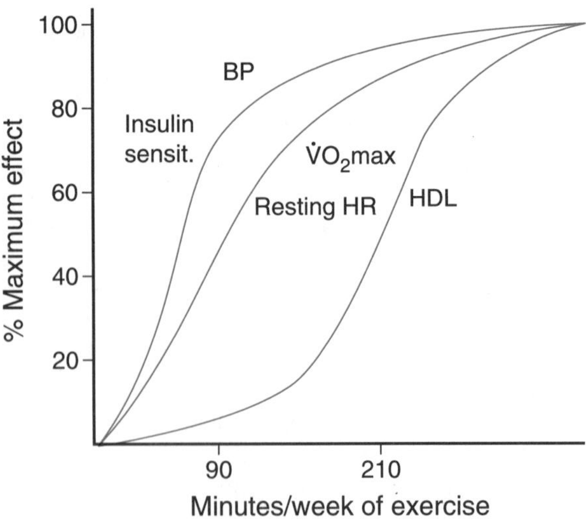

FIGURE 14.2 Proposed dose-response relationships between amount of exercise performed per week at 60% to 70% maximum work capacity and changes in blood pressure (BP) and insulin sensitivity (curve to the left side), which appear most sensitive to exercise; maximum oxygen consumption ($\dot{V}O_2max$) and resting heart rate, which are parameters of physical fitness (middle curve); and lipid changes, such as high-density lipoprotein (HDL) (right hand curve).
Reprinted from G.L. Jennings et al. 1991.

Short- and Long-Term Responses to Exercise

In addition to understanding the cause-and-effect connection between physical activity and specific outcomes, Haskell indicated the need to distinguish between short-term (acute) and long-term (training) responses (27). The patterns of responses in the days and weeks following the initiation of a dose of exercise can vary substantially:

- acute responses—Responses occur with one or several exercise bouts but do not improve further.
- rapid responses—Benefits occur early and plateau.
- linear responses—Gains are made continuously over time.
- delayed responses—Responses occur only after weeks of training.

The need for such distinctions can be seen in figure 14.2, which shows proposed dose-response relationships between physical activity, defined as minutes of exercise per week at 60% to 70% of maximal work capacity, and a variety of physiological responses (36):

- Blood pressure and insulin sensitivity are most responsive to exercise.
- Changes in $\dot{V}O_2max$ and resting heart rate are intermediate.
- Serum lipid changes such as increases in high-density lipoprotein (HDL) are delayed.

The dose-response relationship of exercise to positive physiological responses has important implications when exercise is used alone or in concert with medication to control disease; we discuss this further in chapter 18.

"Exercise Lite"

It should be no surprise, given the previous discussion, that it is difficult to provide a single exercise prescription that addresses all issues related to prevention and/or treatment of various diseases. In spite of this there has been a great need to provide a general exercise recommendation to improve the health status of all adults in the United States. The American College of Sports Medicine and the Center for Disease Control and Prevention responded to this need by publishing the "Exercise Lite" guidelines (4): Every U.S. adult should accumulate 30 min or more of moderate-intensity (3-6 METs) physical activity on most, preferably all, days of the week.

These guidelines were based on a comprehensive review of the literature dealing with health-related aspects of physical activity; the dose-response curve in figure 14.3 summarizes the findings. By having the most sedentary group ("A") move up just one level of physical activity shown in figure 14.3, the greatest gains in health-related benefits can be realized.

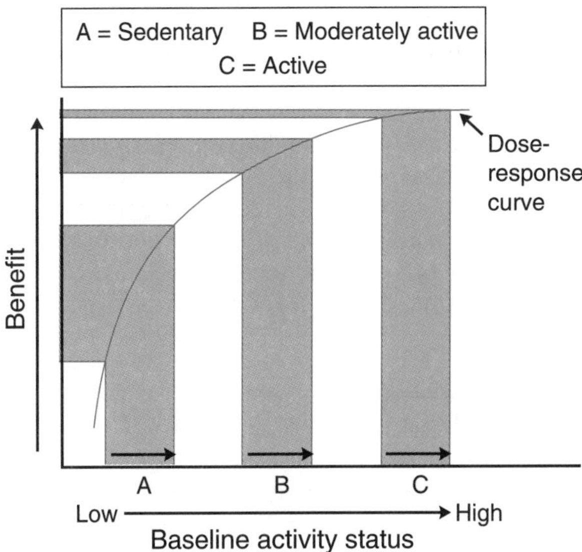

FIGURE 14.3 The dose-response curve represents the best estimate of the relationship between physical activity (dose) and health benefit (response). The lower the baseline physical activity status, the greater will be the health benefit associated with a given increase in physical activity (arrows A, B, and C).
Reprinted from Pate et al. 1995.

The "Exercise Lite" recommendation was based on the finding that caloric expenditure and total time of physical activity are associated with reduced cardiovascular disease and mortality. Furthermore, doing the activity in intermittent bouts as short as 8 to 10 min is a suitable way of meeting the 30-min goal (4, 48). A recent epidemiological investigation suggests, however, that vigorous (> 6 METs) exercise was important in lowering the death rate from all causes; the lower death rate might have been linked to changes in $\dot{V}O_2$max (38).

2 **In Review: The basis of the "Exercise Lite" recommendation is that the health-related benefits of physical activity may be more related to the total number of calories expended than to the intensity level of the exercise. The focus of the "Exercise Lite" exercise prescription is for light-to-moderate activity to be done most, if not all, days of the week for a total of 30 minutes a day.**

The "Exercise Lite" recommendations are appropriate for individuals taking the first step from being sedentary to becoming active. However, individuals who expend more than 2000 kcal per week, or who possess a high $\dot{V}O_2$max, show the lowest death rate from all causes (7, 45). Consequently, there are benefits to be gained not only when a sedentary person becomes active but also as a moderately active person engages in more vigorous exercise that increases functional capacity ($\dot{V}O_2$max). The purpose of this chapter is to lead you through the steps involved in developing an exercise prescription for apparently healthy individuals. But first a brief review of the major principles of training is presented.

EXERCISE TRAINING PRINCIPLES: BASIS FOR PHYSIOLOGICAL CHANGES

The degree to which a tissue such as bone, skeletal muscle, or cardiac muscle functions depends on the activity to which it is exposed. This statement summarizes the two major principles underlying training programs: **overload** and **specificity**.

Overload

The principle of overload describes a dynamic characteristic of living creatures: Use increases functional capacity. If a tissue or organ system is required to work against a load to which it is not accustomed, instead of wearing out and becoming weaker, it becomes stronger. The slang for this principle is "use it or lose it." The corollary of the overload principle is the principle of **reversibility**, which indicates that physiological gains are lost when the load against which a tissue or organ system is working is reduced.

overload — To place greater than usual demands on some part of the body (e.g., picking up more weight than usual overloads the muscles involved). Chronic overloading leads to increased function.

specificity — The principle that states that training effects derived from an exercise program are specific to the exercise done (endurance vs. strength training) and the muscle fiber types involved.

reversibility — A corollary to the principle of overload; loss of a training effect with disuse.

The variables that contribute to an overload in an exercise program include the intensity, duration, and frequency of the exercise. As we will see, it is the combination of these elements that results in a sufficient amount of total work, or energy expenditure, to cause an increase in the functional capacity of the cardiorespiratory (CR) systems.

Specificity

The principle of specificity states that the training effects derived from an exercise program are specific to the exercise done and the muscles involved. For example, a person who runs as a primary form of exercise shows little change in the arm muscles, just as the person who exercises at a low intensity that recruits only Type I muscle fibers will have little or no training effect in the fast-twitch fibers in the same muscle groups. If muscle fibers are not used they cannot adapt, and, consequently, they will not become "trained." The type of adaptation that occurs as a result of training is specific to the type of training taking place (e.g., endurance vs. heavy resistive strength training). Running causes an increase in the number of capillaries and mitochondria in the muscle fibers involved in the exercise and makes them more resistant to fatigue. Strength training causes a hypertrophy of the muscles involved, due to an increase in the amount of contractile proteins, actin and myosin, in the muscle (30, 57).

3 **In Review: Tissues adapt to the load to which they are exposed; to increase the functional capacity of a tissue, it must be *overloaded* (i.e., subjected to a load to which it is not accustomed). The type of adaptation is *specific* to the muscle fibers involved and types of exercise. Endurance exercise increases mitochondria and capillary number, and strength training increases contractile protein and size of the muscle.**

GENERAL GUIDELINES FOR CARDIORESPIRATORY FITNESS PROGRAMS

To apply the principles of overload and specificity to cardiorespiratory fitness (CRF), activities that overload the heart and respiratory systems need to be used in exercise programs. Activities that use the large-muscle groups contracting in a rhythmic manner and on a continuous basis are effective in overloading the CR systems. Activities involving a small-muscle mass and weight training exercises are less appropriate because they tend to generate very high cardiovascular loads relative to energy expenditure (see chapter 4). Activities that improve CRF are high in caloric cost and therefore help to achieve a relative leanness goal. How do you get someone started?

Screen Participants

If the person has not already done so, have him or her fill out one of the health status forms. Chapter 3 provides guidelines for who should and should not seek medical clearance before exercising.

Encourage Regular Participation

Exercise must become a valuable part of a person's lifestyle. It is not something that can be done sporadically; nor will doing it for only a few months or years build up a fitness reserve. Dramatic gains accomplished through fitness activities are lost quickly with inactivity (see pages 71-73). Only people who continue activity as a way of life enjoy its long-term benefits (remember the principle of reversibility).

Provide Different Types of Activities

A fitness program starts with easily quantified activities, such as walking or cycling, so that the proper exercise intensity can be achieved. After a minimum level of fitness is achieved, a variety of activities are included in the program for those who are interested. Chapter 17 outlines three phases of activities: (1) work up to walking briskly for 4 mi per workout; (2) gradually begin jogging, and work up to jogging continuously for 3 mi; and (3) introduce a variety of activities, including exercise to music.

Program for Progression

Given the importance of helping sedentary people become active, the emphasis in any health-related fitness program that includes such individuals should be to *start slowly* and, when in doubt, do too little rather than too much. Participants should begin at work levels that can be easily completed and should be encouraged to *gradually* increase the amount of work they can do during a workout. For example, a sedentary participant who is interested in jogging as a goal should begin a training program by walking a distance that she or he can complete without feeling fatigued or sore. With time, the participant will be able to walk a greater distance at a faster pace without discomfort. After this person can walk 4 mi briskly without stopping, she or he can gradually work up to jogging 3 mi continuously per workout. For the participant who is ready to begin jogging, you might introduce the interval-type workout (walking-jogging-walking-jogging). As individuals adapt to the interval workouts, they will be able to gradually increase the amount of jogging while decreasing the distance walked (see the walking and jogging programs in chapter 17).

Adhere to Format for a Fitness Workout

The main body of the fitness workout consists of dynamic large-muscle group activities at an intensity high enough and a duration long enough to accomplish enough total work to specifically overload the CR systems. Stretching and light endurance activities are included before the workout (warm-up) and after the workout (cool-down) for safety and to improve low-back function.

There are physiological, psychological, and safety reasons for including warm-up and cool-down (18). In general the warm-up and cool-down should consist of

- activities similar to the activities done in the main body of the workout, but done at a lower intensity (e.g., walking, jogging, or cycling below THR);
- stretching exercises for the muscles involved in the activity, as well as those in the midtrunk area; and
- muscular endurance exercises, especially for the muscles in the abdominal region.

These activities help participants ease into and out of a workout and provide activities that help promote a healthy low back. If a workout is going to be shorter than usual, the reduction in time should take place in the main body of the workout, retaining 5 to 10 min for the warm-up and cool-down portions.

Conduct Periodic CRF Tests

Routine health-related physical fitness testing to determine a participant's progress can be motivational and may help alter programs that are not achieving desired results. The HFI can help by setting realistic goals for the next testing session when discussing test results. A rule of thumb would be a 10% improvement in 3 months in the test scores that need to change. Once the person has reached a desirable level, the goal is to maintain that level.

In Review: People interested in a fitness program should be screened for risk factors and encouraged to participate on a regular basis. The program should provide different types of activities, and the individual should start *slowly* and progress *gradually* to higher levels of work. The workout should have a warm-up and a cool-down period, including stretching and muscular endurance exercises for the midtrunk areas. Periodic CRF tests can be used to alter the exercise prescription.

FORMULATING THE EXERCISE PRESCRIPTION

The CRF training effect is dependent on the degree to which the systems are overloaded, that is, upon intensity, duration, and frequency of training. Improvements in CRF have been shown to occur with fitness programs conducted at intensities of 50% to 85% $\dot{V}O_2$max, durations of 20 to 60 min, and frequencies of 2 to 5 days per week (3). The blend of intensity and duration should result in an energy expenditure (total work) of 200 to 300 kcal per session. This latter variable, **total work**, seems to be crucial in developing and maintaining a CRF training effect (3).

Intensity

How hard does a person have to work to provide sufficient overload for the cardiovascular and respiratory systems to increase their functional capacities?

total work — The amount of work accomplished during a workout.

As previously mentioned, gains in CRF have been shown to occur in exercise programs in which the **training intensity** is 50% to 85% $\dot{V}O_2$max (3). It is generally believed that the intensity threshold for a training effect is at the low end of this continuum for those who are sedentary and at the high end of the scale for those who are fit (4). For most people who are cleared to participate in a structured exercise program, 60% to 80% $\dot{V}O_2$max seems to be the optimum range of exercise intensities. Figure 14.4 shows that exercise at the high end of the scale has been associated with more cardiac complications (13, 29). Exercise intensity must be balanced against the duration so that the person can exercise long enough to expend 200 to 300 kcal per session, consistent with achieving CRF and body-composition goals. If the exercise intensity is too high, the person may not be able to exercise long enough to achieve the total work goal.

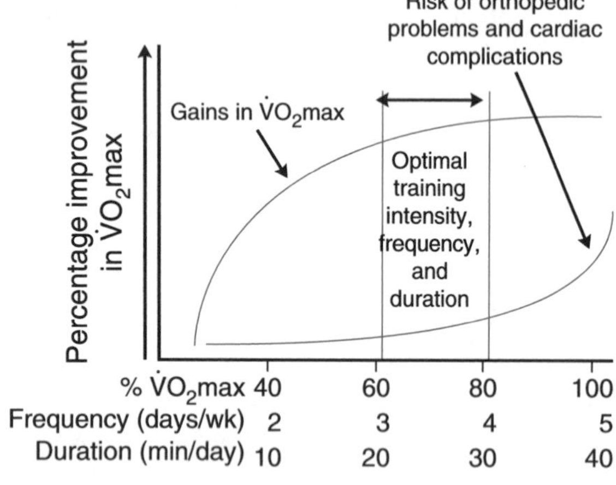

FIGURE 14.4 Effects of increasing the frequency, duration, and intensity of exercise on the increase in $\dot{V}O_2$max in a training program. This figure demonstrates the increasing risk of orthopedic problems due to exercise sessions that are too long or conducted too many times per week. The probability of cardiac complications increases with exercise intensity beyond that recommended for improvements in cardiorespiratory fitness.

From Powers and Howley 1997. Drawing based on Dehn and Mullins 1977, and Hellerstein and Franklin 1984.

Duration

How many minutes of exercise should a person do per session? Figure 14.4 shows that improvements in $\dot{V}O_2$max increase with the **duration** of the exercise session. However, the optimum duration of an exercise session depends on the intensity. The total work accomplished in a session is the most important variable determining CRF gains, once the minimal intensity **threshold** is achieved (5). If the goal is to accomplish 300 kcal of total work in an exercise session in which the individual is working at 10 kcal · min^{-1} (2 L O_2 per min), the session would have to be 30 min long. If the person is working at half that intensity, 5 kcal · min^{-1}, the duration would have to be twice as long. Thirty minutes of exercise can be taken as one 30-min session, two 15-min sessions, or three 10-min sessions. Figure 14.4 also shows that when the duration of strenuous exercise (75% $\dot{V}O_2$max) exceeds 30 min, the risk of orthopedic injury increases (49).

Frequency

Why recommend that someone do 3 to 5 workouts per week, if 2 would suffice? Figure 14.4 shows that gains in CRF increase with the frequency of exercise but begin to level off at 4 days per week (3). People who start a fitness program should plan to exercise 3 or 4 times per week. The long recommended work-a-day-then-rest-a-day routine has been validated on the basis of improvements in CRF, low incidence of injuries, and achievement of weight loss goals (3). Although exercising for fewer than 3 days per week can cause CRF improvements, the participant would have to exercise at a higher intensity, and weight loss goals may be difficult to achieve (49). Exercising for more than 4 days per week for previously sedentary people seems to be too much and results in more dropouts and injuries and less psychological adjustment to the exercise (13, 49).

5 **In Review: CRF is improved with exercise intensities of 50% to 85% $\dot{V}O_2$max. The intensity threshold for a training effect is lower for those who are sedentary. The optimal training intensity for the average individual is approximately 60% to 80% $\dot{V}O_2$max. The duration of an exercise session should balance the exercise intensity to result in an energy expenditure of 200 to 300 kcal. The optimum frequency of training, based on improvements in CRF and a low risk of injuries, is 3 to 4 times per week at a vigorous intensity.**

DETERMINING INTENSITY

How is exercise intensity set for a particular individual? Direct and indirect methods to determine appropriate exercise intensity are reviewed in this section.

Metabolic Load

The most direct way to determine the appropriate exercise intensity is to use a percentage of the measured maximal oxygen consumption. Remember, the optimum range of exercise intensities associated with improvements in CRF is 60% to 80% $\dot{V}O_2max$. The advantage of measuring oxygen consumption to determine exercise intensity is that the method is based on the criterion test for CRF—maximal oxygen consumption. The major disadvantages are the expense and difficulty of measuring oxygen consumption for each individual and trying to suit specific fitness activities to meet the specific metabolic demand for each person.

QUESTION: A 75-kg man completes a maximal GXT, and his $\dot{V}O_2max$ is 3.0 L · min^{-1}. This is equal to 15 kcal · min^{-1} (5 kcal · L^{-1} × 3 L · min^{-1}), 40 ml · kg^{-1} · min^{-1}, and 11.4 METs. At what exercise intensities should he work to be at 60% to 80% $\dot{V}O_2max$?

1. **60% of 3.0 L · min^{-1} = 1.8 L · min^{-1}; 80% of 3.0 L · min^{-1} = 2.4 L · min^{-1}.**
2. **60% of 15 kcal · min^{-1} = 9 kcal · min^{-1}; 80% of 15 kcal · min^{-1} = 12 kcal · min^{-1}.**
3. **60% of 40 ml · kg^{-1} · min^{-1} = 24 ml · kg^{-1} · min^{-1}; 80% of 40 ml · kg^{-1} · min^{-1} = 32 ml · kg^{-1} · min^{-1}.**
4. **60% of 11.4 METs = 6.8 METs; 80% of 11.4 METs = 9.1 METs.**

Answer:

He should use activities that require

1.8 to 2.4 L · min^{-1}

9 to 12 kcal · min^{-1}

24 to 32 ml · kg^{-1} · min^{-1}

6.8 to 9.1 METs

When these values are known, appropriate activities can be selected from tables listing the caloric cost of activities (see appendix C for these tables). However, this is a very cumbersome method for prescribing exercise. Prescribing on the basis of the caloric cost of the activity does not take into consideration the effect that environmental (e.g., heat, humidity, altitude, cold, pollution), dietary (e.g., adequate hydration), and other variables have on a person's response to some absolute exercise intensity. The participant's ability to complete a workout will depend on her or his *perception* of effort associated with the activity, rather than the activity itself. Fortunately, by using specific heart rate values that are approximately equal to 60% to 80% $\dot{V}O_2max$, an exercise prescription can be formulated that takes many of these factors into consideration. These HR values are called the **target heart rate (THR)** range. How is the THR range determined?

THR–Direct Method

As was described in chapters 4 and 11, HR increases linearly with the metabolic load. In the direct method for determining THR, HR is monitored at each stage of a *maximal GXT*. HR is then plotted on a graph against the $\dot{V}O_2$ (or MET) equivalents of each stage of the test. The HFI determines the THR range by taking appropriate **percentages of the maximal $\dot{V}O_2$ (%$\dot{V}O_2max$)** at which the person should train and finds what the HR responses were at those points. Figure 14.5 shows this method being used for a subject with a functional capacity of 10.5 METs. Work rates of 60% to 80% of maximal METs demanded

training intensity — A measure of the effort experienced in a workout, usually expressed as a percentage of maximal heart rate or oxygen consumption.

duration — The length of time for a fitness workout. Guidelines often include 20 to 60 min of aerobic work at a target heart rate; however, more importantly, the total work accomplished (e.g., distance covered) should be emphasized.

threshold — The minimum level needed for a desired effect. Often used to refer to the minimum level of exercise intensity needed for improvement in cardiorespiratory function.

target heart rate (THR) — The heart rate recommended for fitness workouts.

percentage of the maximal $\dot{V}O_2$ (%$\dot{V}O_2max$) — Submaximal oxygen uptake divided by maximal oxygen uptake (e.g., 60% maximal oxygen uptake in a person with a maximal oxygen uptake of 3 L · min^{-1} = 1.8 L · min^{-1} [30 · 0.6]).

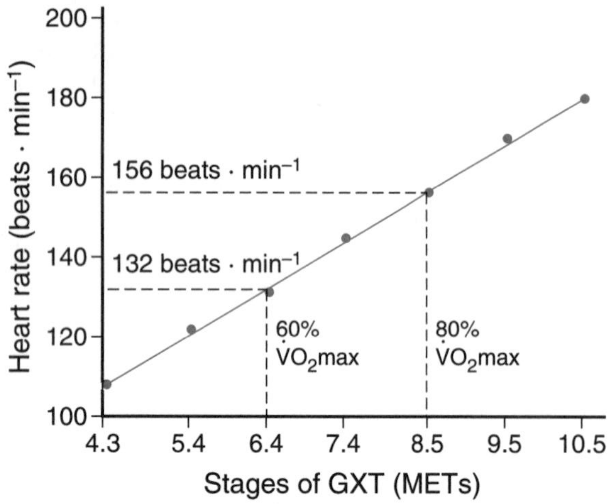

FIGURE 14.5 Direct method of determining the target heart rate zone when maximal aerobic power (functional capacity) is measured during a graded exercise test.
Adapted from ACSM 1980.

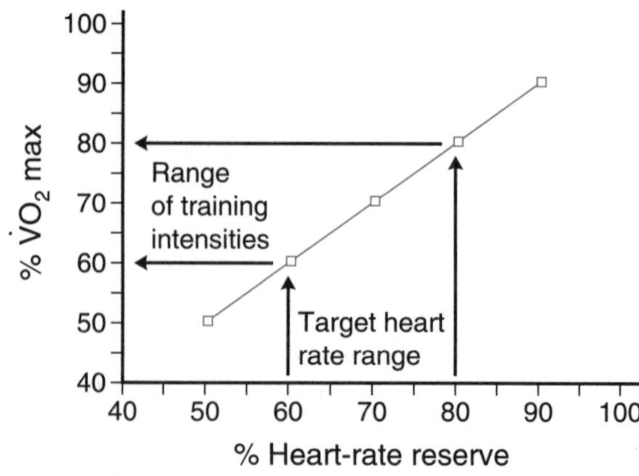

FIGURE 14.6 Relationship of percentage heart rate reserve and percentage of maximal aerobic power ($\dot{V}O_2max$).
Based on Pollock and Wilmore 1990.

HR responses of 132 to 156 beats · min^{-1}, respectively. The HR values become the intensity guide for the subject and represent the THR range (5).

THR–Indirect Methods

In contrast to the direct method, which requires the participant to complete a maximal GXT, two indirect methods have been developed to estimate an appropriate THR.

Heart Rate Reserve Method

The **heart rate reserve (HRR)** is the difference between resting and maximal heart rate. For a maximal heart rate of 200 beats · min^{-1} and a resting HR of 60 beats · min^{-1}, the HRR is 140 beats · min^{-1}. As shown in figure 14.6, the percentage of the HRR is approximately equal to the percentage of $\dot{V}O_2max$. For example, 60% of the HRR is equal to about 60% $\dot{V}O_2max$ (50).

The HRR method of determining the THR range, made popular by Karvonen, requires a few simple calculations (37):

1. Subtract the resting HR from the maximal HR to obtain the HR reserve.
2. Take 60% and 80% of the HR reserve.
3. Add each value to the resting HR to obtain the THR range.

QUESTION: A 40-year-old male participant has a measured maximal HR of 175 beats · min^{-1} and a resting HR of 75 beats · min^{-1}. What is his THR range, calculated by the Karvonen (HRR) method?

Answer:

1. HRR = 175 beats · min^{-1} – 75 beats · min^{-1} = 100 beats · min^{-1}
2. 60% of 100 beats · min^{-1} = 60 beats · min^{-1}; 80% of 100 beats · min^{-1} = 80 beats · min^{-1}
3. 60 beats · min^{-1} + 75 beats · min^{-1} = 135 beats · min^{-1} for 60% $\dot{V}O_2max$; 80 beats · min^{-1} + 75 beats · min^{-1} = 155 beats · min^{-1} for 80% $\dot{V}O_2max$

The advantage of this procedure for determining exercise intensity is that the recommended THR is always between the person's resting and maximal HRs. Although the resting HR is variable and can be influenced by factors such as caffeine, lack of sleep, dehydration, emotional state, and training, this does not introduce serious errors into the calculation of the THR by the Karvonen method (25). Consider the following example:

QUESTION: The 40-year-old subject mentioned previously trains, and his resting HR decreases by 10 beats · min^{-1}. Because maximal HR (175 beats · min^{-1}) is not affected by training, what happens to his THR range?

Answer:

1. The HRR now equals 175 beats · min^{-1} – 65 beats · min^{-1} = 110 beats · min^{-1}
2. 60% of 110 beats · min^{-1} = 66 beats · min^{-1} + 65 beats · min^{-1} = 131 beats · min^{-1}

   80% of 110 beats · min^{-1} = 88 beats · min^{-1} + 65 beats · min^{-1} = 153 beats · min^{-1}

Consequently, the change in resting HR had only a minimal effect on the THR range.

Percentage of Maximal HR Method

Another method of determining THR range is to take a fixed **percentage of the maximal HR (%HRmax)**. The advantage of this method is its simplicity and the fact that it has been validated across many populations (29, 39). Figure 14.7 shows the relationship between %HRmax and $\%\dot{V}O_2max$.

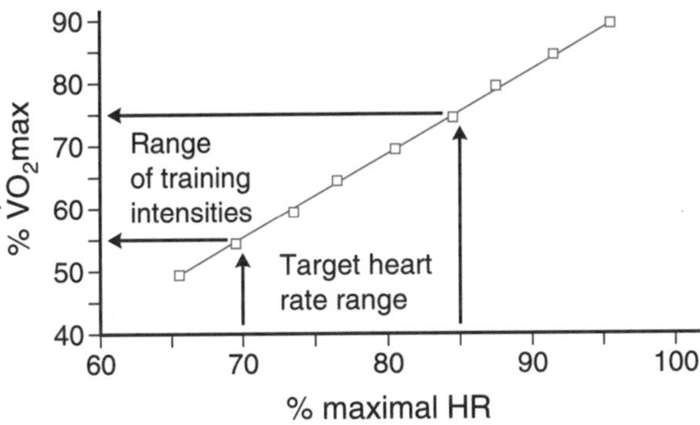

FIGURE 14.7 Relationship of percentage of maximal heart rate and percentage of maximal aerobic power ($\dot{V}O_2max$).
Data from Londeree and Ames 1976.

It is clear that they are linearly related, and the %HRmax can be used to estimate the metabolic load in training programs. The usual guideline used to estimate a reasonable exercise intensity is 70% to 85% HRmax. These HR values are equal to approximately 55% and 75% $\dot{V}O_2max$, respectively, and represent a slightly more conservative intensity prescription than that generated by the HRR method (60% to 80% $\dot{V}O_2max$). The following example shows how to use the %HRmax method of calculating the THR range.

QUESTION: How can I calculate a target heart rate range if I don't know what the resting heart rate is? Use the data from the 40-year-old subject mentioned previously who had a measured maximal HR of 175 beats · min^{-1}.

Answer:

Take 70% and 85% of that value:

70% of 175 beats · min^{-1} = 122 beats · min^{-1}

85% of 175 beats · min^{-1} = 149 beats · min^{-1}

If 55% and 75% of the HRR were used in the Karvonen calculation (to simulate the values for the %HRmax method) for this subject who had a maximal HR of 175 beats · min^{-1} and resting HR of 65 beats · min^{-1}, the THR range would be 125 to 147 beats · min^{-1}, very close to that calculated by the %HRmax method.

Remember, these two indirect methods for estimating exercise intensity provide *guidelines* to use in an exercise program, and small differences between methods are not important. They must be viewed as guidelines only, however, because, as for any prediction equation, there is an error involved in the estimate provided by the equation. For example, two standard deviations of the estimate of $\%\dot{V}O_2max$ determined from HR is ±11.4% $\dot{V}O_2max$ (39). Therefore, for 95% of participants, when we use HR to predict a work intensity that is 60% $\dot{V}O_2max$, the true intensity is somewhere between 48.6% and 71.4% $\dot{V}O_2max$! This is why these calculated THR values should be used as a guideline in helping individuals increase or maintain CRF. The HFI or personal fitness trainer needs other indicators of exercise intensity to compensate for some of the inherent variability in the THR prescription (see later in this chapter).

Relationship of Percentages of $\dot{V}O_2max$, HRR, and HRmax

One area of potential confusion about the calculation of exercise intensity by the two indirect methods is that the percentage value used in the HRR method is about 10% to 15% lower than the values used in the %HRmax procedure for the same work level. Table 14.1 presents values for both of these methods versus work rates expressed as a percentage of maximal oxygen consumption.

Threshold

As was mentioned earlier, the intensity of exercise that provides an adequate stimulus for cardiorespiratory improvement varies with activity level and

heart rate reserve (HRR) — The difference between maximal and resting heart rates.

percentage of the maximal HR (%HRmax) — Submaximal heart rate divided by maximal heart rate (e.g., 70% maximal heart rate in a person with a maximal heart rate of 200 beats · min^{-1} = 140 beats · min^{-1} [200 · 0.7]).

Table 14.1 Relationship of %HRmax, %HRR, and %$\dot{V}O_2$max

%$\dot{V}O_2$max	%HRR[a,b]	%HRmax[c]
50	50	66
55	55	70
60	60	74
65	65	77
70	70	81
75	75	85
80	80	88
85	85	92
90	90	96

[a]HRR is the difference between HRmax and resting HR.
[b]From Pollock & Wilmore 1990.
[c]From Londeree and Ames 1976.

age and spans the range of 50% to 85% V.O_2max. However, for most of the population, the intensity threshold is in the following ranges:

- 60% to 80% of $\dot{V}O_2$max
- 60% to 80% of HRR
- 70% to 85% of HRmax

The threshold is toward the lower part of the range for older sedentary populations, and toward the upper part of the range for younger healthy populations. There is a need to go below this range (i.e., less than 60%$\dot{V}O_2$max) for diseased and extremely deconditioned people and above it (i.e., greater than 80% $\dot{V}O_2$max) for very active people. The middle of the range (70% $\dot{V}O_2$max, 70% HRR, or 80% HRmax) is an *average training intensity* and is appropriate for the typical apparently healthy person who wishes to be involved in a regular fitness program. Participating in activities at this intensity places a reasonable load on the cardiorespiratory system to constitute an overload, resulting in an adaptation over time.

Earlier editions of the ACSM Guidelines presented a sliding-scale method to estimate the *average training intensity*. This method is quite consistent with the previous discussion. An exercise intensity equal to 60% of max METs is taken as the baseline in this calculation. The HFI adds to this a value equal to the subject's maximal METs (e.g., for a person with a functional capacity of 5 METs, the calculation is 60% + 5% = 65%). The 65% value is then multiplied by either the subject's maximal METs or the HRR to obtain the average conditioning intensity. In the previous example, the person would exercise at an average intensity of 3.3 METs (65% of 5 METs). Given that the vast majority of apparently healthy individuals have functional capacities between 8 and 12 METs, the sliding-scale method would yield a value similar to 70% max METs (i.e., 60% + 8 METs = 68% max METs, and 60% + 12 METs = 72% max METs).

Maximal Heart Rate

The indirect methods for determining exercise intensity utilize maximal HR. It is recommended that the maximal HR be measured directly (by maximal GXT) when possible. If it cannot be measured, then any estimation must consider the effect of age on maximal HR. Maximal HR can be estimated by the formula

$$\text{HRmax} = 220 - \text{age}$$

That estimate is a potential source of error for both the HR reserve and the %HRmax methods. For example, given that one standard deviation (SD) of this estimate of maximal heart rate is about 11 beats · min^{-1}, a 45-year-old person's true HRmax may be anywhere between 142 and 208 beats · min^{-1} (±3 SD) rather than the estimated 175. However, 68% (±1 SD) of the population would be between 164 and 186 beats · min^{-1}. If the maximal HR is known (e.g., from a GXT), it should be used to determine THR, rather than using the estimate with its potential error (40). This is another reason for using caution when relying solely on the THR range as an indicator of exercise intensity. Error potential exists both in the estimate of maximal heart rate and in the equations in which various percentages of HRmax are used to predict %$\dot{V}O_2$max (see the earlier discussion).

Use of Target Heart Rate

The concept of an intensity threshold provides the basis for the importance of regular fitness workouts. Low-intensity activity around the house, yard, and office should be encouraged, but specific workouts above the intensity threshold are necessary to achieve optimum CRF results. At the other extreme, a person who pushes him- or herself near maximum does not have a fitness advantage because the same results can be obtained at a lower intensity that is above the threshold.

The THR can be used as an intensity guide for large-muscle group, continuous, whole-body types of activities such as walking, running, swimming, rowing, cycling, skiing, and dancing. However, the same training results may not occur from activities using small-muscle groups or resistive exercises because these exercises elevate the HR much higher for the same metabolic load.

People who are less active and have more risk factors should use the lower part of the THR range. More active people with fewer risk factors should use the upper part of the THR range. The THR can be divided by 6 to provide the desired 10-s THR. If the person's HRmax is unknown, the estimated THR for 10 s, by age and activity level, can be found in table 14.2. People can learn to exercise at their THRs by walking or jogging for several minutes and then stopping and immediately taking a 10-s HR. If the person's HR is not within the target range, then an adjustment is made in intensity (by going slower or faster to try to get within the THR range) for a few minutes and again taking a 10-s count. Using the THR to set exercise intensity has many advantages:

- It has a built-in individualized progression (i.e., as a person increases fitness, harder work has to be done to achieve the THR).
- It takes into account environmental conditions (e.g., a person decreases the intensity while working in very hot temperatures).
- It is easily determined, learned, and monitored.

These recommendations are appropriate for most people, but individuals differ in terms of the threshold needed for a training effect, the rate of adaptation to the training, and how exercise feels to them. The HFI must use *subjective judgment*, based on observation of the person exercising, to determine whether the intensity should be higher or lower. If the work is so easy that the person experiences little or no increase in ventilation and is able to do the work without effort, then the intensity should be increased. At the other extreme, if a person shows signs of doing maximal work and is still unable to reach THR, then a lower intensity should be chosen. In this case the top part of the THR range might be above the person's true HRmax because the 220 − age formula provides only an estimate of the value. The HFI should not rely on the THR as the only method of judging whether or not the participant is exercising at the correct intensity. Attention should be paid to other signs and symptoms of overexertion; Borg's *rating of perceived exertion* might be useful in this regard.

Table 14.2 Estimated 10-s THR for People Whose HRmax Is Unknown

Population	Intensity %$\dot{V}O_2$max	Age (years) 20	30	40	50	60	70	80
Inactive	50	22	21	20	18	17	16	15
with several	55	23	22	21	19	18	17	16
risk factors	60	24	23	22	20	19	18	17
Normal activity	65	25	24	23	21	20	19	18
with few	70	26	25	24	22	21	20	18
risk factors	75	28	26	25	24	22	21	19
	80	29	28	26	25	23	22	20
Very active	85	30	29	27	26	24	23	21
with low risk	90	31	30	28	27	25	24	22

Rating of Perceived Exertion

The Borg rating of perceived exertion (RPE) scale that is used to indicate the subjective sensation of effort experienced by the subject during a graded exercise test (see chapter 11) can be used in prescribing exercise for the apparently healthy individual (9). Exercise perceived as "somewhat hard," a rating of 12 to 14 on the original RPE scale (4 on the revised RPE scale) approximates 60% to 80% of $\dot{V}O_2$max (43, 50). With the RPE, if the maximal heart rate is not known and the THR range is perceived as too low or too high, an RPE rating can provide an estimate of the overall effort experienced by the individual; the exercise intensity can then be adjusted accordingly. Furthermore, as a participant becomes accustomed to the physical sensations experienced when exercising at the THR range, there will be less need for frequent pulse rate measurements.

6 **In Review: The optimal exercise intensity for a CRF training effect can be described in a variety of ways: 60% to 80% $\dot{V}O_2$max, 60% to 80% heart rate reserve, 70% to 85% maximal heart rate, and 12 to 14 on the RPE scale.**

EXERCISE RECOMMENDATIONS FOR THE UNTESTED MASSES

Certain general recommendations can be made for any person wanting to begin a fitness program. Although the HFI might wish to have each individual

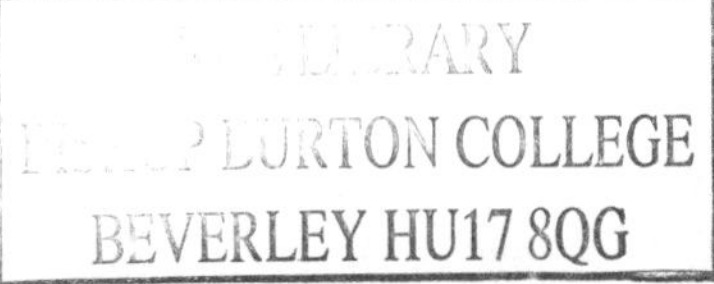

go through a complete testing protocol before beginning exercise, that simply is not realistic. In addition, people without known health problems who follow the general guidelines mentioned before can begin to exercise at low risk. In fact, continuing not to exercise places a person at a higher risk for CHD than if he or she begins a modest exercise program. Figure 14.8 summarizes the recommendations for achieving health, fitness, and performance goals.

EXERCISE PROGRAMMING FOR THE FIT POPULATION

Exercise recommendations written for people who possess reasonably high levels of fitness tend to be associated with less risk, and the participant requires less supervision. In fact, people in this group may focus on performance, in contrast to health and fitness, as the primary goal. A wide variety of programs, activities, races, and competitions are available to address the needs of this group.

The THR range will be calculated as described before, but very fit individuals will work at the top part of the range (> 80% of $\dot{V}O_2max$, or > 85% of HRmax). As was mentioned earlier, a less fit person can start working out at the low end of the range and still experience a training effect. The more fit individual needs to work at the top end of the range to maintain a high level of fitness.

Training for competition demands more than the training intensity needed for CRF. Individuals who do interval-type training programs have peak HRs close to maximum during the intervals. The recovery period between the intervals should include some work at a lower intensity (near 40% to 50% of functional capacity) to help metabolize the lactate produced during the interval (15) and to reduce the chance of cardiovascular complications that can occur when a person comes to a complete rest at the end of a strenuous exercise bout (50).

For people who participate in sports that are intermittent in nature but that still require high levels of aerobic fitness for success, a running/jogging program is a good way to maintain general conditioning when not participating in the primary sport. However, given the specificity of training, there is no substitute for the real activity when conditioning for a sport.

As figure 14.8 shows, people interested in performance who work at the top end of the THR range, exercise 5 to 7 or more times per week, and for longer than 60 min each exercise session are doing much more than the person interested in fitness, and it should be no surprise that they tend to experience more injuries. When this is coupled with the inherent risks associated with competitive activities, it is clear that alternative activities should be planned for that can be done when participation in the primary activity is not possible. This reduces the chance of becoming detrained when injuries do occur.

EXERCISE PRESCRIPTIONS USING COMPLETE GXT RESULTS

In the previous sections, the exercise recommendation was made on the basis of little or no specific

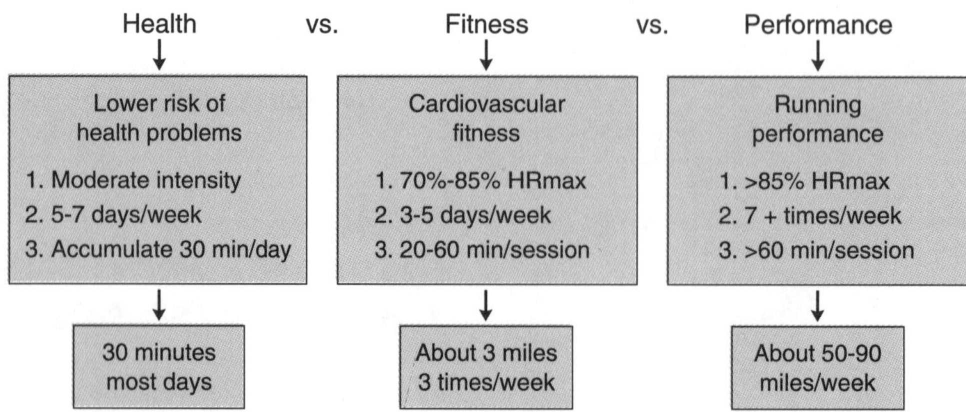

FIGURE 14.8 Contrasting recommendations for achieving health, fitness, and performance goals.

information about the person involved. In many adult fitness programs, potential participants have had a general medical exam or a maximal GXT with appropriate monitoring of the HR, BP, and possibly ECG responses. Unfortunately, this information is sometimes not used in designing the exercise program; instead, the measured maximal HR is used in the THR formulas and the rest of the data are ignored. This section outlines the steps that should be followed when making the exercise recommendation based on information about the person's functional capacity and the cardiovascular responses to graded exercise. The HFI is not directly involved in the clinical evaluation of a GXT, but an understanding of the steps and the procedures used to make clinical judgments clearly enhances communication between the HFI and the Program Director$_{SM}$, Exercise Specialist$_{SM}$, and physician. The following information on Using GXTs for Exercise Prescription and Programming was written with this intent.

Using GXTs for Exercise Prescription and Programming

Steps in GXT analysis for exercise prescription

1. Analyze the person's history and list the known risk factors for CHD; also, identify those factors that might have a direct bearing on the exercise program, such as orthopedic problems, previous physical activity, current interests, and so forth.
2. Determine if the functional capacity is a true maximum or if it is sign- or symptom-limited. Express the functional capacity in METs, and record the highest HR and RPE achieved without significant signs or symptoms.
3. If it was monitored, itemize the person's ECG changes as indicated by the physician.
4. Examine the HR and BP responses to see if they are normal.
5. List the symptoms reported at each stage.
6. List the reasons why the test was stopped (e.g., ECG changes, falling systolic pressure, dizziness).

Steps in designing an exercise program on the basis of a GXT

1. Based on the overall response to the GXT, make a decision to either refer for additional medical care or initiate an exercise program.
2. Identify the THR range and approximate MET intensities of selected activities needed to be within that THR range.
3. Specify the frequency and duration of activity needed to meet the goals of increased cardiorespiratory fitness and weight loss.
4. Recommend that the person participate in either a supervised or unsupervised program, be monitored or unmonitored, do group or individual activities, and so forth.
5. Select a variety of activities at the appropriate MET level that allow the person to achieve THR. Consider environmental factors, medication, and any physical limitations of the participant when making this recommendation.

PROGRAM SELECTION

Exercise program options include exercising alone, in small groups, in fitness clubs, and in clinically oriented settings. The HFI must consider a variety of factors before recommending participation in a supervised or unsupervised program.

Supervised Program

The risk factors, the response to the GXT, the health and activity history, and personal preference influence the type of program in which an individual should participate. Generally, the higher the risk, the more important it is that the person participate in a supervised program. People at high risk for CHD and those who have diseases such as diabetes, hypertension, asthma, CHD, and so on should be encouraged to participate under supervision, at least at the beginning of an exercise program. The personnel in the supervised program are trained to provide the necessary instruction in the appropriate activities, to help monitor the participant's response to the activity, and to administer appropriate first aid or emergency care.

Supervised programs run the gamut from those conducted within a hospital for patients with CHD and other diseases to programs conducted in fitness clubs for people at low risk for CHD. In general, as a person moves along the continuum from "in-patient" to "out-patient," less formal monitoring is required. In addition, the background and training of the personnel tend to vary. The exercise programs aimed at maintaining the fitness level of the CHD patients who went through a hospital-based program have medical personnel and emergency equipment appropriate for the population being served. Supervised fitness programs for the apparently healthy have an HFI who can focus more on the appropriate exercise, diet, and other lifestyle behaviors needed to increase positive health.

The supervised program offers a socially supportive environment for individuals to become and stay active. This is important, given the difficulty of changing lifestyle behaviors. The group program allows for more variety in the types of activities to be used (e.g., group games) and reduces the chance of boredom. To be effective in the long run, the program should try to wean the participants from the group in a way that encourages them to maintain their activity patterns when they are no longer in the program.

Unsupervised Program

In spite of the risks just described, the vast majority of people at risk for or already having CHD participate in unsupervised exercise programs. Reasons for this include the limited number of supervised programs, the level of interest of the participant and physician in such programs, and the financial resources required to bring them about.

Participation in an unsupervised exercise program requires clear communication of correct information from the HFI or physician about how to begin and maintain the exercise program. The emphasis in beginning an unsupervised exercise program is on low intensity, at or below 60% functional capacity (70% HRmax), because the threshold for a training effect is lower in deconditioned people. The goal is to increase the duration of the activity, with exercise frequency approaching every day. This reduces the chance of muscular, skeletal, or cardiovascular problems caused by the exercise intensity and increases muscle function with the expenditure of a relatively large number of calories. In addition, the regularity of the exercise program encourages a positive habit. The outcome of such programs results in the individual being able to conduct her or his daily affairs with more comfort and sets the stage for people who would like to exercise at higher levels.

In an unsupervised exercise program, the person should be provided explicit information about the intensity (THR), duration, and frequency of exercise so that no doubt remains about what should be done. For example, the exercise recommendation might read, "Walk 1 mi in 30 min each day for 2 weeks. Monitor and record your heart rate." The person must be told how to take the pulse rate and be encouraged to follow through on the recording.

Updating the Exercise Program

During participation in an endurance training program, an individual's capacity for work increases. The best sign of this is that the "regular" exercise is no longer sufficient to reach THR; clearly the person is adapting to the exercise. Taking the HR during a regular activity session provides a sound basis for upgrading the intensity or duration of the exercise session.

The exercise program, including the THR, should be periodically updated. The need to update is greater for those with a lower initial level of fitness and a greater number of risk factors. An individual who has a low functional capacity because of heart disease; orthopedic limitations; or chronic inactivity, which might include prolonged bed rest, has difficulty reaching a true maximum on a first treadmill test, and she or he experiences the greatest improvements in the shortest period of time in a fitness program. This individual benefits from frequent retesting because the test allows progress (or the lack thereof) to be monitored, and it may give new information that influences the exercise prescription. If the person has had a change in medication that influences the HR response to exercise, a special need exists for a reevaluation of the exercise program.

For people who reach a true maximum in the first test, actual THR will change little during a fitness program because the maximal heart rate is affected very little by regular endurance exercise. However, they still benefit from an evaluation of the overall exercise program on a regular basis, given that their activity interests may change or they may develop orthopedic problems that did not exist before. The reevaluation allows the HFI to probe for information that may enable her or him to refer the person for treatment at a time when treatment will do the most good. Such contact increases the chance that the person will stay involved in an activity program—which is the most important factor in maintaining aerobic fitness.

7 **In Review: Exercise recommendations for the general public emphasize low intensity and regular participation; see the "Exercise Lite" program described earlier. Exercise performed at 60% to 80% $\dot{V}O_2$max, for 20 to 30 min, 3 or 4 times per week increases and maintains CRF. Exercise recommendations for very fit individuals emphasize the top end of the training intensity (>80% $\dot{V}O_2$max) and frequent (almost daily) participation. The potential for injury is greater for such performance-driven workouts. For those having a comprehensive, diagnostic GXT with ECG being monitored, all test results are used to select an optimal *and safe* exercise prescription.**

Participants with multiple risk factors for CHD and those with existing diseases would benefit from participation in a supervised program. Most individuals will participate in an unsupervised program, necessitating clear communication about the exercise prescription and safety concerns.

ENVIRONMENTAL CONCERNS

Target heart rate is used as an indicator of the proper exercise intensity in health-related fitness programs. However, there are environmental factors such as heat, humidity, pollution, and altitude that can cause HR and the perception of effort to increase during an exercise session. This could shorten the exercise session and reduce the chance of expending sufficient calories and experiencing a training effect. Fortunately, by decreasing the exercise intensity we can "control" these environmental problems to provide a safe and effective exercise prescription. The purpose of this section is to discuss the effects different environmental factors have on the exercise prescription and what we can do about them.

Environmental Heat and Humidity

Chapter 4 described the increases in body temperature that occur with exercise, the heat-loss mechanisms called into play, and the benefits of becoming acclimatized to the heat. Our core temperature (37 °C, or 98.6 °F) is within a few degrees of a value that could lead to death by heat injury. As described in chapter 21, however, to prevent a progression from the least to the most serious heat injury, individuals should recognize and attend to a series of stages from heat cramps to heat stroke. Although treatment of these problems is important, prevention is a better approach.

Each of the following factors influences susceptibility to heat injury and can alter the HR and metabolic responses to exercise:

- *fitness*—Fit people have a lower risk of heat injury (19), can tolerate more work in the heat (16), and acclimatize to heat faster (11).
- *acclimatization*—Seven to 10 days of exercise in the heat increases our capacity to sweat, initiates sweating at a lower body temperature, and reduces salt loss. Body temperature and HR responses are lower during exercise, and the chance of salt depletion is reduced (11).
- *hydration*—Inadequate hydration reduces sweat rate and increases the chance of heat injury (11, 58, 59). Generally, during exercise the focus should be on replacing water, not salt or carbohydrate stores.
- *environmental temperature*—Exercising in temperatures greater than skin temperatures results

in a heat gain by convection and radiation. Evaporation of sweat must compensate if body temperature is to remain at a safe value.

- *clothing*—As much skin surface as possible should be exposed to encourage evaporation, taking care to protect the skin from too much exposure to the sun with sunblock. Materials should be chosen that will "wick" sweat to the surface for evaporation; materials impermeable to water will increase the risk of heat injury and should be avoided.
- *humidity* (water vapor pressure)—Evaporation of sweat is dependent on the water vapor pressure gradient between skin and environment. In warm and hot environments, the relative humidity is a good index of the water vapor pressure, with a lower relative humidity facilitating the evaporation of sweat.
- *metabolic rate*—During times of high heat and humidity, decreasing the exercise intensity decreases the heat load, as well as the strain on the physiological systems that must deal with it.
- *wind*—Wind places more air molecules into contact with the skin and can influence heat loss in two ways: If there is a temperature gradient for heat loss between the skin and the air, wind will increase the rate of heat loss by convection. In a similar manner, wind increases the rate of evaporation, assuming the air can accept moisture.

Recommendations for Fitness

The members of a fitness program should be educated about all of the heat-related factors just mentioned. The HFI might suggest

- information on heat-illness symptoms (e.g., cramps, lightheadedness) and how to deal with them (see chapter 21);
- exercising in the cooler parts of the day to avoid heat gain from the sun or from building or road surfaces heated by the sun;
- gradually increasing exposure to high heat and humidity to safely acclimatize over a period of 7 to 10 days;
- drinking water before, during, and after exercise and weighing in each day to monitor hydration;
- wearing only shorts and a tank top to expose as much skin as possible, but being careful to use a strong sunblock to reduce the chance of skin cancer; and
- taking HR measurements several times during the activity and reducing exercise intensity to stay in the THR zone.

The last recommendation, regarding THR, is most important. HR is a sensitive indicator of dehydration, environmental heat load, and acclimatization. Variation in any of these factors will modify the HR response to any fixed submaximal exercise. It is therefore important for fitness participants to monitor HR on a regular basis and slow down to stay within the THR zone. The RPE can also be used in circumstances of extreme heat to provide an index of the overall physiological strain being experienced by the participant.

Implication for Performance

Any athlete performing in an environment that is not conducive to heat loss is at an increased risk of heat injury. This has been a major problem for football where clothing and equipment prevent heat loss; but the increased number of people participating in 10K races, marathons, and triathlons has shifted our focus of attention (22, 35). In the latter cases, the athlete has a very high metabolic rate while exercising in direct exposure to the sun. In 1985 in response to this problem and on the basis of sound research, the American College of Sports Medicine developed a position stand, "The Prevention of Thermal Injuries During Distance Running" (2). The elements in this position stand are consistent with what was presented earlier in the chapter.

Environmental Heat Stress

The preceding discussion mentioned high temperature and relative humidity as factors increasing the risk of heat injuries. To quantify the overall heat stress associated with any environment, a **wet-bulb globe temperature (WBGT)** guide has been developed (2). This overall heat-stress index is composed of the following measurements:

- **dry-bulb temperature** (T_{db})—Ordinary measure of air temperature taken in the shade
- **black-globe temperature** (T_g)—Measure of the radiant heat load measured in direct sunlight
- **wet-bulb temperature** (T_{wb})—Measurement of air temperature with a thermometer whose mercury bulb is covered with a wet cotton wick (making it sensitive to the relative humidity [water vapor pressure] and providing an index of the ability to evaporate sweat)

The formula used to calculate the WBGT temperature shows the importance of the wet-bulb temperature, being 70% (0.7) of the WBGT index, in determining heat stress (2). This is related to the role the wet-bulb temperature plays in estimating the ability to evaporate sweat, the most important heat-loss mechanism in most situations. The formula is

$$WBGT = 0.7\ T_{wb} + 0.2\ T_{g} + 0.1\ T_{db}$$

The risk of heat stress is given by the following color-coded flags on race courses:

Red flag = High risk
WBGT = 23 to 28 °C (73 to 82 °F)

Amber flag = Moderate risk
WBGT = 18 to 23 °C (65 to 73 °F)

Green flag = Low risk (of heat injury)
WBGT less than 18 °C (less than 65 °F)

White flag = Low risk (of **hyperthermia**,but possibility of **hypothermia**)
WBGT less than 10 °C (less than 50 °F)

Figure 14.9 provides another estimate of heat stress, using just temperature and relative humidity. Because this figure does not include radiant heat load (globe temperature), it should be used conservatively in estimating heat load.

Exercise and Cold Exposure

Exercising in the cold can create problems if certain precautions are not taken. As mentioned in the "white flag" category of heat stress, a WBGT of 10 °C (50 °F) or less is associated with hypothermia. Hypothermia is a decrease in body temperature that occurs when heat loss exceeds heat production. In cold air, there is a larger gradient for convective heat loss from the skin; cold air also is "dry" (has a low water vapor pressure) and facilitates the evaporation of moisture from the skin to further cool the body. The combined effects can be deadly, as shown in Pugh's report of three deaths during a walking competition in very cold temperatures over a 45-mi distance (53).

Factors related to hypothermia include *environmental factors*, such as temperature, water vapor pressure, wind, and whether air or water are involved; *insulating factors*, such as clothing and subcutaneous fat; and the capacity for sustained *energy production*. Each of these factors is discussed in the following paragraphs.

Environmental Factors

Conduction, convection, and radiation are dependent on a temperature gradient between the skin and the environment; the larger the gradient, the greater the rate of heat loss. What is surprising is that the environmental temperature does not have to be below freezing to cause hypothermia. There are other environmental factors that interact with temperature to create the dangerous condition by facilitating heat loss, namely, wind and water.

Windchill Index. The rate of heat loss at any given temperature is directly influenced by wind speed. Wind increases the number of cold air molecules coming into contact with the skin, increasing the rate of heat loss. The **windchill index** indicates what the "effective" temperature is for any combination of temperature and wind speed (see figure 14.10) and allows you to properly gauge the conditions for a variety of wind velocities and temperatures. Keep in mind

wet-bulb globe temperature (WBGT) — Heat stress index that considers dry-bulb, wet-bulb, and black globe temperatures.

dry-bulb temperature — The temperature of the air measured in the shade by an ordinary thermometer.

black-globe temperature — A measure of radiant heat energy; measurement taken in the sunlight to evaluate the potential to gain or lose heat by radiation.

wet-bulb temperature — Air temperature measured with a thermometer whose bulb is surrounded by a wick wetted with water; an indication of the ability to evaporate moisture from the skin.

hyperthermia — An elevation of the core temperature; if unchecked it can lead to heat exhaustion or heat stroke and death.

hypothermia — Below-normal body temperature.

windchill index — The coldness felt on exposed human skin by a combination of temperature and wind velocity.

(%) Relative humidity	Temperature 60	65	70	75	80	85	90	95	100
0									
10	59	62	64	67	69	72	74	77	79
20	59	62	65	68	70	73	76	79	82
30	59	62	65	68	72	75	78	81	84
40	59	63	66	69	73	76	79	83	86
50	59	63	67	70	74	76	81	85	88
60	60	63	67	71	75	79	83	87	91
70	60	64	68	72	76	81	85	88	93
80	60	64	69	73	78	82	86	91	95
90	60	65	69	74	79	84	88	93	98
100	60	65	70	75	80	85	90	95	100
			Caution		Extreme caution				

FIGURE 14.9 Exercise in the heat (apparent temperatures). To read the chart, find the air temperature on the top, then find the humidity on the left. Find the apparent temperature where the columns meet.
Reprinted from Franklin et al. 1990.

that if you are running, riding, or cross-country skiing into the wind, you must add your speed to the wind speed to evaluate the full impact of the windchill. For example, cycling at 20 mi · hr^{-1} into calm air at 0 °F has a windchill value of -35 °F! However, wind is not the only factor that can increase the rate of heat loss at any given temperature.

Water. You can lose heat 25 times faster in water compared to air of the same temperature. Unlike air, water offers little or no insulation where the skin meets the water, so heat is rapidly lost from the body. Movement in cold water would increase heat loss from the arms and legs, so the recommendation is to stay as still as possible in long-term immersions (32).

Insulating Factors

The rate at which heat is lost from the body is inversely related to the insulation between the body and the environment. The insulating quality is related to the thickness of subcutaneous fat, the ability of clothing to trap air, and whether or not the clothing is wet or dry.

Body Fat. Subcutaneous fat thickness is an excellent indicator of total body insulation per unit surface area through which heat is lost (28). For example, a fat man was able to swim for 7 hr in 16 °C water with no change in body temperature; but a thin man had to leave the water in 30 min with a core temperature of 34.5 °C (54). For this reason, long-distance swimmers tend to have more body fat than short-course swimmers; the higher body fatness provides more buoyancy, requiring less energy to swim at any set speed (31).

Clothing. Clothing can extend our natural subcutaneous fat insulation, allowing us to endure very cold environments. The insulation quality of clothing is given in "clo" units, where 1 clo unit is the insulation needed at rest (1 MET) to maintain core

	Actual thermometer reading (°F)											
Wind speed (mi · hr^{1})	50	40	30	20	10	0	−10	−20	−30	−40	−50	−60
	Equivalent temperature (°F)											
Calm	50	40	30	20	10	0	−10	−20	−30	−40	−50	−60
5	48	37	27	16	6	−5	−15	−26	−36	−47	−57	−68
10	40	28	16	4	−9	−21	−33	−46	−58	−70	−83	−95
15	36	22	9	−5	−18	−36	−45	−58	−72	−85	−99	−112
20	32	18	4	−10	−25	−39	−53	−67	−82	−96	−110	−124
25	30	16	0	−15	−29	−44	−59	−74	−88	−104	−118	−133
30	28	13	−2	−18	−33	−48	−63	−79	−94	−109	−125	−140
35	27	11	−4	−20	−35	−49	−67	−82	−98	−113	−129	−145
40	26	10	−6	−21	−37	−53	−69	−85	−100	−116	−132	−148
(Wind speeds greater than 40 mi · hr^{1} have little additional effect)	Little danger (for properly clothed person)				Increasing danger			Great danger				
					Danger from freezing of exposed flesh							

FIGURE 14.10 Windchill index.
Reprinted from Sharkey 1974.

temperature when the environment is 21 °C (70 °F), the relative humidity = 50%, and the air movement is 6 m · hr^{-1} (10). As the air temperature falls, clothing with a higher clo value must be worn to maintain core temperature because the gradient between skin and environment is increasing. Figure 14.11 shows the insulation needed at different energy expenditures across a broad range of environmental temperatures, from −60 to +80 °F (10). It is clear that as energy production increases, insulation must decrease to maintain core temperature. When clothing is worn in layers, insulation can be removed as needed to maintain core temperature. By following these steps, sweating, which can rob the clothing of its insulating value, will be minimized. If the clothing becomes wet, the insulating quality decreases because the water can now conduct heat away from the body about 25 times better than air (32). A primary goal, then, is to avoid wetness due to either sweat or weather. This problem is exacerbated by the cold environment's very dry air, which causes a greater evaporation of moisture. When this problem of cold, dry air and wet clothing is coupled with windy conditions, the risk is even greater. The wind not only provides for greater convective heat loss, as described in the windchill section, but it also accelerates evaporation (23).

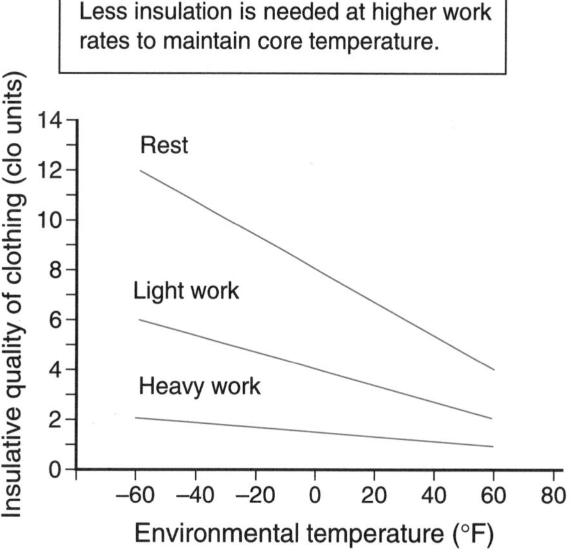

FIGURE 14.11 As work intensity increases, less insulation is needed to maintain core temperature.
Data from Burton & Edholm 1955.

Energy Production

Energy production can modify the amount of insulation needed to maintain core temperature and prevent hypothermia (see figure 14.11). When thin (less than 16.8% fat) male subjects were immersed in cold water, the drop in body temperature that occurred at rest was prevented when they did exercise at an energy expenditure of about 8.5 kcal · min^{-1} (41, 42).

Table 14.3 shows the progression of signs and symptoms of hypothermia that occur as body temperature decreases (62). It is important to deal with these problems "on site" rather than wait until the person can be taken to an emergency room. Following Sharkey (60), one should

- get the person out of the cold, wind, and rain;
- remove all wet clothing;
- provide warm drinks, dry clothing, and a warm, dry sleeping bag for a mildly impaired person;
- keep the person awake; if semiconscious, undress the person and put him or her into a sleeping bag with another person; and
- find a heat source, such as a campfire.

Table 14.3 Clinical Symptoms of Hypothermia

Core temperature (°C)	Symptoms and signs
37	Feeling of cold; skin cooling; decreased social interaction
36	Goose pimples
35	Shivering; muscle tension; fatigue
34.5	Deep cold Numbness Loss of coordination Stumbling Dysarthria Muscle rigidity
32	Disorientation Decreased visual acuity
31-30	Semicoma—coma
28	Ventricular fibrillation and cardiovascular death

Reprinted from Hart and Sutton 1987.

Effect of Air Pollution

Air pollution includes a variety of gases and particulates that are products of the combustion of fossil fuels. The smog that results when these pollutants are in high concentration can have detrimental effects on health and performance. The gases can affect performance by decreasing the capacity to transport oxygen, increasing airway resistance, and altering the perception of effort required when the eyes burn and the chest hurts.

Physiological responses to these pollutants are related to the amount, or "dose," received. The major factors determining the dose are the

- concentration of the pollutant,
- duration of the exposure to the pollutant, and
- volume of air inhaled.

The volume of air inhaled is clearly large during exercise, and this is one reason why physical activity is curtailed during times of peak pollution levels (17). The following discussion focuses on the major air pollutants: ozone, sulfur dioxide, and carbon monoxide.

Ozone

The **ozone** in the air we breathe is generated by the reaction between ultraviolet (UV) light and emissions from internal combustion engines. There is evidence that a single 2-hr exposure to a high ozone concentration, 0.75 ppm (parts per million), decreases $\dot{V}O_2max$; and recent studies show that a 6- to 12-hr exposure to a concentration of only 0.12 ppm (the U.S. air-quality standard) produces a decrease in lung function and an increase in respiratory symptoms. Interestingly, people can adapt to ozone exposure, showing diminished responses to subsequent exposures during the "ozone season." Concern about long-term lung health suggests, however, that it would be prudent to avoid heavy exercise during the time of day when ozone and other pollutants are elevated (17).

Sulfur Dioxide

Sulfur dioxide (SO_2) is produced by smelters, refineries, and electrical utilities that use fossil fuel for energy generation. SO_2 does not affect lung function in normal individuals, but it causes bronchoconstriction in asthmatics—a response influenced by the temperature and humidity of the inspired air. Nose breathing is encouraged to "scrub" the SO_2, and drugs like cromolyn sodium and ß-agonists can partially block the asthmatic's response to SO_2 (17).

Carbon Monoxide

Carbon monoxide (CO) is derived from the burning of fossil fuel, coal, oil, gasoline, and wood, as well as from cigarette smoke. Carbon monoxide can bind to hemoglobin (HbCO) and decrease the capacity for oxygen transport. The carbon monoxide concentration in blood is generally less than 1% in nonsmokers but may be as high as 10% in smokers (56). As mentioned in chapter 4, beyond a HbCO concentration of 4.3% there is a 1% reduction in

$\dot{V}O_2max$ for each 1% increase in the HbCO concentration. In contrast, when one exercises at about 40% $\dot{V}O_2max$, the HbCO concentration can be as high as 15% before endurance is affected. The cardiovascular system simply has a greater capacity to respond with a larger cardiac output when the O_2 concentration of the blood is reduced during submaximal work (33, 55, 56). This, of course, requires a higher HR for the same work task, and a participant needs to reduce the intensity of exercise during exposure to CO to stay in the THR range. Because it takes about 2 to 4 hr to remove half the CO from the blood once the exposure has been removed, CO can have a lasting effect on performance (17). Unfortunately, it is difficult to predict what the actual CO concentration will be in any given environment. Because we must consider the previous exposure to the pollutant, as well as the length of time and rate of ventilation associated with the current exposure, the following guidelines are provided for exercising in an area with air pollution (56):

- Reduce exposure to the pollutant prior to exercise because the physiological effects are time and dose dependent.
- Stay away from areas where one might receive a "bolus" dose of CO: smoking areas, high traffic areas, and urban environments.
- Do not schedule activities during the times when pollutants are at their highest levels: 7 to 10 A.M. and 4 to 7 P.M., due to traffic.

Effect of Altitude

An increase in altitude decreases the partial pressure of oxygen and reduces the amount of oxygen bound to hemoglobin. As a result, the volume of oxygen carried in each liter of blood decreases. As mentioned in chapter 4, maximal aerobic power steadily decreases with increasing altitude, so that by 2300 m (7500 ft) the value is only 88% of that measured at sea level. This means that an activity that demanded 88% of $\dot{V}O_2max$ at sea level now requires 100% of the "new" $\dot{V}O_2max$.

More than maximal aerobic power is affected by altitude exposure. Any submaximal work rate is going to demand a higher HR at altitude compared to sea level (shown in figure 14.12). The reason is quite simple. Because each liter of blood has less oxygen at altitude, more blood is required to deliver the same quantity of oxygen to the tissues. Consequently, the HR response is elevated at any given submaximal work rate. To stay within the THR range, a person must decrease the intensity of the exercise when at altitude. Just like exercise in high heat and humidity, the THR allows the modification of the intensity of the activity relative to any additional environmental demand (34).

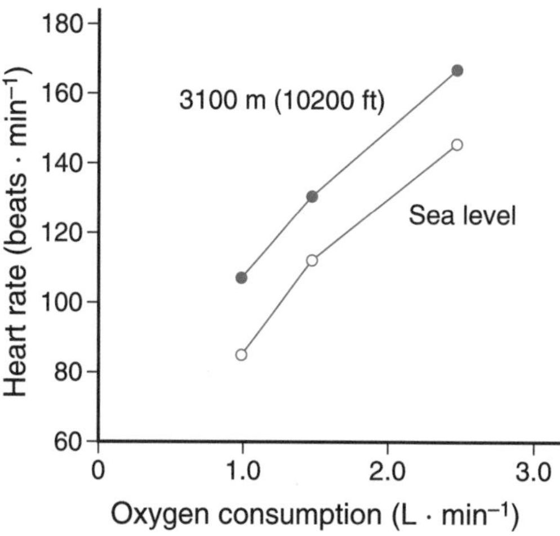

FIGURE 14.12 The effect of altitude on the heart-rate response to submaximal exercise.
Based on data of R. Grover et al. 1967.

8 **In Review: In conditions of high heat and humidity, decrease the work rate to stay in the target heart rate zone. Acclimatize to heat over 7 to 10 days to reduce the risk of heat injury. Drink water before, during, and after exercise and exercise in the early morning to reduce environmental heat load. When exercising in cold weather, wear clothing in layers and remove layers to minimize sweating and stay dry. Avoid exercising at times and in places in which air pollution is a problem. When exercising at altitude, decrease work intensity to stay in the target heart rate zone.**

ozone — An active form of oxygen formed in reaction to UV light and as an emission from internal combustion engines; exposure can decrease lung function.

sulfur dioxide — A pollutant that can cause bronchoconstriction in people with asthma.

carbon monoxide — A pollutant derived from the incomplete combustion of fossil fuels; binds to hemoglobin to reduce oxygen transport and thus reduce maximal aerobic power.

Case Studies

In the following case studies you are given general information about an individual, data on risk factors, and the results of an exercise test. Analyze each case, spell out the risk factors, and react to the responses of the person to the test (whether normal or not). Then, on the basis of your analysis, make some recommendations for the individual relative to an exercise program, risk-factor reduction program, and so forth. See appendix A for a suggested response.

14.1

Paul is a Caucasian male, 36 years of age, 88 kg, and 178 cm tall, and he has 28% body fat. Blood chemistry values indicate that total cholesterol = 270 mg/dl and HDL cholesterol = 38 mg/dl. His mother died of a heart attack at the age of 63, and his father had a heart attack at the age of 68. He is sedentary and has engaged in no endurance training program since college. The following are the results of a *maximal* GXT conducted by his physician.

Test: Balke, 3 mi · hr^{-1}; 2.5% per 2 min

Grade %	METs	SBP mm Hg	DBP mm Hg	HR b/ min	ECG	Symptoms
	Rest	126	88	70	normal	—
2.5	4.3	142	86	142	normal	—
5	5.4	148	88	150	normal	—
7.5	6.4	162	86	160	normal	—
10	7.4	174	84	168	normal	—
12.5	8.5	186	84	176	normal	—
15	9.5	194	84	190	normal	calf tight
17.5	10.5	198	84	198	normal	fatigue

14.2

Mary is a 38-year-old Hispanic-American female, 170 cm tall, and 61.4 kg, and she has 30% body fat. Blood chemistry values indicate a total cholesterol of 188 mg/dl and a HDL cholesterol of 59 mg/dl. Her resting blood pressure is 124/80. Family history indicates that her father suffered a nonfatal heart attack at the age of 67. She has smoked 1 pack-a-day of cigarettes for the past 13 years, and her lifestyle is sedentary. The following is the result of her submaximal cycle ergometer test.

Test: YMCA cycle test

Work rate (kpm · min^{-1})	Heart rate (min 2)	Heart rate (min 3)
150	118	120
300	134	136

Note. Pedal rate = 50 rev · min^{-1}; predicted HRmax = 182 beats · min^{-1}; seat height = 6; and 85% HRmax = 155 beats · min^{-1}

Source List

1. American College of Sports Medicine (ACSM) (1980)
2. ACSM (1985)
3. ACSM (1990)
4. ACSM (1993b)
5. ACSM (1995)
6. American Heart Association (1992)
7. Blair et al. (1989)
8. Blair et al. (1995)
9. Borg (1982)
10. Burton & Edholm (1955)
11. Buskirk & Bass (1974)
12. Corbin & Lindsey (1991)
13. Dehn & Mullins (1977)
14. Dionne et al. (1991)
15. Dodd, Powers, Callender, & Brooks (1984)
16. Drinkwater, Denton, Kupprat, Talag, & Horvath (1976)
17. Folinsbee (1990)
18. Franks (1983)
19. Gisolfi & Cohen (1979)
20. Goodman & Gilman (1975)
21. Grover, Reeves, Grover, & Leathers (1967)
22. Hanson & Zimmerman (1979)
23. Hardy & Bard (1974)
24. Hart & Sutton (1987)
25. Haskell (1978)
26. Haskell (1985)
27. Haskell (1994)
28. Hayward & Keatinge (1981)
29. Hellerstein & Franklin (1984)
30. Holloszy & Coyle (1984)
31. Holmer (1979)
32. Horvath (1981)
33. Horvath, Raven, Dahms, & Gray (1975)
34. Howley (1980)
35. Hughson et al. (1980)
36. Jennings et al. (1991)

37. Karvonen, Kentala, & Mustala (1957)
38. Lee, Hsieh, & Paffenbarger (1995)
39. Londeree & Ames (1976)
40. Londeree & Moeschberger (1982)
41. McArdle, Magel, Gergley, Spina, & Toner (1984)
42. McArdle, Magel, Spina, Gergley, & Toner (1984)
43. Noble, Borg, Cafarelli, Robertson, & Pandolf (1982)
44. Paffenbarger & Hale (1975)
45. Paffenbarger, Hyde, & Wing (1986)
46. Paffenbarger, Hyde, & Wing (1990)
47. Paffenbarger et al. (1993)
48. Pate et al. (1995)
49. Pollock et al. (1977)
50. Pollock & Wilmore (1990)
51. Powell, Thompson, & Caspersen (1987)
52. Powers & Howley (1997)
53. Pugh (1964)
54. Pugh & Edholm (1955)
55. Raven (1980)
56. Raven et al. (1974)
57. Saltin & Gollnick (1983)
58. Sawka, Francesconi, Young, & Pandolf (1984)
59. Sawka, Young, Francesconi, Muza, & Pandolf (1985)
60. Sharkey (1990)
61. Siscovick et al. (1984)
62. Sutton (1990)

CHAPTER

15

Exercise Prescription for Strength, Endurance, and Bone Density

Vernon Bond

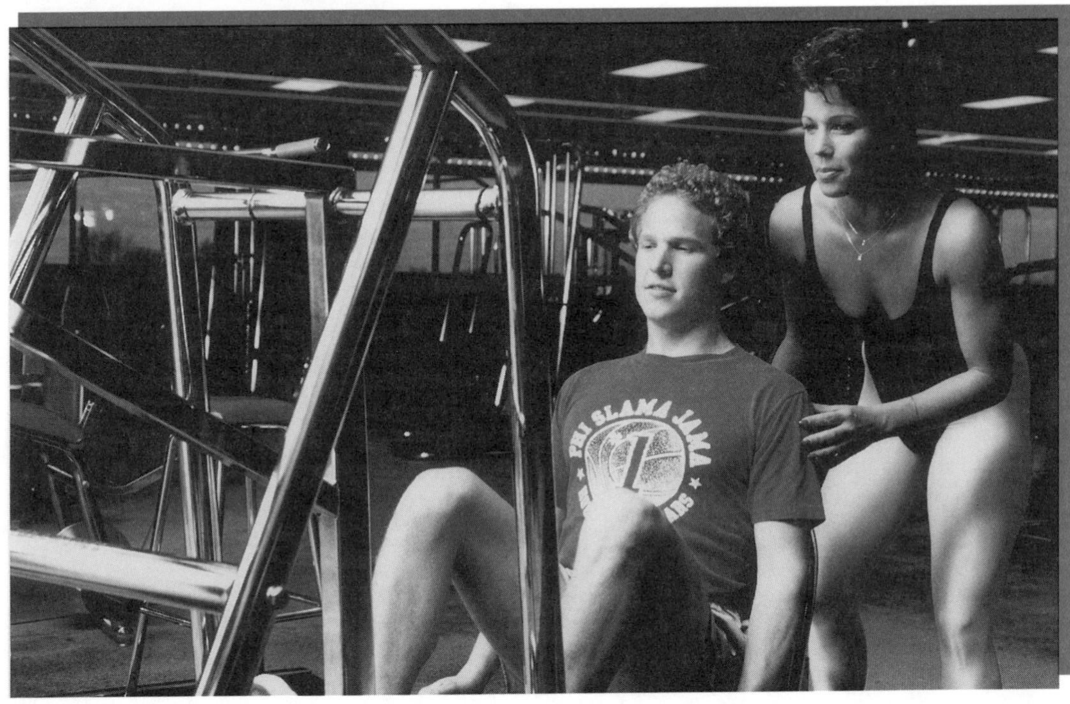

OBJECTIVES

The reader will be able to:

1. **Explain the principles of overload, specificity, and progression and how they relate to resistance training.**
2. **Describe the adaptations of muscle to aerobic and anaerobic training.**
3. **Describe the following methods of resistance training: isometric, dynamic (constant resistance, variable resistance, and circuit training), isokinetic, and plyometric.**
4. **Compare the effectiveness of the different methods of resistance training.**
5. **Describe the following systems of resistance training: super set, pyramid set, and split routine.**
6. **Describe a resistance training program for increasing or maintaining bone mass.**
7. **Contrast the training program used for strength gains versus maintenance of strength and describe the symptoms of overtraining.**
8. **Identify the physiological principles related to warm-up and cool-down exercises.**
9. **Describe the basic precautions taken in a weight room area to ensure participant safety.**
10. **Demonstrate an understanding of the relationship among number of repetitions, intensity, number of sets, and rest with regard to resistance training programs for strength and endurance.**

Resistance training is a systematic program of exercise for development of the musculoskeletal system. A lack of adequate muscular fitness (strength and endurance) and a decrease in bone density with increasing age are health concerns of the general population. As a health fitness instructor (HFI) you must be able to design a program for developing the musculoskeletal system. This chapter focuses on the basic principles of how to design programs to increase or maintain muscle strength, endurance, and bone density.

TRAINING CONSIDERATIONS FOR INCREASING MUSCLE STRENGTH/ENDURANCE AND BONE DENSITY

In designing an exercise program to achieve gains in strength, endurance, and bone density, the program should stress the following three basic principles:

- Overload
- Specificity
- Progression

Overload

The overload principle is the basis of the strength training program and states that to develop the musculoskeletal system, it must experience loads to which it is not accustomed. The overload principle may be achieved by varying the training intensity (amount of resistance), **repetitions** (number of lifts), and **sets** (number of times the desired total number of repetitions is performed).

Specificity

You must train the specific muscles for which increases in strength and endurance are desired. For example, if the goal is to improve the strength of the muscles involved in the bench press, then the training should focus on developing those muscles. In other words, the overload principle should be applied to the muscles in the upper body (triceps, pectoralis major, pectoralis minor) as opposed to the muscles in the lower part of the body. Muscular fitness development is also specific to the training intensity. Figure 15.1 shows that weight training with high resistance and low repetitions results in the greatest strength gains, whereas weight training using low resistance and high repetitions results in the greatest improvement in muscular endurance, with less increase in muscle strength and size. Thus, weight training to develop strength focuses primarily on development of the anaerobic system, and exercises to increase endurance rely on development of the aerobic system. Review chapter 4 for a discussion of the anaerobic and aerobic systems.

Progression

When the muscle adapts to a given load there is no further increase in muscle strength and endurance. Most weight training programs consist of **progressive resistance exercises**. Progressive resistance exercise means that as strength and endurance are increased, the load against which the muscle works must be periodically elevated for strength and endurance gains to continue (39).

1 **In Review:** **Increases in muscle size and strength result from resistance training programs that apply the overload principle: A muscle will increase in strength only when the load is greater than that to which it is accustomed. To increase the strength and endurance of a particular muscle group, exercises should be done that concentrate on those muscles specifically. Gains in strength and endurance are highly specific to the training intensity. For the best gains in strength the training intensity should be high with low repetitions. For optimal gains in endurance the training intensity should be low with high repetitions. For systematic increases in strength and endurance with training, the program must consist of progressive resistance exercise in which the load is steadily increased as the muscle becomes stronger.**

AEROBIC AND ANAEROBIC ADAPTATIONS WITH TRAINING

The mechanism responsible for developing muscular strength and endurance is not completely understood. However, some of the metabolic and morphological changes that occur with regular training have been established. For example, aerobic training leads to a greater capillary density in muscle and an increased ability of the muscle to generate energy (ATP) with oxygen, which increases muscular endurance. In contrast, anaerobic training produces increased muscular strength and a greater tolerance for acid-base imbalances during high-intensity exercise. Table 15.1 contrasts the skeletal muscle

repetitions — The number of muscle contractions executed during each set of exercises.

sets — The number of times the desired number of repetitions are performed.

progressive resistance exercise — A descriptive term for strength training programs in which a muscle adapts to a resistance, and a greater resistance is then chosen to overload the muscle and continue to increase strength.

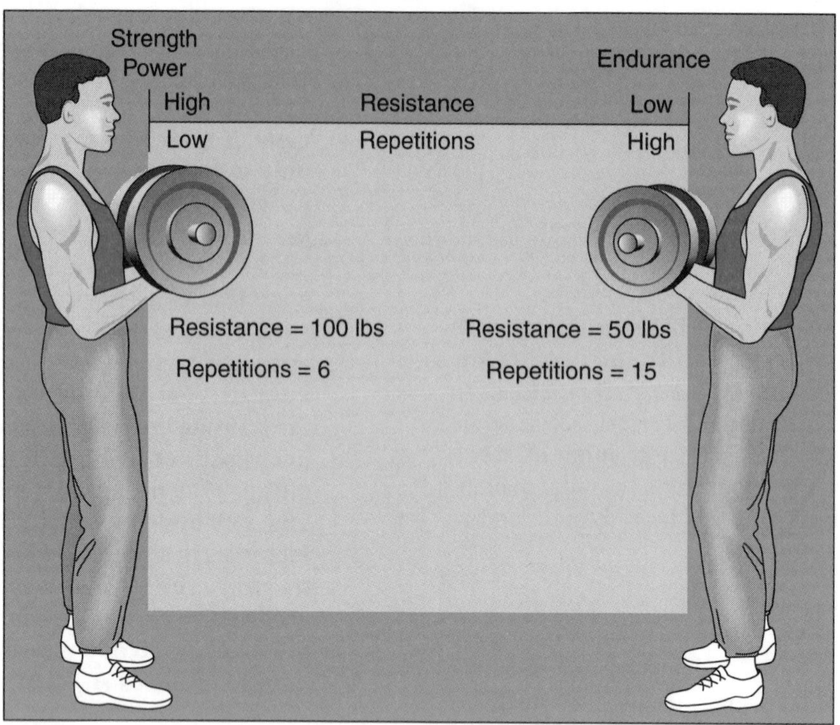

FIGURE 15.1 The strength/endurance continuum. Strength is achieved by using low repetitions/high weight, and endurance is achieved by using high repetitions/low weight.

Modified from Powers and Dodd, *Total fitness: Exercise, nutrition and wellness*. Copyright © 1996 by Allyn and Bacon. Adapted by permission.

Table 15.1 Skeletal Muscle Adaptations to Anaerobic (Strength) and Aerobic (Endurance) Training

Variable	Strength training	Endurance training
Size of muscle	Increases	No change or increases slightly
Number of muscle fibers	No change	No change
Strength	Increases	No change or increases slightly
Muscle fatigue	Rapidly	Slow
Aerobic power	Increases slightly	Increases
Anaerobic power	Increases	Increases slightly
Capillary density	No change or decreases	Increases
Mitochondria number	Decreases	Increases
Oxidation of fat and carbohydrate	No change	Increases
Glycolytic enzymes	Increases	No change
Oxidative enzymes	No change	Increases

adaptations to physical conditioning that occur as a result of resistance (anaerobic) or endurance (aerobic) exercise.

Muscle Adaptations to Aerobic Training

Repeated use of a muscle during endurance training produces changes in the muscle fiber, capillary supply, mitochondria function, and oxidative enzymes. Activities such as low-intensity weight training rely primarily on the slow-twitch fibers. Bassett (7) reported in a review paper of exercise training and muscle adaptations that the percentage of slow-twitch fibers is not altered by endurance training. However, with endurance training the slow-twitch fibers have been reported to become 7% to 22% larger in diameter than the corresponding fast-twitch fibers (15).

Slow-twitch fibers tend to be more highly vascularized than fast-twitch fibers, in accordance with their greater reliance on blood flow for oxidative metabolism (7). Endurance training stimulates an increase in the number of **capillaries** surrounding the muscle fiber. With endurance training the microvascular density has been shown to increase 15% to 40% (2, 25, 28). Increased capillary density enhances the exchange of gases, heat, waste products, and nutrients. The slow-twitch fibers contain the compound **myoglobin** that aids in shuttling the oxygen molecules from the cell membrane to the mitochondria. Although myoglobin's contribution to oxygen delivery is not completely understood, it is known that elevated levels of myoglobin enhance the oxidative capacity of the muscle. Endurance training has been shown to increase muscle myoglobin content by 80% in animals (44). It is not known, however, if endurance training stimulates similar increases of myoglobin in humans.

During aerobic work the mitochondria provide the muscles with the ATP needed for muscle contraction and relaxation. The ability of the muscle to use oxygen and produce energy depends on the number and size of the mitochondria. Both mitochondria size and density are increased with aerobic exercise. This results in a greater oxygen utilization capacity within the muscle and contributes to an increase in muscle endurance. **Succinate dehydrogenase** is one of the key enzymes in the mitochondria used to generate energy. The activity of succinate dehydrogenase (SDH) can increase as much as 300% with aerobic training.

When endurance exercise is performed the muscles rely on the utilization of glycogen and fat for energy production. However, the glycogen levels are often depleted during continuous work such as endurance activity, and the muscles may become fatigued. With aerobic training the muscles become more efficient in burning fat, and the onset of fatigue is delayed because glycogen is not used as rapidly during exercise.

Muscle Adaptations to Anaerobic Training

Activity that emphasizes near maximal force production, such as high-intensity weight lifting, relies on the **ATP-CP system** and anaerobic glycolysis to provide the needed energy. Short duration, maximal effort exercise increases ATP-CP enzyme activity (creatine phosphokinase and myokinase) and glycolytic enzymes (phosphofructokinase and phosphorylase). Whether or not these changes allow the muscle to perform more anaerobic work remains unanswered (44). It is well established that training at near maximal effort in weight lifting causes muscle hypertrophy and enhances performance by improving strength. It was mentioned in chapter 12 that the hydrogen ion concentration is elevated during anaerobic work and causes muscle fatigue. Buffers (such as bicarbonate and muscle phosphate) combine with the hydrogen ion to reduce the fiber's acidity, thus delaying the onset of fatigue during anaerobic work (44). Studies have shown that with anaerobic training the muscle's buffering capacity is increased by 12% to 50% (41). With this increased buffering capacity, more lactic acid can accumulate during high-intensity strength training without causing fatigue.

2 **In Review: Aerobic training increases the muscle's capacity to use considerably more fat as an energy source, sparing glycogen. Aerobic training increases capillary and mitochondria density in skeletal muscle. This facilitates oxygen delivery and the generation of ATP for endurance work. Anaerobic training increases the ATP-CP enzymes and improves the muscle's buffering capacity, which delays the onset of muscle fatigue. These adaptations facilitate gains in muscle strength during high-intensity resistance training.**

WEIGHT TRAINING METHODS

Various resistance training methods have been used to develop muscular strength and endurance. These include isometric (static contraction) and dynamic

capillary (capillaries) — The smallest blood vessel; the link between the end of the arteries and the beginning of the veins.

myoglobin — A compound that aids in shuttling oxygen to the mitochondria.

succinate dehyrogenase — A key enzyme involved in the generation of energy through the aerobic system.

ATP-CP system — Immediate source of energy for cellular function provided through the anaerobic energy system.

modes of training. A warm-up and cool-down should be conducted before and after the training session, as discussed later in the chapter.

Isometric (Static) Training

Isometric resistance training refers to a muscular contraction where no change in muscle length takes place. This type of resistance training is usually performed against an immovable object such as a wall or weight machine. The concept of isometric training gained interest in the 1950s when the work of Hettinger and Muller (26) showed strength gains of 5% per week from using one daily 6-s isometric contraction at two-thirds of maximal force. Strength gains requiring such little time and effort were quite appealing. Later studies concluded, however, that although isometric training led to static strength gains, the gains were substantially less than 5% per week (20).

The advantage of isometric training is that no specialized equipment is required; thus, the cost factor of this training method is minimal. A disadvantage of isometric training is that the muscle development is joint-angle specific as opposed to strengthening the muscle throughout a full range of motion. If isometric training is performed at a joint angle of 90°, strength will be increased at this angle but not necessarily at other angles of that joint (19). The joint-angle specificity appears to have a carryover effect of ± 20° of the training joint angle (30). To increase strength throughout the range of motion, the same exercise must be performed at varying joint angles (e.g., 20°, 40°, 60° of limb range of motion). Increases in strength from isometric training are influenced by the number of repetitions performed, duration of the contractions, intensity of the contraction, and frequency of training. Table 15.2 presents the general guidelines for designing isometric training programs to increase strength and endurance.

To bring about gains in maximal strength the isometric program should consist of maximal static contractions. Submaximal isometric contractions will lead to an increase in strength, but the greatest increase will be in muscle endurance. Hettinger and Muller (26) reported that only one 6-s contraction per day was necessary to produce maximal gains in strength. The majority of isometric training

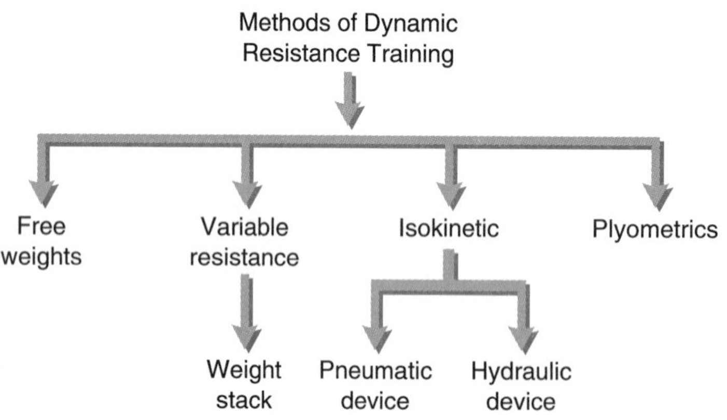

FIGURE 15.2 Examples of dynamic resistance training methods and devices.
Modified from Wilmore and Costill 1994.

Table 15.2 Guidelines for Designing Isometric Training Programs

Training goal	Intensity	Duration	Repetitions	Frequency
Strength	100% MVC[a]	3-10 s/contraction	5-10	5 days/week
Endurance	≤60% MVC	Until fatigued	1/session	5 days/week

Note. [a]Maximum voluntary contraction.
Adapted from Heyward 1991.

studies have used contractions of 3 to 10 s and a relatively small number of repetitions. The training frequency (i.e., the number of training sessions per week) needed to cause increases in isometric strength gains has also been examined. To bring about increases in maximal strength the optimal isometric program should consist of maximal isometric contractions performed on a daily basis (26). To develop muscle endurance with isometric training, the effort of muscle contraction should be 60% of maximal voluntary contraction or less performed daily.

The static nature of an isometric-type muscle contraction may lead to breath holding (called the **Valsalva maneuver)** that reduces venous return to the heart and causes an increase in systolic and diastolic blood pressures. Therefore, the Valsalva maneuver should be avoided, especially by individuals with cardiovascular problems; and a regular breathing pattern (exhale while lifting, inhale while lowering) should be established for all types of resistance training programs.

Dynamic Training Methods

Dynamic methods of resistance training involve a shortening of the muscle with the joint moving through a full range of motion. Modes include **constant resistance** (free weights), **variable resistance**, isokinetic devices, and plyometrics (see figure 15.2). Circuit training is another form of dynamic resistance training that is becoming increasingly popular.

Constant Resistance (Free Weights)

With free weights, such as barbells and dumbbells, the resistance or weight lifted remains constant throughout the dynamic range of motion (44). An example of dynamic exercise with a constant resistance is the arm curl using dumbbells; the dumbbell's weight is constant, although the lifter's leverage varies during the exercise and she or he can notice some points in the range of motion that seem to be easier as well as some that seem to be harder. At the easier points, the muscles are not required to contract to their maximum, in part because of the lifter's leverage or mechanical advantage; however, the lifter often elects to accelerate the movement at these points (33). Figure 15.3 shows how strength varies throughout the range of motion when using free weights (constant resistance).

Variable Resistance

To overcome the limitation of the constant-resistance exercise mode, mechanical devices have been designed that vary the resistance throughout the range of motion. For variable resistance training equipment, there is a moving connection (e.g., a cam) between the resistance and the point of force application. As the weight is lifted, the variable-resistance

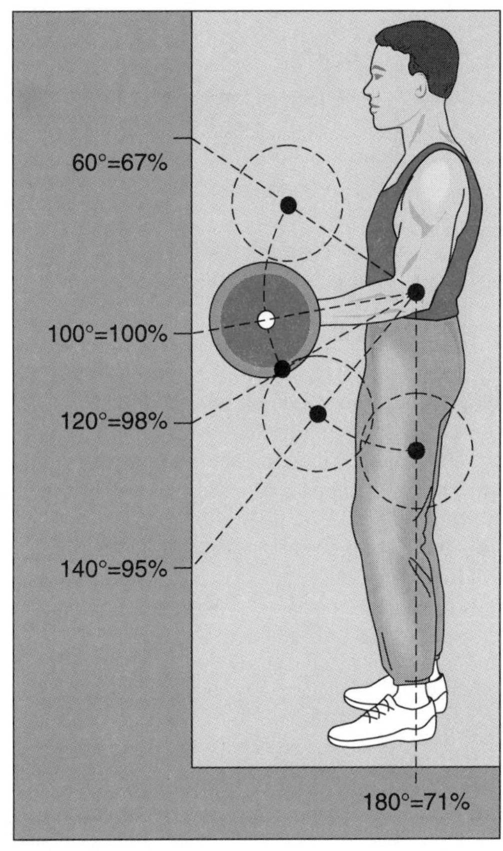

FIGURE 15.3 Variation in strength relative to the angle of the elbow flexors during the two-arm curl. Strength is optimized at an angle of 100°.
Reprinted from Wilmore and Costill 1994.

> Valsalva maneuver — Increased pressure in the abdominal and thoracic cavities caused by breath holding and extreme effort.
>
> constant resistance — A load that remains the same throughout a complete range of motion during a muscle contraction.
>
> variable resistance — A condition in which the intensity of the load varies as the angle of the joint changes throughout the range of motion.

mode of exercise attempts to match the force capability of the skeletal lever system throughout the range of motion by use of the **cam** device (see figure 15.4). Variable resistance machines are available for many of the skeletal muscle groups (e.g., pectoralis major, quadricps femoris).

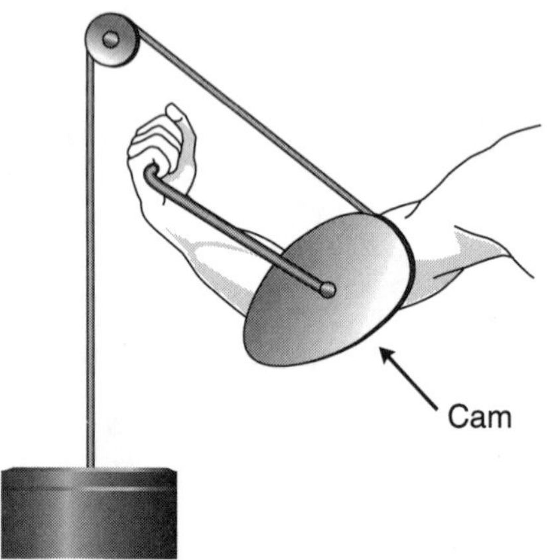

FIGURE 15.4 Illustration of a variable resistance device developing strength in the biceps muscle group in which a cam alters the resistance through the range of motion. The odd-shaped cam compensates for the variations in muscular tension at different joint angles. It does this by changing the lever arm of the machine so that the load varies accordingly. This variation in load provides for maximal or at least near maximal muscular tension throughout the full range of motion.
Modified from Wathen and Roll 1994.

Circuit Training

Another dynamic resistance training program termed **circuit training** is becoming increasingly popular. Circuit training programs are designed to increase muscle strength, endurance, and power (23) and usually consist of 6 to 15 stations per circuit (see figure 15.5).

The circuit should be repeated two to three times so that the total number of minutes of continuous exercise is 20 to 30 min. Each exercise station should consist of a load that fatigues the muscle within approximately 30 s. The exerciser should rest for a period of 15 s between each station. Circuit training programs are usually done 3 days per week, and the gains in strength and endurance compare favorably with those of other dynamic weight training programs (45).

Principles of Dynamic Resistance Training

One of the first dynamic constant resistance training programs was advocated by DeLorme and Watkins (17). In setting forth their method of training for strength development, they first established the idea of the **repetition maximum** (RM). A repetition maximum is the maximal load that a muscle group can lift over a given number of repetitions before fatiguing. A 1-RM is the greatest weight that can be lifted once, using correct form. In general for every reduction of 2.5% of your 1-RM, you can probably do one more repetition. So if your 1-RM is 100 lb, and you want to do 10 repetitions, multiply 10 by 2.5% of your 1-RM. The result is 25 lb (25% of 100 lb). So if you drop 25 lb from your 1-RM of 100 lb, you should be able to lift 75 lb for 10 repetitions (37).

In DeLorme and Watkins' (17) program they used a 10-repetition maximum (10-RM, i.e., the maximal load that can be lifted over 10 repetitions). For each muscle group to be trained, the exercise program consisted of a total of 30 repetitions per training session divided into 3 sets of 10 repetitions each as follows (34):

- Set 1 = 10 repetitions at a load of 1/2 10-RM
- Set 2 = 10 repetitions at a load of 3/4 10-RM
- Set 3 = 10 repetitions at a load of 10-RM

A set is the number of repetitions performed consecutively without resting (in this case, 1 set = 10 repetitions [34]). In the 1960s much research was conducted to determine the optimum number of sets and repetitions/set to develop strength (8) and muscular endurance (12,13) using dynamic resistance training. Table 15.3 presents general guidelines for the exercise intensity, sets, repetitions, and frequency used in developing strength and endurance through dynamic constant/variable resistance training. The results of the research suggest that significant gains in strength can be achieved using a training frequency of 3 to 5 days per week with 3 sets of 6- to 10-RM. While the training frequency is important to maximal strength gains, the research studies do not show any difference between 5- and 3-day training sessions (6). For increased gains in muscular endurance the program should be of lower intensity with higher repetitions. For example a program emphasizing gains in muscle endurance may consist of 3 sets working at 50% of your 1-RM for 30 repetitions.

Advantages of dynamic constant/variable resistance training include the ability to train the muscles through a complete range of motion while providing visual feedback. Disadvantages of this type of training mode include the equipment cost (quite expensive), the space required (can be relatively large), and convenience (varying constant resistance

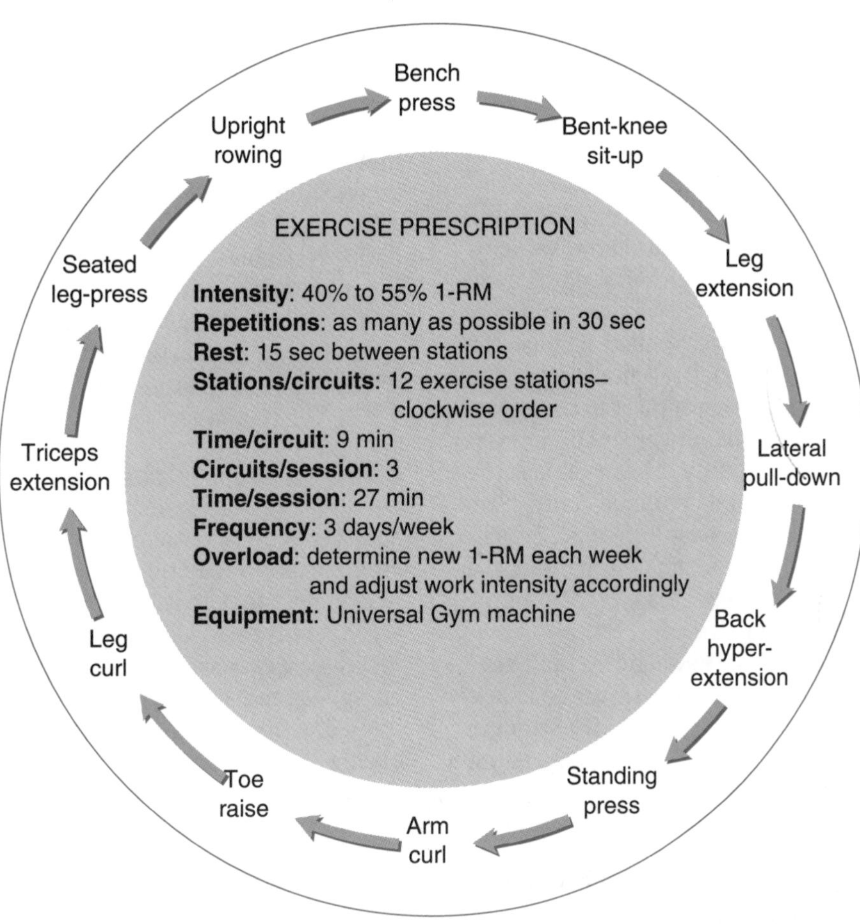

FIGURE 15.5 Sample circuit weight training program.
Adapted from Heyward 1991.

Table 15.3 Guidelines for Designing Constant and Variable Resistance Training Programs

Training goal	Sets	Intensity	Repetitions	Frequency
Strength	3	6-RM or 85% 1-RM	6-10	3-5 days/week
Endurance	3	15-RM or 60% 1-RM	15 or >	3-5 days/week

Note. RM = repetition maximum.
Adapted from Heyward 1991.

cam— A mechanical device that varies resistance throughout the range of motion during muscle contraction.

circuit training— A sequence of different exercises done one after the other in the same workout.

repetition maximum— The maximal load that a muscle group can lift over a given number of repetitions before fatiguing.

exercises [e.g., bench press with free weights] often require a partner for safety).

Isokinetic Training

The term **isokinetic** refers to a muscular contraction performed at a constant angular limb velocity. Unlike other types of resistance training, there is no set resistance to meet; rather, the velocity of movement is controlled. Any force applied against the equipment results in an equal reaction force. The reaction force mirrors the force applied to the equipment throughout the range of movement of an exercise, making it theoretically possible for the muscle(s) to exert a continual, maximal contraction (19). Because isokinetic exercise offers accommodating resistance that is maximal throughout the range of motion, some believe this type of training leads to optimal strength gains.

Two questions inherent to isokinetic training have yet escaped unequivocal answers: What is the optimal training speed—fast or slow? Do strength increases obtained at a particular training speed carry over to speeds above and below it (19)? Although several studies have investigated the first of the two questions, no conclusive answer to the question has been obtained. Moffroid and Whipple (36) reported that gains in peak torque with fast-speed training ($108° \cdot s^{-1}$) was superior to slow-speed training ($36° \cdot s^{-1}$). However, two other studies have shown that slow-speed training produces greater gains in peak torque than fast-speed training (22, 38). Furthermore, other research suggests that there is no evidence to favor either slow or fast speeds when considering gains in peak torque (29). While it is not clear as to what velocity should be used in isokinetic strength training, speeds from 24 to $180° \cdot s^{-1}$ have been recommended (27). The second question concerns whether increases in peak torque carry over to velocities different from the training velocity. Studies indicate that fast-velocity training (108 to $239° \cdot s^{-1}$) causes significant increases in torque below the training velocity (9, 36).

Table 15.4 presents the recommended training intensity, sets, repetitions, and frequency for isokinetic training to increase strength and endurance. Advantages of isokinetic training include accommodating resistance that offers maximal effort throughout a full range of joint motion and visual feedback of the performance. The major disadvantage of isokinetic training is the cost of equipment, making this training method less available than others.

Plyometric Training

Another type of resistance training for developing strength is plyometric training. **Plyometric** refers to exercises that enable a muscle to reach maximal force production in as short a time as possible (1). Plyometric exercises use the force of gravity to store energy in the muscles. This energy is then used immediately in an opposite reaction, so the natural elastic properties of the muscle produce kinetic energy (3). Jumping from a 3-ft stool to the ground and immediately springing back up to another stool is an example of plyometric training for increasing leg strength. This type of training uses the stretch reflex and the accompanying stretch-shortening cycle to elicit more powerful concentric contractions (43). Research indicates that the faster a muscle is stretched with rapid eccentric loading, the more powerful its concentric contraction becomes (18). Due to the high intensity of plyometric training, it should be used only 1 to 3 days/week for 15 to 20 min per session. Because of the potential for muscle injury with this type of training, however, it is not recommended for programs focusing on increasing muscular fitness for general health. Plyometric training sessions should be supervised by individuals with experience in plyometric training.

Table 15.4 Guidelines for Designing Isokinetic Training Programs

Training goal	Sets	Intensity	Repetitions	Contracting speed	Frequency
Strength	3	Maximum contraction	2-15	$24\text{-}180° \cdot s^{-1}$	3-5 days/week
Endurance	1	Maximum contraction	Until fatigued	$\geq 180° \cdot s^{-1}$	3-5 days/week

Adapted from Heyward 1991.

3 **In Review:** Resistance training to increase muscle strength and endurance can use isometric (static) or dynamic methods of training. Dynamic methods of resistance training include the use of constant resistance, variable resistance, circuit training, isokinetic devices, and plyometrics. Isometric training effects are limited to the joint angle at which the training occurred. Constant resistance programs use free weights with movements taken throughout a joint's range of motion. Variable resistance programs use special equipment to alter the resistance throughout a range of motion. Circuit training programs are designed to increase muscle strength, endurance, and power (23) and usually consist of 6 to 15 exercise stations per circuit. Isokinetic training occurs at a constant limb velocity, with maximal force exerted throughout the joint's range of motion. Plyometric training places a muscle in a stretched position (eccentric contraction) prior to a concentric contraction; injury potential is high with this type of training.

COMPARING WEIGHT TRAINING METHODS

Isometric (static) and dynamic resistance training all cause gains in muscle strength and endurance. Because the amount of work performed varies among the methods of training, however, it is difficult to compare training methods and determine the most efficient method to develop strength and endurance. Table 15.5 presents the advantages and disadvantages of isokinetic, static, dynamic constant (free weights), and variable resistance training methods.

Static Versus Dynamic Training

Although the comparisons of strength gains between isometric training and dynamic training are difficult to make due to test specificity, a review of the literature suggests that the better-quality dynamic resistance programs are more effective than the standard isometric programs for increasing strength (4). In contrasting static and dynamic training Clarke (12) reported the following:

1. Dynamic training is preferable to isometric training because dynamic training tends to be

Table 15.5 Advantages and Disadvantages of Varying Resistance Training Methods

	Comparative rating			
Criterion	Isokinetic	Static	Free weights	Variable resistance
Rate of strength gain	Excellent	Poor	Good	Good
Rate of endurance gain	Excellent	Poor	Good	Good
Strength gain over range of motion	Excellent	Poor	Good	Good
Time per training session	Good	Excellent	Poor	Poor
Expense	Poor	Excellent	Fair	Fair
Ease of performance	Good	Excellent	Fair	Good
Ease of progression assessment	Poor	Good	Good	Good
Adaptability to specific movement patterns	Excellent	Poor	Good	Good
Least possibility of muscle sorness	Excellent	Good	Poor	Poor
Least possibility of injury	Excellent	Good	Poor	Poor
Skill improvement	Excellent	Poor	Good	Good

Adapted from Lamb 1984.

isokinetic — A muscular contraction performed at a constant angular limb velocity.

plyometric — Training method in which a muscle is suddenly stretched (eccentric contraction) prior to a maximal concentric contraction.

superior for the development of strength and endurance.
2. Motivation is generally superior with dynamic training because of the visual feedback when one achieves a weight lifting goal.
3. Static training may be effective in developing strength and endurance with simpler equipment in contrast to dynamic training, and no partner is needed for safety purposes in spotting.

Dynamic Constant/Variable Resistance Training Versus Isokinetic Training

Isokinetic-type training combines dynamic full range of motion with the exertion of maximal force. Therefore, one might speculate that isokinetic training is superior to other forms of dynamic (constant resistance, variable resistance) training in developing muscular strength and endurance. Studies comparing traditional methods of training with isokinetic training are limited, but peak force gains of 47%, 29%, and 13% for isokinetic, dynamic, and isometric training methods, respectively have been reported (42). However, before we can conclude that isokinetic training is superior, more research is needed.

4 **In Review: Dynamic resistance training is more effective in developing muscle strength and endurance in comparison to static training, although static training is less expensive and does not require partner work. There is not enough data to conclude that dynamic isokinetic training is superior in causing strength gains in comparison to dynamic methods of constant and variable resistance training.**

SYSTEMS OF RESISTANCE TRAINING

Most resistance training systems were originally designed by individuals who were experienced in resistance training (power lifters, body builders). Many resistance training systems have become popular not due to scientific research but rather to the popular belief of the practitioners concerning gains in muscle strength and size. Certainly more research is needed regarding all types of training systems. Three of the most common training systems used in resistance training include:

- Super set system
- Pyramid system
- Split routine system

Super Set System

A **super set** requires the performance of two exercises in a sequence, followed by a rest interval. A super set exercises one muscle group to fatigue and then immediately works the antagonistic group to fatigue. For example, you might do a set of biceps curls followed immediately by a triceps exercise. Another example of a super set exercise would be the leg extension (quadriceps) followed by a leg curl (hamstring). Super sets are usually used with one-joint exercises (37) with a short rest between sets.

Pyramid System

The **pyramid** system is used by many weight lifters interested in strength gains. In the pyramid system the first set is started with a light load, perhaps 10-RM. The resistance is progressively increased over several sets so that fewer and fewer repetitions can be performed until only 1-RM can be performed. This should be followed by 4 or 6 repetitions with a lighter weight to cool down. In contrast, the pyramid system may start the first set with a heavy load (1-RM), and then with each following set the load is decreased with increased repetitions (reverse pyramid system). In resistance training using the reverse pyramid system, an adequate warm-up is crucial prior to starting the first set with a heavy load. Figure 15.6 illustrates the concept of the pyramid system.

Split Routine

In a **split routine** system different body parts are trained on alternate days. A typical split routine system entails training the arms, legs, and abdomen on Monday, Wednesday, and Friday and the chest, shoulders, and back on Tuesday, Thursday, and Saturday. This system requires training to be done 6 days per week. However, the training intensity can be maintained at a higher level when compared to training programs involving all muscle groups in a single session done 3 or 4 times per week.

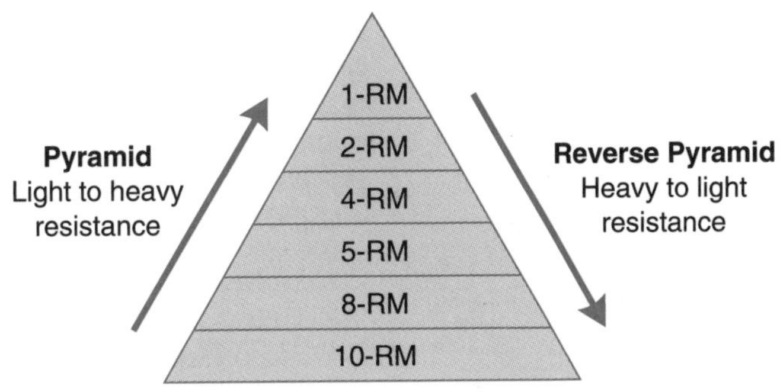

FIGURE 15.6 A light-to-heavy, or ascending, pyramid system consists of performing sets progressing from light to heavy resistance. In a heavy-to-light, or reverse, pyramid system, sets are performed starting with heavy and progressing to light resistance.
Modified from Fleck and Kraemer 1987.

5 **In Review: Three of the most common training systems used in resistance training to increase strength are the super set system, the pyramid system, and the split routine system. The super set system consists of exercising muscle groups in opposition to each other. The pyramid system starts with a light resistance, and, as the sets increase, so does the resistance until 1-RM is achieved. Conversely, the reverse pyramid system starts the first set using a heavy resistance and then progressively decreases the resistance with increased repetitions. The split routine system emphasizes training different body parts on alternate days of the week. This system requires 6 days of training per week.**

WEIGHT TRAINING AND BONE MINERAL DENSITY

Osteoporosis is a disease characterized by an increased loss of bone mass. When bone density is compromised, the bones become weaker and are at an increased risk of fractures. It has been projected that over 5 million fractures of the hip, spine, and wrist will occur in women over the age of 45 and will account for more than $45 billion in direct health care costs over the next 10 years (11). Of course, when men who are at risk of osteoporosis are included, the magnitude of this health care issue becomes even larger.

Physical activity has been proposed as one strategy to reduce fractures by increasing bone mass and by preventing falls through improved functional ability. Cross-sectional studies show that athletes, especially those who are strength trained, have greater bone mineral densities than nonathletes (10). Participation in load-bearing physical activity that increases muscle strength may prove to be beneficial to bone mass. A few longitudinal studies have been performed using resistance exercise as the stimulus for new bone formation. These studies report variable results, with some studies showing gains in bone mineral density (16) and others showing little or no changes consequent to training (24). A summary of the exercise variables common to the training program of athletic populations found to have high bone mineral density values is presented in table 15.6. This table is intended to be a guideline for designing resistance exercise programs to promote increases in bone mass.

Until further studies are performed, the guidelines described in table 15.6 must be viewed as preliminary because they arise from the observation of the strong correlation between muscular strength and

super set — The condition of exercising one muscle group to fatigue, then immediately exercising the opposing muscle group to fatigue.

pyramid set — A mode of resistance training in which the load is either increased or decreased following each set of repetitions.

split routine — A mode of resistance training in which varying muscle groups are exercised on alternate days.

Table 15.6 Recommended Resistance Training Program for Stimulating Bone Growth, Based Upon the Training Regime of Athletes Who Demonstrate Increased Bone Density

Variables	Exercise recommendations
Exercise intensity	1- to 10-RM
Exercise sets	3-6
Repetitions/set	10
Exercise selection	Bench press, shoulder press, squats, deadlifts
Exercise goal	Muscle strength and size

Modified from Conroy and Earle 1994.

bone mineral density, rather than from a documented cause-and-effect relationship (14).

In Review: Osteoporosis is a disease characterized by bone loss that increases the risk of bone fractures. There is some evidence that load-bearing physical activity such as resistance training can attenuate and possibly prevent the loss in bone mass (see table 15.6 for program recommendations).

TRAINING MAINTENANCE AND OVERTRAINING

Most research studies indicate that three training sessions per muscle group per week is the minimum frequency that causes maximum gains in strength. Once the strength training goal has been achieved, can an individual discontinue or decrease the training program and maintain her or his strength gains? In the absence of training, the muscles gradually become smaller and weaker. However, once the strength goal is reached, the program of training can be reduced to one or two brief workouts per week and sufficient strength will be maintained.

Some individuals become obsessed with training and work at levels to which the body cannot adapt. This is called **overtraining** and is often referred to as "staleness." Overtraining may be defined as excessive volume or intensity of training, or both, resulting in chronic fatigue. Yet because fatigue is experienced naturally with training, how do we identify overtraining? The first sign of overtraining is characterized by a sudden decline in performance that cannot be remedied by a few days of rest and dietary manipulation (10). The overtraining syndrome can manifest itself in both physical and psychological symptoms. Physical symptoms of overtraining include the following:

- Decreased body weight
- Decreased appetite
- Sleep disturbances
- Elevated resting heart rate
- Elevated resting blood pressure
- Muscle tenderness
- Nausea

Unfortunately, these physical symptoms can be highly individualized thus making it relatively difficult to identify overtraining.

The psychological response to overtraining may be characterized by mood disturbances. The symptoms may include decreased motivation, confidence, and concentration and raised levels of tension, depression, anger, fatigue, anxiety, and irritability. Often the psychological symptoms of overtraining are observed before the physical symptoms (31).

In Review: Three-day per week resistance training programs to increase strength can be reduced to one or two brief workouts per week to maintain strength gains. Overtraining is characterized by a decline in performance that cannot be remedied by a few days of rest. Overtraining can manifest itself in both physical and psychological symptoms. Often the psychological symptoms of overtraining are observed before the physical symptoms.

EXERCISE WARM-UP AND COOL-DOWN

Warming up prior to moderate- and high-intensity physical activity is a general recommendation in exercise training programs. **Warm-up** refers to exercise conducted prior to a performance or workout session, whether or not muscle or body temperature is elevated (40). Warm-ups are generally classified under one of two categories, though overlap often exists between these categories (35):

1. General warm-up—Examples of this type of warm-up include calisthenics, stretching, jogging, and so forth that are unrelated to the

specific neuromuscular actions of the exercise (review chapters 13 and 16 for stretching techniques).

2. Specific warm-up—This type of preliminary exercise "rehearses" the actual mode of exercise used in the workout. Performing low-resistance lifts on the bench press machine is an example of a specific warm-up for the actual maximal effort used in a workout.

The theoretical benefits of warm-up are separated into physiological, psychological, and safety-related (40). Physiological benefits include faster enzymatic reactions at higher body temperatures. This may alter metabolism to favor less lactate production and, consequently, less fatigue. The warm-up procedures can increase arousal, which is good up to a point, and provide the optimal "mental set" for improved performance (40). Often warm-up has been stressed in training rooms as a practice to prevent injuries. Franks (21) concluded in a review, however, that there is little evidence that warm-up prevents injuries. On the other hand, there is evidence that warm-up prior to high-intensity exercise increases cardiovascular blood flow and increases the heart's adaptive response to stress (5).

The **cool-down** is a brief period of low-intensity exercise following the workout. Immediately after moderate- and high-intensity work, blood tends to pool in the lower extremities. With the pooling of blood, there is a decrease in the volume of blood returning to the heart (decreased cardiac output), and symptoms such as lightheadedness and dizziness may appear. Because muscle movements help return blood back to the heart, it is important to continue some form of low-intensity exercise following the workout. While the muscles are still at or higher than normal body temperature following a workout, stretching exercises can be done to improve or maintain a joint's range of motion (see chapter 16).

8 **In Review: A warm-up period should precede the formal workout to increase body temperature and vascular blood flow. These changes enhance the metabolic and cardiovascular responses to high-intensity exercise. A cool-down period consisting of low-intensity exercise should follow the workout to maintain an adequate return of blood back to the heart. This will prevent the possible symptoms of lightheadedness and dizziness after the exercise session.**

WEIGHT TRAINING SAFETY TIPS

It is a good idea to have a medical clearance before starting a new exercise program. The medical clearance becomes more important as factors such as age and risk factors increase. The following are recommended safety guidelines for weight training:

- Warm up before exercise.
- Cool down after exercise.
- Wear clothing that allows freedom of movement.
- Avoid collision with other lifters and spotters.
- Use collars on plate-loading equipment such as dumbbells.
- Perform lifts using strict exercise form and control the speed of movement.
- Do not hold your breath during a lift.
- Do not bounce weights off your body. If you must bounce the weight this means the load is too heavy.
- Do not perform lifts in which you could be trapped under the weight without a spotter.
- Always use a load that is within your means to lift.
- Make sure you are in a stable and controlled position before the lift.

9 **In Review: Safety precautions should be practiced during exercise training. This may include a medical clearance prior to the exercise program and following safety precautions in the exercise room (see list above).**

overtraining — A condition in which the training (intensity, duration, frequency) is so great that it results in chronic fatigue and a consequent decrease in physical performance.

warm-up — Physical activity of light to moderate intensity prior to a workout.

cool-down — A period of light activity following moderate to heavy exercise. The cool-down period is important because it allows the leg muscles to continue to pump blood back to the heart, whereas stopping immediately after exercise causes pooling of the blood in the legs and a lack of venous return.

EXERCISE PRESCRIPTION OVERVIEW FOR WEIGHT TRAINING

For general fitness the weight training program should focus on developing the entire body as opposed to focusing on one select body part. One exercise per body part is adequate for beginning weight training. The weight training workout should start with the largest muscles first (e.g., chest/back) and proceed to the smaller muscle groups (e.g., biceps, triceps). The large muscles need more energy and often depend on the small muscles for assistance. If the small muscles are fatigued, the participant might have difficulty in performing the large-muscle exercises properly.

A warm-up and cool-down period should be carried out before and after the workout. At the beginning of the weight training program, the load should be light so the exercise can be performed easily throughout the entire range of motion to help prevent muscle soreness. As the training period progresses, the load should be increased gradually.

The weight training program should consider the appropriate exercise intensity, repetitions, sets, frequency, and rest intervals. Resistance training to develop primarily strength should use between 1- to 5-RM per set; training to develop primarily strength and muscle size should use between 6- to 12-RM per set; and training to develop local muscle endurance should use between 20 to 50 repetitions at 60% 1-RM or less per set. The exercise sets performed during each training session also depend on the training goal (keeping in mind the RM per set). For strength training the selected set of repetitions should be 4 to 8 sets/session. Weight training programs for increasing muscle strength and size should repeat the selected training load and repetitions for 3 to 6 sets/session. For developing muscular endurance the selected load and repetitions should be performed using 2 to 4 sets/session. Between each set of repetitions performed, the exerciser should rest. The following rest period between sets of repetitions is recommended for the specific training goals:

Training Goal	*Rest Interval Between Sets*
Strength	*2 to 4 min*
Muscle size	*1 to 2 min*
Muscle endurance	*30 to 90 s*

Skeletal muscle usually requires 2 or 3 days of rest to recover after training. Exercising a muscle 3 days per week with 48 to 72 hr of rest between training sessions is appropriate for most beginning weight training programs. As the weight training program progresses, the training frequency may increase to 4, 5, or 6 days a week, but no muscle group should be trained every day. Once the muscle adapts to the training overload, the resistance must be gradually increased to stimulate further gains in strength and endurance (apply the principle of progressive resistance exercise). The progressive resistance program should alternately increase repetitions and resistance. For example, at the start of a program an individual may begin with a resistance that can be performed for 8 repetitions. When the individual can complete 12 repetitions, the resistance should be increased by 5% or less. It is not recommended to increase the resistance by more than 10% between successive training sessions. Table 15.7 recommends an exercise prescription for a beginning dynamic resistance training program for strength or endurance. Note that once the strength goal has been reached in the training program, the frequency of training can be reduced to 1 to 2 days per week to maintain the achieved muscle strength or endurance gains.

To help guide the training progression it is important for a participant to record the workout during each training session. Thus, the daily **training log** is the guide to successful progressive resistance exercise training such as weight lifting. Form 15.1 shows an example of a personal weight training log used in monitoring the exercise progression. The log consists of recording the training week, repetitions, weight, and sets for each training session. The log also provides space for general training comments. For example, the log shows that at week 4 triceps training was done to achieve strength gains and that the individual's workout consisted of a 3-day training session, at a load of 50 lb, with 6 repetitions per set for 3 sets. A comment during the fourth week of training was that slight muscle soreness was experienced in the middle portion of the triceps.

10 **In Review: Training frequency of 3 days per week with a day of rest between training sessions is appropriate for the beginning weight training program. Training goals to primarily increase muscle strength, muscle size and strength, and**

training log— A daily plan monitoring the training frequency, intensity, and sets performed.

FORM 15.1

Weekly 3 to 5 Day Weight Training Log

Name John Doe	**Day 1**			**Day 2**			**Day 3**			**Day 4**			**Day 5**			**Training goal**
Week of training 4th	Wt	Rep	Set	Wt	Rep	Set	Wt	Rep	Set	Wt	Rep	Set	Wt	Rep	Set	Comments
Triceps extension	50	6	3				50	6	3				50	6	3	Slight soreness in midportion of triceps
Biceps curl	55	6	3				55	6	3				55	6	3	
Abdominal curl	No wt	35	3				No wt	35	3				No wt	35	3	
Leg extension	180	6	3				180	6	3				180	6	3	
Leg curl	100	6	3				100	6	3				100	6	3	
Lat pulldown	60	6	3				60	6	3				60	6	3	
Chest press	90	6	3				90	6	3				90	6	3	
Back extension	45	6	3				45	6	3				45	6	3	

Wt = weight
Rep = repetitions

Table 15.7 Suggested Exercise Prescription for Beginning Dynamic Resistance Training Program to Develop Muscle Strength and Endurance for General Health

Training goal: Muscle strength				
Weeks	Frequency	Sets	Repetitions	Resistance
1-3	2 days/week	2/session	6-10/set	12-RM
4-20	3 days/week	3/session	6-10/set	6-RM
20+ (maintenance)	1-2 days/week	3/session	6-10/set	6-RM
Training goal: Muscle endurance				
Weeks	Frequency	Sets	Repetitions	Resistance
1-3	2 days/week	2/session	15/set	40% 1-RM
4-20	3 days/week	3/session	15+/set	60% 1-RM
20+ (maintenance)	1-2 days/week	3/session	15+/set	60% 1-RM

Note. RM = repetition maximum.

endurance vary in the training intensity, sets, repetitions, and rest intervals, respectively. At the beginning of the training program the level of resistance should be such that approximately 8 repetitions/set can be performed. As the muscle adapts, the resistance must be progressively increased. A training log to monitor the training progression is essential for a successful progressive resistance training program.

After determining the goal of the weight training program and the exercise prescription, the appendix to this chapter can be used for selecting exercises to develop the major muscle groups.

Case Studies

You can check your answers by referring to appendix A.

15.1

You are giving a tour of a new weight training club and are to provide basic information on both free weights and the variable resistance machines as far as strength gains, ease of use, safety, and so on. Provide an outline of your remarks.

15.2

Summarize the basics of a workout routine aimed at improving muscle strength compared to muscle endurance.

Source List

1. Allerheiligen (1994)
2. Andersen (1975)
3. Asmussen & Bonde-Peterson (1974)
4. Atha (1981)
5. Barnard, Gardner, Diaco, MaCalpin, & Kattus (1973)
6. Barnham (1960)
7. Bassett (1994)
8. Berger & Hardage (1967)
9. Caiozzo, Perrine, & Edgerton (1981)
10. Chilibeck, Sale, & Webber (1995)
11. Chrischilles, Sherman, & Wallace (1994)
12. D. Clarke (1973)
13. H. Clarke (1974)
14. Conroy & Earle (1994)
15. Costill et al. (1976)
16. Dalsky et al. (1988)
17. DeLorme & Watkins (1948)
18. Desmedt & Godaux (1977)
19. Fleck & Kraemer (1987)
20. Fleck & Schutt (1985)
21. Franks (1983)
22. Gettman, Ayres, Pollock, & Jackson (1978)
23. Gettman & Pollock (1981)
24. Gleeson, Protas, LeBlanc, Schneider, & Evans (1990)
25. Hermansen & Watchtlova (1971)
26. Hettinger & Muller (1953)
27. Heyward (1991)
28. Inger (1979)
29. Katch, Pechar, Pardew, & Smith (1975)
30. Knapik, Mawdsley, & Ramos (1983)

31. Kramer (1994)
32. Lamb (1984)
33. Liemohn & Sharpe (1992)
34. Mathews & Fox (1976)
35. McArdle, Katch, & Katch (1996)
36. Moffroid & Whipple (1970)
37. O'Connor, Simmons, & O'Shea (1989)
38. Oteghen (1975)
39. Powers & Dodd (1996)
40. Powers & Howley (1994)
41. Sharp, Costill, Fink, & King (1986)
42. Thistle, Hislop, & Moffroid (1967)
43. Wathen & Roll (1994)
44. Wilmore & Costill (1994)
45. Wilmore et al. (1978)

Appendix

Resistance Training Exercises for the Upper and Lower Extremities

Upper Body

Bench Press

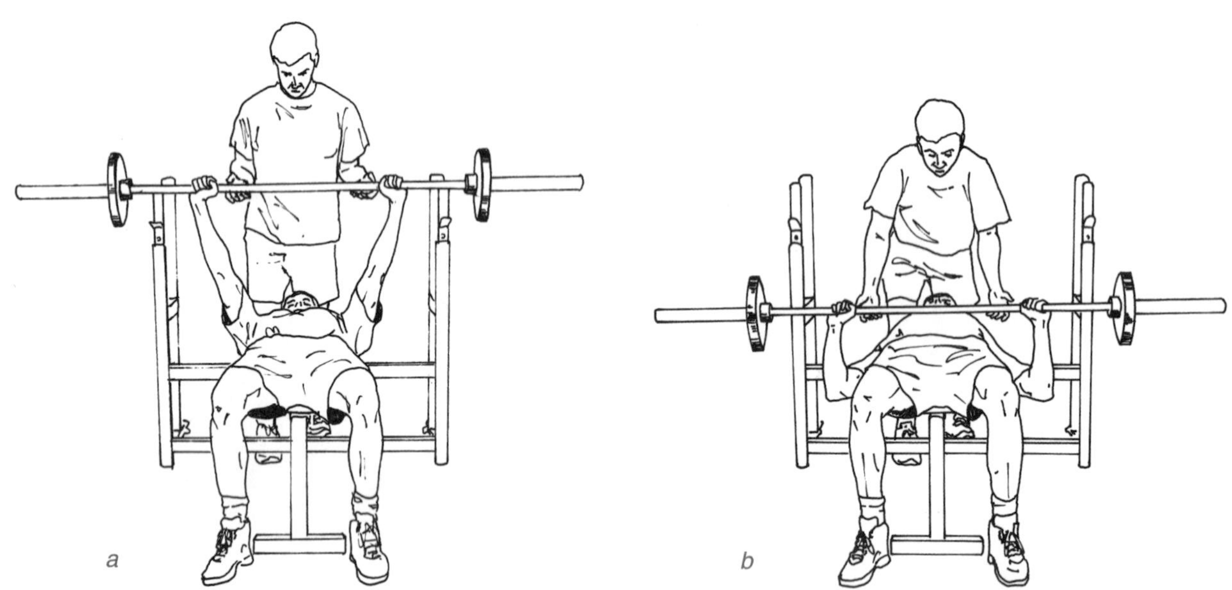

a *b*

Purpose: To develop the pectoralis major, anterior deltoid, and triceps muscles.
Directions: Lie flat on the bench; hold the weight bar directly above your shoulders, arms straight, and feet on the floor (*a*). Inhale as you lower the bar to touch the chest (*b*). Exhale as you press the weight bar back up to the starting position (*a*).

Note. Have a spotter at the head end of the bench.

Arm Curl

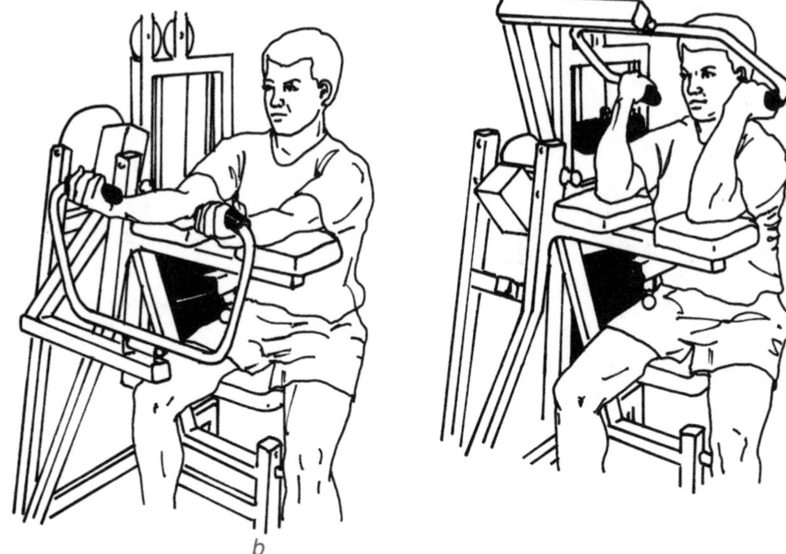

a *b*

Purpose: To develop the biceps brachii and brachioradialis muscles.
Directions: Grasp the exercise handles on the arm curl machine with a palms-up grip. With the elbows on the pads, and the arms extended (*a*), exhale as you slowly pull your arms toward your shoulders (*b*). Inhale as you slowly extend the arms and lower the weights to the starting position (*a*).

Triceps Extension

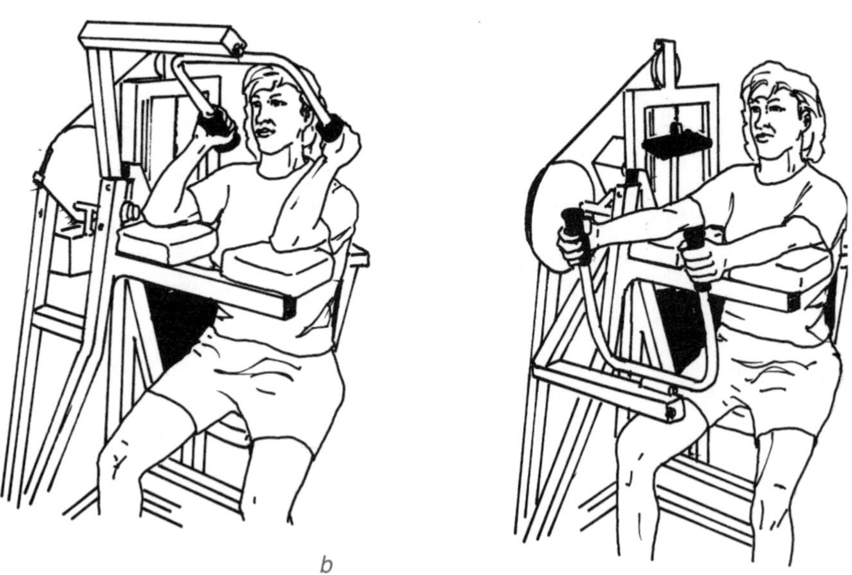

a *b*

Purpose: To develop the triceps muscles.
Directions: Grasp the exercise handles on the arm extension machine with a palms-lateral grip. Sit with the elbows bent and against the pad (*a*). With the elbows against the pads, exhale as you push out (*b*) and inhale as you slowly return the weights to the starting position (*a*).

Shoulder Shrug

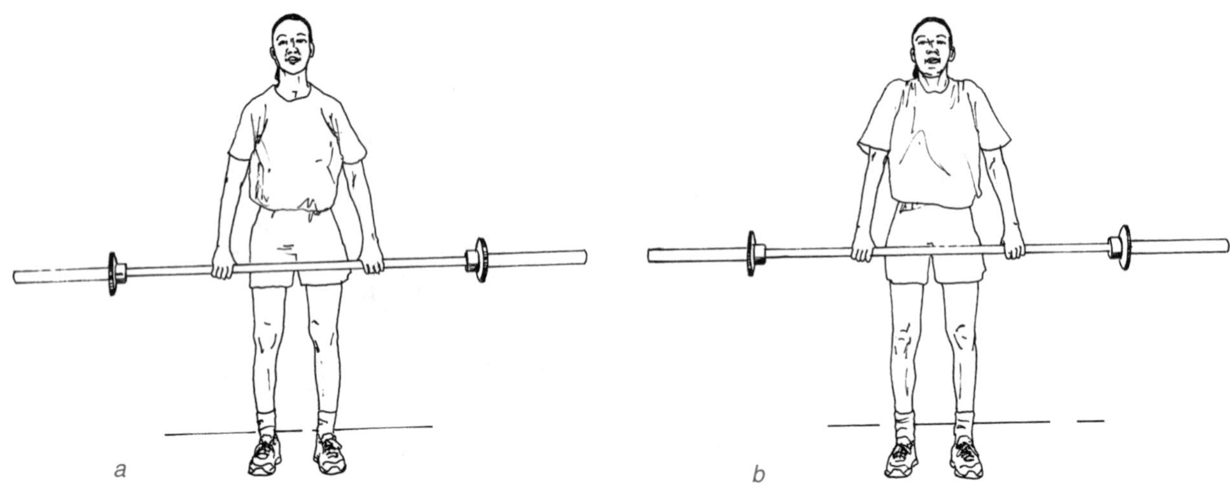

Purpose: To develop the trapezius and levator scapulae muscles.
Directions: Stand with a barbell hanging at arms length in front of your body (*a*). Inhale as you lift or shrug your shoulders to the highest upward position without bending the arms (*b*). Exhale as you slowly lower the bar to the starting position (*a*).

Abdominal Curl

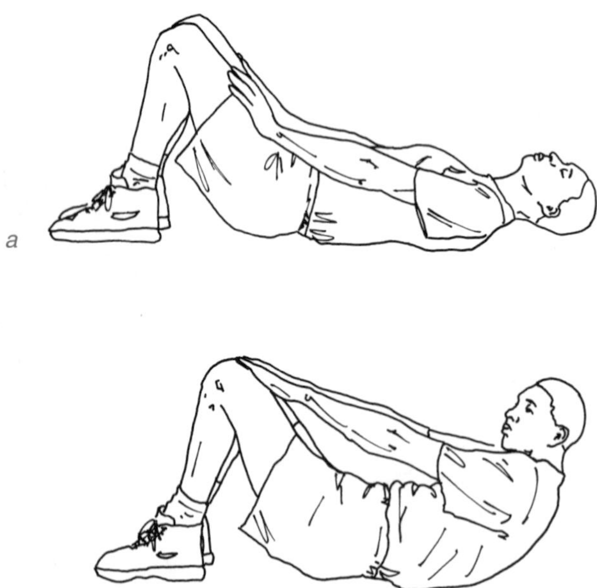

Purpose: To develop the rectus abdominis and oblique muscles.
Directions: Lie flat on your back. Bend the knees and place your feet flat on the floor. Exhale as you curl up slowly with fingers moving up to the knees (*a*). At the upper limit of this movement, hold this position for approximately 1 s (*b*). Slowly release the contraction, and inhale as you return to the starting position (*a*).

Lower Body

Leg Extension

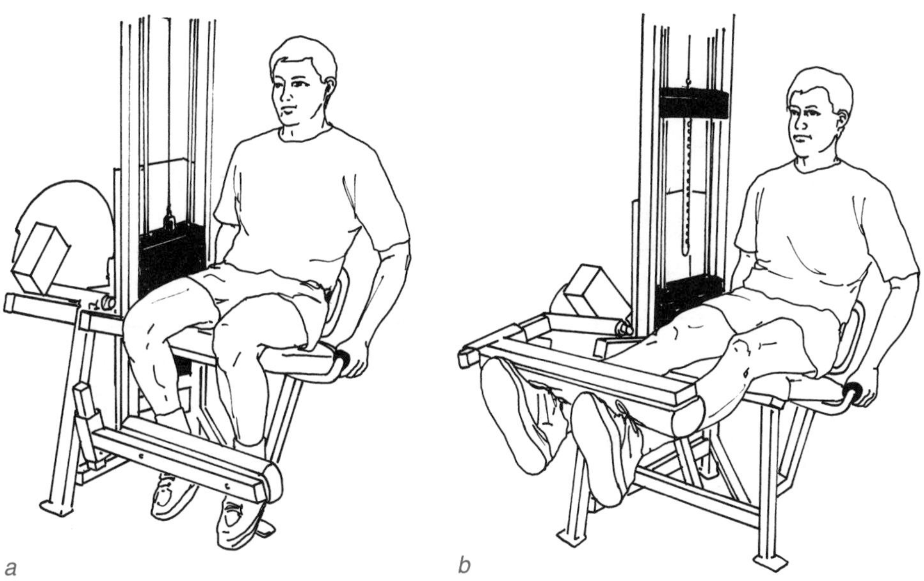

a b

Purpose: To develop the quadriceps muscle group.
Directions: In the seated position with the knees bent (*a*), exhale as you extend your legs (do not hyperextend the knees) (*b*). Inhale and allow the knees to slowly bend with the legs returning to the starting position (*a*).

Knee Flexion

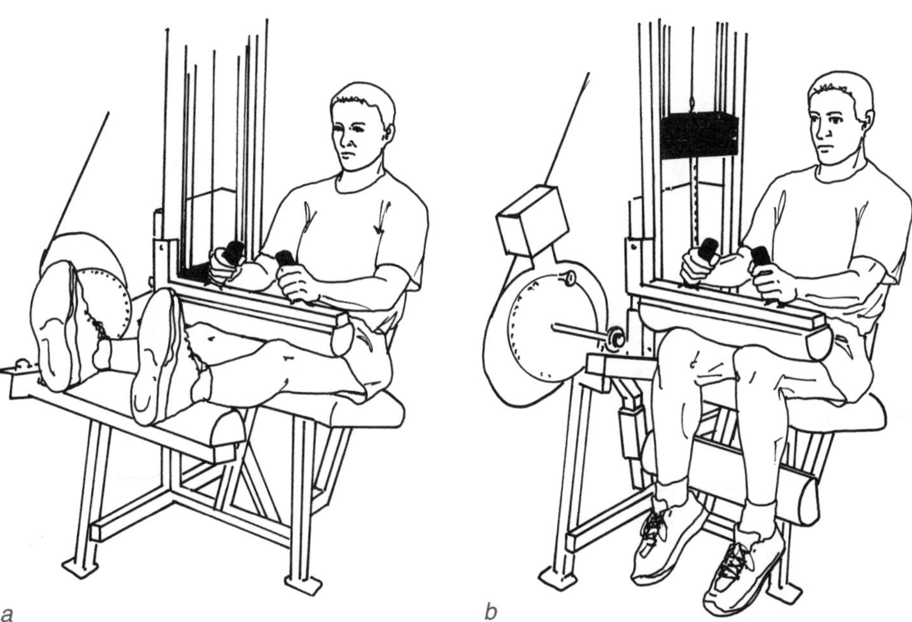

a b

Purpose: To develop the hamstring muscle group.
Directions: In the seated position with the knees extended (*a*), exhale as you bend your knees to full flexion (*b*). Inhale and allow the knees to slowly extend with the legs returning to the starting position (*a*).

CHAPTER

16

Exercise Prescription for Flexibility and Low-Back Function

Wendell Liemohn

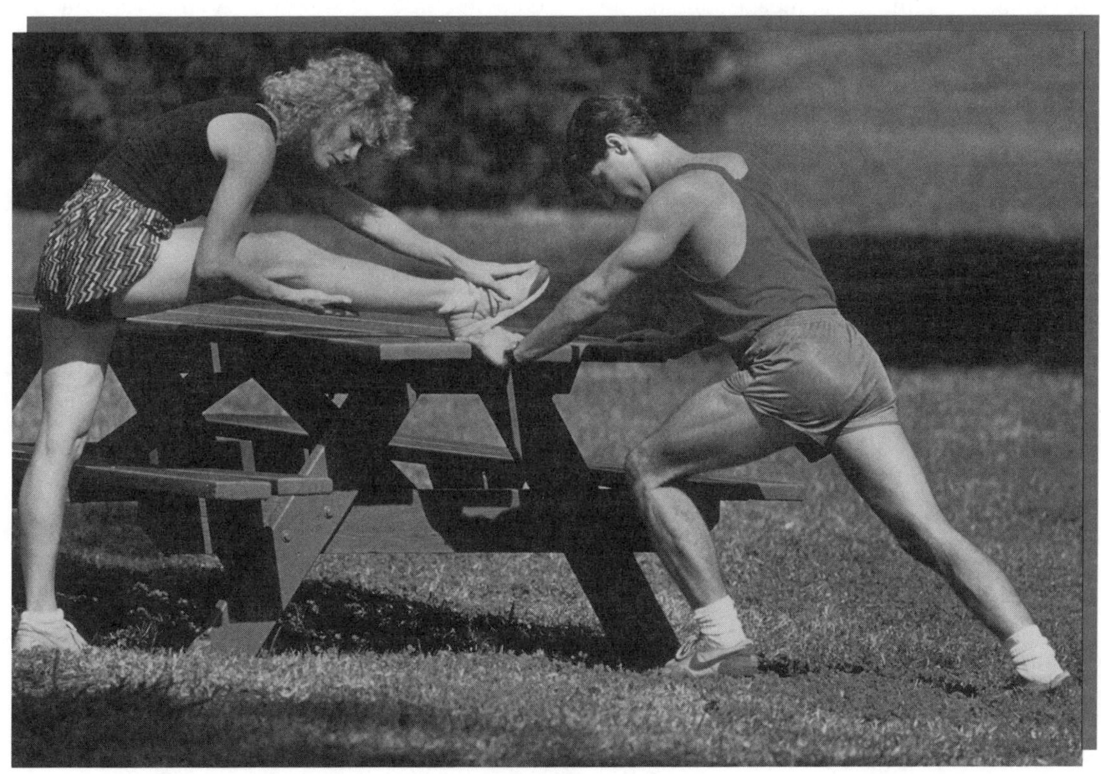

© Camerique

OBJECTIVES

The reader will be able to:

1. **Describe a motion segment, the shock absorbers of the spine, and the role of the facet joints.**
2. **Differentiate between functional and structural spinal curves and describe limitations that either may impose on exercise programs for the afflicted individual.**
3. **Explain why it is important that the muscles of the trunk should be able to control pelvic positioning.**
4. **Differentiate between the low-back problems typically seen in adults and those seen in youth.**
5. **Explain why full sit-ups should not be done.**
6. **Explain how the muscles of the trunk can work together as a dynamic corset and how they can be strengthened.**
7. **Describe how the anatomical limitations of range of motion (ROM) should be a factor as you prescribe ROM exercises for your clients.**

Low-back pain (LBP) is one of the most common complaints among adults in the United States; it accounts for more lost person-hours than any other type of occupational injury and is the most frequent cause of activity limitation in individuals under age 45. The discussion of LBP in this chapter begins with a review of select anatomical and biomechanical concepts of the trunk and spine. The types of LBP seen in adults versus those seen more often in youth are then explored. A discussion follows on potential stresses to the spine and how they can produce symptoms related to LBP. The last section describes exercises that can be used to improve flexibility and low-back function.

ANATOMY OF THE SPINE

The spine is depicted in figures 5.2 and 5.9. In our discussion of LBP the emphasis is on the five lumbar vertebrae stacked on the sacrum; the latter is also the posterior wall of the pelvis. When LBP is discussed, the fundamental unit of the lumbar spine is the **motion segment**; it consists of two vertebrae and their intervening **disc** (figure 16.1). Although the bodies of the vertebrae and their intervening disc are usually discussed, the posterior elements are sometimes neglected. The posterior elements of the vertebrae include the superior and inferior articular processes; each of their junctions is referred to as a **facet joint**. In addition to assisting in supporting loads on the spine, the facet joints control the amount and the direction of spinal movement.

A series of ligaments provide additional reinforcement for the spine; these ligaments include the anterior and posterior longitudinal ligaments running

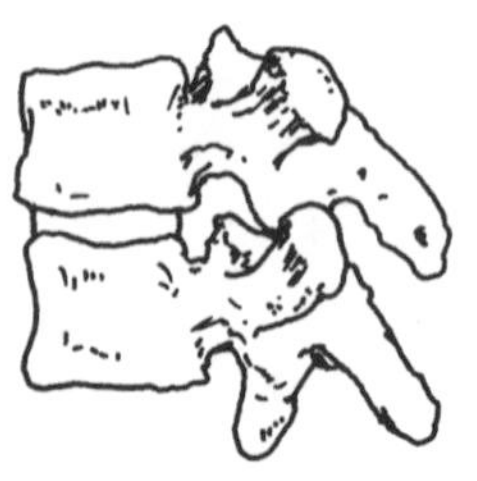

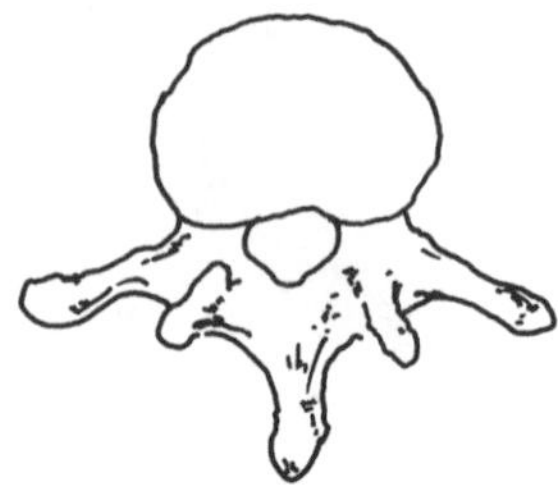

FIGURE 16.1 Lumbar vertebral motion segment. Note how the facet joint (i.e., the junction of the superior and inferior articular processes) is positioned to provide stability and control the amount and direction of movement.

the length of the spine on the bodies of the vertebrae as well as the intervertebral discs, the ligamentum flavum providing support immediately posterior to the spinal cord, the interspinous and supraspinous ligaments connecting the spinous processes, and the facet joint ligaments that span the synovial joints formed by the superior and inferior articular processes. These ligaments have pain receptors; therefore, a sprain to any of them could signal a potential back problem.

The discs enable the spine to be more mobile (figure 16.2). Each intervertebral disc consists of a centrally placed nucleus (nucleus pulposus) surrounded by a sheath of connective tissue fibers (annulus fibrosis); a disc is somewhat analogous to a jelly donut (the disc's nucleus and periphery, respectively). Intervertebral discs act as spacers and shock absorbers; when compressive forces are placed on the spine (e.g., carrying a load), the nucleus of the disc exerts pressure in all directions to help absorb the force. The disc most vulnerable to injury is the one between the fifth lumbar vertebra and the sacrum (i.e., L5–S1 disc); the next most often injured disc is the one between L4 and L5. Except for their periphery the discs do not have pain receptors; however, if the nucleus of a disc breaks through its normal boundaries, the disc's peripheral pain receptors will be activated. (The pain receptors in the ligaments of the spine can also quickly tell the body when something is wrong in a ligament or in an adjacent damaged disc that exceeds its normal confines.) If a disc is diseased and/or injured, its ability to withstand stress is adversely affected and the motion segment to which it belongs becomes unstable. The disc is avascular (i.e., without a blood supply); its nutrition is enhanced by motion occurring in the spine (e.g., motion enables the disc to absorb nutrients through the vertebral end plate). This is one reason why long-term bed rest is an inappropriate prescription for LBP. Smoking has also been found to similarly decrease nutrition to the disc (1).

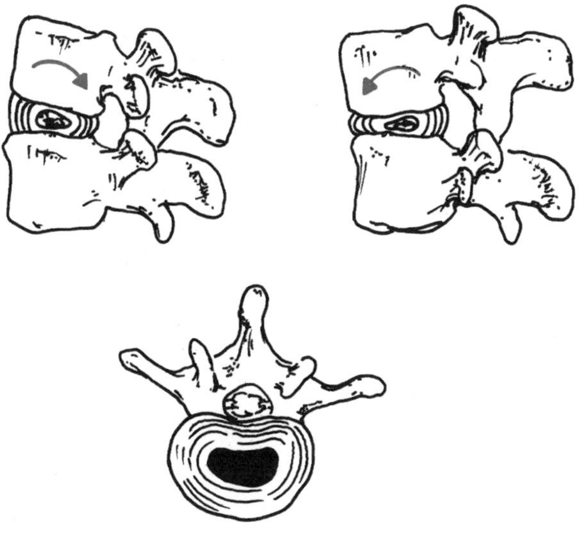

FIGURE 16.2 Discs allow flexibility and act as shock absorbers. In adults most low-back problems start in the disc.

The curvatures of the spine as viewed from the side are described as lordotic when they are concave and **kyphotic** when they are convex; cervical and lumbar curves are normally lordotic (e.g., the indentation at the small of the back) and the thoracic curve is kyphotic (see figure 5.10). Exaggerations of these curves are not desirable. For example, an increased anterior (or forward) pelvic tilt would increase the lordotic curve in the lumbar area; this posture increases stresses on the connective tissue structures as well as the musculature of the spine. A small lumbar lordotic curve is natural, and along with the cervical lordosis and thoracic kyphosis curves, assists the discs in cushioning compressive forces occurring to the spine in activities of daily living. Some believe that an excessive lordosis is a risk factor for low-back pain, but not all research supports this contention. It should be noted that factors such as being overweight, wearing high heels often, or lack of appropriate muscle length or strength can affect the degree of lordosis. With respect to the latter, tightness in the hip flexors (e.g., the iliopsoas) can increase the lordotic curve by causing an anterior pelvic tilt; conversely, tightness in the hamstrings can reduce the lordosis (see figures 5.10 and 13.5).

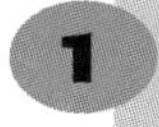

In Review: The fundamental unit of the spine is the motion segment; it consists

motion segment — Fundamental unit of the lumbar spine; made up of two vertebrae and their intervening disc.

disc — Located between vertebrae; acts as a shock absorber and can be involved in low-back pain.

facet joint — Junction of the superior and inferior articular processes of the vertebrae.

kyphotic — Describes the condition of kyphosis, a convex curvature of the spine (e.g., the thoracic curve).

of two vertebrae and their intervening disc. The spinal discs absorb shock to the spine by exerting pressure in all directions to help absorb the force. Most back problems begin in the disc; the disc most often injured is the one between L5–S1. Natural curvatures of the spine assist the discs in cushioning compressive forces. Although the facet joints aid in supporting loads, one of their prime responsibilities is controlling the amount and direction of spinal movement.

SPINAL MOVEMENT

The reader should refer to chapter 13 for a general review of spinal movement constraints. This section discusses flexion, spinal curvature, extension, and lateral movement.

Flexion

The flexion movements seen in curl-up and crunch-type exercises were discussed in chapter 5. To reiterate, in these exercises each lumbar vertebra rotates from its backward tilted position to a neutral or **end-ROM** (straightened lumbar) position. After the lumbar spine is straightened in the up movement of the curl-up or crunch, for example, no further spinal flexion can take place. If the crunch movement is continued until a full sit-up position is reached, the movement must occur at the hip joint. Then the muscles crossing this joint (e.g., psoas and iliacus) would be the prime movers as the abdominals contract statically. A full sit-up could be particularly harmful to the individual with weak abdominal muscles; under these circumstances the pull of the psoas muscles places extreme compressive forces on the discs of the lumbar motion segments of the vertebral column. Bilateral leg raises could be similarly detrimental to the discs.

Functional/Structural Spinal Curves

Spinal curves are called **functional** if the curve can be removed by assuming a posture that takes away the force responsible for the curve. Figure 16.3 provides an example of how leg posture affects the pull of the psoas musculature on the lumbar spine (figure 16.3a); when the paired psoas are relaxed (figure 16.3b), the lordotic curve is reduced. Habitually tight hip flexors, however, will cause an anterior tilt of the pelvis and thus reduce ROM at the hip joint; if this happens a functional curve may become **structural**. A structural curve would not be amenable to

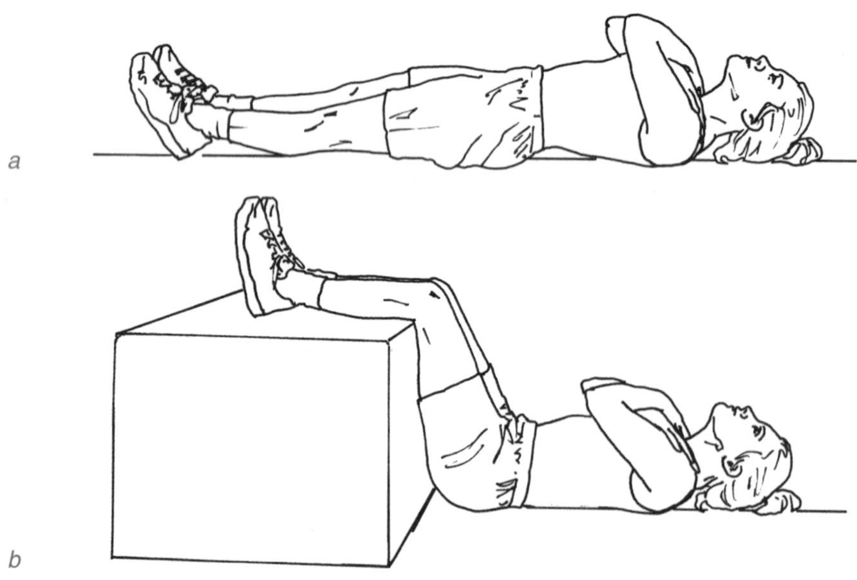

FIGURE 16.3 When the supine posture is assumed the pull of the psoas muscle can produce an exaggerated lordotic curve (*a*). When the legs are supported, the psoas relaxes and the lordotic curve flattens if it is a functional curve (*b*). However, if the lordosis were a structural curve, a curve similar to that seen in (*a*) would be seen in (*b*) despite the absence of muscle tension.

easy reduction; such curves result from an unhealthy posture assumed over a period of years. For example, if the individual in figure 16.3 had a structural lumbar lordosis, the lordotic curve would be retained regardless of whether the legs were supported.

It should be understood that a person with a structural lumbar lordosis would have extreme difficulty in doing crunches because of lack of mobility in the **lumbosacral** area. Although this person might be able to do sit-ups by using the hip flexors *if* the feet were held, this could exacerbate the problem. It would be far better if the exercise leader would provide a substitute abdominal exercise such as isometric holds for an individual with this mobility problem.

Extension

As discussed in chapter 13, spinal extension movements/postures are less often used than spinal flexion ones in most activities of daily living; therefore, it should not be any surprise that with aging there is often a greater loss in extension ROM than flexion ROM. For example, an individual sitting for long hours each day at a computer terminal may assume a "slumping" position for much of this time; an increase in thoracic kyphosis, round shoulders, and a decrease in lumbar lordosis might be the result (see figure 13.1). If this individual does not extend the spine or retract the shoulders periodically, the capability of doing these movements may be lessened and the poor posture may become structural. From a mechanical perspective, slumping forward also puts more stress on the discs of the lumbar spine. Sitting postures are usually more stressful on the spine than standing postures because the lordotic curve is usually diminished; when this happens the individual may "hang" on his or her ligaments (i.e., posterior ligaments of the lumbar spine) or use the back musculature to hold this posture. The slump posture shown in figure 13.1 is an example of a person hanging in end-ROM. Hanging in end-ROM can cause lengthening of ligaments and an increase of the compressive forces placed on intervertebral discs. Keeping the spine in a neutral position (i.e., midway between maximum flexion and extension) is much more desirable.

Lateral Flexion and Rotation

Because some of the most forceful stresses are placed on the spinal discs in movements that combine bending and rotation, exercises involving these movements should *always* be done under muscle control. In other words, exercises involving intervertebral movement should not be done ballistically (i.e., jerkily); instead, the movement should be done in one continuous, smooth motion. If the movement results from momentum rather than muscle control, the exerciser's movements may exceed normal end-ROM. If this happens connective tissue structures such as spinal ligaments or discs may be damaged.

Lateral Curvatures

When the spine is viewed from the back, ideally a straight vertical line is seen (see figure 13.4); however, minor lateral deviations are prevalent and may be related to something so nominal as hand dominance. In young individuals with scoliosis (an abnormal lateral curvature of the spine) bracing is the mainstay of nonoperative therapy (see figure 16.4). However, because bracing is rarely effective for adults, internal fixation devices such as Harrington rods are often surgically implanted (3). The exercise program for the scoliotic patient with either external bracing or internal fixation would have to ascribe to the limitations that either device presents on ROM and general mobility.

Therapeutic exercise alone is not very effective in correcting scoliotic curves. Moreover, inappropriate exercise prescription can make a scoliotic condition worse. Therefore it is imperative that exercise leaders obtain advice from a physical therapist, an orthopedic surgeon, or other appropriate medical personnel before giving or prescribing exercises in an attempt to straighten or correct a scoliotic curve.

end-ROM — Point at which further movement stress may stretch ligaments and/or other soft tissue structures such as discs.

functional (spinal curve) — Ability to remove a spinal curve (e.g., lordotic curve) by assuming a different posture.

structural curves — Refers to the lack of ability to remove a spinal curve in normal movement due to chronically shortened musculotendinous units and/or ligaments; in this case a functional curve becomes structural.

lumbosacral — Area encompassing the lumbar vertebrae and the sacrum.

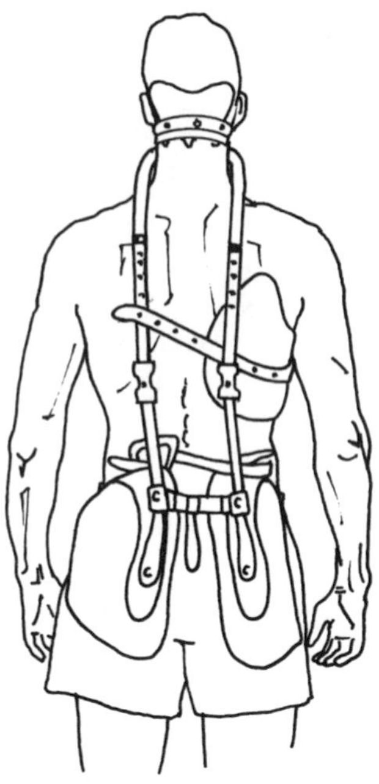

FIGURE 16.4 Milwaukee brace. This brace is used to correct a scoliotic curve; corsets made out of synthetic materials such as plastic may also be used.

2 In Review: **Functional curves can be removed by assuming a posture that reduces the force causing the curve. Structural curves usually develop over a period of years and are not amenable to easy reduction.**

MECHANICS OF THE SPINE AND HIP JOINT

For this discussion the reader is encouraged to refer to figures 5.10 and 13.5. The muscles crossing the hip joint can be viewed as guy wires bracing the pelvis; if any of these guy wires are too tight, the abdominal musculature cannot control pelvic positioning. Because the sacral portion of the pelvis is the foundation for the "kinetic chain" of 24 vertebrae stacked on it, pelvic positioning is important to the integrity of the spine. For example, tightness in the hamstrings can severely affect the ability of the pelvis to be tilted anteriorly and thus pelvic ROM is diminished. If the body were subsequently subjected to an unplanned stress (e.g., stepping in a hole or slipping on ice), body parts are obligated to give with the resulting movement. If the hamstrings cannot give, connective tissue structures of the spine may have to absorb the stress. If there is tearing or other damage to spinal ligaments, discs, or both, a step toward having an acute low-back problem has been made.

3 In Review: **The pelvis serves as the foundation for the spine, so the ability of the muscles of the trunk to control pelvic positioning is essential to having a healthy back. It is essential that neither the hip flexors nor hip extensors are too tight.**

LOW-BACK PAIN: A REPETITIVE MICROTRAUMA INJURY

Even though some individuals might remember a specific movement that they believe caused their low-back problem, this is not generally the case. Rather, it is the analogy of the straw that breaks the camel's back that usually better describes the occurrence of a low-back problem.

Low-Back Problems Seen in Adults

It has been contended that most cases of acute low-back pain in adults are caused by damage of some sort to the intervertebral discs (4). It should be realized that this damage would seldom be caused by just *one* movement; LBP is typically caused by a succession of the same type of movements occurring over a period of time. Because of this, LBP is often called a repetitive microtrauma condition.

If one takes a paper clip and bends it once, it is still quite strong; however, its molecular makeup has been changed and it will never be the same again. The paper clip can be further bent and remain strong, but with each successive bend it becomes weaker; with continual bending it eventually breaks. Similarly, one could use poor biomechanics in lifting an object; however, the one maneuver is not apt to cause a back problem. If poor biomechanics in lifting objects are repeated hundreds of times, however, connective tissue structures of the spine can weaken like the paper clip and eventually yield to even a nominal stress. It might not be until this time that acute symptoms are noted.

Cumulative repetitive microtrauma affects the disc's homeostasis, and eventually it adversely alters the disc's pivotal responsibility as a shock absorber of the spinal unit. For example, minor tears in the periphery of the disc can be painful and can be a forewarning of more serious problems. Eventually the jellylike nucleus may leak out of its normal confines and cause an unstable motion segment; when this occurs specific movements may be exceedingly painful and the condition will get worse unless appropriate interventions are made. Thus what started as a minor problem can evolve into a major one. The key is to never let the problem get started; maintaining good physical fitness and strengthening the trunk musculature with appropriate exercises are keys to preventing LBP.

Low-Back Problems Seen in Youth

In youth low-back problems are not typically seen in the disc as in adults but rather in the part of the vertebrae posterior to the spinal cord, including the superior and inferior articular processes (refer to figure 16.1). The part of a vertebra between the superior and inferior articular processes is called the **pars interarticularis**. Stress to this area can lead to complications such as **spondylolysis** or **spondylolisthesis**. The former condition is essentially a stress fracture in the pars interarticularis; sometimes it evolves into a complete fracture on both sides of a spinous process, either because the bone does not unite properly and/or it fails to withstand the stress to which it is subjected. Then the condition is called spondylolisthesis and an anterior slipping of the body of the vertebra over the vertebra below is apt to occur. This injury usually occurs at the lumbosacral junction (i.e., L5 slipping over S1).

Although the causes of spondylolisthesis might include genetic ties, stresses resulting from participation in activities such as weight lifting or gymnastics also could be the cause. Appropriate coaching and guidance in athletic activities for youth is very important for avoiding unhealthy stresses on growing bones. It should be noted that not all cases of spondylolysis and spondylolisthesis necessarily begin before skeletal maturity; although the exact age of onset might be unknown, many professional football linemen have this condition (6). Spondylolisthesis has been cited as the most likely cause of LBP in patients under 26 years of age, but it is rarely the sole cause of LBP in individuals over 40 (3).

4 **In Review: Low-back pain is often referred to as a repetitive microtrauma injury because its development occurs over a period of time as opposed to being the result of one traumatic incident. Low-back problems seen in adults usually originate in the disc; in youth low-back problems usually originate in the posterior elements of the vertebrae.**

EXERCISE CONSIDERATIONS: PREVENTIVE AND THERAPEUTIC

"Stepped-up" versions of the exercises viewed as being therapeutic can often be used as prophylactic (preventive) exercises. Ideally ROM, strength, or both, should be improved before their deficiencies cause a problem.

Range of Motion and Low-Back Function

As discussed in chapter 13, ROM deficiencies in the spine and its supporting structures have been viewed as prognostic indicators of low-back pain. Good ROM can decrease the probability of a low-back problem; once LBP occurs, good ROM can be a factor in reducing the severity of the problem.

As displayed in figure 5.9, a limited degree of spinal mobility in the sagital plane (e.g., flexion, extension) and the coronal plane (e.g., lateral flexion) is present in the cervical and lumbar segments. Although rotation is restricted in the lumbar and thoracic regions, a considerable amount is present

pars interarticularis — Part of vertebra between its upper elements (superior articular process and transverse process) and its lower elements (inferior articular process and spinous process).

spondylolysis — A stress fracture in the pars interarticularis.

spondylolisthesis — Condition in which the vertebral body and transverse processes slip anteriorly (forward) on the vertebral body below; common for L4 to slip over L5.

in the cervical region, particularly between C1 and C2.

Extension of the spine is an issue often ignored or misinterpreted in exercise programs. Although it is acknowledged that ballistic-extension movements of the spine (and ballistic-rotation movements) are totally inappropriate, as discussed in chapter 13, slow and controlled extension movements are appropriate and should be included in exercise programs.

Trunk Strength and Low-Back Function

Other things being equal, individuals with good ROM and good trunk strength and endurance are less apt to have LBP. Although the popular literature often indicts weakened abdominal musculature as a prime cause of LBP, the back musculature is proportionately weaker than the abdominal musculature in low-back patients (2). Nevertheless, the strength of the abdominal muscles are also vital to the maintenance of a healthy spine.

For research purposes sophisticated testing equipment to assess trunk strength may be desirable. For nonclinical settings, however, and clinical settings not having the latter equipment, a back-raise test that combines strength and endurance is frequently used (figure 16.5). When trunk extension exercises are done to develop back extensor muscle strength, a key to remember is never to exceed one's normal lordosis when doing the trunk raise (i.e., do not hyperextend the spine).

Although the back musculature may be disproportionately weaker in LBP patients, it is still imperative that the abdominal muscles are not neglected. For example, the rectus abdominis is in a position to control the tilt of the pelvis directly (figure 13.5); this is a most important consideration in maintaining a healthy spine. Development of the rectus

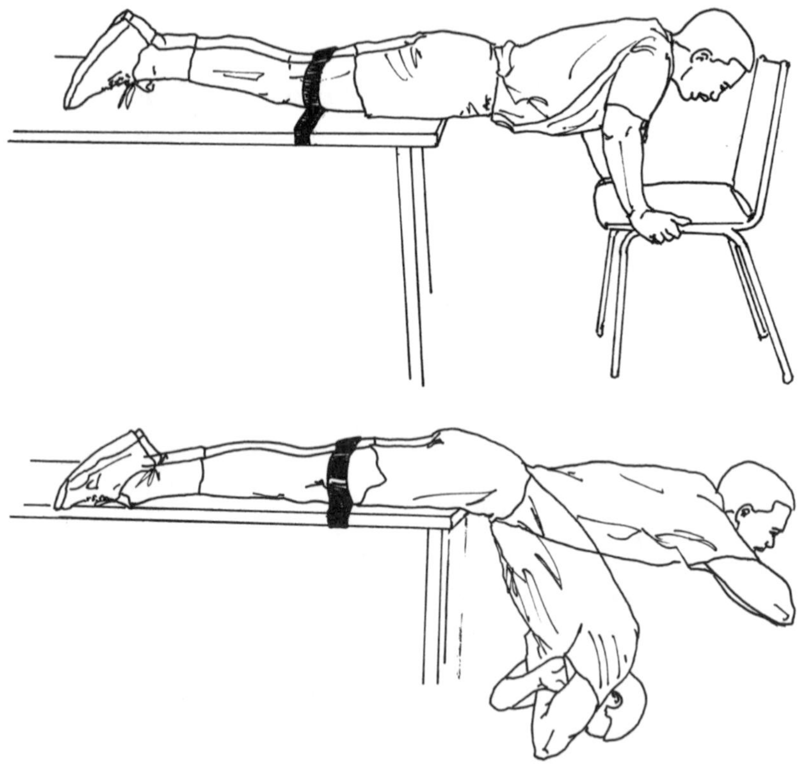

FIGURE 16.5 Back extension strength/endurance. This activity can be used as a test or as an exercise. When it is used as a test the individual being tested pushes up from the chair until the trunk is horizontal; the subject then folds the arms behind the neck and maintains the position as long as possible by isometric contraction of the erector spinae musculature. (Originally 4 min was used as the maximum hold time; however, because in recent research it was found that most subjects could hold this position for 4 min, no time limit is now recommended.) Although the same maneuver could be used to develop strength, raising the trunk from the "head down" position to the horizontal position could also be done (no chair needed). The key to remember if the activity is done dynamically is to never extend the trunk beyond one's normal lordosis (i.e., do not hyperextend the spine).

abdominis is emphasized in crunch-type activities. To repeat the discussion appearing earlier in this chapter as well as in chapter 5, if the trunk is lifted more than 30° the hip flexors (e.g., the paired psoas) come into play. Unfortunately many individuals thought that by bending the knees the role of the psoas muscles was reduced; this is not so, particularly if the feet are supported. If developing the hip flexors is desirable, other exercises can be used that will not compromise low-back function; the point is, *never* do a full sit-up!

5 **In Review: If full sit-ups are done, the hip flexors perform the final portion of the movement because the abdominal muscles contract statically, regardless of the knee position.**

It should also be realized that in standard crunch-type activities the rectus abdominis does most of the work and the lateral abdominal muscles are seldom called into play. The lateral abdominal muscles (i.e., transversus abdominis, internal and external obliques) should also be developed because by their attachments both anteriorly (i.e., where they ensheathe the rectus abdominis) and posteriorly (i.e., where they attach to extensive connective tissue structures of the spine that ensheathe the erector spinae), the lateral abdominal muscles can enhance both anterior and posterior muscle groups. Strong lateral abdominal muscles are in a position to brace and splint the trunk; this can help prevent undesirable rotary motion in addition to protecting the back as heavy objects are lifted. The lateral abdominal musculature may be the most important trunk musculature with which to obtain and maintain a healthy low back.

6 **In Review: Maintaining ROM is an important consideration in maintaining a healthy spine; ROM is also important in therapeutic exercise. In individuals with low-back problems, the back musculature are often proportionately weaker than the abdominal musculature; in part this might be due to neglect of extensor muscle strength in exercise programs. The trunk musculature can work together as a dynamic corset; the lateral abdominal muscles "tie" the flexors and extensors of the spine together and their development is exceedingly important.**

PROPHYLACTIC EXERCISES FOR ENHANCING LOW-BACK FUNCTION

Even though many injuries and diseases of the low back can be treated conservatively with therapeutic exercise, the diversity and complexity of low-back problems are such that they preclude making a simple diagnosis and presenting an exercise regimen for that diagnosis. Moreover, arming a person with a set of therapeutic exercises who did not concurrently understand the nuances of different low-back conditions could be dangerous. Because it is beyond the scope of this chapter to provide the reader with the background on these countless nuances, the emphasis in this discussion is on the presentation of sound exercises that enhance low-back function. Be that as it may, it should be no surprise that some of the exercises presented in this section are sometimes used by therapists with low-back patients.

Exercises to Enhance Flexibility

This chapter's appendix describes exercises recommended for flexibility of the low back. The guy-wire concept discussed in chapter 13 (see figure 13.5) is helpful to consider when exploring exercises for low-back flexibility. Although the trunk musculature (e.g., the abdominals and the erector spinae) are crucial to controlling pelvic positioning, their ability to control the pelvis is reduced or negated if either the hip flexors or the hip extensors are too tight. The bottom line is that having good hip-joint mobility is fundamental to having a healthy spine. Several exercises that can be used to improve ROM in joints and structures relevant to the low back are presented in the chapter appendix beginning on page 325.

Exercises to Develop the Trunk Musculature

Exercises for the development of the back musculature of the trunk are delineated in the appendix to this chapter. A key point to remember in doing spinal extension movements is that exercisers should not exceed their normal lumbar lordosis when moving into extension.

Posterior pelvic tilts and crunches are basic to the exercise programs of many individuals for the development of the abdominal musculature. As previously mentioned, when individuals do these exercises the rectus abdominis often does most of the work and the lateral abdominal muscles are involved minimally. Exercises that will enhance the development of the lateral musculature include diagonal crunches and isometrics. Besides doing the diagonal curl dynamically, it can be done isometrically by using challenging lengths of isometric holds (e.g., 5 to 30 s). Although isometric exercises may be considered passé for limb movements because of lack of specificity of training, in reality isometrics are most specific to the stabilization of the spine (5). With strong lateral abdominals it is much easier to stabilize and brace the spine; if the spine has a "strong" brace, it will be much less susceptible to the repetitive microtrauma that can lead to serious cases of LBP.

7 **In Review: Maintenance of good hip-joint ROM is essential for a healthy spine. Never exceed the normal lordotic curve when doing active back extension exercises. The ROM capabilities of the trunk are quite nominal; keep this in mind when setting up exercise programs for clients. Isometric holds can nicely supplement regular crunches as well as diagonal crunches.**

Case Studies

You can check your answers by referring to appendix A.

16.1

An exercise leader is using a double-leg lowering task with a group of relatively fit adults, ostensibly to improve the strength of the abdominals. When questioned about the use of this exercise, he advises you that physical therapists have often used a similar activity to test the abdominal strength of their patients, even those who are symptomatic for low-back pain. Discuss the appropriateness/inappropriateness of the use of such an exercise.

16.2

An exercise leader is utilizing the sit-and-reach (or standing toe-touch) exercise presumably to improve hip-joint flexibility. Because he or she is aware that ballistic stretches are usually contraindicated, the exercise leader strongly admonishes his or her group to perform the exercise with slow and easy stretches. Discuss the appropriateness/inappropriateness of these directions.

16.3

An exercise leader prescribes oblique (diagonal) curls which require the exerciser to maintain a 15-second isometric contraction after at least one shoulder blade is raised from the exercise surface. Discuss the appropriateness/inappropriateness of this activity.

Source List

1. Battie et al. (1991)
2. Biering-Sorensen (1984)
3. Borenstein & Wiesel (1989)
4. Cailliet (1988)
5. Nachemson, Andersson, & Schultz (1986)
6. Sinaki, Lutness, and Ilstrup, et al. (1989)
7. Sullivan, Dejulia, & Worrell (1992)

APPENDIX

Flexibility, Strength, and Endurance Exercises to Improve Low-Back Function

Flexibility Exercises to Improve ROM

In performing hip flexor stretches, a key point to keep in mind is to stretch to symmetry; *after* symmetry is achieved, work on improvement in flexibility in both limbs.

Hip Flexor Stretch (Standing)

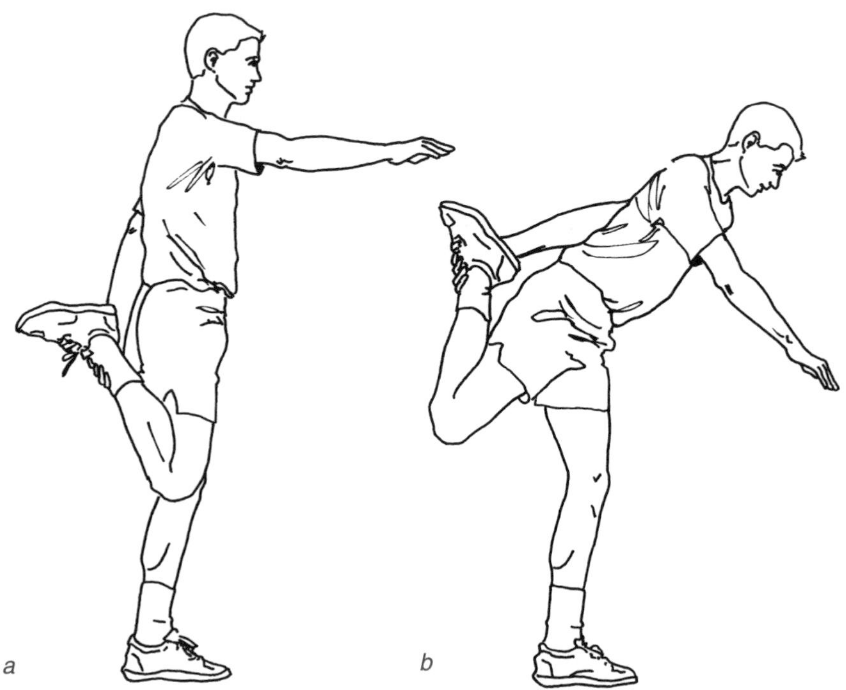

Grasp contralateral ankle and raise leg while keeping trunk straight (*a*). Note incorrect technique of individual on the right (*b*); tilting the pelvis precludes stretching the hip flexors.

Hip Flexor Stretch (Supine)

Assume Thomas test position and pull contralateral leg back as far as possible; this posterior rotation of the pelvis can place added tension on the hip flexors.

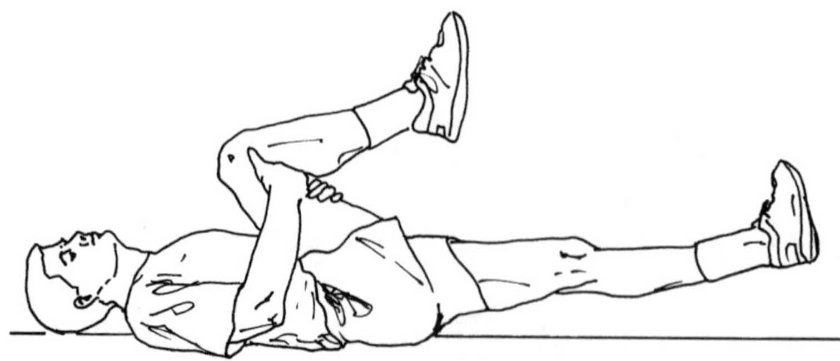

Hip Extensor Stretches

Cailliet Stretch

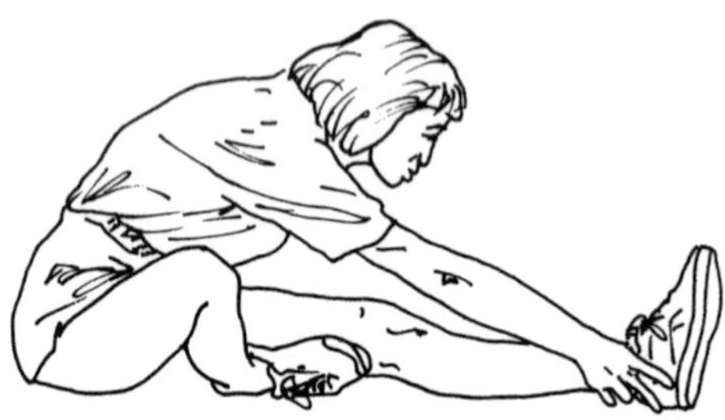

Exerciser should lean forward until tension is felt in the hamstrings; then hold this position 15 to 20 s. Repeat sequence for each leg 3 to 4 times. If the hamstrings are tight (e.g., sacral angle less than 80°), more stress would be placed on structures of the spine. This is not desirable. The back should be kept straight and the movement emphasis should be at the hip joint.

Step/Chair Stretch

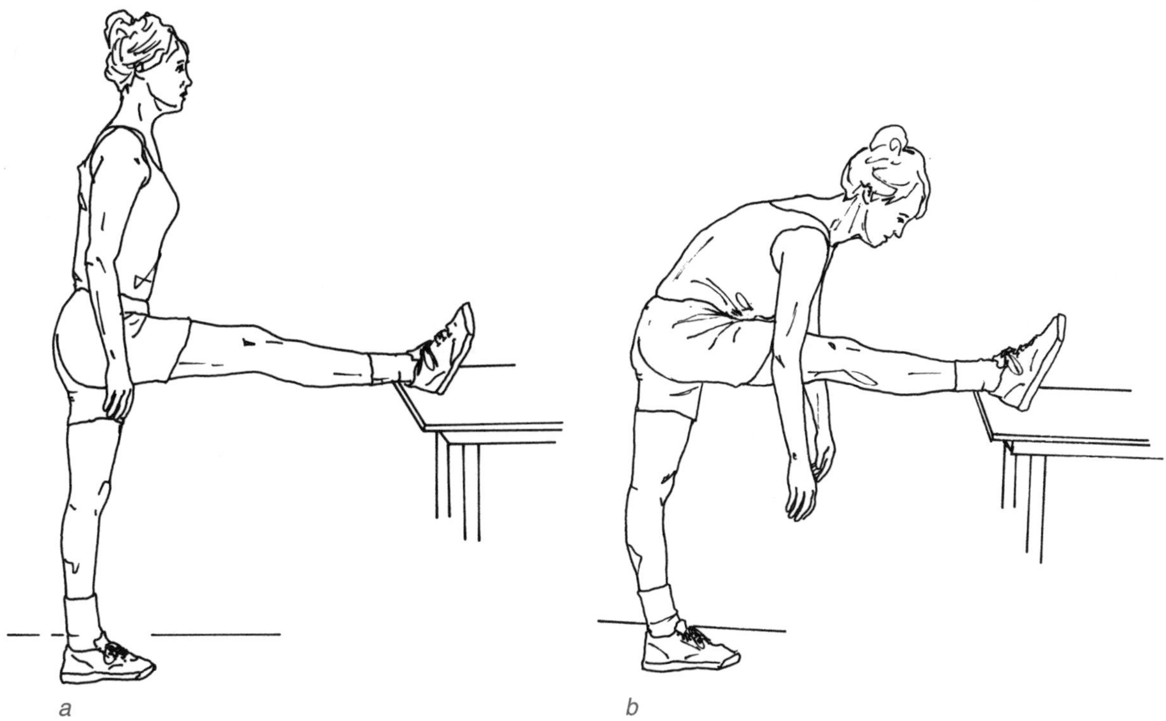

This stretch can be more effective if the trunk is "splinted" and the movement emphasis is at the hip joint rather than using the more slouched posture also depicted (*b*). In (*a*) the hamstrings can be isolated in the stretch if the movement is made only at the hip joint. Although the hamstrings can also be stretched in (*b*), the soft tissue structures of the lower back are also stretched. A more appropriate stretch for the lower back is presented in the next figure.

Trunk Flexion Exercise

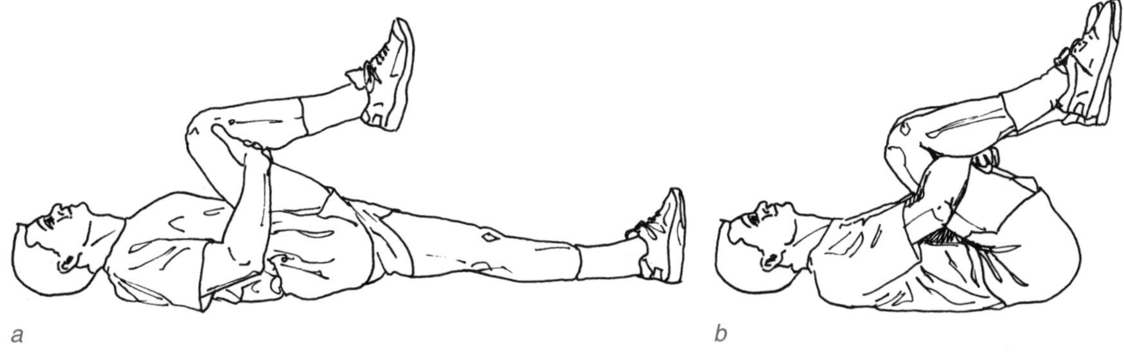

Pull one (*a*) and eventually both (*b*) knees toward shoulder(s).

Trunk Extension Exercise

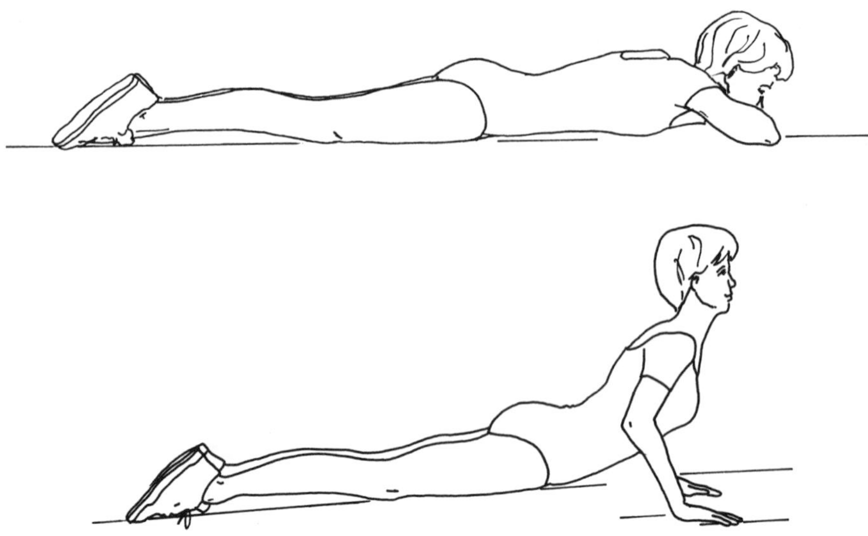

Place hands under shoulders and slowly extend arms while keeping pelvis in contact with floor (keep back muscles relaxed).

Trunk Flexion Strength and Endurance Exercises

Posterior Pelvic Tilt

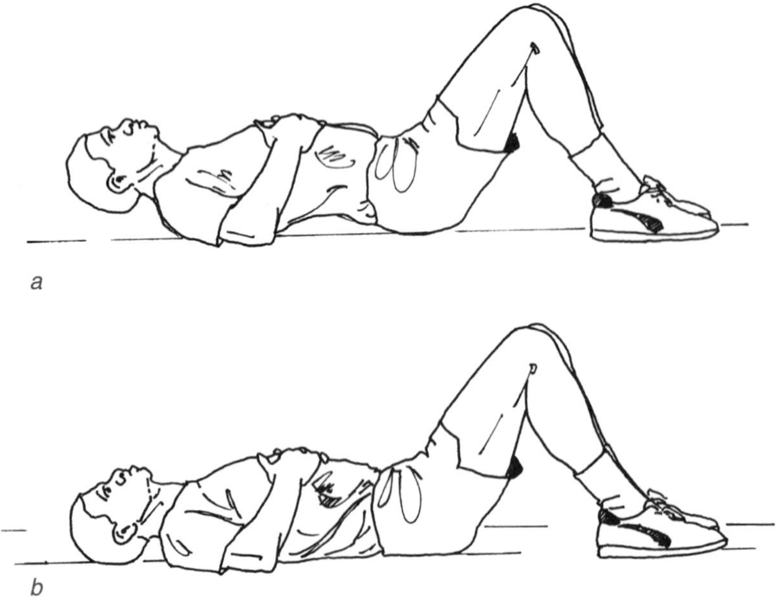

This exercise can be done by itself or as the first phase of a crunch. Posteriorly rotate the pelvis from starting position (*a*) until the low back is snug against the floor (*b*).

Crunch/Partial Curl

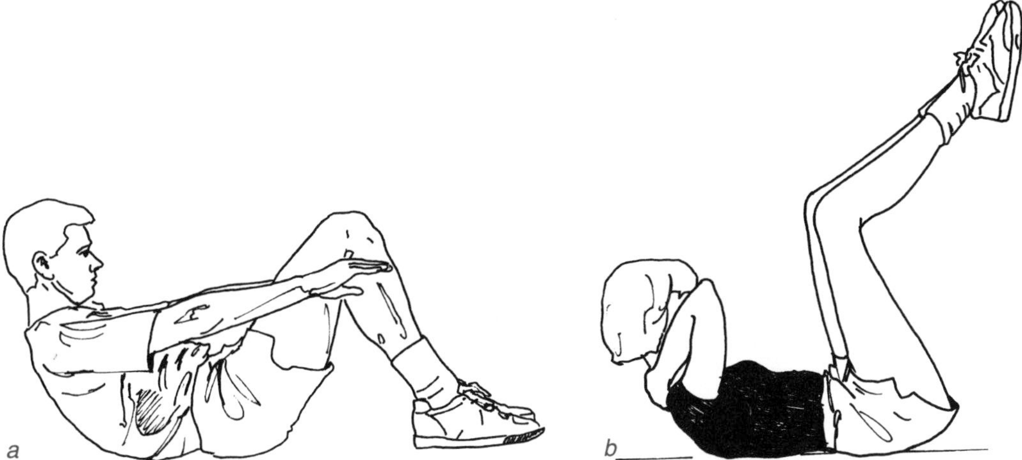

Once the shoulders are raised from the floor the normal lordosis has been straightened and movement should cease (*a*). If the movement is continued, it will occur at the iliofemoral joint and the movers will be the hip flexors as the abdominal muscles contract isometrically to stabilize the trunk. The crunch can also be performed with the thighs vertical (*b*). A minimum of 10 to 15 repetitions should be the goal. Two or three sets may be repeated and/or isometric holds of 5 s or more can be incorporated with the up position.

Diagonal/Oblique Curl

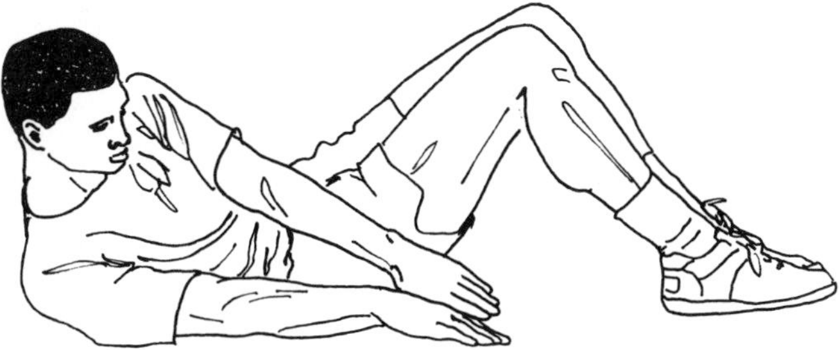

This exercise ensures greater involvement of the internal and external oblique musculature. A minimum of 10 to 15 repetitions should be the goal. Two or three sets may be repeated and/or isometric holds of 5 s or more can be incorporated with the up position.

Chapter 17

Exercise Leadership for Health and Fitness

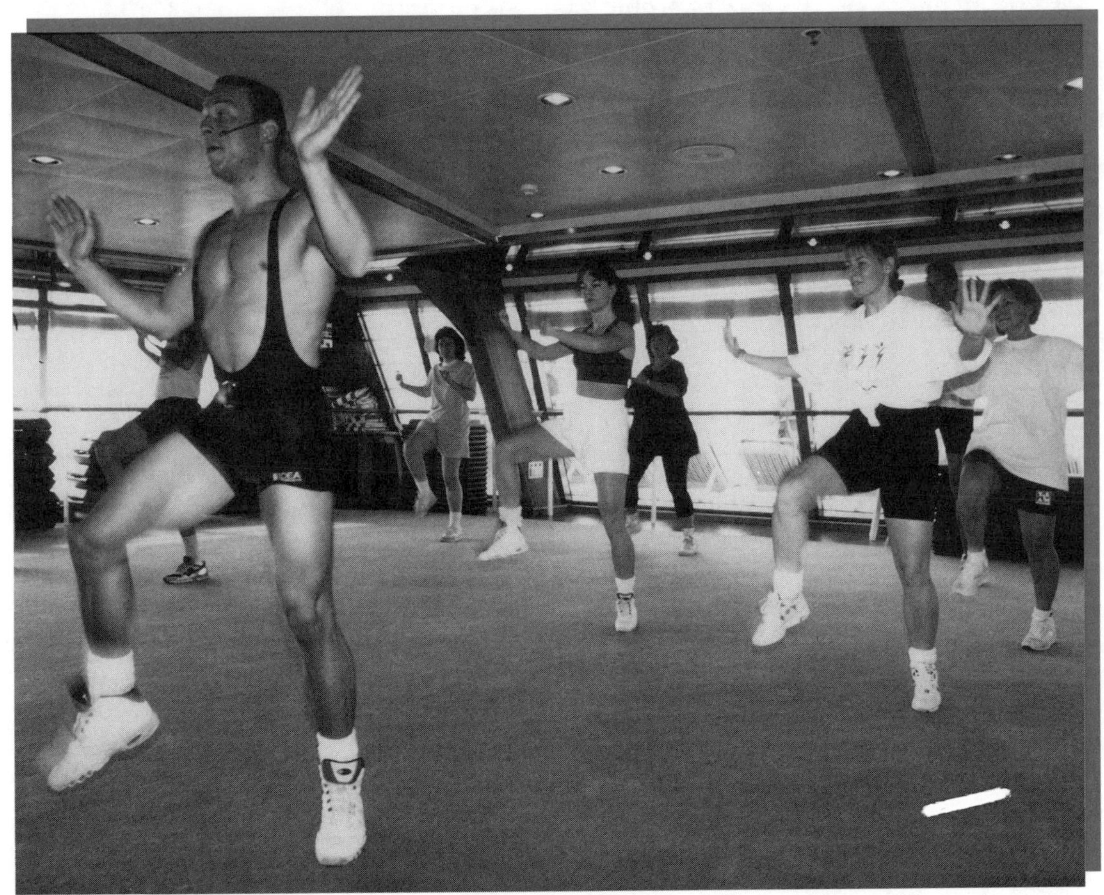

© W. Lynn Seldon

OBJECTIVES

The reader will be able to:

1. Distinguish between guidelines for moderate-intensity exercise programs recommended for everyone and systematically structured exercise programs for people interested in improving functional capacity.
2. Describe the factors related to a high and low probability of participation.
3. Describe the characteristics of a good exercise leader.
4. Indicate how exercise intensity is monitored in an exercise session.
5. Describe safety and clothing considerations relative to walking and jogging programs.
6. Explain the balance between duration and intensity in a typical walking program, and indicate activities used in walking programs to improve enjoyment and adherence.
7. Outline appropriate walk-jog-walk intervals used at the beginning of a jogging program.
8. Describe exercise recommendations for cycling that result in cardiorespiratory fitness improvements.
9. List the elements of games that provide effective fitness benefits.
10. Describe the activities done in a swimming pool, other than lap swimming, that can be an effective part of an aerobic exercise program.
11. Provide recommendations for beginners starting low- and high-impact dance exercise programs, and indicate the typical kinds of exercises included in such programs.
12. Recommend appropriate beginning goals for people using exercise equipment.
13. Describe a circuit training program using aerobic and strength training equipment.

The purpose of a fitness program must be kept uppermost in the health fitness instructor's (HFI's) mind. The HFI is trying to help people include appropriate physical activity as a vital part of their lifestyles. This assumes that the participants understand what type of physical activity is appropriate, have sufficient skills to achieve satisfaction from the activities, and have the intrinsic motivation to continue to be active for the rest of their lives. Thus HFIs try to help people increase their physical fitness levels in ways that are psychologically, mentally, and socially relevant and appealing.

EFFECTIVE LEADERSHIP

Individuals need to do 30 min of moderate-intensity physical activity daily for health goals. To obtain and maintain cardiorespiratory fitness, a person must participate in vigorous, dynamic aerobic exercise at least 3 days per week. Yet, about one in four Americans is completely sedentary, and about 40% do irregular exercise less than recommended. Only about one in five meets the moderate-intensity guideline, one in four does some stretching, and less than 15% are involved in regular vigorous aerobic or strengthening exercises (16). At the same time, over half of the people who start a formal exercise program drop out within a few months (2).

> **1 In Review: Moderate-intensity exercise (30 min daily) is recommended for all people. Vigorous aerobic exercise should be done at least 3 days a week to improve functional capacity.**

Figure 17.1 summarizes the factors related to a high probability and a low probability of participation. What must be clear to the HFI and the exercise leader is that there are a wide variety of factors

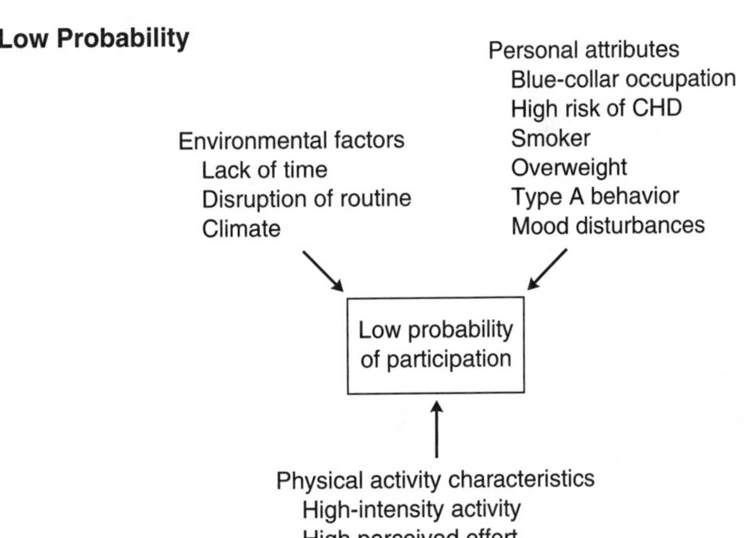

FIGURE 17.1 High and low probability of participation.

affecting people's involvement in personal or supervised exercise programs. In general, better educated, self-motivated individuals who enjoy physical activity and believe in the health outcomes associated with physical activity are more likely to exercise on a regular basis. In contrast, individuals with a high risk of CHD who also hold blue-collar jobs are less likely to be involved in formal exercise. It would appear that the people with the greatest need to exercise are the least likely to become involved. More than personal characteristics, however, are involved in the decision.

2 **In Review: Different environmental factors, personal attributes, and physical activity characteristics can predict the probability of an individual's participating in an exercise program. See figure 17.1.**

Support from one's spouse or partner, family, physician, and peers seems to drive involvement, but this must be viewed against the variable of perceived convenience of facilities. People with poor time-management and goal-setting skills are less likely to be successful. What does this say about the HFI's role in providing exercise leadership? It is clear that exercise leadership involves much more than exercise!

Henry Kissinger is cited as saying that a leader is one who can take people from where they are to where they have not been (14). This is very true for the exercise leader, who must counter the negative influences bearing on the portion of the population most in need of physical activity. We normally think that an HFI

- *screens* individuals relative to health status;
- *evaluates* various fitness components;
- *prescribes* activities at the appropriate intensity, duration, and frequency consistent with test results and personal goals;
- *leads* individuals or groups in appropriate activities;
- *monitors* participants' responses within an exercise session;
- *modifies* activities depending on environmental and other factors;
- *records* progress and problems;
- *responds* to emergencies; and
- *refers* problems to appropriate health professionals.

Leadership, however, means more than simply taking a class through its paces. HFIs also must make the participant feel welcome, motivate the person or group, and be a friend. To do all these things, the exercise leader must develop interpersonal skills. A summary of these leadership abilities is in the box below.

Since 1980 a variety of organizations have developed certification and education programs to promote exercise programming in preventive and rehabilitative settings. One of the earliest to do so was the American College of Sports Medicine (ACSM). Qualification in these certification areas requires the applicant to have a specific knowledge base and demonstrate specific behaviors. The current certification programs (1) include

Relationship-Oriented Abilities Associated With Effective Leadership

Listening skills
Attention to individual needs
Concern regarding integration of new participants
Acceptance to group interaction
Educational skills
Motivational skills with participants and staff
Rapport and empathy leading to sensitivity
Consistency/honesty/tactfulness
Skilled at opening avenues of communication between participants and staff

Reprinted from Oldridge, 1988, Qualities of an exercise leader. In *Resource manual for guidelines for exercise testing and prescription*. By permission of Lea & Febiger.

- **Exercise Leader$_{SM}$**—Qualified to lead exercise "on the floor";
- **Health/Fitness Instructor$_{SM}$**—Qualified in exercise testing, prescription, and leadership in preventive programs;
- **Health/Fitness Director®**—Qualified as an HFI and responsible for management of preventive programs;
- **Exercise Test Technologist$_{SM}$**—Qualified in exercise testing in preventive and rehabilitative programs;
- **Exercise Specialist$_{SM}$**—Qualified in exercise testing, prescription, and leadership for all populations, with a focus on clinical exercise programs for high-risk individuals and individuals with cardiac, respiratory, or metabolic diseases; and
- **Program Director$_{SM}$**—Qualified as an exercise specialist and responsible for administration, community education programs, research and development, and so forth in preventive and rehabilitative programs.

These certifications are considered the standard by many in the fitness and cardiac-rehabilitation areas. However, there are a variety of other respected certification programs:

- American Council on Exercise (ACE)—Aerobics Instructor, Personal Trainer, and Lifestyle & Weight Management Consultant (ACE; 5820 Oberlin Drive, Suite 102; San Diego, CA 92121-3787)
- Aerobics and Fitness Association of America (AFAA)—AFAA Fitness Practitioner™ (AFAA; 15250 Ventura Boulevard, Suite 200; Sherman Oaks, CA 91403)
- Disabled Sports USA—Adapted Fitness Instructor certification for adapted physical education teachers and personal fitness trainers (Disabled Sports USA; 451 Hungerford Drive, Suite 100; Rockville, MD 20850)
- National Strength and Conditioning Association—Certified Strength and Conditioning Specialist (C.S.C.S. Agency; P.O. Box 83469; Lincoln, NE 68501)
- YMCA—YMCA Exercise Instructor, YMCA Exercise Instructor Trainer, and their advanced counterparts (YMCA of the USA; 101 North Wacker Drive; Chicago, IL 60606-7386)

In addition to these certification programs, certifications for unique aspects of exercise leadership will be presented later in this chapter. Next, the responsibilities of the HFI are examined in greater detail.

Role Model

The authors of this book clearly support the notion that the HFI should be an inspiring role model for his or her clients. The idea of an overweight, out-of-shape exercise leader is one whose time has passed. A leader must plan appropriate activities, evaluate the progress of the participants, provide incentives, and so forth; but the leadership associated with many exercise programs is in the form of quiet, subtle value statements that do not require words. The HFI's presence and behaviors, consistent with a healthy

leadership — The ability to influence and motivate people in a group to make decisions and to act on the basis of those decisions.

Exercise Leader$_{SM}$ — A person who is certified by the American College of Sports Medicine as qualified to lead exercise "on the floor."

Health/Fitness Instructor$_{SM}$ — A person who is certified by the American College of Sports Medicine as qualified in exercise testing, prescription, and leadership in preventive programs.

Health/Fitness Director® — A person who is certified by the American College of Sports Medicine as qualified for management of preventive programs.

Exercise Test Technologist$_{SM}$ — A person certified by the American College of Sports Medicine to conduct graded exercise stress tests for a variety of populations.

Exercise Specialist$_{SM}$ — A person certified by the American College of Sports Medicine to work in exercise rehabilitation settings with high-risk or diseased populations.

Program Director$_{SM}$ — A person certified by the American College of Sports Medicine to be responsible for administration, community education programs, research and development, and so forth, in preventive and postcardiac rehabilitative health fitness programs.

lifestyle, add much meaning and value to her or his words and programs.

Program Planning

All activity programs must have daily, weekly, and monthly plans to provide appropriate activities, meet the needs of the participants, and reduce the possibility of boredom. This planning allows the HFI to judge the usefulness of the activity and encourage systematic modification from one month to the next. If the HFI is working with individuals who exercise on their own, then the need for specific exercise recommendations becomes obvious. The value of the feedback received from these individuals depends on the information they were given at the start of their program. The following considerations can be applied to both group and individual exercise programs.

Vary the Program

Variety should be a cornerstone of every exercise program. Some elements are a part of each exercise session: warm-up and stretching, a stimulus phase, and a cool-down. The variety comes in the form of different exercises used in each part of a session, short educational messages presented to the class while they are stretching or cooling down, or the use of games to add spice to routine exercises. The most important thing is to plan the activity sessions far enough in advance to minimize repetition and maximize variety.

Accommodate Individual Differences

A participant should be able to choose from a variety of activities. A program must address the needs, interests, and limitations of the group being served. The choice of equipment, activities, and the pace of the class must be considered when planning for young/old, less fit/very fit, and more skilled/less skilled participants (11). Offer different options from which people may choose (e.g., 1-lb vs. 5-lb weights, low-impact vs. high-impact moves, 1-mi vs. 3-mi jogs).

Maintain Control

The exercise leader must have control over the exercise session. This is especially true in the use of games (e.g., indoor soccer), where the intensity is not as easily controlled as in jogging. Control implies an ability to modify the session as needed to meet the target heart rate (THR) and total work goals of each individual. Some people will have to slow down; others may need encouragement to increase their intensity. The element of control (at a distance) for people who exercise without direct supervision can be provided by using written guidelines about what to do and when to move from one stage to the next. In addition, specific information should be provided about symptoms that indicate inappropriate responses to exercise.

Monitor Progress and Keep Records

Keeping track of a participant's response to the exercise session will give clues about that individual's adaptation to that particular session and about overall, day-to-day changes. This information is important for updating exercise prescriptions and answering specific questions the participant may raise. Each exercise class should have regular pauses to check HR and determine whether individuals are close to their THRs. Rather than keeping track of a large number of 10-s THRs, ask each participant to indicate the number of beats over or under the 10-s goal. This increases the participant's awareness of the THR and indicates how the intensity of the exercise should be adjusted to stay on target.

Each person's HR response is probably the best and most objective indicator of his or her adjustment to an exercise session, but do not stop with that. Elicit information about how the participant feels in general; ask about any new pains, aches, or strange sensations. Record keeping should include a daily attendance check, a weekly weighing, a regular BP check (if appropriate), and a column asking for comments (e.g., THR, any aches or pains). An example of such a form is the Daily Activity Form (see form 17.1). This information allows the HFI to make better recommendations about the participants' exercise programs and refer them to appropriate professionals if needed.

The point we have emphasized throughout this section on exercise leadership is the need for the leader to help the participant. The Behavioral Strategies list on page 338 suggests ways for HFIs to become better leaders.

> **3** **In Review: The effective fitness professional must develop relationship-oriented abilities, serve as a role model for others, understand the importance of variety, accommodate differences, control the environment for safety, and monitor and record clients' progress.**

FORM 17.1

Daily Activity Form

Name: ______________________ Target weight: ______________ Target heart rate zone: ______________

Week	*Day*	*Weight*	*Resting BP*	*Resting HR*	*Exercise HR*	*RPE*	*Signs*	*Symptoms*	*Comments*
1	Mon	____	____	____	____	____	____	____	____
	Wed	____	____	____	____	____	____	____	____
	Fri	____	____	____	____	____	____	____	____
2	Mon	____	____	____	____	____	____	____	____
	Wed	____	____	____	____	____	____	____	____
	Fri	____	____	____	____	____	____	____	____
3	Mon	____	____	____	____	____	____	____	____
	Wed	____	____	____	____	____	____	____	____
	Fri	____	____	____	____	____	____	____	____
4	Mon	____	____	____	____	____	____	____	____
	Wed	____	____	____	____	____	____	____	____
	Fri	____	____	____	____	____	____	____	____

Behavioral Strategies of the Effective Exercise Leader

1. Show a sincere interest in the participants. Learn why they have gotten involved in your program and what they would really like to achieve.
2. Be enthusiastic in your instruction and guidance.
3. Develop a personal association and relationship with each participant.
4. Consider the various reasons why adults exercise (i.e., health, recreation, weight loss, social, personal appearance) and allow for individual differences.
5. Initiate participant follow-up (e.g., postcards or telephone calls) when several unexplained absences occur in succession. Novice exercisers should be advised that an inevitable slip in attendance does not imply failure.
6. Practice what you preach. Participate in the exercise sessions yourself. Good posture and grooming are essential to projecting the desired self-image. Cigarette smoking should be prohibited, and drinking soda or eating candy on the gymnasium floor should also be unacceptable.
7. Honor special days (e.g., birthdays) or exercise accomplishments with extrinsic rewards such as T-shirts, ribbons, or certificates.
8. Attend personally to orthopedic and musculoskeletal problems. Provide alternatives to floor exercise.
9. Counsel participants on proper foot apparel and exercise clothing.
10. Avoid constant references to complicated medical or physiological terminology, but don't ignore it altogether. Concentrate on a few selected terms to provide a little education at a time.
11. Arrange for occasional visits by personal physicians.
12. Provide a constant flow of newspaper or magazine articles to the participants on topics related to physical activity and other pertinent information.
13. Encourage an occasional visitor or participant to lead activity.
14. Have a designated area for participant counseling. Avoid trying to converse with clients while performing another task simultaneously.
15. Display your continuing education certifications and educational degrees. You are more likely to be successful at modifying behavior if you are perceived to be an expert.
16. Introduce "first-time" exercisers on the gymnasium floor or in the locker room. This orientation will encourage a sense of belonging to the group.
17. Reinforce participants by complimenting them on their appearance as they are exercising. Your conversation during exercise can also serve as a distractor from any unpleasant sensations that they may be experiencing.
18. Consider entering city- or business-sponsored road races to pace your participants. Exercise leaders can also show their interest and enthusiasm by cheering clients at community fitness events.

Reprinted from Franklin et al. 1990.

In Review: Asking for participants' heart rate, perceived exertion (RPE), and any unusual responses to the exercise are ways to monitor exercise intensity during an exercise session.

PROGRESSION OF ACTIVITIES

Sedentary people who want to begin a fitness program should follow a logical sequence of fitness activities. Moderate-intensity activities are encouraged for everyone, but a systematic program of activities should be provided to help participants achieve an increase in functional capacity. The following paragraphs summarize our recommendations on how this can be accomplished.

Phase 1: Regular Walking

The first phase, for sedentary individuals, is to get them in the habit of including exercise as a part of their weekly patterns. The major fitness goal is to be able to increase the exercise that can be done comfortably, so no emphasis on intensity is necessary at this point. The person starts with the distance that can be walked easily without pain or fatigue, then gradually increases the distance and pace until about 4 mi can be walked briskly every other day. People with an orthopedic limitation can substitute a weight-supported activity such as cycling, rowing, or swimming.

Phase 2: Recommended Work Levels for a Change in Fitness

Once Phase 1 is accomplished, the person is taught about recommended levels of work for fitness changes (see chapter 14). A work-relief, interval training program is introduced—jogging is the work, and walking is the relief. So the person walks, jogs a few steps, then walks, and so forth. Gradually, jogging covers more distance than walking, until the person can jog continuously for 2 to 3 mi at target heart rate (THR). Interval training can also be used by people interested in cycling and swimming (see later in this chapter). People interested in aerobic dance should transition from the walking program to a low-intensity, low-impact class.

Phase 3: Variety of Fitness Activities

The first two phases are generally recommended for everyone (with alternative activities for people who cannot or choose not to jog—such as cycling, dancing, or running in water). Phase 3, on the other hand, is quite individualized, based on the person's interests. The purpose is to promote the continued activity habit by participation in an activity that the person naturally enjoys. Some people prefer to continue to stretch, walk, and jog; some prefer to exercise alone; and others (the majority) enjoy working out with others. Some people like cooperative and relatively low-level competitive activities, and others like the thrill of competition. Some enjoy a variety of different movement forms; others enjoy repeating the same type of activity. The HFI must provide an atmosphere where people feel free to try new things without embarrassment and allow individuals to choose from among a variety of options for their fitness activities.

WALK/JOG/RUN PROGRAMS

While walking, at least one foot is in contact with the ground at all times. In jogging and running more muscular force is exerted to propel the body completely off the ground, causing a nonsupport phase. The distinction between jogging and running is not as clearly defined. Some people view the speed as being the difference, but no single criterion for speed is commonly accepted. Others distinguish between the two by the intent of the participant—a jogger is simply interested in exercise, whereas a runner trains to achieve performance goals in road races.

General Safety Considerations

There are a variety of safety factors common to both walking and jogging that should be mentioned before we begin a presentation of how to institute walking and jogging programs.

Footwear

Any comfortable pair of good, well-supported shoes can be worn for a beginning walking program. The serious walker and all joggers should invest in appropriate shoes having well-padded heels that are higher than the soles and a fitted heel cup. The shoes should be flexible enough to bend easily. The same kind of socks that will be worn while exercising should be worn during the fitting to ensure a comfortable and proper fit. Only the serious competitive runner needs racing shoes, which are a lighter weight and offer less cushioning.

Clothing

The weather conditions and vigorousness of the activity determine the amount and type of clothing to be worn. Warm weather dictates light, preferably cotton, loose-fitting clothing. Nothing should be worn that prevents perspiration from reaching the outside air. A brimmed hat should cover the head on hot, sunny days. For the jogger, long pants are probably not needed until the temperature (wind-chill factor considered) drops below 40 °F.

In cold weather the walker or jogger should dress in layers for the flexibility of removing or adding clothing when necessary. Wool and the new polypropylene fabrics are good choices for extreme cold, but most joggers have a tendency to overdress. A hat, preferably a wool stocking cap, that can be pulled down over the forehead and ears and gloves or mittens also should be worn. Cotton socks worn as mittens are useful not only to keep hands warm but also to act as "wipers" for the sniffling nose that often accompanies cold-weather walking and jogging.

Surface

The surface for walkers is not as crucial as it is for joggers, although some walkers (especially those with orthopedic problems) should exercise on a soft surface such as grass or a running track with a shock-absorbent surface. Many people prefer exercising off of the track for visual stimulation and interest, but regular jogging on hard surfaces such as concrete or blacktop can lead to stress problems in the ankle, knee, and hip joints and in the lower back. Joggers need to observe special precautions when running on the road: Jog facing traffic, assume cars at crossroads do not see joggers, and beware of cracks and curbs. Running cross country usually means running on a softer surface, but joggers must be aware of the uneven terrain and the increased potential for ankle injuries.

Safety Tips

Educate your participants that for safety when walking or jogging, they should

- move toward the oncoming traffic;
- yield the right of way to cars;
- listen to music only while exercising on a very quiet street, and always listen for and be aware of traffic;
- choose well-lighted streets or running tracks on school grounds; and
- walk or jog with a partner if you must exercise at night.

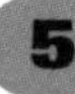

5 **In Review: Walkers and joggers should have supportive and flexible shoes and should wear clothing that accommodates weather conditions and exercise intensity. They should follow rules of the road and walk or jog in safe areas at safe times.**

Walking

The advantages of walking include its convenience, practicality, and naturalness. Walking is an excellent activity, especially for people who are overfat and poorly conditioned and whose joints cannot handle the stresses of jogging.

As with all exercise programs, the participants begin with warm-up activities and perhaps some static stretching before the actual walk. The walk should begin at a slow speed and gradually increase to a pace that feels comfortable to the participant. The arms should swing freely, and the trunk should be kept erect with a slight backward pelvic tilt. The feet should be pointing forward at all times. Many walkers have taken to malls, which provide air-conditioned comfort, safety, and a smooth surface and are usually within a short, convenient drive.

Walking programs can progress by increasing the distance and/or the speed. Participants should gradually increase their distances until they can easily walk 4 mi at a brisk pace. Thinking about jogging or achieving the THR in an aerobic dance class is not necessary until the 4-mi walking goal can be reached. The Walking Program on page 341 is graduated and leads to an activity level needed for individuals who want to start a jogging program.

How do you make walking interesting for a class of 30 to 40 participants? An exercise leader must emphasize variety to keep interest high in such situations. Some ways you might do this are to

- have participants follow the leader over hill and dale, up and down steps or slopes, with the walking speed changing from time to time;

Walking Program

Rules

1. Start at a level that is comfortable to you.
2. Be aware of new aches or pains.
3. Don't progress to the next level if you are not comfortable.
4. Monitor your heart rate and record it.
5. It is healthful to walk at least every other day.

Stage	*Duration*	*Heart rate*	*Comments*
1	15 min	______	______________________
2	20 min	______	______________________
3	25 min	______	______________________
4	30 min	______	______________________
5	30 min	______	______________________
6	30 min	______	______________________
7	35 min	______	______________________
8	40 min	______	______________________
9	45 min	______	______________________
10	45 min	______	______________________
11	45 min	______	______________________
12	50 min	______	______________________
13	55 min	______	______________________
14	60 min	______	______________________
15	60 min	______	______________________
16	60 min	______	______________________
17	60 min	______	______________________
18	60 min	______	______________________
19	60 min	______	______________________
20	60 min	______	______________________

Reprinted from Franks and Howley 1989.

- have the group do "line-walking" on a track, in which the person at the end of the line must walk faster to catch up to the front of the line, which, as a whole, moves at a steady pace—giving each person an interval-type workout;
- add a ball to the front of the line-walking line, and have participants pass it to the side or overhead until it reaches the end of the line, at which time the last person dribbles to the front and restarts the process;

- vary the activity used to reach the front of the line-walking line, with people skipping, jogging, and so on;
- vary the length of the line-walking line so that "teams" can be formed, and control the overall pace by balancing the teams and checking the THR;
- plan a game of "tag" in a gym or field where all participants must walk, with the leader exerting control by defining the boundaries; and
- establish a distance goal for a 15-week walking class—such as "we will walk from here to Nashville" (a total of 180 mi walked over the 15 weeks)—and use a large map to monitor each participant's progress from week to week, using stick pins. Award T-shirts or hold a country-western party when everyone finishes. Longer distances can be used along with the class total of miles walked to focus on group accomplishments.

6 **In Review: Walking programs should begin at a slow speed and gradually increase the speed to a comfortable pace. Distance should be increased gradually until 4 mi can be walked at a brisk pace. The previous list details activities that improve enjoyment and, consequently, adherence to the program.**

Jogging

No single factor determines when an individual can begin jogging. A person who can walk about 4 mi briskly but is unable to reach the THR range by walking should consider a jogging program to make additional improvements in CRF. A slow to moderate walker whose HR is within the THR zone should increase the distance and/or speed of walking rather than begin jogging. Also, the ability of the individual's joints to withstand the additional stresses of jogging should be considered. Remember, walking may be the first and only activity for a large number of people, and it is more important that they stay active than move up the scale to more intense activities.

The techniques of jogging are basically the same as walking. Jogging requires a greater flexion of the knee of the recovery leg, and the arms are bent more at the elbows. The arm swing is exaggerated slightly but should still be in the forward/backward direction. The heel makes the first contact with the ground; then the foot immediately rolls forward to the ball of the foot and then to the toes. As speed increases, the landing foot may contact the ground closer to a flat-footed position. Breathing is done through both the nose and mouth. Common faults of the beginning jogger include breathing with the mouth closed, insufficiently bending the knee during the recovery phase, and swinging the arms across the body.

Many people begin jogging at too high a speed, which results in an inability to continue for a sufficient length of time to accomplish the desired amount of total work; often this causes people to dislike jogging. This problem can be prevented by jogging at a speed slow enough to allow conversation and using work-relief intervals, which for beginners is slow jogging for a few seconds, then walking, then slow jogging, and so forth. Participants should be reassured that they will be walking less and/or jogging more as they become more fit. An example of such a progression is shown in the Jogging Program on page 343.

7 **In Review: Stages 1 through 5 of the Jogging Program are appropriate walk/jog intervals to use at the beginning of a jogging program.**

After a person has progressed to the point where 2 or 3 mi can be jogged continuously within the THR zone, several approaches to a jogging program are available. A person can just go out and jog 3 or 4 times a week, with the only plan being to exercise at an intensity that will elevate the HR to the training zone for a predetermined minimum length of time (or distance), with the option to go longer (or farther) on days when so desired. Other people do better with a specific program to follow that gives progressive speed and distance goals, even if they do not have plans for competition.

As for the walking class mentioned earlier, the HFI should include variety in a jogging program, and the same types of modifications cited earlier for the walking program would be appropriate. In addition, in some communities where there are established exercise or fitness trails, one can combine walking/jogging with specific exercises for all parts of the body. "Fun runs" are often held in many communities; the goal is to finish the distance, and a small prize is usually awarded.

Joggers who are not fast enough to compete successfully in road races may enjoy other types of competition, such as prediction runs, in which speed

Jogging Program

Rules

1. Complete the Walking Program before starting this program.
2. Begin each session with walking and stretching.
3. Be aware of new aches and pains.
4. Don't progress to the next level if you are not comfortable.
5. Stay at the low end of your THR zone; record your heart rate for each session.
6. Do the program on a work-a-day, rest-a-day basis.

Stage 1	Jog 10 steps; then walk 10 steps. Repeat five times and take your heart rate. Stay within THR zone by increasing or decreasing walking phase. Do 20 to 30 min of activity.
Stage 2	Jog 20 steps; walk 10 steps. Repeat five times and take your heart rate. Stay within THR zone by increasing or decreasing walking phase. Do 20 to 30 min of activity.
Stage 3	Jog 30 steps; walk 10 steps. Repeat five times and take your heart rate. Stay within THR zone by increasing or decreasing walking phase. Do 20 to 30 min of activity.
Stage 4	Jog 1 min; walk 10 steps. Repeat three times and take your heart rate. Stay within THR zone by increasing or decreasing walking phase. Do 20 to 30 min of activity.
Stage 5	Jog 2 min; walk 10 steps. Repeat two times and take your heart rate. Stay within THR zone by increasing or decreasing walking phase. Do 30 min of activity.
Stage 6	Jog 1 lap (400 m, or 440 yd) and check your heart rate. Adjust pace during run to stay within the THR zone. If heart rate is still too high, go back to the Stage 5 schedule. Do 6 laps with a brief walk between each.
Stage 7	Jog 2 laps and check heart rate. Adjust pace during run to stay within the THR zone. If heart rate is still too high, go back to Stage 6 activity. Do 6 laps with a brief walk between each.
Stage 8	Jog 1 mi and check heart rate. Adjust pace during the run to stay within THR zone. Do 2 mi.
Stage 9	Jog 2 to 3 mi continuously. Check heart rate at the end to ensure that you were within THR zone.

Reprinted from Franks and Howley 1989.

does not determine the winner. The purpose of a prediction run is to see which jogger comes closest to her or his predicted time of finishing, which is declared before the race. A "handicapped" run requires joggers to know and declare their previous fastest times for the distance. A percentage (80% to 100%) of the time difference between the fastest runner's declared time and each other runner's time is subtracted from each runner's actual finish time. For example, suppose runner A's fastest previous time is 18 min for 3 mi; runner B's, 19 min; and runner C's, 20 min. Forty-eight s (0.8 [80%] × 60-s difference between A and B) is subtracted from B's finish time, and 96 s (0.8 × 120-s difference) is subtracted from runner C's. Suppose runner A completes the race in 17:50, runner B in 18:30, and C in 20:10. The adjusted finish times would be runner A = 17:50 (actual time), runner B = 17:42 (18:30 – 48), and runner C = 18:34 (20:10 – 96). Runner B is the winner. Another method of handicapping a race is to stagger the start according to each jogger's previous best time, with the slowest runner starting first, the fastest last. The first one over the finish line is the winner. Teams can be formed in which each four-member team, for example, could have one runner from each of four groups classified by running speed.

Competitive Running

In almost all communities there are road races sponsored by track clubs and service organizations as a means of raising funds, many for worthy purposes. Each entrant pays a registration fee, and most of the races have gender and age divisions, with prizes awarded to the top finishers, both overall and in each division. Usually every finisher receives an award such as a certificate or T-shirt. The race distances range between 1 mi (often considered a "fun run") and 100 mi, but the most common are the 5K (3.1 mi) and 10K (6.2 mi). Remember that fitness participants should not be pressured to enter road races by those who enjoy them. The HFI should consider entering races with interested participants to help them select a starting spot and establish a pace and to provide encouragement. This may help them make a good transition from a jogging group to an individualized jogging program.

It must be remembered that those who train for performance goals will be working at the top part of the THR range, 6 to 7 days per week, and for more than 30 to 40 min per exercise session. Such programs are bound to result in more injuries, and the HFI should encourage participants pursuing such goals to have an alternative activity that they can enjoy when they are recovering from injuries.

CYCLING

Riding a bicycle or stationary exercise cycle is another good fitness activity. Some people who have problems walking, jogging, or playing sports may be able to cycle without difficulty. The Cycling Program on page 345 follows the guidelines for making CRF improvements (see chapter 14). Although bicycles and terrain vary widely, checking THR allows the cyclist to adjust the speed so that she or he is working at the appropriate intensity. Generally, a person covers three to four times the distance cycling compared to jogging (e.g., a person works up to 3 mi jogging or 9 to 12 mi cycling per workout). The seat should be comfortable, and its height should be adjusted so that the knee is slightly bent at the bottom of the pedaling stroke.

8 **In Review: In general, one should cycle three to four times the distance compared with jogging for an equivalent caloric expenditure and cardiorespiratory workout.**

GAMES

One of the wonderful characteristics of children that is often lost in adulthood is a sense of playfulness. A child does not feel a need to justify spending time playing a game just for the fun of it. One of the attributes that seems to be present in coronary-prone behavior is the inability to appreciate play for its own sake. Perhaps one of the things a good fitness program can do for people is provide them with activities that increase both fitness *and* playfulness.

For games to be an effective part of a fitness program, certain elements must be present:

- *competition*—Competition is not to be avoided, but little emphasis should be put on winning; the game should not be used to exclude people from participating.
- *cooperation*—Having small groups solve problems together to accomplish fitness tasks can be enjoyable and healthy.
- *enjoyment*—Enjoyment requires a balance of cooperation and competition, continued participation by everyone, and the chance for everyone to be a winner.
- *inclusion*—A key ingredient for a fitness game is that everyone is included. This may mean modifying the rules.
- *skill*—Some fitness games may require certain minimum levels of skill that can be taught as part of the fitness program.

Cycling Program

Rules

1. Adjust the seat so that it is comfortable for you.
2. Use either a regular bicycle or a stationary exercise cycle.
3. If you are starting at Stage 1, simply get used to riding 1 or 2 mi. Don't be concerned about time or reaching the lower end of your THR zone.

Stage	*Distance (mi)*	*THR (%HRmax)*	*Time (min)*	*Frequency (days/week)*
1	1-2	—	—	3
2	1-2	60	8-12	3
3	3-5	60	15-25	3
4	6-8	70	25-35	3
5	6-9	70	25-35	4
6	10-15	70	40-60	4
7	10-15	80	35-50	4-5

Reprinted from Franks and Howley 1989.

- *vigor*—The main body of the workout should include games in which all participants are continuously active in the THR range.

Special Considerations

The warm-up and cool-down activities of most games can be done by participants at any fitness level. The more vigorous games, however, usually involve high-intensity bursts, stopping, starting, and quickly changing directions. They are not recommended for the early stages of a fitness program. Some additional stretching and easy movements in different directions should be included as part of the warm-up for games. Obviously the space, number of people, equipment, and so forth have to be considered in the selection of activities. The leader must emphasize safety and should change the rules immediately when something is not working. A variety of games should be offered, so that people with different skill levels can participate. When large groups are involved in activities, the activities should be changed frequently to maintain interest. In addition to warm-up and cool-down activities, higher- and lower-intensity activities should be alternated to prevent undue fatigue. People should be encouraged to go at their own pace. THR should be checked periodically to ensure that people are within their ranges.

Fitness Games

The classes of Fitness Games and Activities are summarized on page 346. In general, the level of control varies from that associated with circle and line activities to those with few rules, such as "keep-away." Games can involve diverse muscle groups, using the body weight as a resistance. Simultaneously, games encourage the continued development of balance and coordination, which are not necessarily outcomes of walking, jogging, or exercising with fixed equipment. *On the Ball* (3), a book written specifically to encourage games in a fitness setting, should be a part of every exercise leader's library. In addition, *The New Games Book* (12) provides a playful, fun, and inclusive approach to games for various numbers of people. In games, as with all activities, the HFI needs to include individuals with disabilities by modifying or adapting the activities (6).

Fitness Games and Activities

1. Skills and games with balls of various sizes. The size and type of ball can lead to innovative use—for instance, the cage ball can be used as a substitute for a basketball. Examples of other balls include tennis balls, volleyballs, playground balls, basketballs, medicine balls, handballs, softballs, mush balls, and Nerf balls.
2. Activities with apparatus. Examples include hoola hoops, Frisbees, paddle rackets, skip ropes, skittles, "quoits," surgical tubing, culverts, and play buoys.
3. Chasing games. Examples include tag, chain tag, fox and geese, and dodge ball.
4. Relays with and without apparatus. Examples include running, hopping, rolling, crawling, and dribbling with hands and feet.
5. Stunts and contests. Examples are dual activities such as balancing stunts, foward rolls, backward rolls, strength moves, push-ups, sit-ups, and limited combatives such as rooster fights and partner sparring.
6. Lead-up games for major sport games. Examples are soccer, tennis, basketball, volleyball, handball, and football, often with rules adjusted to fit the level of skill and capacity of the participants.
7. Children's games. Activities include skittle ball, four square, and bounce ball.

Adapted from Giese, 1988, Organization of an exercise testing session. In *Resource manual for guidelines for exercise testing and prescription*. By permission of Lea & Febiger.

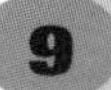

In Review: Effective games for a fitness program should be enjoyable, inclusive, vigorous, cooperative, competitive, and skill-related.

AQUATIC ACTIVITIES

Aquatic activities can be a major part of a person's exercise program or can be the needed relief from other forms of exercise, especially when a person is injured. The intensity of the activity can be graded to suit the needs of the least and the most fit, from the recent postmyocardial infarction patient to the endurance athlete. HR can be checked at regular intervals to see whether THR has been reached, and a caloric expenditure goal can be achieved, given the high-energy requirement associated with aquatic activities. Individuals with orthopedic problems who cannot run, dance, or play games can exercise in water. The water supports the person's body weight, and problems associated with weight-bearing joints are minimized.

Target Heart Rate

One consistent finding is that the maximal HR response to a swimming test is about 18 beats · min^{-1} lower than that found in a maximal treadmill test. This suggests that for swimming, THR should be shifted downward (2 beats less for a 10-s count) to achieve the 60% to 80% $\dot{V}O_2max$ goal associated with an endurance training effect (9).

Progression

Swimming activities can be graded not only by varying the speed of the swim but also by varying the activity. A postmyocardial infarction patient with an extremely low functional capacity benefits from simply walking through the water. People with recent bypass surgery benefit from moving the arms as they walk across the pool. Following are examples of the types of activities that can be used in aquatic exercise programs. The reader is referred to the books *Water Fitness After 40* by Ruth Sova (15) and *Water Exercise* by Martha White (17) as well as to the Aquatic Exercise Association (P.O. Box 497, Port

Washington, WI 53074) for information on certification programs for this specialty.

Side-of-Pool Activities

A wide variety of activities can be done while holding on to the side of the pool with one or both hands. These range from simple movements of the legs to the side, front, or back to practicing a variety of kicks that can ultimately be used while swimming. Range-of-motion-type movements in the pool are a good way to warm up before undertaking the more vigorous activities of walking or jogging across the pool.

Walking and Jogging Across the Pool

A person with a low functional capacity can begin an aquatic program by simply walking across the shallow end of the pool. The water offers resistance to the movement while supporting the body weight, resulting in a reduced downward load on the ankles, knees, and hips. The arms can be involved in the activity to simulate a swimming motion; this increases the range of motion of the arms and shoulder girdle. The speed and form of the walk can be changed as the person becomes accustomed to the activity. The person can walk with long strides with the head just above the water or do a side step across the pool. Lastly, the person can practice jogging across the pool with the water at chest height. Remember to check to see whether THR has been achieved.

Flotation Devices

People with limited skill can use flotation devices (e.g., a life jacket or kickboard). The extra resistance offered by the jacket compensates for the extra buoyancy it provides. The participant should stop periodically to determine whether THR has been reached.

Lap Swimming

The participant must be skilled to use swimming as a substitute activity for running or cycling. An unskilled swimmer operates at a very high energy cost, even when moving slowly, and may become too fatigued to last through the whole workout. But this doesn't mean that swimming should be eliminated as an option in personal fitness programs. A person can learn to swim over a period of several months, gradually adjusting during that time to the exercise. After learning to swim, the person becomes able to use swimming as the primary activity, even if elementary strokes are used. Increasing the number of activities a person can do increases the chance that the person will remain active when something interferes with a primary activity.

Lap swimming should be approached the same way as lap running: warming up with stretching activities, starting slowly, taking frequent breaks to check the pulse rate, and gradually increasing the distance. Remember, the caloric cost of swimming compared to the cost of running is about a 1:4 ratio. If jogging a total distance of 1 mi is a reasonable goal in someone's physical activity program, then swimming 400 m (one-quarter mile) is equivalent in terms of energy expenditure. The Swimming Program on page 348 describes a series of stages that could be included in an endurance swimming program, beginning with walking across the pool. All steps assume that a warm-up has preceded the activity and that a cool-down follows.

The HFI should not view the stages in the Swimming Program as discrete steps that must be followed in a particular order. Two stages can be combined, or games can be introduced, to make the walk-and-jog and width swims more enjoyable. The major point to keep in mind is to gradually increase the intensity and duration of the aquatic activities.

10 **In Review: Various aquatic activities include doing upright activities (e.g., walking and jogging across the pool, using flotation devices) as well as swimming. Exercises can also be done holding on to the side of the pool, such as moving the legs from front to back or practicing a paddle kick.**

EXERCISING TO MUSIC

Moving to the rhythm of music is an enjoyable way to participate in exercise. One can join a group at a fitness club, do individual workouts with a personal fitness trainer, or exercise at home with videotapes.

Advantages

Exercise to music provides an enjoyable fitness activity for many participants—young and old, male

Swimming Program

Rules

1. Start at a level that is comfortable for you.
2. Don't progress to the next stage if you are not comfortable with the current one.
3. Monitor and record your heart rate.

Stage 1	In chest-deep water, walk across the width of the pool four times and see if you are close to THR. Gradually increase the duration of the walk until you can do two 10-min walks at THR.
Stage 2	In chest-deep water, walk across and jog back. Repeat twice and see if you are close to THR. Gradually increase the duration of the jogging until you can complete four 5-min jogs at THR.
Stage 3	In chest-deep water, walk across and swim back (any stroke). Use a kick-board or flotation device if needed. Repeat this cycle twice and see if you are at THR. Keep up this pattern of walk-swim to do about 20 to 30 min of activity.
Stage 4	In chest-deep water, jog across and swim back (any stroke); repeat and check THR. Gradually decrease the duration of the jog and increase the duration of the swim until four widths can be completed within the THR zone. Accomplish 20 to 30 min of activity per session.
Stage 5	Slowly swim 25 yd, rest 20 s. Slowly swim another 25 yd, and check THR. On the basis of the heart rate response, change the speed of the swim and/or the length of the rest period to stay within the THR zone. Gradually increase the number of lengths you can swim (e.g., three, then four) before checking THR.
Stage 6	Increase the duration of continuous swimming until you can accomplish 20 to 30 min without a rest.

Reprinted from Franks and Howley 1989.

and female. Since the mid-1970s aerobics has evolved from the traditional high-intensity and low-impact classes to a variety of specialized classes to fit everyone's tastes and fitness levels. The use of water, steps, slides, tubing, resistance balls, martial arts, and boxing provide numerous opportunities to cross-train or learn new techniques. Fortunately, certification and continuing education programs to support this expansion have developed in conjunction with these trends (see later in this chapter).

Getting Motivated

Working out to music is a great way to motivate people to continue exercising. The variety of tempos and rhythms of the different songs keeps the workout exciting and challenging for participants. Familiar lyrics often distract from the feeling of fatigue. Music makes routine exercises fun, and the class setting helps to promote camaraderie and regular participation.

Achieving Target Heart Rate

Aerobic dance programs can develop all the fitness components. The recommended frequency, intensity, and total work (see chapter 14) can be achieved in exercise-to-music programs and cause gains in $\dot{V}O_2$max (18). THR can be monitored easily following a music segment, but beginners need to be cautioned about doing too much too soon. A recent review indicated that THR can be achieved with either low- or high-impact routines. Although the energy cost of high-intensity, high-impact aerobic dance is higher than that of low-impact programs for the same routines and music, the activities are not very different in terms of caloric expenditure when multidirectional movements are included in the low-impact routines (18).

Low Skill Requirement

Movement to music can be adapted to any skill level because no competition is involved. The only rule is to keep moving at a pace needed to achieve THR. The routines can also be adapted for all ages. Most aerobics classes provide participants with an appropriate workout routine within a safe environment (assuming instructors are certified and emphasize safe exercises). Warm-ups are structured to provide low-impact movements and dynamic stretching prior to the 30-40 min of the cardiovascular portion of the workout. Gradual progression within each session, as well as from one workout to the next, is provided to enhance enjoyment.

The HFI should be familiar with the types of aerobic dance programs offered in his or her community because some (e.g., Jazzercize®) may require more knowledge and skill of "dance" movements than other forms. HFIs should also be aware of the programs that would be appropriate for different age, skill-level, and interest groups.

Disadvantages

Injury is always a potential risk in fitness programs, and aerobic dance is no different. One review found that about 44% of students and 76% of instructors reported injuries resulting from aerobic dance, with the injury rate being 1 injury per 100 hr of activity for students, and 0.22 to 1.16 injuries per 100 hr for the instructors. The severity of the injuries, however, were such that only once in 1092 to 4275 hr of participation did an individual have to seek medical attention (5). It is our recommendation that people should participate in aerobic dance programs *only after* they can walk about 4 mi *without discomfort.* They should move from low-intensity, low-impact sessions to more strenuous sessions using THR as a guide. Furthermore, introductory classes to step or other specialized forms of aerobics should be taken to develop the skills needed for participation in the regular classes.

It is not uncommon for individuals to experience muscle soreness, as well as a variety of acute soft-tissue injuries, due to regular participation in aerobic activities. In addition, evidence shows that chronic conditions may develop due to improper form, or simply doing large numbers of repetitions of a specific exercise. These can include

- chronic shoulder soreness from too many overhead pulls,
- elbow or wrist pain from the use of hand-held weights in aerobics classes,
- Achilles tendonitis and plantar fasciitis from high-impact forces and improper step techniques,
- groin pulls and shin splints from improper slide technique,
- low-back problems from exercising with weak abdominals (anterior pelvic tilt) and doing improper stretching, and
- knee problems from using a step that is too high.

It is also common for instructors and participants to experience some hearing losses from music played too loud. See chapter 21 for advice on how to prevent and deal with acute and chronic problems associated with participation in exercise.

Here are some suggestions to minimize the risk of injury in exercise-to-music classes:

1. Warm up with low-impact activity and dynamic stretching, and cool down with static stretches of the following muscles: calf, anterior tibialis, quadriceps, hamstrings, hip flexors, low-back area, and shoulders.
2. Avoid hypertension of the neck.
3. Avoid forward flexion of the spine unless supported by a bent knee balanced directly over the heel.
4. Practice correct standing posture (i.e., pelvis in neutral position, buttocks tight, head and chin up, shoulders back).
5. Avoid deep-knee bends; don't take a squat to where the thighs are below parallel and the knees are over the toes rather than placed properly over the middle of the foot.
6. Wear good shoes with good cushioning and support.
7. Work all muscle groups evenly to achieve a balanced workout.
8. Do not stop in the middle of a routine to prevent venous pooling in the lower legs.
9. The leader should practice routines to ensure that movement transitions are smooth, safe,

and easy to follow. Teach basic movements before using them in combination.

10. Monitor the class at all times. Use eye contact, emphasize safe movements by making corrections while leading, and check target heart rate or RPE regularly.

Music Selection

Selection of music for different phases of the exercise session sets the tone for the appropriate intensity of warm-up, aerobic phase, and cool-down (8, 10). The music can vary, depending on choice, from top-40 hits to instrumental Muzak. The warm-up starts slowly, with the music tempo about 100 beats · min^{-1}. The cardiorespiratory endurance phase includes increasingly intense aerobic exercises at a faster pace (no more than 160 beats · min^{-1}) while the muscle conditioning phase (typically including abdominal work) is set to a slower tempo (usually 118 to 130 beats · min^{-1}). Step classes are limited to 118 to 125 beats · min^{-1}, and slide classes are restricted to < 140 beats · min^{-1}. In the final cool-down, the music tempo and volume are decreased to invoke a relaxing conclusion.

The leader should consider purchasing music selections from one of the many aerobic music companies in the fitness market. They sell professionally mixed music selections with appropriate tempos for each class. Not only are the tapes made for specific classes (e.g., step, slide, low-impact), but most companies pay the licensing fees that protect the instructor from suits related to fraud. The music should be changed periodically to provide variety.

Components

There are no set routines; the program can be individualized by the instructor. Suggested components of an exercise session include a full-body warm-up (including low-impact and dynamic flexibility exercises); exercises for cardiorespiratory endurance using a variety of muscle groups; an active standing recovery cool-down; exercises for muscular endurance and strength for the arms, legs, and abdominals; and a final cool-down.

An easy progression for beginners would include 25 to 30 min of mostly flexibility activities, with light muscular and cardiorespiratory endurance activities. A more advanced program would last 45 to 60 min, with longer duration for all of the fitness components. The phases of an exercise-to-music class are discussed next.

Warm-Up

For a gradual progression, the program should begin with low-impact movements and dynamic stretching for the whole body. Dynamic flexibility includes exercises such as arm circles, side bends, back rolls, half-knee bends, stationary lunges, toe taps, and Achilles curls. The warm-up should continue for 5 to 10 min, gradually bringing the heart rate up and preparing the body for the cardiorespiratory workout to come.

Cardiorespiratory Endurance

In this segment, movements concentrate on the large muscles of the legs, with arm movements adding flair and extra cardiorespiratory intensity (arm movements are optional). This segment is specific to the type of class. For the high-intensity/low-impact classes, marches, step-touches, hops, strides, skips, knee lifts, hamstring curls, jumping jacks, step-hops, cross-over steps, toe-heel kicks, and so forth are used to elevate the heart rate within the target heart rate zone. The instructor can individualize the style from a calisthenics workout to a funky dance routine.

If the class utilizes a step or slide the leader should be knowledgeable and trained in that form of movement to provide safe instruction. It is most important for an aerobics instructor to hold a national certification and be able to lead a class with smooth transitions before instructing a class on her or his own.

The duration of the cardiorespiratory section is 15 to 40 min, with THR taken about every 15 min. The intensity of this segment can be increased by using more vigorous arm movements or higher hops (power jumps), and it can be decreased by lowering the arms, slowing the pace, and walking rather than jogging through the movement. It is recommended that one stay within the safety guidelines for speed of music, height of step, and width of slide. This element of control will enhance the participant's safety.

Recovery Cool-Down

A 2 to 5 min active-standing cool-down should follow the cardiorespiratory segment. It should begin by lowering the intensity of the previous activities (e.g., walking) to decrease the heart rate. Dynamic stretches should be repeated, followed by static stretches.

Muscular Endurance

Once the recovery cool-down is completed, the muscular endurance exercises can be performed for

10 to 20 min. It is recommended that these activities begin with exercises done in the standing position, with a gradual movement to the floor. Many classes end with abdominal work in the supine position.

Final Cool-Down

The final cool-down consists mainly of static stretches done lying on the floor. The stretches are held for at least 10 s. Incorporate every muscle group, especially those specifically worked on in the class, with special focus on the hamstrings and low back.

Aerobic Dance Organizations

Here are some of the many aerobic dance organizations that provide opportunities to be certified as well as educational and professional support materials:

- Aerobex, Fort Sanders West, 270 Fort Sanders West Boulevard, Knoxville, TN 37922
- Aerobics and Fitness Association of America (AFAA), 15250 Ventura Boulevard, Suite 200, Sherman Oaks, CA 91403
- American Aerobics Association International, International Sports Medicine Association (AAAI/ISMA), P.O. Box 15016, Richboro, PA 18954
- American Council on Exercise (ACE), 5820 Oberlin Drive, Suite 102, San Diego, CA 92121-3787
- Jazzercize, 2808 Roosevelt Boulevard, Carlsbad, CA 92008

11 **In Review: Beginning dance exercisers should be able to walk 4 mi without discomfort before participating in aerobic dance programs. Components of an exercise session include a full-body warm-up; exercises for cardiorespiratory endurance using a variety of muscle groups; an active-standing recovery cool-down; exercises for muscular endurance and strength for the arms, legs, and abdominals; and a final cool-down.**

EXERCISE EQUIPMENT

The traditional walk, jog, run, and dance programs offered by an exercise leader have been supplemented in many fitness clubs by exercise equipment. The equipment includes treadmills, cycle ergometers, ski machines, rowers, climbing ergometers, and stepping devices. The variety of equipment can help a participant stay with an exercise program as well as provide feedback about the number of calories used. Participants with orthopedic limitations can choose weight-supported activities (e.g., cycle ergometers). People training for specific performance goals can do so in air-conditioned comfort, although air conditioning may be a problem for participants who plan to engage in races scheduled for hot days; and the issue of acclimatization to a hot environment must be addressed for reasons of performance and safety (see chapters 14 and 21).

If a participant plans to buy exercise equipment for home use, the HFI can help with the decision by encouraging experimentation with all types of equipment and, within each type (e.g., rowing machines), as many brands as possible. The cost of the equipment may appear high in the short term, but it may be a wise investment in the long run in terms of health care costs, provided it is used.

Generally, fitness clubs provide a variety of strength training equipment (e.g., Nautilus or Universal Gym) that can be used as part of an overall workout or as a separate strength training workout on another day. Recommendations for gains in muscular strength and endurance were presented in chapter 15. The emphasis at the start of a program must be on endurance, low resistance, and high repetitions. As strength and interest increase, some participants may shift the emphasis to high-resistance, low-repetition workouts. It is important to work all the major muscle groups evenly, rather than to concentrate on gaining strength only in a few.

12 **In Review: Appropriate beginning goals for people using exercise equipment are to emphasize endurance, low resistance, and high repetitions. Encourage beginners to use a variety of equipment and to be sure to work all major muscle groups.**

CIRCUIT TRAINING

Circuit training can be an effective way to conduct an exercise program. The point is to maximize the variety of exercise, distribute the work over a larger muscle mass than could be accomplished with a single form of exercise, and include exercises for all aspects of a fitness session. Circuits can include the following:

- Moving from one piece of exercise equipment to another with a brief rest period between each. A person might exercise for 5 to 10 min (or 50 to 100 kcal) on a cycle ergometer, then on a treadmill, then on a rower, then on a bench step, and so on.
- A typical workout for muscular strength and endurance, in which one "set" is done on a specific machine before moving to the next, and the rotation is repeated 2 to 3 times (see chapter 15).
- A circuit set up around the perimeter of a large room with signs posted in discrete locations describing specific exercises that the participant should do during one trip around the circuit. The circuit could include warm-up activities; flexibility activities; strengthening exercises using body weight as a resistance; and, of course, aerobic activities. Beginning, intermediate, and advanced goals specifying the number of repetitions (or duration) can be posted at each station. Build in a station to check the THR following the aerobic exercise stations.

Good examples of walk/jog/run circuits have been in place for the past decade. Many communities have set up jogging trails that have signposts along the way indicating specific exercises to do at each stop. They can be found in many cities, and they provide a break in the regular routine of steady jogging or running while focusing attention on flexibility and strengthening exercises.

13 **In Review: Circuit training programs offer variety and can include exercises in all aspects of fitness (e.g., cardiorespiratory, muscle strength/endurance, flexibility). The preceding list suggests a few circuit training possibilities.**

Case Studies

You can check your answers by referring to appendix A.

17.1

You are making a presentation to a group of adults who have their own neighborhood walking program. What topics should you address to emphasize safety and comfort?

17.2

A participant who has been involved in your walking program for the past 10 weeks asks your advice regarding an aerobic dance class. What would you recommend?

Source List

1. American College of Sports Medicine (1995)
2. Dishman (1990)
3. Franklin, Oldridge, Stoedefalke, & Loechel (1990)
4. Franks & Howley (1989b)
5. Garrick & Requa (1988)
6. Giese (1988)
7. Kasser (1995)
8. Kisselle & Mazzeo (1983)
9. Londeree & Moeschberger (1982)
10. Mazzeo (1984)
11. McSwegin & Pemberton (1993)
12. New Games Foundation (1976)
13. Oldridge (1988)
14. Peters & Waterman (1982)
15. Sova (1995)
16. U.S. Department of Health & Human Services (1996)
17. White (1995)
18. Williford, Scharff-Olson, & Blessing (1989)

CHAPTER

18

Exercise Prescriptions for Special Populations

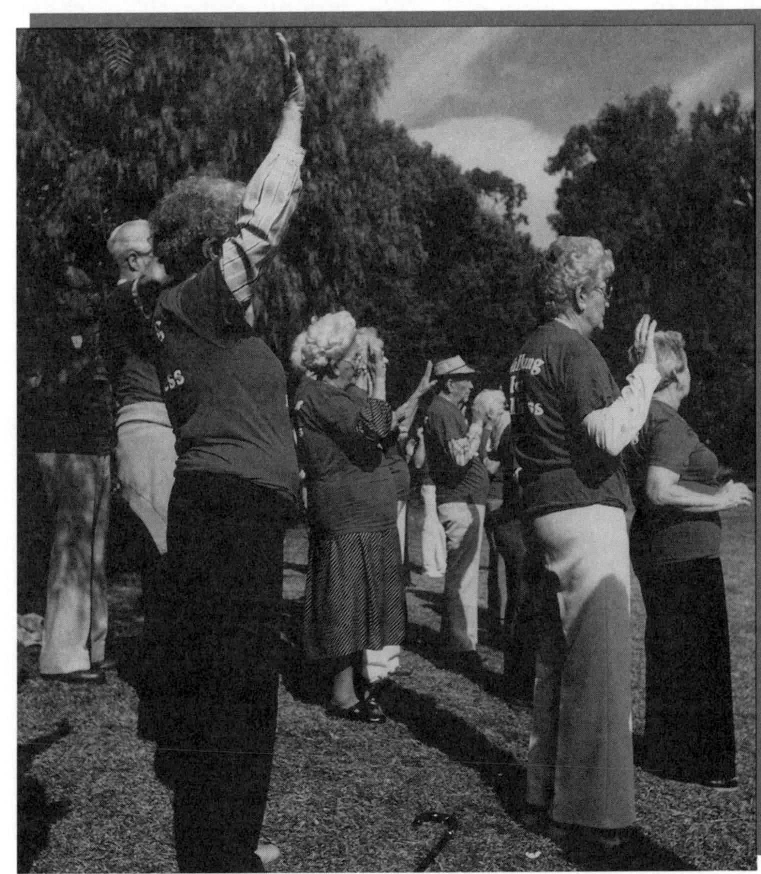

The reader will be able to: **OBJECTIVES**

Modify the exercise prescription for the following populations and controlled diseases and disabilities:

1. Children.
2. Elderly.
3. Pregnant women.
4. Orthopedic limitation.
5. Type I diabetes.
6. Type II diabetes.
7. Asthma.
8. Hypertension.
9. Seizure disorder.
10. Chronic obstructive pulmonary disease.
11. Cardiac disease.

Physical activity is needed for optimum growth and development in early childhood, it is an essential ingredient in the development of general motor ability and sport skills in middle and late childhood, and it is important in lowering the risk of a wide variety of chronic diseases throughout adult life. In addition, physical activity is both a nonpharmacological intervention and a part of the rehabilitation process for people with a wide variety of diseases. Consequently, it is important for health fitness instructors (HFIs) to be able to prescribe physical activity across the life span. This chapter provides a brief introduction to how exercise is used for special populations and for specific diseases. Several of these summaries have been adapted from Powers and Howley's *Exercise Physiology* (54).

EXERCISE PRESCRIPTION FOR CHILDREN

The incidence of childhood obesity has been increasing since the mid-1970s, and these children often have elevated blood pressure, blood lipids, and plasma insulin (22). Concern for the fitness of our children and youth, however, goes back over 100 years. Park's (51) historical review of the topic of fitness and fitness testing indicates that the early leaders in physical education in the latter part of the 19th century were convinced of the connection among exercise, fitness, and health. Not surprisingly, fitness testing was a part of the process. Initially, testing was concerned more with anthropometry, strength, and sometimes a physical exam. Tests of motor ability were also developed, but it was a long time before a national test battery of fitness tests became a reality.

The driving force in the promotion of fitness in the first half of the 20th century was war or the threat of war, due to the concern caused when a large number of young men could not pass an induction exam into the armed forces. In the early 1950s a new alarm was sounded when a study showed that a large percentage of American children could not pass basic flexibility and power tests. In response to this concern, President Eisenhower established the President's Council on Youth Fitness. Soon after that, the American Association of Health, Physical Education, and Recreation published its Youth Fitness Test, with fitness test items such as the pull-up, sit-up, shuttle run, standing broad jump, 50-yd dash, softball throw for distance, and the 600-yd run-walk. This test battery emphasized "skill-related" fitness with an emphasis on muscular power (51).

In the early 1980s the publication of *Healthy People* and *Promoting Health/Preventing Disease: Objectives for the Nation* shifted the focus to health-related fitness. In support of this health-related focus, the American Alliance of Health, Physical Education, Recreation and Dance published the *Health-Related Physical Fitness Test Manual* with the emphasis on testing fitness components related to health, including the 1-mi run for cardiorespiratory fitness, skinfold measurements to evaluate body composition, and the sit-and-reach and the sit-up to evaluate low-back function. Following this publication, the introduction of criterion-referenced standards was advocated in order to focus on health-related goals rather than maximal performance (51). The criterion-reference standard for cardiorespiratory fitness is 42 ml · kg^{-1} · min^{-1} for males ages 5 to 17 years. For females the standards are 40 ml · kg^{-1} · min^{-1} for ages 5 to 9, with a decrease of 1 ml · kg^{-1} · min^{-1} per year until age 14 at which the standard becomes 35 ml · kg^{-1} · min^{-1} (21). In short, these standards are not very different from those recommended for adults. Currently, the trend is to emphasize the physical activity behavior more than the fitness test scores. The major question is, what kinds of physical activities should children do?

Childhood is a period in which most motor skills (e.g., throwing, jumping, running, riding, swimming) develop. Children are inherently active, and one of the most important elements adults must provide is an opportunity to play. This need for children to develop motor skills must be kept in mind when attending to fitness goals (76). Relative to adults, children are similar in terms of

- $\dot{V}O_2$max in ml · kg^{-1} · min^{-1} (endurance tasks can be performed well), and
- creatine phosphate + ATP (children can deal well with very brief, intense exercise).

Children are lower in terms of

- capacity to generate ATP via glycolysis (children have a lower capacity to do intense activity lasting 10 to 90 s),
- ability to dissipate heat via evaporation and acclimatize to heat (children have an increased potential of heat-related illness), and
- economy of walking and running (children require more oxygen to walk or run at the same speed; standard equations listed in chapter 7 for estimating energy expenditure of walking and running cannot be used).

Children are better in terms of

- achieving a steady state in oxygen uptake (children experience a smaller oxygen deficit and faster recovery; they are well suited to intermittent activities).

Cardiorespiratory Fitness

Measuring $\dot{V}O_2$max in children using both the cycle ergometer and the treadmill has a sound historical foundation (9, 56). The GXT format is used for children, and one must match the characteristics of the test (initial grade/speed on the treadmill, increments per stage) to the child in the same way as for the adult. Treadmill testing may be easier due to the role that children's shorter attention span can play in completing a cycle protocol. In addition, local muscle fatigue may shorten a cycle ergometer test prior to maximum aerobic power being reached. If a cycle is used for young children, adjustments must be made to the handlebars, seat height, crank length, and resistance scale (76). Table 18.1 lists the ACSM's recommendations of suitable treadmill and cycle ergometer protocols to follow when testing children (4).

In general, the same exercise prescription for cardiorespiratory fitness for adults (see chapter 14) can be used for children. However, there is some disagreement about whether the standard prescription will result in an increase in $\dot{V}O_2$max. The prescription may be effective in increasing $\dot{V}O_2$max in pubescent and postpubescent children but less so in younger children (57, 76). This suggests that attention be directed toward health-related benefits of aerobic exercise rather than simply on $\dot{V}O_2$max. When the focus is on health-related benefits, the use of a wide variety of continuous physical activities (e.g., cycling, running, in-line skating), team sports (e.g., basketball, soccer), individual and dual sports (e.g., tennis, racquetball), and recreational activities (e.g., hiking) can contribute to energy expenditure and its associated benefits. Parents, schools, and communities must provide (a) opportunities for children to have safe places to walk, run, and cycle; (b) organized programs to learn and play sports; and (c) the focus on personal achievement rather than on winning at all costs.

Strength

Muscular strength and endurance of children can be improved by participating in formal weight training

Table 18.1 Protocols Suitable for Graded Exercise Testing of Children

Modified Balke Treadmill Protocol				
Subject	Speed ($mi \cdot hr^{-1}$)	Initial grade (%)	Increment (%)	Stage duration (min)
Poorly fit	3.00	6	2	2
Sedentary	3.25	6	2	2
Active	5.00	0	2.5	2
Athlete	5.25	0	2.5	2

McMaster Cycle Test			
Height (cm)	Initial load (W)	Increments (W)	Step duration (min)
<120	12.5	12.5	2
120-139.9	12.5	25	2
140-159.9	25	25	2
≥160	25	50 (boys) 25 (girls)	2

Reprinted from American College of Sports Medicine 1995.

programs. Safety precautions must be taken, however, because children are anatomically, physiologically, and psychologically immature (57, 76). The following guidelines are offered (4, 57):

- Trained personnel should supervise each session.
- Teach proper lifting techniques, with no breath holding.
- Stress controlled lifting techniques; avoid ballistic movements.
- Perform 1 or 2 sets of 8 to 10 different exercises (with 8 to 12 reps per set), and include most major muscle groups.
- Limit training sessions to 2 times per week to encourage other activities.
- Do not use a resistance that cannot be lifted at least 8 times; overload by first increasing the number of repetitions and then the absolute resistance.
- Do not perform exercises to the point of momentary muscle fatigue due to risks to developing bone and joint structures.

1 **In Review: Health-related goals can be realized by involving children in a wide variety of recreational and sport activities in a safe and supportive environment. The focus should be on achieving health-related goals rather than simply increasing $\dot{V}O_2$max. Strength training can be used as an effective part of an exercise program for children. The emphasis is on safety, with a minimum of 8 to 12 reps being done for each of 8 to 10 exercises involving most of the major muscle groups. Exercises should not be done to the point of momentary muscular fatigue.**

EXERCISE PRESCRIPTION FOR THE ELDERLY

Maximal aerobic power decreases in the average population after the age of 20 at the rate of about 1% per year (17). However, this decrease is due to both inactivity and weight gain as well as to an "aging effect." Studies show that this rate of decline can be reduced by regular physical activity and that middle-age men who maintain their activity and body weight show only half the expected change in $\dot{V}O_2$max over a 22-year period (39). Unfortunately, most people experience the steady decline in $\dot{V}O_2$max with age, so that by the time they are ready to retire, their ability to engage in normal physical activities has been compromised. This reduced capacity for work can lead to a vicious cycle, resulting in lower and lower levels of cardiorespiratory fitness that may not allow them to perform activities of daily living. This, of course, affects older adults' quality of life and independence, and they may end up having to rely on others. Regular physical activity is useful in combating not only this downward spiral of cardiorespiratory fitness but also osteoporosis and the related hip fractures that can lead to more inactivity and also death (61).

Osteoporosis is a loss of bone mass that is responsible for 1.2 million fractures annually. *Type I osteoporosis* is related to fractures of the vertebrae and the distal radius in 50- to 65-year-olds, and it is eight times more common in women than men. *Type II osteoporosis*, experienced by those age 70 and above, results in hip, pelvic, and distal humerus fractures and is twice as common in women (35). Osteoporosis is more common in women over 50 due to the lack of estrogen after menopause. If estrogen treatment is instituted early in menopause, it may prevent bone loss. If the treatment is initiated years after menopause, however, it cannot replace the lost bone; it will only maintain existing bone (35, 43). To prevent the problem, attention is focused on adequate dietary calcium (33) and exercise (61). Dietary calcium is important in preventing and treating osteoporosis. Because most women take in less than the Recommended Daily Allowance (RDA; see chapter 8), they must focus more attention on taking in an adequate amount of calcium (33).

Bone structure is maintained by the downward force due to gravity (upright posture) and the lateral forces generated by muscle contraction. Unfortunately, although research has shown that exercise programs can slow or reverse bone loss, the optimal training program to prevent osteoporosis has yet to be defined (23, 62). Weight-bearing activities (such as walking and jogging) are better than bicycling and swimming for maintaining spine and hip mineral, but for the low fit or people with previous fractures, the latter activities are recommended (61). Two to 3 hr of exercise a week may reduce or reverse the bone mineral loss that occurs with age (23, 61).

Since about 1980 research has documented the capacity of the elderly to experience a training effect similar to that of younger men and women. Such a capacity is important when one considers the need of older adults to maintain their health status and independence for as long as possible. These conclusions are based on data collected in cross-sectional studies comparing older athletes to their sedentary counterparts and from longitudinal studies in which training programs have been implemented. A brief summary of the findings from these studies follows (31).

Cross-sectional studies have shown that, in contrast to older sedentary individuals, endurance-trained older athletes have

- half the expected decrease in $\dot{V}O_2$max;
- higher HDL cholesterol and lower triglycerides, total cholesterol, and LDL cholesterol;
- enhanced glucose tolerance and insulin sensitivity; and
- greater strength, reaction time, and a lower risk of falling.

Cross-sectional comparisons could be biased, however, due to the potential for a strong genetic factor that might drive an individual to pursue an active life. Longitudinal studies control for this by comparing a group involved in systematic training to a control group over many months to see how each changes. The results from these studies parallel those mentioned above:

- Endurance training increases $\dot{V}O_2$max in a manner similar to younger individuals, but more time may be required for the training effect to occur (10). The increase in $\dot{V}O_2$max is due to both peripheral (skeletal muscle) and central (cardiovascular) adaptations (66). Interestingly, the training effect can be brought about by lower intensities of exercise than that required for younger subjects.
- Endurance training causes favorable changes in blood lipids, but the changes seem to be linked to a reduction in body fatness, rather than exercise, per se.
- Endurance training lowers blood pressure to the same degree as shown for younger individuals with hypertension.
- Endurance training improves glucose tolerance and insulin sensitivity.
- Endurance training increases or maintains muscular endurance and bone density. Resistance training results in large increases in strength, which may play an important role in reducing the risk of falls.

With respect to making exercise recommendations for fitness, Smith (60) indicated the need to distinguish among the older population as follows:

- Athletic old—greater than 55 years of age; $\dot{V}O_2$max = 9 to 10 METs
- Young old—55 to 75 years of age; $\dot{V}O_2$max = 6 to 7 METs
- Old old—greater than 75 years of age; $\dot{V}O_2$max = 2 to 3 METs

The $\dot{V}O_2$max values of the "athletic old" allow for a variety of activities that would be similar to those suitable for the ordinary younger and more sedentary population. The "young old" subject's $\dot{V}O_2$max of 6 to 7 METs is similar to that of a cardiac patient, and the structure and routine of this individual's exercise program would not be too different from that of the cardiac patient. However, prescribing activities for the "old old" group, whose members have extremely low functional capacities, demands creativity in terms of both exercise testing and prescription (60).

Smith and Gilligan's chair-step test (61) provides an interesting substitute for traditional treadmill and cycle ergometer testing of the elderly. In this test the person remains seated on a chair and alternates leg lifts to raise the heel of the foot 6, 12, or 18 in., pausing momentarily on a step. The recommended cadence results in work increments of only 0.5 METs. Although exercise prescription follows the procedures described in chapter 14, the HFI must implement unique, low-intensity, controlled exercises focusing on the low end of the MET scale, with support (63). The "old old" individual can do these exercises while lying, seated, or holding onto a chair while standing. The exercises include foot, leg, and arm movements that will increase flexibility and muscular endurance and expend calories. Given the rapid increase in the number of individuals in this age group, the HFI would be wise to develop competence with such exercise programs.

2 **In Review: Regular exercise slows the rate at which $\dot{V}O_2$max decreases with age. Exercise helps maintain strength, bone density, and independence and reduces the chance of a bone break. Exercise is useful in decreasing blood pressure and improving glucose tolerance in the elderly. Exercise recommendations can vary from the standard prescription similar to that for younger, sedentary individuals for the "athletic old" to closely supervised programs for the "old old."**

EXERCISE PRESCRIPTION FOR PREGNANT WOMEN

Pregnancy places special demands on a woman, given the developing fetus's needs for calories, protein, minerals, vitamins, and, of course, the physiologically stable environment necessary to process these nutrients. The fitness program must be evaluated against these diverse needs. The process should begin with a thorough medical examination by the woman's physician to rule out complications that would make exercise inappropriate and to provide specific information about signs or symptoms to watch for during the course of the pregnancy. Examples of absolute contraindications for aerobic exercise during pregnancy include Type I diabetes, history of two or more spontaneous abortions, multiple pregnancy, smoking, and excessive alcohol intake. Relative contraindications include a history of premature labor, anemia, obesity, Type II diabetes, and very low fitness prior to pregnancy (73). Clearly, to protect mother and fetus, a consultation with a physician is important prior to the initiation of an exercise program.

What are reasonable recommendations to follow when a pregnant woman wishes to exercise? In general, moderate exercise does not appear to interfere with oxygen delivery to the fetus, and the HR response of the fetus shows no signs of "distress." For women in excellent condition before pregnancy, exercise does not appear to have any negative or positive effects in terms of fetal outcome (44, 45). Guidelines have been developing since the mid-1980s but not without some disagreement. In an earlier set of guidelines from the American College of Obstetricians and Gynecologists, fixed criteria (e.g., don't exercise over a HR of 140 beats · min^{-1}) were provided with the emphasis on taking a conservative approach to exercise prescription. The most recent guidelines (see page 359) recognize, however, that research support for such restrictions does not exist. The guidelines emphasize the need to avoid doing exercise in the supine position after the first trimester and to modify intensity according to symptoms and not push on to exhaustion. Weight-supported activities are encouraged due to the lower risk of injury, and attention is focused on the need for hydration to maintain body temperature in the normal range associated with exercise. The latter recommendation is different from earlier guidelines to limit the increase in maternal body temperature to 38 °C. Research suggests that normal exercise-induced increases in body temperatures carry little risk to the fetus (20). Although heart rate has been used to set exercise intensity, the fact that the relationship between heart rate and $\dot{V}O_2$ may change over the course of pregnancy suggests that the rating of perceived exertion (RPE; see table 11.5) may be a better choice (4).

Recommendations for Exercise in Pregnancy and Postpartum

There are no data in humans to indicate that pregnant women should limit exercise intensity and target heart rates because of potential adverse effects. For women who do not have any additional risk factors for adverse maternal or perinatal outcome, the following recommendations may be made:

1. During pregnancy, women can continue to exercise and derive health benefits even from mild-to-moderate exercise routines. Regular exercise (at least three times per week) is preferable to intermittent activity.
2. Women should avoid exercise in the supine position after the first trimester. Such a position is associated with decreased cardiac output in most pregnant women; because the remaining cardiac output will be preferentially distributed away from splanchnic beds (including the uterus) during vigorous exercise, such regimens are best avoided during pregnancy. Prolonged periods of motionless standing should also be avoided.
3. Women should be aware of the decreased oxygen available for aerobic exercise during pregnancy. They should be encouraged to modify the intensity of their exercise according to maternal symptoms. Pregnant women should stop exercising when fatigued and not exercise to exhaustion. Weight-bearing exercises may under some circumstances be continued at intensities similar to those prior to pregnancy throughout pregnancy. Non-weight-bearing exercises such as cycling or swimming will minimize the risk of injury and facilitate the continuation of exercise during pregnancy.
4. Morphologic changes in pregnancy should serve as a relative contraindication to types of exercise in which loss of balance could be detrimental to maternal or fetal well-being, especially in the third trimester. Further, any type of exercise involving the potential for even mild abdominal trauma should be avoided.
5. Pregnancy requires an additional 300 kcal/day in order to maintain metabolic homeostasis. Thus, women who exercise during pregnancy should be particularly careful to ensure an adequate diet.
6. Pregnant women who exercise in the first trimester should augment heat dissipation by ensuring adequate hydration, appropriate clothing, and optimal environmental surroundings during exercise.
7. Many of the physiologic and morphologic changes of pregnancy persist 4 to 6 weeks postpartum. Thus, prepregnancy exercise routines should be resumed gradually based on a woman's physical capability.

Reprinted from American College of Obstetricians and Gynecologists 1994.

3 **In Review: A pregnant woman should consult with her physician before starting an exercise program. Endurance exercise can be done during pregnancy without complication to mother and fetus. Regular exercise (at least three times per week) is preferable to intermittent activity. See the box on page 359 for recommendations.**

EXERCISE PRESCRIPTION FOR CONTROLLED DISEASES/DISABILITIES

Physical inactivity is regarded as a risk factor not only for coronary heart disease (CHD) but for hypertension, glucose intolerance (adult-onset diabetes), elevated serum lipids (cholesterol and triglycerides), low HDL cholesterol, and hyper-reactivity to stress (11). Because each of these problems is, in itself, a risk factor for CHD, physical activity, both directly and indirectly, decreases the risk of CHD. In fact, one of the main nonpharmacological interventions used to treat hypertension, adult-onset diabetes, hyperlipidemia, and stress is to systematically increase a person's physical activity (11).

In chapter 14 we presented the basics of exercise prescription, with the emphasis on the apparently healthy individual. In addition, the work of Jennings et al. (34) (see figure 14.2) showed that some problems such as insulin sensitivity and hypertension are more easily changed by regular exercise than others (e.g., blood lipids). It is clear that the optimum exercise prescription needed to address the problems just mentioned has yet to be developed (32). In spite of this HFIs should certainly be aware of the limitations associated with certain diseases and within certain populations and how exercise can be used to improve or maintain health and fitness.

Orthopedic Limitations

Orthopedic limitations (e.g., ankle, knee, or hip pain when walking or jogging) must be considered on a case-by-case basis when designing an exercise program. The exercise recommendation still indicates working within the THR range, but the participant should be advised to stay at the low end of the THR range while the problem exists. The emphasis should be on light work interspersed with rest periods. The type of activity recommended is somewhat dependent on the interests and abilities of the participant; however, weight-supported activities (e.g., cycle ergometer, rowing) and aquatic activities tend to reduce the chance of aggravating the problem. Chapter 21 outlines procedures to follow in caring for chronic injuries. The participant should be informed of proper procedures for warm-up, cool-down, and immediate care of the affected body part following an activity session.

In Review: People with orthopedic limitations should exercise at the low end of the THR range and emphasize weight-supported activities.

Diabetes

Diabetes is a disease characterized by a chronically elevated blood glucose concentration. It is the third largest cause of death by disease in the United States, with more than 12 million people having the disease. Diabetes causes blindness, kidney disease, heart disease, stroke, and peripheral vascular disease that can lead to the amputation of a leg or foot (5). Diabetics are classified into two groups on the basis of whether the diabetes is caused by a lack of **insulin** (Type I diabetes) or by a resistance to insulin (Type II diabetes) (see table 18.2). **Type I, insulin-dependent diabetes**, occurs primarily in young persons, with the rapid development of signs or symptoms, including

- frequent urination,
- unusual thirst,
- extreme hunger,
- rapid weight loss,
- weakness and fatigue,
- irritability,
- nausea, and
- vomiting (5).

To counter the pancreas's lack of natural insulin, Type I diabetics are dependent on injected insulin to maintain the blood glucose concentration within normal limits.

About 90% of all diabetics have **Type II, non-insulin dependent diabetes**, which occurs later in life than Type I diabetes and is linked to obesity (12). The Type II diabetic displays a resistance to insulin, which is usually available in adequate amounts. However, some may require injectable insulin or an oral medication that stimulates the pancreas to produce additional insulin. The primary treatment of Type II diabetics includes diet and exercise to reduce body weight and help control blood

Table 18.2 Differences Between Type I and Type II Diabetes

Characteristics	Type I insulin dependent	Type II non-insulin dependent
Another name	Juvenile-onset	Adult-onset
Proportion of all diabetics	~10%	~90%
Age at onset	<20	>40
Development of disease	Rapid	Slow
Family history	Uncommon	Common
Insulin required	Always	Common, but not always
Pancreatic insulin	None, or very little	Normal or higher
Ketoacidosis	Common	Rare
Body fatness	Normal/lean	Generally obese

Note. From Berg 1986 and Cantu 1982.

glucose. Before describing the role that exercise plays in the treatment of diabetes, let's review the means by which the blood glucose concentration is regulated at rest and during exercise.

Control of Blood Glucose at Rest and During Exercise

Blood glucose is the primary fuel for the brain, and the concentration of blood glucose is maintained within close limits to ensure a constant supply. If the concentration of blood glucose is falling, the pancreas releases the hormone **glucagon** to stimulate the liver to release glucose and bring the blood level back to normal. If the blood glucose concentration is too high (e.g., following a meal), the pancreas releases insulin, which, when bound to receptors at various tissues, allows glucose to be taken up at a faster rate to be used as a fuel or stored for later use. The blood glucose concentration then returns to normal.

During exercise additional glucose must be released from the liver to replace that taken up by muscle, which uses it as a fuel for energy production. To facilitate this, the plasma insulin level decreases during exercise and the glucagon level increases. These changes favor the mobilization of glucose from the liver. What must be noted is that during and following exercise, the muscles have an increased sensitivity to the available insulin; that is, for any insulin level, blood glucose is taken into the muscle faster *during* and *following* exercise. This increased sensitivity is what makes exercise useful in the treatment of diabetes, in that it reduces the need for insulin and helps to lower the blood glucose concentration. However, there is more to the story.

Exercise and Insulin

Knowing that exercise increases the rate at which glucose leaves the blood, one can see that it can be a useful part of the treatment to maintain blood glucose control because less insulin is required. All of this depends, however, on whether the diabetic's blood glucose is "in control." Having it in control means that *prior* to exercise the diabetic has eaten the proper quantity of carbohydrates and injected the proper amount of insulin to keep the blood glucose concentration close to normal values. The Type I diabetic who is in control maintains normal values during exercise because the liver production of glucose is balanced by the increased uptake by the muscles. On the other hand, too little or too much insulin injected before exercise can cause problems. The diabetic with an inadequate level of insulin experiences only a small increase in glucose utilization by muscle but has the "normal" increase in glucose release from liver; this causes a **hyperglycemia**,

orthopedic — Skeletal problem, disease, or deformity.

insulin — A pancreatic hormone, secreted into the blood, that influences carbohydrate metabolism by stimulating the transport of glucose into cells.

Type I, insulin-dependent diabetes — Form of diabetes in which the individual must take daily insulin injections because the pancreas is not producing insulin.

Type II, non-insulin dependent diabetes — Occurs later in life than Type I diabetes and is linked to obesity. The Type II diabetic displays a resistance to insulin, which is usually available in the body in adequate amounts.

glucagon — Hormone released from the pancreas that helps to mobilize glucose from the liver and fat from adipose tissue; opposes the action of insulin.

hyperglycemia — An elevation of blood glucose that can occur in the diabetic who does not achieve a proper balance between carbohydrate intake and injected insulin.

an elevation of the plasma glucose. When an insulin-dependent diabetic starts exercise with too much insulin, blood glucose is used by muscle faster than it is released from the liver; this causes a very dangerous condition called **hypoglycemia**, a low blood glucose concentration (55). This information is important in understanding the use of exercise as part of a program to help diabetics control the blood glucose concentration. Type I diabetics are primarily the ones confronted with the problem of a variable insulin level because they must inject the insulin themselves; Type II diabetics tend to have normal or slightly elevated insulin levels naturally. Because of this we discuss each type of diabetes separately.

Type I Diabetes

For many years the treatment for Type I diabetics was based on the triad of insulin, diet, and exercise (13). However, consider the difficulty a sedentary Type I diabetic has at the start of an exercise program. Dietary carbohydrate and injected insulin would not only have to achieve a balance between each other, but they would also have to be balanced against an exercise session whose intensity and duration would demand a variable amount of the body's carbohydrate store. Such regimentation is difficult for some to follow, and, given the variability in how a diabetic's blood glucose might respond to exercise on a day-to-day basis, the use of exercise as a primary tool in maintaining metabolic control has been diminished (6). Yet, these same authorities recognize the fact that many Type I diabetics believe that participating in exercise and sports is a normal part of life and that they must deal with the complications brought on by exercise. What steps should the Type I diabetic follow in starting an exercise program?

The Type I diabetic should have a careful medical exam before starting an exercise program because strenuous exercise can aggravate any retina, kidney, or peripheral nerve problems that are already present. The exam might include a graded diagnostic exercise test if the person is over 30 years of age or has had diabetes for 15 years or more. In addition, peripheral nerve damage may block signals coming from the foot, so that serious damage may occur before it is perceived. The diabetic should wear supportive shoes during exercise, and the exercise should not aggravate existing problems (18, 26).

The primary concern to address when exercise is prescribed for the Type I diabetic is the avoidance of hypoglycemia. This is achieved through careful self-monitoring of the blood glucose concentration before, during, and after exercise and varying carbohydrate intake and insulin depending on the exercise intensity and duration and the fitness of the individual (18):

- Before exercise, if the blood glucose concentration is less than 80 to 100 mg/dl, carbohydrates should be consumed. If it is above 250 mg/dl, exercise should be delayed until it is below 250 mg/dl.
- One should not exercise at the time of peak insulin action, which varies with the type of insulin (short or intermediate acting, continuous infusion). The insulin should be injected in a nonexercising muscle group or into a skinfold, and the quantity of insulin injected is usually decreased, the extent depending on the type of insulin.
- Glucose should be monitored frequently during exercise (every 15 min for beginners, less often for experienced participants), immediately after exercise, and 4 to 5 hr after exercise.
- Additional carbohydrate should be consumed during recovery from exercise. Hypoglycemia might occur following exercise if this is not done because dietary carbohydrate is also being used to replace the depleted muscle glycogen store.

The exercise prescription for the Type I diabetic must also consider other problems associated with this disease: autonomic neuropathy, peripheral neuropathy, retinopathy, and nephropathy. Individuals with autonomic nervous system dysfunction may have abnormal heart rate and blood pressure responses to exercise. People with peripheral nerve damage may experience pain, impaired balance, weakness, and decreased proprioception. Damage to the retina is common in people with diabetes, and it is aggravated by increased blood pressure or any jarring action directed at the head. Kidney damage is also a common experience for people with Type I diabetes. This can lead to altered blood pressure responses that can affect the retina. It should be no surprise that the exercise prescription for the diabetic must address these problems if they are present. Suggestions include (18)

- performing a submaximal exercise test and setting the exercise intensity in terms of heart rate and rating of perceived exertion (RPE) responses based on the blood pressure response to the test;
- choosing non-weight-bearing, low-impact activities (e.g., water exercise, cycling);
- avoiding heavy weight lifting and the Valsalva maneuver (breath holding) to minimize the

blood pressure response; light weight lifting is acceptable when blood pressure responses are normal.

In addition, the Type I diabetic should increase fluid intake, carry a readily available form of carbohydrate and adequate identification, and follow the buddy system by exercising with someone who can help in an emergency. Participation in exercise on a daily basis helps to maintain insulin sensitivity. In conclusion, although exercise may not be viewed as a primary factor in maintaining the blood glucose concentration in the normal range, the fact that Type I diabetics who stay physically active have fewer diabetic complications is reason enough to pursue the active life (28).

5 **In Review: Type I diabetics should have a thorough medical exam, possibly including a stress test, before starting the exercise program. Educate the diabetic about control and self-monitoring of blood glucose. The diabetic may have to increase carbohydrate intake and/or decrease the amount of insulin *prior* to activity to maintain the glucose concentration close to normal *during* the exercise. The extent of these alterations is dependent on a number of factors, including the intensity and duration of the physical activity, the blood glucose concentration prior to the exercise, and the physical fitness of the individual.**

Type II Diabetes

Type II diabetes occurs later in life (greater than 40 years of age), and patients generally have a variety of CHD risk factors in addition to glucose intolerance, including hypertension, hyperlipidemia, and obesity (13, 69). There is some epidemiological evidence that Type II diabetes is linked to a lack of physical activity and low fitness, independent of obesity (42). As a result, these individuals need a thorough physical exam before starting an exercise program. However, in contrast to the Type I diabetic's potential trouble with trying to maintain blood glucose control at the start of an exercise program, exercise is a primary recommendation for the Type II diabetic to help deal with the obesity that is usually present as well as to help control blood glucose. The combination of exercise and diet may decrease or eliminate the need for insulin or the oral medication taken to stimulate insulin secretion (29). With Type II diabetics representing about 90% of the whole population of diabetics, it is not surprising to find such individuals in adult fitness programs. It is important that clear communication exists between the participant and the exercise leader to reduce the chance of a "surprise" hypoglycemic response. Even though Type II diabetics do not experience the same fluctuations in blood glucose during exercise as do Type I diabetics, Type II diabetics taking insulin or oral medication may have to reduce the dosage to maintain their glucose concentration, as does the Type I diabetic (55).

The exercise prescription for the Type II diabetic is similar to that described in chapter 14 for improving $\dot{V}O_2max$: dynamic aerobic activity, done at 50% to 70% $\dot{V}O_2max$, for 20 to 60 min, three to five times per week (daily if on insulin therapy) (18, 75). Strength training with light weights is also recommended (18, 64). Following are some important points:

- The frequency should be as high as five to seven times per week to promote a sustained increase in insulin sensitivity and to facilitate weight loss and weight maintenance.
- Little is gained by working at or above the top end of the intensity recommendation. Those exercising at 50% $\dot{V}O_2max$ experience the same improvement in insulin sensitivity as those exercising at 70% $\dot{V}O_2max$ (15).

For any overweight, deconditioned individual, it is better to do too little than to do too much at the start of an exercise program. In addition, for the Type II diabetic it may be more important to do daily activity to maintain the increased insulin sensitivity effect, which is short-lived (69). By starting with light activity and gradually increasing the duration, diabetics can exercise each day. Daily activity provides an opportunity to learn how to control blood glucose while minimizing the chance of a hypoglycemic response. In addition, a habit of exercise may develop that is crucial if one is to realize long-term improvement in glucose tolerance. Furthermore, the combination of intensity, frequency, and duration mentioned above has been shown to directly benefit those with borderline hypertension, a condition often associated with Type II diabetes. Consistent with the recommendations for the Type I diabetic,

hypoglycemia — Dangerous low blood sugar condition, attended by anxiety, perspiration, delirium, or coma.

clear identification and a readily available source of carbohydrate should be carried along during an exercise session. In addition, it is reasonable to recommend that the buddy system be followed.

Exercise is only one part of the treatment; diet is the other. The American Diabetes Association (7) states five goals related to nutrition therapy for the diabetic:

1. Maintain near-normal blood glucose levels by balancing diet and insulin.
2. Achieve optimal serum lipid levels.
3. Provide adequate calories to attain reasonable weight.
4. Prevent long-term complications associated with diabetes.
5. Improve overall health through optimal nutrition, using the Dietary Guidelines for Americans and the Food Guide Pyramid as guides (see chapter 8).

The emphasis in the latter is on a low-fat (<30%), high-carbohydrate diet to achieve nutrient goals for protein, vitamins, and minerals. The low-fat diet has been shown to be useful in achieving weight loss and blood lipid goals as well as diabetic control.

The combination of the recommended diet and regular exercise not only improves the diabetic's chance of maintaining control over blood glucose, it lowers body fat and weight, increases HDL cholesterol and $\dot{V}O_2$max, and improves self-concept (12, 69). These changes will reduce the overall risk associated with CHD (55).

6 **In Review: Type II diabetics may have a variety of risk factors in addition to their diabetes, including hypertension, high cholesterol, obesity, and inactivity. An exercise prescription emphasizing moderate-intensity, long-duration activity that is done almost every day will maximize the benefits related to insulin sensitivity and weight loss. The dietary recommendation is for a low-fat diet, similar to what is recommended for all Americans for good health, with the additional goals of achieving an appropriate body weight and normal serum glucose and lipid levels.**

Asthma

Asthma is a respiratory problem characterized by labored breathing (dyspnea) and a shortness of breath accompanied by a wheezing sound. It is due to a spasmodic contraction of the smooth muscle around the bronchi, a swelling of the mucosal cells lining the bronchi, and an excessive secretion of mucous. Asthma attacks can be initiated by allergic reactions, exercise, aspirin, dust, pollutants, and emotions (49). Before presenting the guidelines to follow in providing recommendations for exercise, we need to outline the causes of and ways to prevent an asthma attack.

A variety of factors, such as dust, chemicals, antibodies, and exercise cause asthma attacks by increasing the calcium level in the **mast cells** lining the bronchial tubes, resulting in a release of chemical mediators such as histamine. These chemical mediators cause

- bronchoconstriction, leading to a narrowing of the airway, and
- an inflammation (swelling) of the bronchial tubes.

Most people do not experience an asthma attack on exposure to the above factors; a "sensitivity" or hyperirritability of the respiratory tract is a necessary prerequisite to initiate the asthma attack (49).

Prevention and Relief of Asthma

A variety of drugs and procedures are used to either prevent the asthma attack or provide relief when one occurs. For people with allergies, simple avoidance of the allergen prevents the attack. If exposure is unavoidable, immunotherapy helps the person become less sensitive to the allergen. Drugs are now available to alter the activity of the mast cells, which is where the asthma attack begins, as well as relax the bronchiolar smooth muscle that decreases the airway diameter. Drugs to prevent or alleviate asthma symptoms include

- *cromolyn sodium*, which reduces chemical mediator release from the mast cells;
- *beta-receptor agonists* (β_2-agonists), epinephrine-like drugs that cause a relaxation of bronchiolar smooth muscle as well as a decrease in chemical mediator release by stimulating ß-adrenergic receptors; and
- *theophylline*, a caffeine-like compound that relaxes bronchiolar smooth muscle.

The net result of using these drugs is that both the inflammation response and the constriction of the bronchiolar smooth muscle are blocked. With that background, let's discuss exercise-induced asthma.

Exercise-Induced Asthma

A form of asthma of particular interest to the HFI is **exercise-induced asthma (EIA)**. The attack is initiated by exercise and can occur 5 to 15 min (early phase) or 4 to 6 hr (late phase) following exercise. Approximately 80% of asthmatics experience EIA, versus only 3% to 4% of the nonallergic population (68). Interestingly, 67 members (11%) of the 1984 Olympic team had EIA, and 41 of them (61%) won Olympic medals (41, 68), showing that EIA can be controlled.

The following have been identified as causes of EIA: cold air, hypocapnia (low PCO_2), respiratory alkalosis, and specific intensities and durations of exercise. Scientists are now studying the role that cooling and drying of the respiratory tract have on the initiation of EIA. When large volumes of dry air are inhaled during the exercise session, moisture is evaporated from the surface of the airways, which becomes cooled (24, 47, 59). When dry air removes water from the surface of the mast cells, an increase in osmolarity occurs, and this triggers the influx of calcium that leads to the increased release of chemical mediators and the narrowing of the airways (24, 40, 41, 59). This proposed mechanism has received support from observations showing that EIA can be prevented by breathing warm, humidified air.

The chance that an exercise-induced bronchospasm will occur is related to the

- type of exercise done,
- time since the previous bout of exercise,
- interval since medication was taken, and
- temperature and humidity of the inspired air.

It has been observed that running causes more attacks than cycling or walking, which cause more attacks than swimming (59). Exercise prescriptions should be guided by observations that

- attacks are associated with strenuous, long-duration exercise, and
- exercising within 60 min of a previous EIA attack reduces subsequent bronchospasms (24, 41, 59).

This suggests that a warm-up within an hour of more strenuous exercise would reduce the severity of an attack; this proposition is supported by strong evidence (48). How should exercise be prescribed for someone with EIA?

The asthmatic should follow a medication plan to *prevent* the occurrence of an EIA attack. This is done by the physician working with the individual to fine-tune the medications to prevent the problem without interfering with the person's response to exercise. In a majority of cases EIA can be prevented when β_2-agonists are used prior to athletic performance (16). Cromolyn sodium is also effective in inhibiting the early- and late-phase responses and can be used in conjunction with a β_2-agonist (46).

The HFI should structure the exercise session to include a conventional warm-up and mild to moderate activity organized into 5-min segments. Swimming is better than other types of exercise because the air above the water tends to be warmer and contain more moisture. A scarf or face mask can be used to help trap moisture when exercising outdoors in cold weather. The participant should carry an inhaler with a β_2-agonist and use it at the first sign of wheezing (27, 40, 52). As for the diabetic, the buddy system is a good plan to follow in case a major attack occurs.

In Review: People with asthma who engage in exercise should pretreat with medication, warm up, perform 5-min intermittent bouts of light to moderate activity, carry a β_2-agonist, and follow the buddy system.

Hypertension

The risk of coronary heart disease increases with increases in either diastolic or systolic blood pressure (37). Hypertension, defined as systolic pressure of ≥140 mmHg or diastolic pressure of ≥90 mmHg, is a major health problem in the United States involving over 50 million people (38). Typically hypertension

asthma — A respiratory problem characterized by labored breathing (dyspnea), coughing, mucous discharge from the mouth, and a shortness of breath accompanied by a wheezing sound. May be initiated by exercise, allergies, or other irritants.

mast cells — A cell in the bronchial tube that releases histamine and other chemicals in response to certain stimuli; involved in an asthmatic attack.

exercise-induced asthma (EIA) — A form of asthma induced by exercise that can occur 5 to 15 min (early phase) or 4 to 6 hr (late phase) following exercise.

is treated with drugs, but this form of treatment has its own risks, both medically and personally. Studies indicate that death rates are higher for hypertensives with ECG abnormalities who were treated with diuretic medications than for those treated with other medications. Furthermore, simply classifying a person as a "patient" due to the presence of hypertension increases symptoms of other diseases and can actually alter a person's lifestyle (38). For example, a person who finds out he or she is hypertensive may give up some activities because of a fear of making the condition worse. Consequently, although there is little disagreement that people with blood pressures of $>180/>105$ mmHg should be treated with medication, many believe that for those with mild hypertension, 140 to 180/90 to 104 mmHg, the nonpharmacological interventions discussed next should be considered (3, 30, 37, 38, 74).

The presence of mild hypertension must be verified by several independent measurements taken days apart (74). If mild hypertension is identified, the person needs a complete physical exam to determine whether other risk factors are present that would increase the overall risk of CHD. Although a decision might be made to medicate someone with multiple risk factors (e.g., smoking, high cholesterol, obesity), Kannel (37) pointed out that getting a hypertensive patient to quit smoking confers more immediate benefit against CHD risk than any known medication. It should be no surprise that dietary, weight-control, and exercise recommendations would be included in any nonpharmacological treatment package (8, 11, 30, 74).

Dietary change includes a reduction in sodium intake that has been shown to independently reduce systolic and diastolic blood pressures by approximately 5 and 3 mmHg, respectively (8, 30, 38). Obesity is linked to hypertension, and a review of various studies indicated that a loss of 1 kg of weight resulted in a decrease in systolic and diastolic pressures of 1.6 and 1.3 mmHg, respectively (30, 38). Lastly, participation in an endurance exercise program has been shown to cause decreases in systolic and diastolic pressures of 10 mmHg (3, 30, 38).

The standard American College of Sports Medicine exercise prescription for improving $\dot{V}O_2max$ (see chapter 14) is also effective in reducing blood pressure in previously hypertensive individuals. In addition, endurance exercise at moderate intensities (40% to 70% $\dot{V}O_2max$) has also been shown to reduce blood pressure (3, 30). Moderate-intensity exercise should be done frequently and for durations long enough to result in the expenditure of a large number of calories. Furthermore, for those with higher blood pressures who are taking medication, such an exercise program can also be used along with changes in diet, smoking, and body weight to lower blood pressure. In these cases, blood pressure should be checked frequently to allow medications to be reduced as needed. The gradual establishment of appropriate diet and exercise habits improves the chance that a person will maintain an appropriate blood pressure once it has been normalized. If a person is being treated with beta-adrenergic blocking drugs, the ordinary calculation of the THR using the 220 – age formula to estimate the maximal HR should not be used because beta-blocking drugs lower the maximal HR (see chapter 22). Using an RPE rating of 10 to 12 on the original scale (2 on the revised scale) to establish moderate-intensity exercise (40% to 60% of $\dot{V}O_2max$) is a reasonable alternative (2).

8 **In Review: Nonpharmacological treatment of mild hypertension (140 to 180/90 to 104 mmHg) includes changes in diet (including sodium intake), smoking, body fatness, and exercise. Moderate-intensity exercise (at 40% to 60% of $\dot{V}O_2max$; 10 to 12 on the original RPE scale) is recommended. The patient's blood pressure should be evaluated regularly to alter medication if necessary.**

Seizure Susceptibility

Individuals with controlled seizure disorders (e.g., epilepsy) are able and encouraged to lead normally active lives. In many cases the individual is aware of the unique circumstances that might trigger a seizure and can avoid the situation. The HFI should be aware of any member of an exercise group that has a seizure disorder. Recommendations include participation in a variety of activities with little or no restriction. Suggestions for safety include exercising with a partner who can physically support and aid the individual in case of a seizure in potentially dangerous situations, such as jogging on a road or swimming.

9 **In Review: People with controlled seizure disorders can participate in a variety of activities with little or no restriction, however, the buddy system should be used for safety.**

Chronic Obstructive Pulmonary Disease

Chronic obstructive pulmonary diseases (COPDs) cause a reduction in airflow that can dramatically affect one's ability to perform daily activities. These diseases include chronic bronchitis, emphysema, and bronchial asthma, alone or in combination. Each of the following diseases causes an obstruction to airflow, but the underlying reason is different for each (14, 36, 58):

- Bronchial asthma—bronchial smooth-muscle contraction and increased airway reactivity
- Chronic bronchitis—persistent production of sputum due to a thickened bronchial wall with excess secretions
- Emphysema—loss of elastic recoil of alveoli and bronchioles and enlargement of those pulmonary structures

COPD is considerably different from the controlled asthmatic condition discussed previously. Asthma is reversible; chronic bronchitis and emphysema are not. The patient with developing COPD perceives an inability to do normal activities without experiencing dyspnea, but tragically, by the time this occurs the disease is already well advanced (14).

Testing and Evaluation

A patient with COPD receives a thorough medical examination as well as a variety of tests to help classify the degree of disability associated with the disease. One of the most important pulmonary function tests is the FEV_1, a measure of the maximum volume of air that can be moved in one second. Unfortunately, due to the progressive nature of this disease, by the time the person is aware of symptoms, the FEV_1 is already less than 60% of the predicted value (36). Exercise tests are also used to assess people with COPD. The tests may be the standard graded exercise test (GXT) or a simple 6- or 12-min walk on a flat surface. During the GXT, cardiovascular, pulmonary, metabolic, and power-output measurements are obtained and used to evaluate the severity of disability on a 4-point scale. Table 18.3 presents the standards for each of the four grades of disability (36).

COPD is characterized by a gradual decrease in the ability to exhale, and because of the narrowed airways, a "wheezing" sound is made. The person with COPD experiences a decreased capacity for work, which may influence employment; he or she may also experience an increase in psychological problems, such as anxiety regarding the simple act of breathing and depression related to a loss of sense of self-worth (14, 36, 50).

Rehabilitation

Given the complex problems associated with this disease, it should be no surprise that treatment of COPD includes more than simple medication and O_2 inhalation therapy. A typical COPD rehabilitation program has the patient's self-care as its goal, and to achieve that goal, physicians, nurses, respiratory therapists, psychologists, exercise specialists, and clergy are recruited to deal with the various manifestations of the disease process (50, 65). The patient with COPD receives education about the different ways to deal with the disease, including breathing exercises, ways to approach the activities of daily living at home, and how to handle work-related problems. The latter can be so affected that new on-the-job responsibilities may have to be assigned, or if the person cannot meet the requirements, changing jobs or retirement may be the only outcome. To help deal with these problems, counseling by psychologists and clergy may be needed for the patient and her or his family. The extent of these problems is directly related to the severity of the disease. Those with minimal disease may require the help of only a few of these professionals, while others with severe disease may require the assistance of all. It is therefore important to understand that the rehabilitation program is very individualized (50).

The exercise component of the rehabilitation program varies with the level of disability. People with Grade 1 disability (see table 18.3) can follow the normal exercise prescription process. However, additional guidelines are needed for those with Grade 2 or Grade 3 disability. Those with Grade 2 disability are limited to exercises that demand only 60% to

chronic obstructive pulmonary diseases (COPDs) — A term used to describe a number of specific diseases that cause a chronic unremitting obstruction to flow of air in the airways of the lungs. These diseases include chronic bronchitis, emphysema, and bronchial asthma, alone or in combination. Each disease causes an obstruction to airflow, but the underlying reason is different for each. COPD can dramatically affect one's ability to perform daily activities.

Table 18.3 Guide to Grading COPD (Based on a 40-Year-Old Man)

Grade	Cause of dyspnea	FEV_1 (%pred)	Max $\dot{V}O_2$ (ml · min^{-1} · kg^{-1})	Exercise Max V_E (L · min^{-1})	Blood gases
1	Fast walking and stair climbing	> 60	> 25	Not limiting	Normal PCO_2, S_aO_2
2	Walking at normal pace	< 60	< 25	> 50	Normal P_aCO_2; S_aO_2 above 90% at rest and with exercise
3	Slow walking	< 40	< 15	< 50	Normal P_aCO_2; S_aO_2 below 90% with exercise
4	Walking limited to less than 1 block	< 40	< 7	< 30	Elevated P_aCO_2; S_aO_2 below 90% at rest and with exercise

Note. Max V_E = maximal ventilatory expiration.
Reprinted from Jones et al., 1987, Chronic obstructive respiratory disorders. In *Exercise testing and exercise prescription for special cases*. By permission of Lea & Febiger.

80% of ventilatory capacity and a breathing frequency of 30 breaths · min^{-1}. A THR may be prescribed relative to those goals. The person should do several short-duration exercise bouts each day and, with time, gradually increase the duration of each exercise bout as tolerance improves (36).

Those with Grade 3 disability follow the intermittent-exercise recommendation of the Grade 2 guidelines, but the exercise intensity is very low, and oxygen supplementation may be needed. Breathing exercises are also included. Unfortunately, those with Grade 4 disability are probably in respiratory or cardiovascular failure, and the emphasis is on counseling the person on how to conserve energy to accomplish daily tasks, which may require supplemental oxygen (36).

The goals of the exercise component of the COPD rehabilitation program are very pragmatic: ability to do home or work activities, ability to climb two flights of stairs, and so on (14, 50). Generally, COPD patients achieve an increase in exercise tolerance without dyspnea and an increase in the sense of well-being, but without a reversal of the disease process (50, 58). The changes in the psychological variables are very important in the long run, given that the person's willingness to continue the exercise program is a major factor that will dictate the rate of decline during the course of the disease.

10 **In Review: Chronic obstructive pulmonary disease (COPD) includes chronic asthma, emphysema, and bronchitis.**

These latter two diseases create changes in the lung that are irreversible and result in a gradual deterioration of function. Rehabilitation is a multidisciplinary approach involving medication, breathing exercises, dietary therapy, exercise, and counseling. The programs are individually designed due to the severity of the illness, and the goals are very pragmatic in terms of increasing or maintaining the ability to do the activities of daily living and work.

Cardiovascular Disease

Exercise training is now an ordinary part of the treatment of individuals with CHD. The details of how to structure such programs, from the first steps taken after being confined to a bed to the time of returning to work and beyond, are spelled out clearly in books such as *Exercise in Health and Disease* (53) and *Rehabilitation of the Coronary Patient* (70). This section is meant as a brief introduction to various aspects of such programs.

Populations in Cardiac Rehabilitation Programs

Cardiac rehabilitation programs include patients who have experienced angina pectoris, myocardial infarctions (MI), coronary artery bypass graft surgery

(CABGS), and angioplasty (25). **Angina pectoris** refers to the chest pain that is due to ischemia of the ventricle resulting from an occlusion of one or more of the coronary arteries. The pain appears when the oxygen requirement (work) of the heart (estimated by the double product, i.e., systolic BP · HR) exceeds a value that coronary blood flow cannot meet. Nitroglycerin can prevent an angina attack or relieve the pain by relaxing the smooth muscle in veins to reduce venous return and, thus, the work of the heart. Angina patients may also receive a beta- (ß-) adrenergic blocking drug like propranolol (Inderal®) to reduce the HR and/or BP responses to work; the angina symptoms would then occur at a later stage into work (see chapter 22 for medications). Exercise training supports this drug effect, in that as the person becomes trained, the HR response and double product are reduced at any work rate. More strenuous tasks can then be done without experiencing chest pain.

Myocardial infarction (MI) patients have actual heart damage (loss of ventricular muscle) due to the occlusion of one or more of the coronary arteries. The degree to which left-ventricular function is affected depends on the mass of the ventricle permanently damaged. MI patients usually take medications (ß-blockers) to reduce the work of the heart and control the irritability of the heart tissue so that dangerous *arrhythmias* (irregular heart beats) do not occur. Generally, these patients experience a training effect similar to those who did not have an MI (25).

Coronary artery bypass graft surgery (CABGS) patients have had surgery to bypass one or more blocked coronary arteries. In this procedure a blood vessel is sewn into existing coronary arteries above and below the blockage. Those with chronic angina pectoris prior to CABGS find a relief of symptoms, with 50% to 70% having no more pain. Generally, with an increased blood flow to the ventricle there is an improvement in left-ventricular function and the capacity for work (71). These patients benefit from systematic exercise training because most are deconditioned prior to surgery as a result of activity restrictions related to chest pain. The cardiac rehabilitation program also helps the patient differentiate angina pain from chest-wall pain related to the surgery. The overall result is a smoother and less traumatic transition back to full function.

Some CHD patients undergo a special procedure, **percutaneous transluminal coronary angioplasty**, to open occluded arteries. In this procedure the chest is not opened; instead, a balloon-tipped catheter (a long slender tube) is inserted into the coronary artery, where the balloon is inflated to push the plaque back toward the arterial wall. These patients tend not to have as severe disease as those who undergo CABGS (67).

Testing

Testing of patients with CHD is much more involved than for the apparently healthy person described in chapter 11. There are classes of CHD patients for whom exercise or exercise testing is inappropriate and dangerous (4). For those who can be tested, a 12-lead electrocardiogram (ECG) is monitored at discrete intervals during the GXT while a variety of leads are displayed continuously on an oscilloscope. Blood pressure, RPE, and various signs or symptoms are also noted. The criteria for terminating the GXT focus on various pathological signs (e.g., S-T segment depression) and symptoms (e.g., angina pectoris) rather than on achieving some percentage of age-adjusted maximal HR. On the basis of the response to the GXT, the person may be referred for additional testing: use of radioactive molecules to evaluate perfusion (^{201}thallium) and the capacity of the ventricle to eject blood (^{99}technetium), or direct *angiography,* in which a radiopaque dye is injected into the coronary arteries to determine the blockage directly (53).

Exercise Program

The basic cardiac rehabilitation exercise program resembles the one mentioned earlier for the apparently healthy; it includes warm-up with stretching, endurance exercise at a THR, muscle-strengthening activities, and a cool-down period. However, due to the fact that CHD patients are generally very deconditioned, only light exercise is required to achieve

angina, angina pectoris — Severe cardiac pain that may radiate to the jaw, arms, or legs. Angina is caused by myocardial ischemia, which can be induced by exercise in susceptible individuals. Exercise should be stopped, and the person should be referred for medical attention.

coronary artery bypass graft surgery (CABGS) — Surgery to bypass one or more blocked coronary arteries. In this procedure a blood vessel is sewn into existing coronary arteries above and below the blockage.

percutaneous transluminal coronary angioplasty — A procedure in which a catheter is inserted in a blocked artery and a balloon is inflated to push the plaque back toward the wall to open the artery.

their THR. In addition, because these patients are on a wide variety of medications, some of which will decrease maximal HR, the THR zone is determined from their GXT results; the 220 – age formula is not used. The patients usually begin with intermittent moderate-intensity exercise (1 min on, 1 min off) and gradually increase the duration of the work period. Given that CABGS and post-MI patients have had direct damage to their hearts, the exercise should facilitate, and not interfere with, the healing process. As you might guess, given the nature of the patients and the risks involved, cardiac rehabilitation programs take place in hospitals and clinics where there is direct medical supervision and the capacity to deal with emergencies should they occur. After a patient completes an 8- to 12-week Phase II program, the person may continue in a Phase III program away from the hospital, with less supervision but the same capacity to respond to emergencies (53). What are the benefits of such programs to the patient with CHD?

Benefits of Rehabilitation Programs

There is no question that CHD patients have improved cardiovascular function as a result of exercise programs. This is shown in higher $\dot{V}O_2$max values; higher work rates achieved without ischemia, as shown by angina pectoris or S-T segment changes; and an increased capacity for prolonged submaximal work (53, 70). The improved lipid profile (lower total cholesterol and higher HDL cholesterol) is a function of more than the exercise alone, given that weight loss and the saturated-fat content of the diet can modify these variables (8). It must be mentioned that a cardiac rehabilitation program should not be viewed simply as an exercise program. It is a multi-intervention effort involving exercise, medication, diet, and counseling.

11 In Review: Cardiac patients take diagnostic GXTs prior to participation in an exercise program. The prescription is based on the signs and symptoms monitored during the test. The exercise program is similar to that of the apparently healthy individual, with moderate-intensity intermittent exercise done at a prescribed THR. Exercise prescriptions may need to be adjusted weekly.

Case Studies

You can check your answers by referring to appendix A.

18.1

A Type I diabetic is about to begin a 3-hr hike up a nearby mountain. Should the insulin dose be decreased or increased?

18.2

A 38-year-old woman with asthma would like to enter your fitness program. What kinds of questions would you ask her during your screening interview? What kind of exercise program would you recommend?

SOURCE LIST

1. American College of Obstetricians and Gynecologists (1994)
2. American College of Sports Medicine (ACSM) (1990)
3. ACSM (1993a)
4. ACSM (1995)
5. American Diabetes Association (ADA) (1985)
6. ADA (1990)
7. ADA (1994)
8. American Heart Association Committee Report (1982)
9. P.-O. Åstrand (1952)
10. Babcock, Paterson, & Cunningham (1994)
11. Bassett & Zweifler (1990)
12. Berg (1986)
13. Berger & Kemmer (1990)
14. Berman & Sutton (1986)
15. Braun, Zimmermann, & Kretchmer (1995)
16. Brysasco & Crimi (1994)
17. Buskirk & Hodgson (1987)
18. Campaigne & Lampman (1994)
19. Cantu (1982)
20. Carpenter (1994)
21. Cureton & Warren (1990)
22. Deprés, Bouchard, & Malina (1990)
23. Drinkwater (1994)
24. Eggleston (1986)
25. Franklin, Hellerstein, Gordon, & Timmis (1986)
26. Franz (1987)

27. Gerhard & Schachter (1980)
28. Giacca, Shi, Marliss, Zinman, & Vranic (1994)
29. Gudat, Berger, & Lefèbvre (1994)
30. Hagberg (1990)
31. Hagberg (1994)
32. Haskell (1994)
33. Heaney (1987)
34. Jennings, Deakin, Korner, Meredith, Kingwell, & Nelson (1991)
35. Johnson & Slemenda (1987)
36. Jones, Berman, Bartkiewig, & Oldridge (1987)
37. Kannel (1990)
38. Kaplan (1994)
39. Kasch, Boyer, Van Camp, Verity, & Wallace (1990)
40. Katz (1986)
41. Katz (1987)
42. Kriska, Blair, & Pereira (1994)
43. Lindsay (1987)
44. Lotgering, Gilbert, & Longo (1984)
45. Lotgering, Gilbert, & Longo (1985)
46. Mahler (1993)
47. Makker & Holgate (1994)
48. McKenzie, McLuckie, & Stirling (1994)
49. Middleton (1980)
50. Miracle (1986)
51. Park (1989)
52. Pierson, Covert, Koenig, Namekta, & Shin Kim (1986)
53. Pollock & Wilmore (1990)
54. Powers & Howley (1990)
55. Richter & Galbo (1986)
56. S. Robinson (1938)
57. Rowland (1990)
58. Shephard (1976)
59. Sly (1986)
60. Smith (1984)
61. Smith & Gilligan (1987)
62. Smith, Smith, & Gilligan (1990)
63. Smith & Stoedefalke (1978)
64. Soukup & Kovaleski (1993)
65. Stockdale-Woolley, Haggerty, & McMahon (1986)
66. Tate, Hyek, & Taffet (1994)
67. Tommaso, Lesch, & Sonnenblick (1984)
68. Voy (1986)
69. Vranic & Wasserman (1990)
70. Wenger & Hellerstein (1984)
71. Wenger & Hurst (1984)
72. Wolfe, Brenner, & Mottola (1994)
73. Wolfe et al. (1989)
74. World Health Organization (1986)
75. Young (1995)
76. Zwiren (1993)

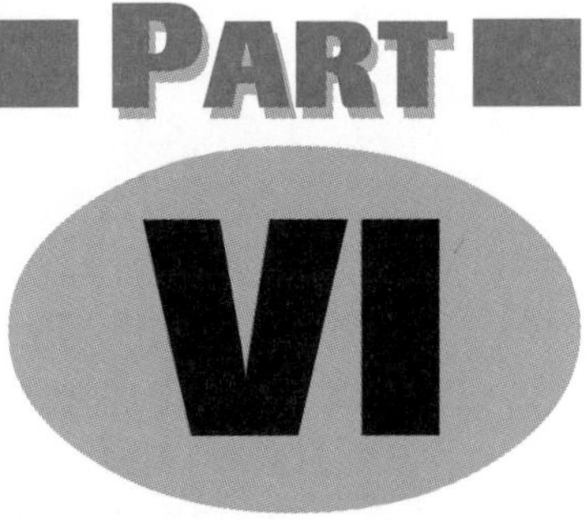

Part VI

Exercise Programming Considerations

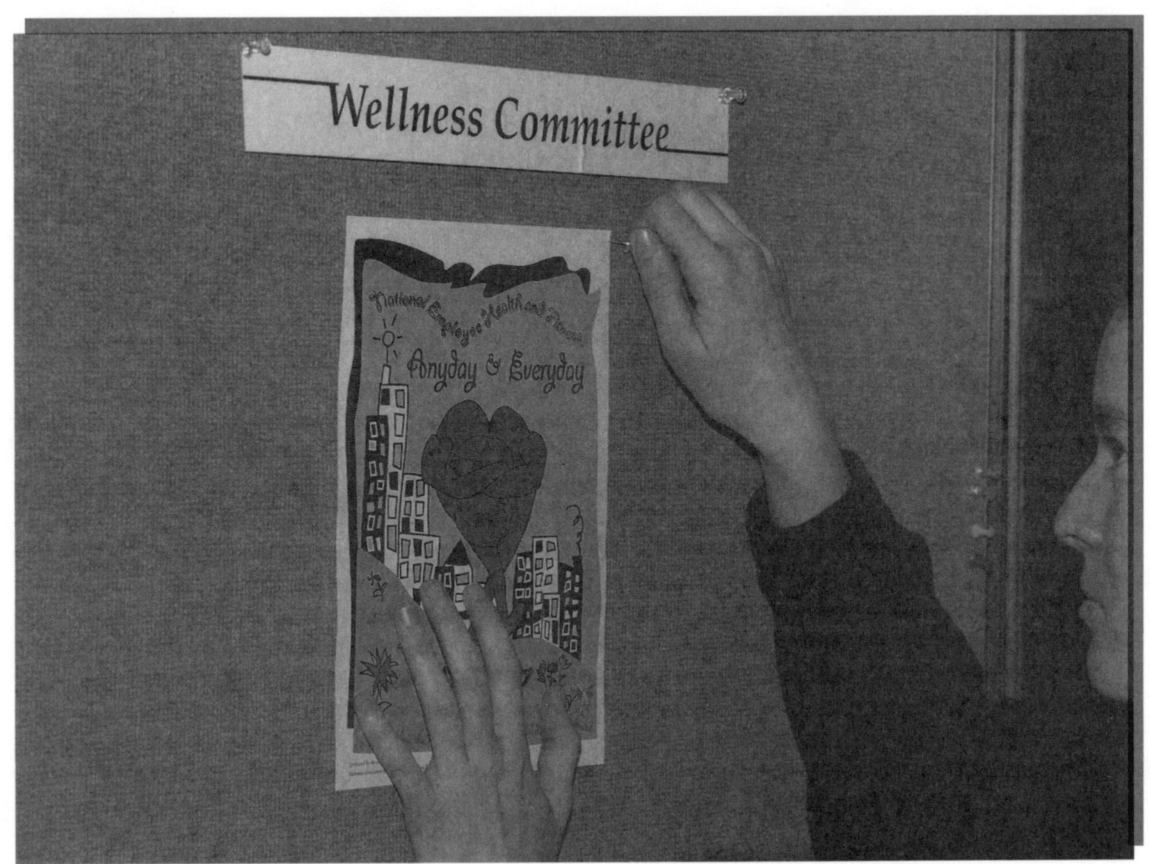

© Chris Brown

Part VI

Prior parts of the handbook have dealt with assessment and exercise prescription for components of physical fitness. This section includes other elements needed for a comprehensive and effective fitness program. Chapters 19 and 20 deal with psychological aspects of personality and stress, and ways to help motivate individuals to adopt a healthy lifestyle. Chapter 21 summarizes the prevention and treatment of injuries. Chapter 22 reviews analysis of the electrocardiogram and current medications used for cardiovascular problems. Finally, chapter 23 describes the processes used in program administration.

CHAPTER

19

Human Behavior/ Psychology, Stress, and Health

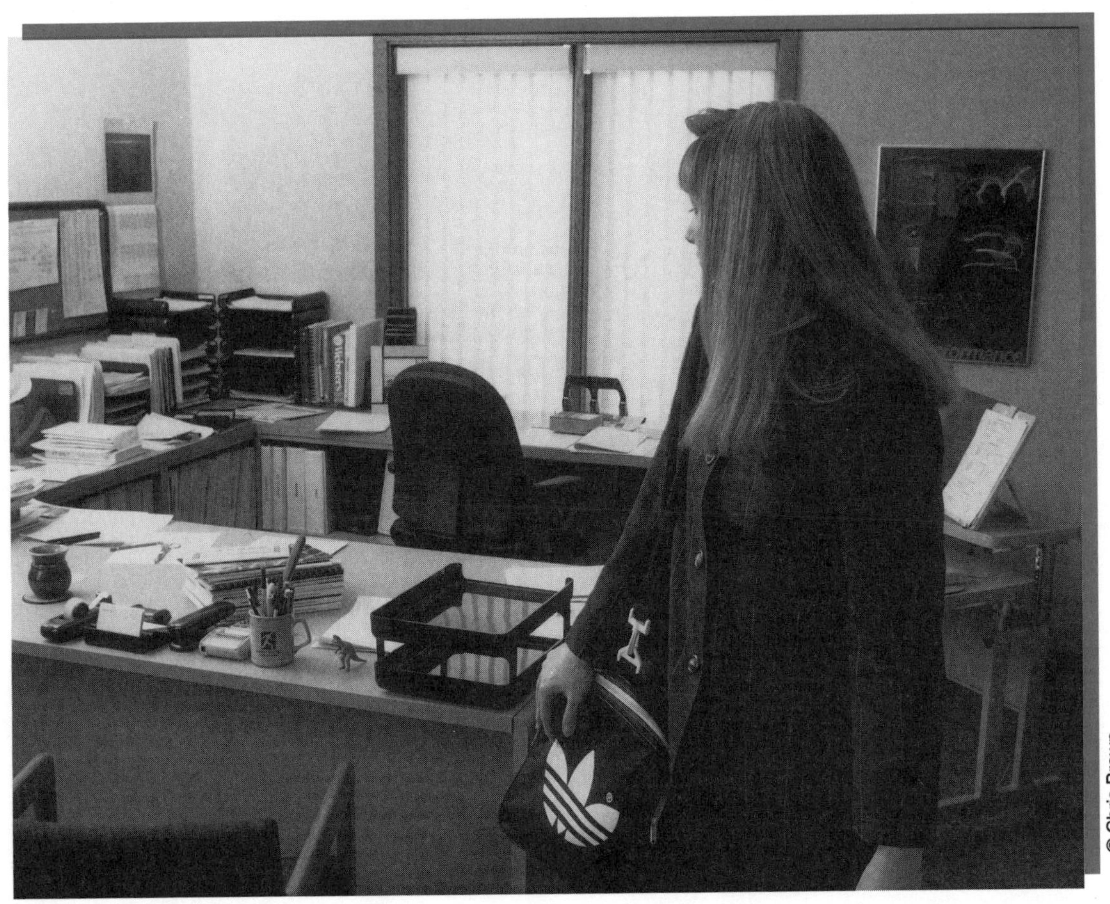

© Chris Brown

The reader will be able to: **OBJECTIVES**

1. Describe how the HFI deals with different personalities in an exercise setting.
2. Explain how to enhance motivation to begin and continue exercise.
3. List techniques to communicate with individuals in group programs.
4. Describe the components of stress.
5. Explain how physical activity may affect stress.
6. Describe the positive and negative aspects of stress and how aging may affect response to stressors.
7. List ways to minimize unhealthy stress levels.
8. Identify techniques that can be used in an exercise program to facilitate skill development in muscular relaxation.

This book emphasizes physical fitness; yet physical, mental, psychological, social, and spiritual aspects of life are all intertwined. This chapter deals with stress, an area that bridges the psychological and physiological aspects of fitness (see 6).

After a review of exercise, fitness, and mental health, Brown (4) reported that 25% of the U.S. population may be functioning at less than optimal levels as a result of stress and stress-related emotions such as anxiety and depression. Robinson (10) reported that in the United States, two thirds of visits to primary-care physicians are stress related; 112 million people take medication for stress, and industry loses more than $150 billion annually on stress-related problems. Exercise and fitness play an important role in promoting positive mental health and preventing the negative consequences of stress.

RELAXATION/AROUSAL BALANCE

The healthy life involves the ability to relax and disregard irrelevant stimuli during quiet times. The fit person can also work and play with vigor and enthusiasm. **Relaxation** (parasympathetic nervous system dominance) and **arousal** (sympathetic nervous system dominance) are both enhanced by physical conditioning. One of the keys to a healthy life is a balance between arousal and relaxation. People who are *always* relaxed and easygoing do not usually accomplish very much. In contrast, people who at all moments have the go-get-'em attitude toward every single aspect of life exhibit "coronary-prone" behavior. This chapter describes the relationships among personality, physical activity, stress, and health. Dealing extensively with all psychological aspects of fitness is beyond the scope of this chapter. People with pathological traits or behaviors (i.e., mental illness) should be referred to appropriate health or psychological professionals. We are examining mental health in terms of different levels of *normal* personality and stress, with an emphasis on their implications for fitness programs.

PERSONALITY-RELATED VARIABLES AND PHYSICAL ACTIVITY PROGRAMMING

Providing definitive comments about the psychophysiological effects of a specific external stimulus is impossible because individuals perceive and react to the same situation differently. The same movie may evoke anger, laughter, or no emotion at all from three different people. Playing in front of a crowd might cause best or worst performances in different people.

Part of the different perception of and reaction to the same situation is related to personality. Although completely characterizing someone's personality or predicting exactly how that personality will interact with physical activity or other stimuli is not possible, some generalizations aid the health fitness instructor (HFI) and personal fitness trainer (PFT) in working with the many different types of individuals enrolled in fitness programs.

Type A and Type B Behavior

There is general agreement that one's personality and ability to cope with stress are related to one's risk for coronary heart disease (CHD). The exact characteristics, however, that cause the higher risk are difficult to enumerate or measure. One attempt to do this separates people's behaviors into Type A and Type B. **Type A behavior** (i.e., the go-getter, hard-driving, time-conscious, hostile, impatient person) is coronary-prone behavior. A Type A person has a greater stress response to psychological stressors (9). Therefore, this person should learn to relax, should be cautious about overdoing exercise, and should be engaged in more relatively noncompetitive activities. The Type A person often has to learn to deal with anger and hostility. The person with **Type B behavior** (easygoing, nonaggressive, "laid-back"), on the other hand, may need to be more stimulated and motivated to begin and continue with the exercise program.

Anger

Some evidence suggests a relationship between **anger** and CHD. People who keep their anger "bottled up" inside rather than expressing it (e.g., talking to a close friend about it) have increased risk of CHD. Three recommendations can be made to help people cope with anger:

1. Try to develop positive attitudes toward self, others, and the world in general, so that anger is less frequent.
2. Express emotions, such as anger, rather than denying the emotions or keeping them inside.
3. Develop the kinds of relationships with others in which emotions can be shared.

By being open about her or his own feelings (e.g., "that really made me angry yesterday") and by being sensitive about the fitness participants' moods (e.g., "you seem upset today"), the HFI can help people acknowledge their emotions.

relaxation — To loosen or make less stiff or gain relief from work or tension.

arousal — The act of becoming excited, causing a stress response (i.e., a greater physiological response than is needed to perform the task). Arousal often occurs in competitive situations.

Type A behavior — A label denoting a person who is hard-driving, time-conscious, and impatient. Some evidence suggests that this type of behavior is a secondary risk factor of CHD. Type A is the opposite of Type B.

Type B behavior — The opposite of Type A behavior; easygoing, nonaggressive, and "laid-back."

anger — A strong emotion of displeasure or antagonism, which is often excited by a sense of injury or insult and frequently paired with a desire to retaliate.

Aggression, Assertiveness, Hostility, and Denial

Aggression, assertiveness, hostility, and denial may all, for different reasons, cause a person to do too much. Individuals who are **aggressive** or hostile may overdo exercise because they get so involved in the activity that they don't pay attention to signs of discomfort or danger. Some people try to deny that they have pain and thus tend to do too much. One of the distinctions between **assertiveness** and aggression or hostility is that the assertive person pursues objectives firmly, yet remains sensitive to others; whereas the aggressive or hostile person tends to be less concerned with others' feelings. The HFI needs to protect other members of the group from aggressive or hostile behavior.

Anxiety, Depression, and Fear

Many individuals, often including postcardiac patients, have high levels of **anxiety**, **fear**, and **depression**. People who are unduly worried or afraid need support. They must be able to ease into activity and be shown that positive results can occur with minimum risks; gradually they can be introduced to higher levels of exercise. The feeling of lack of control is often a part of anxiety, fear, or depression; a person who is becoming physically active and adopting other healthy behaviors may have increased perception of control over her or his own life.

Rationalization

One of the difficult skills in working with people is to be able to differentiate between the actual reason for behavior and the **rationalization** that is given that sounds "better" than the real reason. It will not be possible to help a person commit to exercise or other healthy behaviors until the real reasons for the current behaviors are known. The HFI hears many excuses for why someone can't develop healthy activities or discontinue unhealthy behaviors. One technique to help the person deal with the underlying reasons for her or his inactivity is to keep asking questions aimed at uncovering the truth behind what is making it difficult to change. Chapter 20 provides assistance for helping people modify behavior.

Rejection

Rejection is relevant in two ways for the HFI. Some people in the fitness program have rejected exercise in the past or feel that active people have rejected them (e.g., they were the last ones chosen to play games). The HFI must be sensitive to this feeling and help the person feel included and welcome. On the other hand, the HFI should realize that he or she will not be 100% successful in helping people become active. Some potential fitness participants will reject fitness programs despite the HFI's best efforts to help them stay active; it is important for the HFI not to take that rejection personally.

Catharsis

Some people use exercise to experience a **catharsis**, a cleansing agent for the mind and emotions. Fitness activities are used to erase the cluttered state and allow the person to start fresh following the exercise. After a minimum level of fitness is reached, the fitness program should accommodate activities that allow individuals to "let go." Chapter 17 describes a variety of activities, including group games, that might be utilized in this type of atmosphere.

Euphoria

Numerous reports show that some people experience a special emotional state (e.g., "runner's high") while exercising. This state of **euphoria** resembles a deep religious experience or some of the emotional states achieved by drugs. It cannot be planned, nor can it serve as the basis for motivation because not all people will experience it. However, people can develop a positive addiction to exercise as they achieve the common state of feeling good as a result of appropriate exercise. One of the HFI's main purposes is to help people progress to the fitness levels where they become addicted to exercise in the sense that they look forward to their regular workouts. As with all healthy behaviors, however, it is possible to go to the extreme; so that instead of a healthy addiction to exercise as a part of one's life, some may become obsessed and overemphasize its importance, spending time exercising that should be spent on other parts of their lives (e.g., time with family and friends, attention to work). The HFI assists at both extremes, helping inactive people become active and discouraging exercise fanatics from spending excessive amounts of time in physical fitness activities.

1 **In Review: A number of psychological traits may promote or interfere with healthy exercise. Various personality**

traits, such as Type A behavior, anger, and hostility, increase the risk of health problems. Other emotional problems, such as anxiety and depression, may result from health problems and low fitness levels. Individuals with these characteristics need special, sensitive attention in exercise situations.

Understanding the different responses to physical activity, including rationalization, rejection, catharsis, and euphoria, will assist HFIs in helping individuals with their exercise program.

Motivation

The HFI is concerned with the **motivation** for exercise at two levels. First, how can we get people to begin a fitness program? What kind of contact can be made with people in our community to encourage them to begin fitness programs? The public has been educated about healthy behaviors (e.g., most people agree that they should exercise on a regular basis). However, convenient programs that provide personal contact with and guidance from exercise professionals are needed to complement information about the healthy life. The second level of motivation deals with the things that can be done to get people to continue to exercise as a part of their lifestyle. Individual attention, realistic goals that are periodically tested, options for group participation, involvement of spouse or important others, contracts, and programs that minimize injury all seem to help people commit to continuing in their fitness programs. Chapter 20 identifies the characteristics of people who tend to drop out of fitness programs and suggests ways to enhance regular exercise behavior. Whether the HFI is motivating a participant to begin or to continue activity, fitness has to achieve priority status (like eating and sleeping) in a person's life. Efforts at increasing self-motivation must have that end in sight at all times. Thus, external (extrinsic) rewards must be viewed as a temporary means to change behavior, but the behavior can only be maintained over the long haul with internal (intrinsic) motivation.

Empathy

It may be difficult for the HFI to understand the feelings of many people who join fitness programs. The HFI must try to understand and appreciate how it feels to have low self-esteem about one's body, to be unable to perform well on many physical tasks, and to be slow at learning new physical skills. The HFI should pay attention to her or his own emotional feelings when in uncomfortable situations. Many potential fitness participants have similar feelings when involved in fitness tests and exercise. An HFI's sensitivity to the emotional feelings of participants (his or her ability to empathize) is part of the individual attention and concern that is important to being an effective motivator.

aggressive — Label given to a person who exhibits high levels of animosity or hostility, often unprovoked, which sometimes results from frustration or a feeling of inferiority.

assertiveness — Pursuing objectives firmly. One of the distinctions between assertiveness and aggression or hostility is that the assertive person is sensitive to others, whereas the aggressive or hostile person tends to be less concerned with others' feelings.

anxiety — Feeling of fear, apprehension, and dread, often without apparent cause.

fear — A distressing emotion aroused by actual or perceived impending pain or danger.

depression — Emotional dejection greater than that warranted by any objective reasons, often with symptoms such as insomnia, headaches, exhaustion, anorexia, irritability, loss of interest, impaired concentration, feelings that life is not worth living, and suicidal thoughts.

rationalization — The process of inventing plausible explanations for acts or opinions that actually have other causes.

rejection — Relative to exercise, some people may have rejected exercise in the past or feel that active, fit people may have rejected them.

catharsis — A cleansing agent for the mind and emotions. Fitness activities are used to erase the cluttered state and allow the person to start fresh following the exercise.

euphoria — An exaggerated sense of well-being.

motivation — An incentive that prompts a person to act with a sense of purpose.

Play and Goal Orientation

One of the key elements in achieving a balance between arousal and relaxation and in defusing the Type A or Type B personality is to help people appreciate a balance of work and play. The Type A individual has difficulty taking time just to play and enjoy an activity that is not directly related to productivity; the Type B person has a problem in settling down to a task and getting it done. People who try to pattern fitness programs after military or athletic models often have the goal orientation without the play. Others who are not discriminating about the selection of activities, as long as everyone is happy, have a play orientation and may achieve the playfulness without achieving fitness goals. The good fitness program achieves this balance by including activities designed to improve all fitness components (**goal orientation**) *and* a playful atmosphere where participating is fun for its own sake (**play orientation**).

Goal and Ego Orientation

Recent research (5) has differentiated between the goal orientation with its emphasis on doing the activity well, with the **ego orientation** of trying to win at all costs. Motivating participants to continue being active is best achieved when the instructor and the participants adopt the goal orientation. They do the activity, trying their best, and are pleased when they can improve their skill. This does not mean that the participants do not try to win when playing a game, but the major emphasis is on the process of playing the game, not on the final score.

Traits and States

The ability to make a distinction between the usual personality characteristics (trait) and the specific, situational personality characteristics (state) is helpful in dealing with people. For example, a person who is normally very quiet and introverted (has that trait) may become an extrovert (be in that state) during competitive games. Or a person who is normally very relaxed (trait) may get anxious (state) during an exercise class.

Generally, personality traits do not change very much or very quickly. An HFI should use an understanding of traits to work with individuals on a long-term basis. Emotional states vary with situations and are more susceptible to change. For example, people who are afraid of or anxious about exercise need to be introduced to activity in a way that helps them become relaxed and unafraid when exercising.

2 In Review: Motivating individuals to begin and continue exercise can be enhanced by a sensitivity to people's personality traits and states. Motivation is enhanced with a fitness program that includes a goal orientation and a balance of play and work approaches to exercise.

UNDERSTANDING THE PERSONALITIES OF PARTICIPANTS

Understanding the different personalities and interests of individual fitness participants will assist the HFI and PFT in providing fitness alternatives in an atmosphere that will motivate participants to adopt and continue healthy lifestyles. Two ways to enhance motivation are being more sensitive to individuals and providing fitness activities that will appeal to people with diverse interests.

The HFI and PFT learn to respond to specific behaviors. For example, participants with Type A, angry, aggressive, or hostile behavior need to be directed to more relaxing, noncompetitive activities. Participants with Type B behavior need to be motivated; and participants who are afraid or anxious need to be encouraged to ease into activities that can be easily learned, taking small steps in trying new activities.

The way the HFI communicates with fitness participants can assist in providing a good atmosphere for the program. Taylor and Miller (13) listed four types of communication skills recommended for the HFI:

- Noncommittal acknowledgment
- Door opening
- Content paraphrasing
- Confrontation

In the first form of communication, noncommittal acknowledgment, the HFI indicates acceptance of the participant by comments like, "I see," or nodding her or his head. In the second, door opening, the HFI asks the participant to continue expressing a thought. In content paraphrasing the HFI may want to repeat what the participant has said in different words to demonstrate that he or she has been listening and to check for accuracy. For example, Diane, a member of your fitness club says, "I can't do the strength routine." You might say, "I see, what seems to be the problem?" Diane: "When I try to lift the bar, the right side goes up, but I can't get the left side up." You: "So you're not able to lift the bar smoothly?" Diane: "That's right." You: "Let's go in the weight room and check it—you may need to start with a lower weight." These first three types of communication are especially helpful for participants who are uncomfortable or withdrawn in the exercise setting. These communication skills are especially helpful in talking with people who are not participating on a regular basis. The HFI can use the suggestions in chapter 20 to help these people become regular exercisers.

The fourth type of communication skill, confrontation, is useful for dealing with participants who are behaving inappropriately. Participants who are disrupting the class or threatening the safety of themselves or other participants should be dealt with directly and firmly. People who are not ready for exercise either physically or mentally should be excused from class and told that they are welcome to return when they are ready and able to participate. Those who disrupt the program by finding fault with everything, being a "clown," doing too much above the recommended intensity, or trying to take over the class often need special individual attention. It is important to spend some additional time with these individuals to help them identify their goals for the program and understand clearly what type of behavior is and is not considered appropriate.

To provide for the many different types of personalities that participants bring to the exercise situation, fitness programs should include options for individual or group, controlled or uninhibited, and competitive or cooperative activities with an "it's okay to choose any of the options" atmosphere.

In Review: An HFI should be able to communicate with individual participants using the four communication skills: noncommittal acknowledgment, door opening, content paraphrasing, and confrontation.

STRESS CONTINUUMS

Personality is related to stress; a person's perception of a stimulus or situation largely determines how stressful the situation is for that person. No uniform agreement exists on definitions of stress terms. For our purposes, a **stressor** is defined as any stimulus or condition that causes physiological arousal beyond what is necessary to accomplish the activity. This excessive arousal is called **stress**.

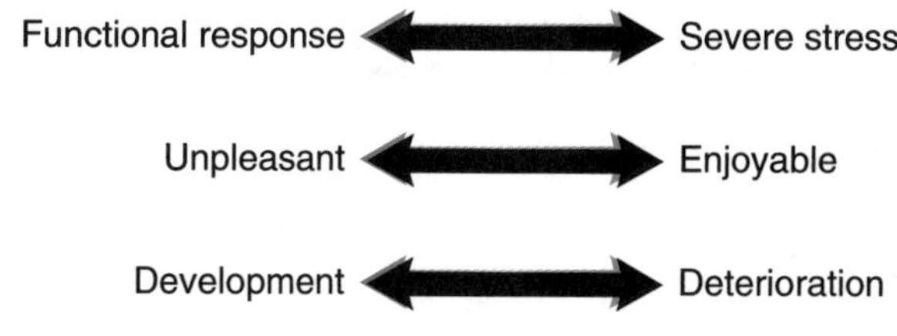

FIGURE 19.1 Stress continuums.

Stress has three major components (see figure 19.1). A complete description of a stressful event includes the amount by which the stress response exceeds the functional demand, how pleasant it is to the individual, and whether it causes development or deterioration. The following sections expand on each of these bases for understanding stress.

Functional-to-Severe Stress Continuum

The physiological response at any one time lies on a continuum from what is essential to provide the energy for that task to an extreme physiological response beyond what is needed. Physiological responses to stress include increased

- heart rate,
- blood pressure,
- catecholamine levels,

goal orientation — The tendency of a person to behave on the basis of her or his goals, with an emphasis on doing the activity well.

play orientation — The tendency of a person to participate in an activity because it is fun, rather than to concentrate on achieving a specific goal.

ego orientation — Trying to win at all costs.

stressor — Any stimulus or condition that causes physiological arousal beyond what is necessary to accomplish the activity.

stress — A physiological or psychological response to a stressor beyond what is needed to accomplish a task.

Table 19.1 Stress Components of Heart Rate (beats · min^{-1})

Component of heart rate	Activity		
	Sitting	Climbing stairs	Running
HR needed to do task	30	50	100
Additional HR due to chronic stress			
Poor aerobic fitness	+15	+20	+40
Excess fat	+5	+15	+20
Additional HR due to acute stress			
Not relaxed	+10	+5	0
Emotional state	+15	+10	0
Total HR	75	100	160

Note. This HR model shows the contribution of the heart rate necessary to do various tasks plus the additional HR response caused by chronic and acute stressors. The actual HR values will vary with the individual depending on body size, fitness level, and type and severity of stressors.

- ventricular arrhythmia,
- levels of free fatty acids and serum cholesterol, and
- platelet adhesion (12).

Table 19.1 illustrates how typical resting and submaximal HRs include not only the HR needed to provide energy for the body but also the increased HR due to chronic stressors (e.g., excess fat) and acute stressors (e.g., emotional states). The same principle applies to psychological attention needed for various tasks. For example, moving in a crowd requires moderate psychological attention. A person under stress will respond to the same situation with high psychological attention (6). Individuals who overreact to stressors have a higher risk of a number of health problems (9).

Unpleasant-to-Enjoyable Stress Continuum

Another aspect of stress is how the stressor is perceived by the individual on a continuum between unpleasant and enjoyable. A person might have similar stress responses to an exciting music concert and to taking the Health Fitness Instructor's Certification examination, but she or he may perceive the concert as being more enjoyable.

Development-to-Deterioration Continuum

The third aspect of stress is what happens to an individual as a result of a stressful experience on a continuum from development to deterioration. What happens to the person under stress is, of course, the main criterion for determining whether the stressful event was positive or negative. The positive stressor results in a healthier, stronger person. The negative stressor leads to a weaker individual. The end result of stress is somewhat independent of the other two aspects of stress previously discussed. For example, a very stressful event (i.e., causing a large stress response beyond what is essential physically) could result in a person being inspired to achieve great things, or it might destroy a person's initiative. On the other hand, conditions that cause small stress responses might lead to steady development or gradually wear down a person's desire to excel. In addition, a person might grow and develop from stressors that are both pleasant (e.g., positive reinforcement) and unpleasant (e.g., deadline to have a project done). Either pleasant or unpleasant stressors might tempt a person to avoid dealing with important areas of life. For these reasons the HFI should be cautious in identifying a specific stressor as being healthy or unhealthy based on the degree of physiological and psychological stress response or how much the individual liked the situation. A better criterion is to determine whether the experience led the person toward higher levels of mental, social, or physical health.

In Review: Excessive response (stress) to a situation (stressor) is described in terms of level of arousal (the functional-to-severe stress continuum); degree of unpleasantness (the unpleasant-to-enjoyable stress continuum); and, most important,

whether it results in a positive or negative shift in health status (the development-to-deterioration stress continuum).

PHYSICAL ACTIVITY AND STRESS

One of the advantages of separating functional stimuli from stressors is that they interact with physical activity differently. Separating the effects of immediate and long-term physical activity on stress responses is also helpful in terms of understanding physical activity and stress.

Response to Acute Exercise and Functional (Environmental) Stimuli

The physiological response to acute physical activity and functional stimuli is additive. Numerous environmental stimuli such as exercise, heat, altitude, and pollution cause a functional increased physiological response (see chapter 14). If more than one of these stimuli is present, the physiological response is greater than if only one stimulus were present. Thus, when people exercise in hot, humid, or polluted conditions, or at high altitude, they must do less exercise to achieve the same physiological response (e.g., target heart rate). The one exception is exercising in the cold because the heat by-product of exercise helps one cope with the cold.

Response to Acute Exercise and Psychological Stressors

The physiological response to acute exercise and psychological stressors varies with the intensity of exercise, but generally it is not additive. Nonfunctional stimuli appear to affect the physiological response at rest and during light exercise but have little effect on the response to moderate or hard exercise. Nonfunctional stimuli also affect a person's decision about when to stop during a maximal task. Thus, if a person is very angry or happy, the heart rate (HR) and blood pressure (BP) at rest and during light exercise may be elevated, and the person may decide to continue exercising longer or quit early. If the person is sad or relaxed, the HR and BP during light work may be depressed, and the decision to stop exercising may come earlier or later than usual. Thus emotional state, such as anxiety about taking the test during a graded exercise test, may affect some of the physiological and psychological measurements taken early in the test as well as the length of time until voluntary exhaustion.

Physical Activity for Stress Reduction

Many professionals have justified exercise programs partly on the basis of stress reduction. Although the claims have often exceeded the evidence, there is some basis for a relationship between stress reduction and acute (immediate) and chronic (long-range) exercise.

Acute Activity and Stress Reduction

Acute exercise results in a positive mood change and has been shown to reduce state anxiety and muscle tension (4). Five factors are related to single bouts of exercise helping to reduce stress:

1. Distraction
2. Perception of personal control
3. Feeling good
4. Interaction with others
5. Physiological changes

As with many other activities, exercise can serve as a temporary distraction from stressors. Stepping away from a problem and then coming back to it at a later time is often helpful. This technique is healthy as long as exercise does not become an avenue of escape from the problem. The ultimate reduction of stress must come from coping with the stressor. One part of the coping strategy, however, can be the distraction of physical activity.

One of the primary concepts in a person's ability to cope with stressors is the perception of personal control. In some cases, exercise enhances this feeling of control. For example, increased practice and skill acquisition causes less stress in playing a game in the presence of others. One of the benefits of a postcardiac program is that it reduces the fear that any exertion will cause another heart attack and leaves the individual feeling more in control of his or her everyday life.

Stress is also reduced by the simple response of a positive mood change. The subjective reports of feeling good after exercise last as long as 6 hr post-exercise (11). Exercise is related to reduction in feelings of depression, anxiety, and tension (11).

Another way acute exercise may reduce stress is by providing a time to have either more or less interaction with others. Stress reduction can result when the exercise session provides a time to be alone for people who experience daily stress from constant contact with other people (e.g., the working parent who must spend almost every waking moment in the presence of others, such as children, spouse, employees, employer, and colleagues, all demanding time and attention). That person can use a walk/jog program as a time to be alone with her or his own thoughts. At the other extreme is the person who has little contact with other people during the typical day and for whom loneliness is a potential stressor. Doing activities and having time to talk with other people in an exercise program can aid that person. The HFI should be aware of the needs of individuals in terms of the amount of social interaction during the exercise sessions.

The physiological changes that take place as a result of exercise can also affect levels of stress. For example, endorphins (i.e., endogenous, morphine-like chemicals) are increased as a result of exercise. One of the effects of this change is to lessen our perception of pain. The increased arousal (sympathetic nervous system) may cause some individuals to feel good. Following exercise people often feel more relaxed (parasympathetic nervous system), with reduced muscle tension.

Chronic Activity and Stress Reduction

The long-term effects of a regular exercise program also provide bases for stress reduction. Reduced arousal prior to, during, and after exposure to stressors; quicker recovery from stressors; and improved emotional reactions to some stressors are related to habitual exercise (2).

Regular acute bouts of exercise provide substantial time when people are less affected by stressors—one additional benefit of physical conditioning. This includes an improved glucose tolerance, positive mood changes, and reduction in tension. Several studies have found that regular physical activity reduces anxiety and depression in individuals who start with high levels of these traits (8).

Increased cardiorespiratory fitness (CRF) and decreased body fat cause individuals to be less stressed throughout the day. Furthermore, these changes reduce the risk of CHD, hypertension, glucose intolerance, and the risk of sudden death.

With increased fitness levels, physical activity itself becomes less of a stressor. For example, numerous studies have shown that a fit person can do the same amount of external work with lower HR, BP, catecholamines, and so forth. Thus the functional response to the work (the energy necessary to accomplish the task) remains the same, but the stress response is reduced.

Some researchers believe, with some support, that increased adaptation to physical activity provides a basis for better adaptation to other stressors. Others believe, with some support, that increased adaptation is specific to different stimuli and stressors. Additional research into this question is needed before definitive claims can be made.

5 **In Review: Exercise and physical stimuli, such as heat or altitude, interact to produce increased cardiorespiratory response at all levels of exercise intensity. Psychological stressors affect physiological and psychological responses at rest and during light work, as well as time to voluntary exhaustion, but have little influence on physiological response to moderate work. Single bouts of activity may reduce stress through distraction, increased perception of control, positive mood shift, interaction with others, and physiological changes in the body. Chronic exercise (conditioning) may reduce stress through a series of acute activities, reduction of chronic stressors, lessening the stress of exercise, reduction of anxiety and depression, and perhaps some cross-adaptation to stressors.**

RELATIONSHIP BETWEEN STRESS AND HEALTH

Stress is important for both positive and negative aspects of health. No discussion of the highest quality of life possible or of serious health problems would be complete without including the relevance of stress.

Positive and Negative Stress

People often think of stress as primarily a negative influence on their lives, but it has many positive features. The presence of a great variety of stimuli and stressors provides the interesting experiences essential to a full life. People develop, learn, grow, and strive for their optimal potential through encountering stress. Even peak experiences, those special emotional moments of the good life that are remembered forever, are usually stressful. Without stress, life would be bland indeed.

The inability to cope with stress is considered a risk factor for many major health problems (e.g., CHD, hypertension, cancer, ulcers, low-back pain, and headaches). Although inability to cope with stress probably is not sufficient to cause any of these problems if no predispositions exist, stress seems to manifest itself wherever the *weak link* is found. So for some people, stress results in a myocardial infarction; for others, it results in hypertension, ulcers, low-back pain, or headaches.

An inability to cope with one stressor can be transferable to other stressors. Many people, because of stressors in other areas of their lives, find themselves getting upset (stressed) over something that normally would not bother them. Two aspects of the inability to cope are perception of and reaction to a potential stressor. Although the positive transfer of adaptation from one stressor to other stressors is an open question, there is little doubt about negative transfer: An inability to cope in one area leads to coping problems in other areas of life.

The health problems caused by lack of exercise can also be sources of stress, and negative physiological and psychological changes (stressors) have also been related to excessive exercise (e.g., exercising more than 5 days per week, longer than 30 min per workout, or at intensities higher than THR [4]). Health problems related to lack of or excess exercise include increased injury risk, soreness, obsession, impatience, strain on relationships, neglect of work, and withdrawal symptoms when one cannot exercise (4, 11).

Aging, Stress, and Health

It is difficult to separate the effects of aging, itself, from things that typically happen as a person gets older. Certain experiences are more likely to have happened (more often) as a person becomes older. Positive aspects of aging include increased opportunities to deal with a variety of stressors. From this, many people develop a varied repertoire of coping behaviors.

On the negative side, the longer a person lives, the more likely it is that he or she will develop a serious health problem (although not living longer does not appear to be an attractive alternative). Some of the special life events that appear to cause stress (e.g., death of a loved one) obviously become more frequent with age. Parents are often affected dramatically when all of the children leave home; retirement is also associated with a period of severe change of lifestyle. Lifestyle patterns developed over decades undergo major modifications, sometimes with additional financial difficulties. Evidence shows that people are more likely to have a number of health problems following a series of stressful life events.

Older people often become less active, causing more deterioration in fitness and performance than would occur naturally simply because of increased age. Careful warm-up, safety precautions, cool-down, and gradual progression in activity become even more important in older populations because of the higher risk of health problems and injury and decreased fitness and performance skills. The good news is that an active lifestyle can slow down the physical deterioration of aging. It's never too late to start, and previously sedentary, elderly individuals show remarkable fitness improvements as a result of initiating fitness programs.

6 **In Review: Stress is a factor in positive health. Stressors are involved in having varied experiences, coping with life's special moments, and accomplishing one's goals. Inability to cope with stress is related to major health problems as a secondary risk factor and can cause problems in other areas of one's life.**

Both too little and too much exercise can be related to stress. In addition, aging provides experiences that may cause more stress as the individual deals with the death of loved ones and changes in living conditions and relationships. Older individuals are often better able to cope with stressors because they have learned coping mechanisms over a lifetime of experience with stress. Physical activity can slow down typical aging deterioration.

RECOMMENDATIONS FOR MAINTAINING HEALTHY STRESS LEVELS

People can do many things to maximize the positive aspects of stress while minimizing stress's negative side. In a fitness program, the HFI can help participants learn to fill their lives with healthy stress.

Seek Exposure to a Variety of Stimuli and Stressors

Simply being exposed to a wide range of experiences helps a person become better educated in coping with and less stressed by new situations. A good fitness program provides a variety of experiences, including cooperative, problem-solving, competitive, individual, partner, and team activities. This variety enriches the participant by improving fitness and improving the ability to cope with different physical and social experiences.

Develop a Range of Coping Abilities

People should observe the different strategies that seem to enhance coping with a potentially stressful situation. Facing the problem, looking at alternatives, talking about the problem with close friends, seeking professional or technical advice when needed, stepping back or away from it for a brief time, and so on, are all behaviors that people use to cope with stress. People should ask themselves which coping behaviors are better suited for particular situations. Do some behaviors help but feel uncomfortable to the individual? In terms of fitness, the variety of activities in a good program require different coping strategies. The HFI should be sensitive to participants who need help just coping with physical activity itself. After easing these people into exercise, the HFI can use a variety of fitness activities and the behavior modification suggestions found in chapter 20 to help them develop coping abilities.

Maintain Social Support

Coping with stressors is often aided by positive connections between an individual and her or his social surroundings: family; close friends and relatives; and groups to which one belongs such as places of worship, clubs, unions, and other social groups. The support for one's health is related to a special kind of relationship in these types of social settings (3).

Develop Optimal Fitness

Developing physical, mental, and social fitness characteristics causes potential stressors to be less threatening. For the person who can do hard physical work, physical stressors are not dreaded. For people who are accustomed to the mental processes that lead to problem solving, having a difficult problem is less stressful. Social fitness can be enhanced by doing such things as establishing meaningful relationships with other people, therein developing a support group that helps one respond positively to stressful situations.

Gain Control of as Much of Life as Possible

Perception of control repeatedly looms as a major element in coping with stress. Therefore, whatever a person can do to help gain control of her or his life diminishes the stress of potentially stressful conditions. Some ways to take control of one's life are to adopt healthy behaviors, gain competence in important areas, be assertive in resisting unreasonable demands, and learn to relax.

One of the by-products of exercising, eating nutritious foods, and refraining from use of harmful drugs, is the feeling that one is taking responsibility for one's own life. Not only do the healthy behaviors reduce stress, but the fact that one has "taken charge" also reduces stress levels. Chapter 20 recommends ways to increase healthy behaviors.

People should give attention to the relationships, tasks, and other things that are important to them, so that they increase their skills in those areas and gain enhanced self-confidence that they can be successful in what they find important. In the fitness program, the HFI helps people improve skills in the activities in which they are interested.

People must learn to recognize unreasonable demands, whether imposed by themselves or by someone else, and to work with others (e.g., boss, spouse) to try to accomplish common goals in a reasonable way within an appropriate time frame; this is essential to good health. The HFI must be careful not to place unrealistic goals or demands for future activities and fitness gains on the participant. The HFI can also help individuals set goals that will not be sources of stress.

Techniques can be learned to help people relax (see next section). Benson (1) and others have demonstrated the benefits of the *relaxation response*, including increased parasympathetic dominance resulting in decreased HR, BP, and muscle tension. The HFI should include relaxation techniques as part of the program, perhaps including a short relaxation period following the cool-down.

7 **In Review:** **Coping with stress can be aided by exposing oneself to many stimuli, developing a social network, and increasing levels of fitness. The concept of gaining control of one's life is important in learning to cope with stress. Gaining control includes exhibiting healthy behaviors, getting rid of unhealthy habits, increasing competence in important areas, becoming assertive related to unreasonable demands, and learning how to relax.**

TEACHING PEOPLE TO RELAX

HFIs can use different methods to increase relaxation including

- biofeedback-assisted relaxation,
- autogenic training,
- breathing strategies,
- quieting-reflex training,
- cognitive restructuring,
- sensory awareness, and
- progressive relaxation.

Biofeedback includes focusing on something (e.g., heart rate, muscle tension) and learning how to decrease it through relaxation. Autogenic training involves learning to relax by concentrating on respiration and feeling heaviness and warmth in different parts of the body, such as the solar plexus and forehead. Participants are asked to think and say to themselves phrases such as "my left leg is feeling heavy," or "my right arm is feeling warm." Imagery is often evoked to help participants visualize or imagine the feeling of heaviness and warmth (e.g., "Imagine that your leg is a 25-lb bag of sand that is flowing from your pelvis out through your toes. As the sand flows out of you, imagine each muscle in your leg relaxing."). Attention to respiration can help one relax. The participant is asked to use primarily the abdomen (rather than the chest) in breathing and to relax during exhalation. Quieting-reflex training involves a combination of other methods, such as self-talk (encouraging an alert mind and a calm body), relaxed breathing, conscious relaxation during exhalation, and imagining a wave of warmth and heaviness. Cognitive restructuring helps the participant become more positive about her- or himself through self-talk. Sensory awareness can be used with other relaxation techniques by helping the person realize that the sensation of pressure from contact with objects (e.g., a ball, the floor, the wall) has diminished during the relaxation.

One very effective technique (progressive relaxation) introduced by Jacobsen (7) is aimed at having people recognize the feelings produced by tension. The HFI should have participants get into comfortable positions with their eyes closed. We recommend that the technique be done with the participants lying on mats, but they can do this technique while sitting. The procedure is to have people tense a specific area of the body, hold for about 20 s, then relax; then tense a larger segment, hold, relax; and so forth. The HFI talks in a calm voice, asking people to feel the tension during the hold period and to feel the tension leave the area during the relax period. The following tense/hold/relax sequence can be used:

Right toes
Left toes
Right foot
Left foot
Right leg below the knee
Left leg below the knee
Right leg below the hip
Left leg below the hip
Both legs below the hips
Abdomen and buttocks
Right fingers
Left fingers
Right arm below the elbow
Left arm below the elbow
Right arm below the shoulder
Left arm below the shoulder
Both arms below the shoulders
Chest
Neck
Jaw
Forehead
Entire head
Entire body

Extend the final whole-body relaxation period; have people feel the tension leaving their bodies, feel their breathing, then be silent for several minutes.

> **8** **In Review:** **Techniques the HFI can use in an exercise program to facilitate a participant's skill development in muscle relaxation include biofeedback-assisted relaxation, autogenic training, breathing strategies, quieting-reflex training, cognitive restructuring, sensory awareness, and progressive relaxation.**

Case Studies

You can check your answers by referring to appendix A.

19.1

Jim Goldberg, a former long-distance runner, is trying to get everyone in his exercise program to run in 10K races on Saturday morning. Jim entered the exercise class as a team in a race coming up, without asking anyone, and is now trying to get 100% of the members to run. You get the feeling that some of the participants would enjoy running but would be embarrassed by their times, and that others prefer to spend their weekend doing other things. What would you do?

19.2

Linda Perez, a single parent with three young children, has an executive position dealing with personnel in the local government. She joined the fitness center several months ago and seemed to enjoy the walking and jogging programs. After she had advanced in her jogging to 3 mi per day, 4 days per week, you suggested that she might enjoy participating in the coed games group 2 days per week. She tried it a couple of weeks and then quit coming to the center. You decide to call her and ask if she would like to come in to talk about why she is no longer active in the program. What do you think might be the problem? How would you proceed with the conversation?

Source List

1. Benson (1975)
2. Bouchard et al. (1994)
3. Breslow (1990)
4. Brown (1990)
5. Duda (1996)
6. Franks (1995)
7. Jacobsen (1938)
8. Landers (1995)
9. Plowman (1994)
10. Robinson (1990)
11. Sime (1990)
12. Sime & McKinney (1988)
13. Taylor & Miller (1988)

CHAPTER

20

Behavior Modification

Janet Buckworth

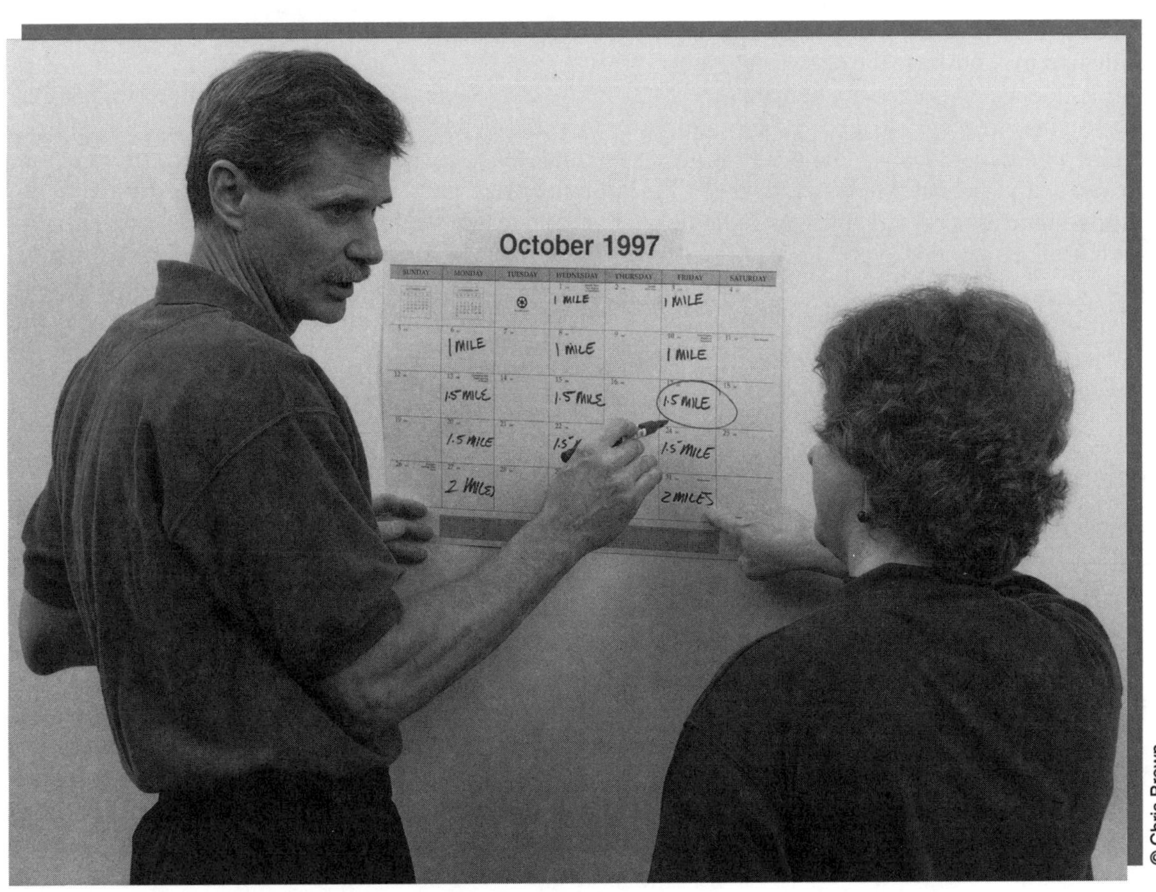

© Chris Brown

The reader will be able to: OBJECTIVES

1 **Describe the transtheoretical model and stages involved in health behavior change.**

2 **Discuss the role of motivation in exercise adoption and adherence and identify six specific behavior change strategies for facilitating the adoption and maintenance of exercise.**

3 **Describe strategies health fitness instructors (HFIs) and personal fitness trainers (PFTs) can use to monitor and support behavior change.**

4 **Describe ways that relapse prevention can be applied to exercise behavior.**

5 **Identify effective communication skills useful in motivating and fostering health behavior change.**

Translating the *desire* to change a health behavior into *action* is a challenge for most people. Individuals may wish to be more active or eat a healthier diet but may not have the knowledge, skills, or motivation to make the necessary behavior modifications and stick to them. To help people adopt and maintain a healthier lifestyle, the health fitness instructor (HFI) and personal fitness trainer (PFT) should understand basic principles of behavior change and develop the skills to put those principles into practice.

This chapter begins with an overview of the transtheoretical model of behavior change. Methods and strategies are then presented from the perspective that change is not an all-or-none proposition but a process with specific stages that can warrant different interventions. For an excellent review of the transtheoretical model applied to exercise, the reader is referred to Prochaska and Marcus (16). Various factors for the HFI to consider as he or she helps participants move through each stage of the model are discussed along with specific strategies for encouraging adoption of and adherence to exercise and other health behaviors. Additional strategies and suggestions for interventions can be found in articles by Franklin (5), King (8), and Knapp (10). The last section in this chapter examines communication skills the HFI should possess to motivate participants and foster health behavior change.

TRANSTHEORETICAL MODEL OF BEHAVIOR CHANGE

There are several theoretical orientations for guiding specific behavior change strategies (10, 18, 19). In other theories, change is typically seen as an all-or-none event in which individuals are expected to respond to interventions and modify their target behavior quickly. The transtheoretical model views change as a *dynamic process* where attitudes, decisions, and actions evolve through different stages over a period of time. This chapter describes this theory and its implications for helping people think about, decide to begin, and continue an active lifestyle.

In the late 1970s and early 1980s, Prochaska and DiClemente developed the transtheoretical model of behavior change by observing smokers trying to quit without professional intervention (16). They discovered that self-changers progressed through specific stages as they tried to decrease or eliminate their high-risk behavior. Although the model was developed based on removing high-risk behaviors, it has been applied to promoting exercise (6, 12, 13).

Concepts

The **transtheoretical model** is a general model of intentional behavior modification. Behavior change is seen as a dynamic process that occurs through a series of interrelated stages that are stable but open to change (6). The individual's readiness to change is emphasized, along with his or her history regarding the target behavior and its influence on current behavior. The problem with most interventions is that they are for people who are prepared to take action (16). According to the transtheoretical model, traditional participant recruitment strategies will not affect people who are not ready to change. Different strategies must be used to persuade people to consider change and then motivate them to take action. Other approaches will be more effective in maintaining adherence to the new behavior.

Levels

There are three levels of the transtheoretical model described next (6, 16). Evaluating the participant in terms of the stage, processes of change, and the level of change dimension enables the selection of individually tailored and stage-specific interventions.

Level 1: Stages of Change

1. *Precontemplation*: In this stage, the potential participant is not seriously thinking about changing a health behavior in the next 6 months or denies the need to change.
2. *Contemplation*: The potential participant is seriously thinking about changing an unhealthy behavior within the next 6 months.
3. *Preparation*: This is a transitional stage in which the individual intends to take action within the next month. Some plans have been made, and the individual tries to determine what to do next.
4. *Action:* This stage is the 6-month period following the overt modification of an unhealthy behavior. Motivation and investment in behavior change are sufficient in this stage, but it is the least stable and busiest stage with the highest risk of relapse.
5. *Maintenance*: Maintenance begins 6 months after the initial behavior has been changed. The longer one is in maintenance, the less risk of relapse.

Level 2: Concepts Hypothesized to Influence Behavior Change

- *Processes of change* are activities used to change behavior. They include changing the individual's experiences, such as seeking out new information, and/or changing the environment. To change the environment, the individual may set up reminders and rewards for the desired behavior.
- *Self-efficacy* is the confidence in one's ability to engage in a positive behavior or abstain from an undesired behavior. This expectation of success predicts progress through the action and maintenance stages.
- *Decisional balance* refers to monitoring potential gains and losses arising from any decision. Perceived gains increase and perceived losses decrease as one moves through the stages described previously.

Level 3: Level of Change Dimension

Identifying the context in which the problem behavior occurs helps determine what people must change to be successful. For example, one person may want to exercise but does not have access to facilities, and another person thinks he does not have the will power to stick with a program. The first person would be helped with a home exercise program, whereas the second would benefit from social support and rethinking discouraging thoughts.

Applying the Transtheoretical Model to Exercise

Applying the transtheoretical model to exercise involves matching the appropriate intervention to an individual according to his or her activity history and readiness for change (2) (see figure 20.1). For example, the goal in working with people in the precontemplation stage is to get them to begin thinking about changing. The benefits of exercise should be strengthened and the costs reduced. Strategies to help develop a personal value for exercise and provide information about the role of exercise in a healthy lifestyle are useful in moving to the next stage (6).

The goal with contemplators is to help them prepare to take action. Marketing and media campaigns

transtheoretical model — A general model of intentional behavior change in which behavior change is seen as a dynamic process that occurs through a series of interrelated stages. Basic concepts emphasize the individual's readiness to change, processes of change, self-efficacy, decisional balance, and the level of the problem.

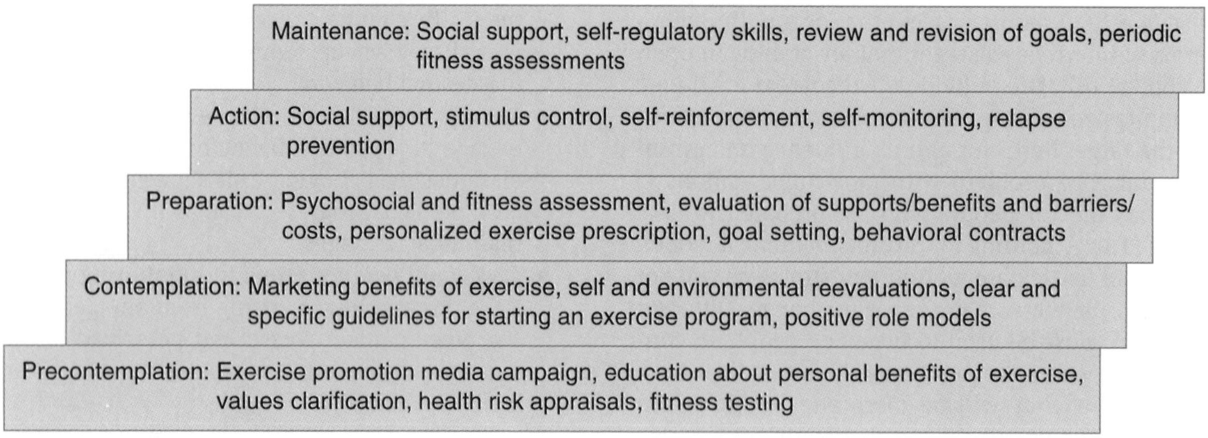

Maintenance: Social support, self-regulatory skills, review and revision of goals, periodic fitness assessments

Action: Social support, stimulus control, self-reinforcement, self-monitoring, relapse prevention

Preparation: Psychosocial and fitness assessment, evaluation of supports/benefits and barriers/costs, personalized exercise prescription, goal setting, behavioral contracts

Contemplation: Marketing benefits of exercise, self and environmental reevaluations, clear and specific guidelines for starting an exercise program, positive role models

Precontemplation: Exercise promotion media campaign, education about personal benefits of exercise, values clarification, health risk appraisals, fitness testing

FIGURE 20.1 Intervention strategies for various stages of change.

promoting exercise along with accurate, easy to understand information about how to start an exercise program can help move contemplators into the action stage. Other factors in the intention to start exercising are role models, perceived barriers and benefits, and psychosocial variables such as self-efficacy. The processes of change, such as self- and environmental reevaluation are critical in these earlier stages of change.

Behavioral factors come into play more in moving from preparation to action and from action into maintenance. Working with a participant who is in the preparation stage must include a thorough assessment and a specific plan for change. Goals should be set that are consistent with capabilities, values, resources, and needs. Perception of self-efficacy predicts adoption and maintenance of exercise and can be increased with mastery experiences. Initial goals should thus be set that will be challenging but assured of being met to foster increased exercise self-efficacy. Environmental and social supports and barriers should also be evaluated and modified to promote the new behavior.

Participants in the action phase are at a high risk of relapse. Social support for exercise in this stage is critical. Another useful strategy is instruction in self-regulatory skills such as stimulus control, reinforcement management, and self-monitoring of progress. Relapse prevention, which is discussed later, is also critical.

Movement from the action phase to the maintenance phase follows a decrease in the risk of relapse and an increase in self-efficacy. The HFI can help the participant reevaluate rewards and goals and plan for ways to cope with potential lapses from relocation, travel, or medical events. Social support and self-regulatory skills continue to be important.

1 **In Review: The transtheoretical model addresses the dynamic nature of behavior change, basing choice of interventions on characteristics of the individual, environment, and the stage of change. Interventions should match the stage the individual is in and the context in which the problem behavior occurs. (See figure 20.1.)**

PROMOTING EXERCISE: TARGETING PRECONTEMPLATORS AND CONTEMPLATORS

Understanding the knowledge, attitudes, and behavioral and social skills associated with adopting a regular exercise program is important in helping people in the early stages of exercise behavior change. People in precontemplation may be uninformed about the long-term consequences of the behavior. They may be demoralized, have low self-efficacy, or feel defensive because of the social pressures to change. They see no personally convincing reason to change, and the pros of the risk behavior seem to outweigh the cons.

Individuals move on to the contemplation stage because of convincing, personal, and timely information (16). This stage is characterized by ambivalence in which the pros equal the cons of exercise. Variables that will support the desire to exercise and enhance motivation can initiate the move to preparation. Specific factors related to the adoption of exercise are presented next, followed by a review of strategies to market exercise and increase motivation.

Factors Influencing Exercise Adoption

Identifying individual, social, and environmental factors related to exercise adoption can aid in the selection of more effective behavior change interventions.

Individual Influences

Generally, individual variables influencing the initiation of exercise are demographics, activity history, past experiences, perception of health status, perceptions regarding access to facilities, time, intensity of exercise, knowledge, aptitudes, beliefs, self-motivation, and self-efficacy (2, 9). Higher education, higher income, gender (male), and younger age are associated with exercise (2, 9), and there is greater adherence with moderate-intensity versus high-intensity exercise prescriptions (2).

Exercise history is an important factor in current exercise behavior. Past participation is linked with physical activity in supervised exercise programs and in treatment programs for patients with coronary heart disease and obesity (2). Past exercise experience can also influence expectations about exercise and self-efficacy, and positive self-efficacy is associated with increased exercise participation (8).

Motivation is another individual variable influencing exercise adoption. People may be motivated to exercise for a variety of reasons such as health, appearance, social outlets, stress management, and competition (10). Self-motivation is the ability to continue a certain behavior without the benefit of external rewards (3). Self-motivated participants are probably good at goal setting, monitoring their progress, and self-reinforcement (10, 18). If self-motivation is low, individuals may need more external reinforcement and encouragement such as group activities and social support to adopt and adhere to exercise.

Perceived behavioral control has been found to be significantly correlated with intention to exercise (1). If participants believe they have more control over the exercise and have choices about when and how to exercise, they are more likely to begin a program. If participants set their own goals, they have a greater chance of success than if goals are assigned to them (11).

Social Influences

Social support from family and friends is usually associated with physical activity (2). Spouses appear to provide a consistent, positive influence on exercise participation (4, 7). Group factors may be particularly important in adhering to regular exercise for older adults and individuals whose motivation for exercise stems more from the social reinforcement than from health or other benefits.

Environmental Influences

Research has found that environmental prompts, social support, and convenience are factors in exercise adoption (8). Environments that prompt increased activity, while offering easily accessible facilities and removing real and perceived barriers, also make maintenance of exercise easier. Examples of specific environmental cues are posters, slogans, post-it notes, placement of exercise equipment in visible places, and recruitment of social support (10).

The convenience of exercise is influenced by the sequence, or chain, of behaviors that must be completed in order to exercise. For example, there is a greater potential for a break in the link if an individual must leave work, drive home, gather up exercise clothes, drive to a facility, park, sign in, and change clothes to exercise than if the individual jogs first thing in the morning in the neighborhood. The longer the behavior chain, the more potential barriers there are to exercise.

The number one reason given for not exercising is lack of time (2). Time can be a true determinant, a perceived determinant, an indication of poor time-management skills, or a rationalization for the lack of motivation to be active (2). Flexibility in an exercise program (e.g., classes offered at many different times of day and evening, a lunch-hour walking group) can help with actual time problems. The HFI can help identify how time is a barrier and then choose appropriate interventions, such as modification of an exercise schedule or referral to a time-management class.

Marketing and Motivational Strategies

Your goal as an HFI or PFT may be to help individuals who have not considered exercise begin thinking about starting a fitness program. For example, the primary goal of a media campaign may be to capture the individual's attention and motivate him or her to contemplate beginning an exercise program or starting another health behavior. This might involve "point-of-decision" informational prompts such as catchy posters next to elevators encouraging people to take the stairs (8). Bulletin boards, pamphlets, flyers, and handouts with upbeat information about the benefits of exercise and practical suggestions for increasing physical activity can also be used to catch the attention of potential exercisers. Handing out passes to an aerobics class at local restaurants is a proactive form of recruitment. Fun runs/walks supporting a local charity may get folks who primarily want to help the organization to begin thinking about exercise for its own sake. Health risk appraisals and fitness testing can also prompt contemplation and enhance motivation to become more active (8).

To increase participation in the early stages of behavior change, the HFI's role is to provide education about why individuals should be more active, describe how to exercise sensibly, and offer motivation to follow through with a personal exercise program (5). Several specific strategies to increase adoption and early adherence are recommended (5, 9, 10, 19):

1. Ask participants about their exercise history. They may need proper information to dispel myths (e.g., the myth, "no pain, no gain") and to develop positive attitudes about exercise.
2. Help participants develop knowledge, attitudes, and skills to support the behavior change. In addition to providing information and self-management skills training, the HFI may use cognitive restructuring to identify discouraging thoughts and replace them with positive statements. For example, these negative statements could be turned into corresponding positive statements:

   Negative Statements

   (a) I'm never going to get in shape.
   (b) I'm fatter than everyone else in the class.
   (c) I've tried to stay with exercise and each time I fail.
   (d) It's just impossible to find time to exercise with my schedule.

   Positive Statements

   (a) Change takes time. I didn't get out of shape overnight, and I am making progress bit by bit.
   (b) Everyone has to start somewhere. Other people have worked long and hard to get where they are.
   (c) Every time I begin a new exercise program, I get closer to sticking with it for good.
   (d) I can take a little time for myself to exercise every day because I deserve it. I'm the one in control.

3. Bolster the participant's exercise self-efficacy. Success-producing learning experiences, such as behavioral rehearsal with proper supervision and positive feedback can enhance self-efficacy. Self-persuasion or verbal persuasion from the HFI can be used to talk participants into increased confidence about exercising. Modeling has also been effective in increasing self-efficacy. The HFI can set up situations in which participants see someone like themselves succeed (e.g., post a newspaper story about seniors who now exercise regularly) or watch a peer who has trouble coping with the task succeed (e.g., the HFI can point out to a new participant that "Lynette also had difficulty jogging 3 mi when she first started the program, but after months of hard work, she can now reach her goal!").
4. Clarify expectations and make sure they are reasonable and realistic. Use guidelines for goal setting to ensure initial successes.
5. Identify potential barriers to behavior change. Barriers can be personal (low exercise self-efficacy), physical (past injuries), interpersonal (peer pressure from sedentary friends to engage in competing behaviors), or environmental (inclement weather or lack of transportation to an exercise facility). Brainstorm with the participant on ways to overcome these barriers.
6. Foster motivation to adopt and maintain an exercise program. Set up incentives to exercise. Incentives can be tangible, such as T-shirts, certificates, water bottles, or recognition on a bulletin board, or intangible, such as a sense of competence. Tangible incentives are useful early in a program. Offer a variety of incentives and foster intrinsic motivation, like a sense of accomplishment or avoidance of obesity, for long-term adherence. The box on page 395 lists strategies to increase motivation.

2 **In Review: Individual, social, and environmental factors motivate people to move from precontemplation to contemplation of an exercise program. A variety of strategies can be employed from**

Motivational Strategies

- Provide positive, behavioral feedback.
- Encourage group participation and group support to offer the opportunity for social reinforcement, camaraderie, and commitment.
- Recruit spouse and peers to support the behavior change.
- Use upbeat, positive music. Make the program enjoyable.
- Provide a flexible routine to decrease boredom and increase enjoyment. Consider alternatives to traditional exercise modes such as games and backpacking to provide a variety of exercise options.
- Provide periodic exercise testing to give information about progress toward goals and the opportunity for positive reinforcement.
- Use behavioral change strategies, such as personal goal setting, contracting, and self-management to foster personal control and perceived competency.
- Chart progress on record cards or graphs. Note and record progress daily to give immediate, positive feedback.
- Recognize goal achievement in newsletters and bulletin boards. Individual effort increases when individual effort is identifiable (11).
- Set up group or individual competitions.
- Offer lotteries based on individual or group accomplishment of a specific goal. Everyone can contribute money; set a winning criteria, such as the first one to walk 15 mi per week for 5 weeks wins, and the winner gets all the money. An alternative is to set a criteria (e.g., attending 20 out of 24 aerobic classes) for participation in a random drawing.

mass media campaigns to fitness testing to motivate individuals to move from contemplation into the action stage. Six strategies to facilitate adopting and maintaining exercise are 1) ask participants about exercise history, 2) help participants develop knowledge, attitudes, and skills to support the change, 3) bolster self-efficacy, 4) set clear and realistic goals, 5) identify barriers to change, and 6) foster motivation.

METHODS OF BEHAVIOR CHANGE

Various strategies have been discussed to illustrate behavior change principles and to describe ways to market and motivate exercise. Once a participant has started an exercise program (action stage), the HFI and PFT play an important role in monitoring and supporting the establishment and maintenance of behavior change.

Assessment

Regardless of the intervention, a comprehensive fitness and psychosocial assessment is necessary to choose and carry out the appropriate behavior change strategy for participants in the action stage. Reassessment should be conducted periodically during maintenance to evaluate the effectiveness of the plan.

First, the problem must be identified and defined in behavioral terms. For example, being overfat is not the problem, but rather the result of overeating and underexercising. The HFI can also help the participant decide what can be realistically changed and what cannot.

Next, examine past attempts at behavior change. Find out what worked, what did not, and why. This information will be useful in goal setting and identifying high-risk situations (see later section).

It is also important to find out if the initiation of the behavior change is voluntary or recommended by someone else. This will give you an idea of the motivation and commitment to change. If a participant is there because a doctor prescribed exercise, you may have to help the participant find personal reasons for exercising. There are a variety of reasons for beginning an exercise program, like health, enjoyment, weight loss, and anxiety reduction, but the initial reasons may not be why someone continues to exercise. Ask the participant what he or she expects to get out of exercise and be prepared to peak the person's interest by presenting additional short- and long-term benefits.

Another useful assessment tool is the decision matrix (14). The participant lists all short- and long-term consequences, positive and negative, of both changing and not changing the behavior. The participant and the HFI then brainstorm about ways to avoid or cope with the projected negative consequences of behavior change.

Self-Monitoring

Most people do not know exactly why they start and stop exercising unless they monitor their activity (9). Part of the assessment can be accomplished by self-monitoring, in which the participant records thoughts, feelings, and situations before, during, and after the target behavior (15). The participant can identify the internal and external cues and behavioral consequences that inhibit and prompt exercise. Barriers and supports also become evident with self-monitoring. Strategies can then be developed to cope with the barriers and make use of the supports. The chain of behaviors encompassing exercise can be evaluated and weak links identified. For example, if the participant discovers she always skips her 5:30 P.M. aerobics class when she oversleeps and doesn't have time to pack her workout clothes before she leaves for work, you can suggest that she pack her workout bag the night before. Immediate benefits and reinforcements tailored to individual preferences can also be established at critical links in the chain (e.g., if she remembers to pack her workout bag the night before, she can push the snooze button for an extra 5 min of sleep the next morning).

Goal Setting

We set goals to accomplish a specific task in a specific period of time. Goals can be as simple and time limited as getting to the intersection before the light turns red to the complicated and encompassing aim of earning an advanced degree. **Goal setting** provides a plan of action that focuses and directs activity and emphasizes a clear link between behavior and outcome.

There are several characteristics of effective goal setting. Goals should be behavioral, specific, and measurable. Plans are easier to make if the goal is stated in behavioral terms. For example, a goal of "walking 4 days per week for 30 to 45 min" is easier to implement than a goal to "get in shape." Specific, measurable goals make it easier to monitor progress, make adjustments, and know when the goal has been accomplished. Goals must also be reasonable and realistic. A goal might be achievable, but personal and situational constraints can make it unrealistic. Losing 2 lb a week through diet and exercise is reasonable, but it is almost impossible for the working mother of three who has minimal time for exercise and cooking. Unrealistic goals set the participant up to fail, which can damage self-efficacy and adherence to the behavior change program.

By using information from the assessment and self-monitoring, the HFI can help the participant set positive, realistic, behavioral goals based on the participant's age, sex, fitness, health, interests, exercise history, skills, and schedule. Both short-term and long-term goals should be included. Short-term goals mobilize effort and direct present actions, but both short- and long-term goals lead to a more effective plan of action (11).

Reinforcement

Social and self-reinforcement are crucial in the action phase, especially since the longer someone has been inactive, the longer it is until exercise itself becomes reinforcing (9). Immediate feedback from exercise can be pain and fatigue, so external, immediate, positive rewards are necessary for beginners. Monitoring progress is rewarding and can involve charting miles walked after each session or instructors giving positive feedback after a difficult class. Positive reinforcement from others can enhance self-esteem, especially when it is feedback from people whom the participant considers to be powerful. Praise is more effective if it is immediate and behaviorally specific (9). "Looking good!" is not as effective as "Sally, you did a great job getting through all the leg lifts today," especially if Sally has been struggling with leg lifts.

Self-reinforcement involves positive reinforcers that are important to the participant. Using special spa soaps and creams only after an aerobic workout or getting tickets to the big game after logging in a certain number of miles are rewards that are personalized and administered by the participant.

Social support should be both tangible, such as transportation to exercise class, and verbal. It can come from the class instructor, exercise partners, and family members. Significant others must be involved in the exercise plan and educated about the differences between support and nagging. Constructive verbal feedback, praise, encouragement, and positive attention will help a family member stick with exercise, while punishing comments, jokes about the person's efforts, or discouraging social comparisons can hinder adherence. Support focuses on what *has* been accomplished ("You're being consistent in your walking to lose weight. I'm proud of you."), whereas nagging harps on what *has not* been accomplished ("You should walk faster to lose weight. Why can't you pick up the pace?").

Friends in an exercise program can provide both social support and cues to exercise. They can be positive role models and part of a buddy system to support the exercise effort. Some participants are more likely to stick with a program if they know someone else is counting on them to be there to work out (8).

Behavioral Contracts

Behavioral contracts are written, signed, public agreements to engage in specific goal-directed behaviors (9) and have been used effectively in increasing exercise adherence (2). Contracts should include clear, realistic objectives and deadlines. They are a way to get the participant involved in the behavioral change program in a way that is motivating, challenging, and public. The public nature of contracts is especially important as public goals are more likely to be met than private or semi-private goals (11).

Contracts can be set by individuals or groups. The benefits of a group contract are the feeling participants can have about not wanting to let others down and the desire to be part of a group. Individual contracts, however, can be tailored to the participant's specific situation and goals.

Consequences of meeting and not meeting the contracted goals should be clear and relevant to the participant. Material reinforcers are good initially but should be faded as natural reinforcers, such as social reinforcement and inherent benefits of exercise, are promoted. Contingency reinforcement can be set up where the participant agrees to do a low-preference activity (e.g., squats) before a high-preference activity (e.g., yoga). Form 20.1 shows a sample contract for a middle-age man starting a walking program.

3 In Review: Assessment is an important first step in the action stage of behavior change. Self-monitoring is useful in determining the antecedents and consequences of the target behavior as well as the potential costs and barriers to behavior change.

Strategies such as goal setting and behavioral contracts must be tailored to the individual participant and should be reevaluated regularly during the maintenance stage. Some of the variables that influence exercise maintenance are enjoyment, convenience, exercise intensity, program flexibility, social support, incentives, rewards, and skills like self-regulation and self-motivation.

RELAPSE PREVENTION

The relapse prevention model is based on relapse in alcohol problems, smoking, and drug abuse in which the goal is to decrease a high frequency, undesired behavior. This model is best applied to voluntary behavior. Although exercise is voluntary, the goal is to increase a low-frequency, desired behavior. Even so, the concepts and techniques of relapse prevention can be used with exercise adherence (10).

goal setting — Goals are desired tasks sought to be accomplished in a specific amount of time. Effective goal setting includes establishing objectives that can be measured, concretely defined, and practically reached.

behavioral contracts — Behavioral contracts are written, signed, public agreements to engage in specific goal-directed activities. Contracts include a designated time frame and clear consequences of meeting and not meeting the agreed upon objectives.

FORM 20.1

Behavioral Contract

Goal: To walk 3 mi without stopping.

Time frame: By May 15.

To reach my goal, I will:

1. Monitor my speed at the high school track during two walks on the weekend.
2. Walk at least 3 days a week during my lunch hour with Bob or Mary.

Goal supporting activities:

1. Keep a spare pair of walking shoes at work.
2. Watch sports on Saturday and Sunday only after I have completed my walks.
3. Reward myself with 30 min on the Internet each time I walk at least 30 min during my lunch hour.
4. Purchase a new modem when I have reached my overall goal.
5. Let my wife know about my plan and have her encourage me to walk on the weekends.

Barriers and countermeasures:

1. Luncheon meetings. I will walk for 30 min before I leave work on days we have meetings during lunch.
2. Rain: I will walk the stairs for at least 30 min during lunch when it rains.

Signed: ______________________________ Date: ______________________________

HFI: ______________________________ Date: ______________________________

This contract will be evaluated every 2 weeks:

Date: ____________________

Revisions:

Date: ____________________

Revisions:

Relapse occurs when people who have been exercising regularly or engaging in other positive health behaviors stop the healthy behavior and go back to the old, unhealthy behavior. It is important to understand the concepts of relapse applied to exercise because relapse is inevitable for many people. The HFI must help participants understand that relapse does not mean failure and devise strategies to cope with temporary setbacks in their behavior change program.

Defining High-Risk Situations

Relapse begins with a **high-risk situation** that challenges an individual's perceived ability to maintain the desired behavioral change. A wedding reception with all her favorite foods can be a high-risk situation for a dieter, and weekend guests can challenge a jogger's motivation to keep up with his afternoon runs. Someone is predisposed to high-risk situations if he or she has a lifestyle imbalance in which "shoulds" exceed "wants." This leads to feelings of deprivation and desires for indulgence. Rationalization, denial, and apparently irrelevant decisions can then occur (10).

Successful coping in a high-risk situation leads to increased self-efficacy and decreased probability of relapse. Not coping or an inadequate coping response leads to decreased self-efficacy and positive expectations about not maintaining the behavior change (e.g., being able to eat like "normal people," having more time to spend with friends). If this leads to an actual "slip," the abstinence violation effect occurs in which the participant perceives he or she has failed. All-or-none thinking, such as the belief that you cannot skip a weekend of jogging and still be a jogger, makes the participant more susceptible to this effect. Feelings of failure lead to self-blame, lowered self-esteem, guilt, perceived loss of control, increased probability of relapse, and possibly giving up (10).

Fostering Coping Strategies for Exercise

Relapse prevention, as described by Marlatt and Gordon (14), attempts to identify and deal with high-risk situations. The strategy begins by educating the individual about the relapse process and enlisting his or her help as an active participant in preventing a relapse (10, 15).

Next are specific strategies to prevent exercise relapse:

1. Identify situations with a high risk of relapse. High-risk situations are incompatible with exercise, such as eating, drinking, overworking, or smoking (19). High-risk situations can also involve relocation, medical events, and travel. Personal high-risk situations can be determined from information gathered during assessment and self-monitoring. Attention should be paid to the exercise behavior itself, the time of day, place, people, moods, thoughts, and the particular situation that can threaten exercise adherence.
2. Revise plans to avoid or cope with high-risk situations. Flexible, short-term goals can be adapted to uncontrollable situational demands. Resetting goals temporarily can decrease the sense of noncompliance and increase a sense of control. ("While my weekend guests are here, I will jog one day in the morning before they get up instead of trying to jog on both Saturday and Sunday afternoons.")
3. Improve coping response by referring participants to classes covering techniques such as time management, relaxation training, assertiveness training, stress management, confidence building, and other efforts to decrease barriers to activity.
4. Provide realistic expectations of potential outcomes from not exercising so the behavioral consequences of relapse are placed in proper perspective.
5. Encourage the participant to expect and plan for relapse. He or she should plan for some alternate modes of exercise, times of day, places, and so forth. If the individual is likely to skip a day of exercise if all the treadmills are in use, suggest using the cycle or stair-climber on those days.
6. Minimize the tendency to interpret a temporary relapse as a total failure. Use cognitive

high-risk situation — An event, thought, or interaction that challenges an individual's perceived ability to maintain a desired behavioral change.

relapse prevention — Relapse prevention was developed by Marlatt and Gordon to identify and deal successfully with high-risk situations by educating the client about the relapse process and using a variety of strategies to foster an effective coping response.

restructuring to change the definition of a missed exercise class from "the end of my exercise program" to "a temporary lapse that most people who exercise experience."

7. Correct a lifestyle imbalance in which "shoulds" outweigh "wants." Make exercise a "want" instead of a "should." Use positive reinforcement and other strategies to make exercise fun.

4 **In Review: Because missing regular exercise is inevitable for many people, the HFI must be prepared to help the participant prevent lapses in an exercise routine from leading to the end of an exercise program. Strategies such as being flexibile in setting goals, realizing that the occasional relapse is just temporary, and building one's self-confidence can help the participant deal successfully with a potential relapse.**

HEALTH FITNESS COUNSELING

The HFI and PFT are called on to provide counseling during assessment, exercise prescription, and ongoing monitoring of exercise participants. Good communication skills are the foundation of effective counseling. For additional information, the reader is referred to Willis and Campbell (19), who provide an excellent chapter on counseling in the fitness profession.

Communication Skills

To be able to communicate well, the HFI must be able to listen effectively and respond empathetically. Listening involves being able to accurately discriminate the feeling and meaning of the speaker's message. Listening is more complicated than simply hearing words. Communication occurs at different levels. There is the actual, objective meaning of the words, or the content of the message; however, tone of voice, loudness or softness of speech, speed, and nonverbal behavior can change the meaning of a statement. A participant who smiles and says, "My program is going really well," is not saying the same thing as the person who mumbles the same words and looks down at her or his shoes. To enhance our understanding of the message, we must be able to attend to the verbal and nonverbal as well as overt and covert messages (19). The HFI should pay attention to facial expressions, body language, and tone of voice in addition to listening to the actual words.

The context of the message, determined by the social and cultural implications of the situation, can create "noise" that will interfere with sending and receiving the message. Noise is also created by the ideas, experiences, expectations, and prejudices of the speaker and listener. Barriers to communication occur not only in the context of the message but also in the way a listener responds. Ordering or commanding, threatening, criticizing, interpreting, interrupting, interrogating, and diverting, often by humor, are responses that shut off understanding and make the speaker feel you do not care.

Do not assume you understand what a person is saying. We react to a communicated message according to our own perceptions of the nature of the message. Use responsive listening to clarify communications and confirm with the speaker that you comprehend the speaker's message. Reflect back what you have heard, and ask questions and make statements that respond to the feeling and meaning of the message. Responsive listening lets the person know you understand what he or she has expressed, helps build a relationship, encourages the participant to keep talking, and clarifies what the person means. Responsive listening is illustrated in the following exchange:

Participant: I'm the only one in this class who can't get the new step routines. (The HFI should observe the tone of voice, eye contact, and posture.)

HFI: You think the other members of the class catch on before you do. That must be really frustrating. (The HFI paraphrased the participant's statement and interpreted probable underlying feelings. Other feelings could be discouragement or a sense of futility or failure. The tendency to want to respond with an offer to teach the participant the steps might not have addressed an underlying lack of confidence. Responsive listening keeps the communications open so the participant can express what kind of help he or she wants.)

Characteristics of an Effective Helper

The role of the HFI as counselor is to help the client achieve his or her health-related goals. It is easier to provide this help when the HFI responds to the client with empathy, respect, concreteness, genuineness, and confrontation:

- ***Empathy*** is an expression of a sensitive understanding of the personal meaning of events and experience to the participant. This is different from knowing what the problem is. You may know that John has 25% body fat because he eats fast food every day and does not exercise. Empathy means you have a sense of what it must be like for him to be overweight and inactive, and you are able to communicate your understanding in a nonjudgmental manner. Even if you are not sure you are empathetic, when the participant perceives that you are trying to understand, he or she will be encouraged to communicate more of the problem. The additional information will help you empathize more and give you clues to the underlying nature of the problems and how to come up with a more realistic intervention plan. The effort to understand also communicates to the participant that you value him or her as an individual.
- *Respect* is a feeling of positive regard for the participant. You display warm acceptance of the participant's experiences and place no conditions on your acceptance and warmth. This means not making judgments. It is often hard for the HFI to respect a person whose behavior (smoking, sedentary lifestyle, high-fat diet) shows a lack of self-respect for one's body. We must prize the person but not necessarily the behavior. When we respect another person, we help that person develop self-respect.
- *Concreteness* is the ability to help the participant be specific about feelings and goals he or she is trying to communicate. Reflective listening enables the participant to become more precise, which is critical in the goal-setting process.
- *Genuineness* is being real in a relationship with another person. In a helping relationship, the counselor is honest and open with the client. Some self-disclosure is appropriate and can help develop trust, but the goal of the relationship is to help the client, not deal with the HFI's personal issues.
- *Confrontation* involves telling the other person that you see things differently from how they are being presented to you. You point out incongruities that are observable facts about which the participant may not be consciously aware. Confrontation should only be used after you have an established relationship.

Other qualities important in effective health counseling are listed on page 402.

Ethical Considerations

There is an ethical dilemma involved in weighing the consequences of persuading people to behave in ways conducive to good health versus the right of individuals to do as they please with their own health as long as it does not impinge on the rights of others (17). "Informed consent" theoretically gives participants a free choice after they have been given all the information needed to make a decision. If an unhealthy lifestyle is based on ignorance or incorrect information, we should provide the necessary information for an informed choice, not aggravate feelings of guilt or failure. But if an individual has chosen an unhealthy lifestyle as a matter of choice and free will, we must accept the "informed refusal," although health care providers seem to have some difficulty doing this. Thus, an awareness of our own value preferences is essential in helping others set goals. We must consider whose values are to be served by the intervention, ours or the potential client's, and respect the choices of others.

Confidentiality is another critical ethical concern for the HFI. In addition to the client information that is clearly confidential, the HFI may become aware of other information the participant wants to keep private. Trustworthiness is an important characteristic of an effective helper and reflects an ethical stand. A participant will trust someone who keeps information confidential, treats him or her with respect, and keeps the relationship professional.

It is also important to recognize your limitations and know when to refer to a professional therapist. It is the role of the HFI to help people change health behavior, but marital problems; eating disorders; and affective disorders, such as depression, are a few of the areas that should be handled by someone trained to work with these issues. We must know our limits and help connect participants with the best resources for handling their unique problems.

5 In Review: Listening to the actual words and the nonverbal message in context is the foundation of good communication skills. To communicate effectively, the HFI should practice reflective listening

empathy — Identification with the thoughts or feelings of another person.

Qualities of an Effective Health Behavior Counselor

- Access to material resources and services
- Knowledge and experience
- Legitimate authority
- Ability to generate expectations of success
- Believable instructions and plans
- Model of healthy behavior
- Patience to help the participant build small changes upon one another
- Ability to enhance the problem-solving skills of the participant
- Flexibility
- Support
- Trustworthiness
- Self-awareness
- Commitment to providing timely, specific feedback

and empathetic responding. Characteristics of an effective helper include empathy, respect, concreteness, genuineness, and confrontation.

Case Studies

You can check your answers by referring to appendix A.

20.1

Dana Carter was given a 3-month membership to your facility by her boyfriend, Mike Johnson, who attends aerobics classes regularly. They are going on a backpacking trip in Colorado this summer, and Mike thought you could help get her ready for the physical strain of the trip. She is a self-proclaimed "couch potato" who went to a couple of aerobics classes with Mike last year, but got so sore she stopped after one week. You have completed a fitness assessment and found she is healthy and just below average in her aerobic capacity. She said her goal is to be prepared for the trip, and she wants to try aerobics again. However, she confides she is afraid she will disappoint Mike because she is "really out of shape." What stage of behavior change is she in, and what strategies could you use to work with her?

20.2

Jack Bishop is a middle-age college English teacher who joined the walking club in your facility 3 months ago after you conducted his fitness and psychosocial assessment. His goal was to "walk around the world" (in terms of total miles walked), and his progress has been marked on the walkers' promotional map at the front entrance. His office is two blocks from your facility, and Jack usually walks on your indoor track before he goes home. You notice his mileage has decreased over the past 2 weeks, and another walker tells you that Jack said, "I won't make it out of the state thanks to term papers and final exams." What stage of behavior change is he in, and what strategies could you use with him?

Source List

1. Courneya & McAuley (1996)
2. Dishman & Buckworth (1996)
3. Dishman & Gettman (1980)
4. Erling & Oldridge (1985)
5. Franklin (1988)

6. Gorely & Gordon (1995)
7. Heinzelmann & Bagley (1970)
8. King (1994)
9. King & Martin (1993)
10. Knapp (1988)
11. Kyllo & Landers (1995)
12. Marcus, Rossi, Selby, Niaura, & Abrams (1992)
13. Marcus & Simkin (1994)
14. Marlatt & Gordon (1985)
15. Marlatt & Parks (1982)
16. Prochaska & Marcus (1994)
17. Ross & Morowsky (1983)
18. Sonstroem (1988)
19. Willis & Campbell (1992)

CHAPTER

21

Injury Prevention and Treatment

Sue Carver

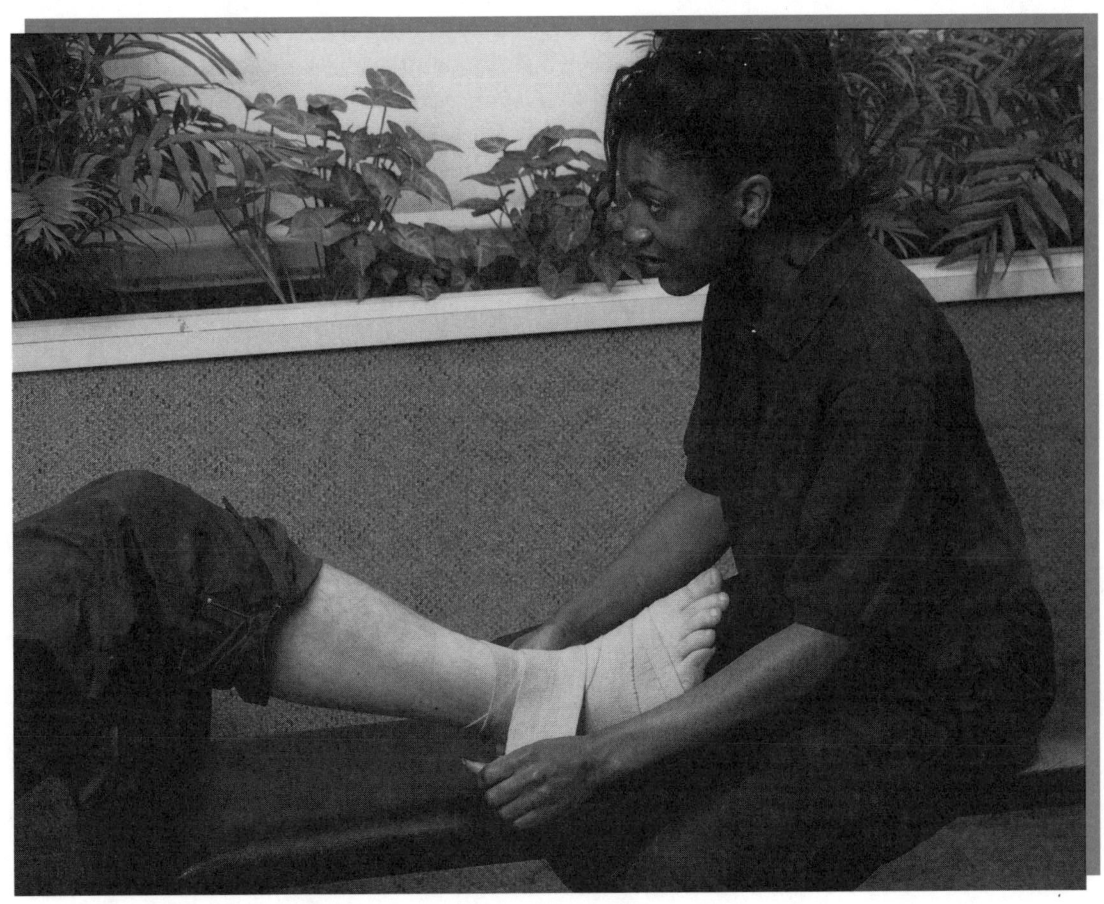

© Chris Brown

The reader will be able to: **OBJECTIVES**

1. Describe ways to minimize injury risk and prevent the transmission of bloodborne pathogens.
2. Describe the signs and symptoms of soft-tissue injuries (sprains, strains, contusions, and heel bruises), how to provide initial treatment of injuries, and when to use heat in long-term treatment.
3. Identify signs, symptoms, and proper treatment measures for bone injuries, wounds, and common skin irritations.
4. Describe the causes of heat-related disorders, how to prevent heat illness, and how to treat a heat-related emergency when it occurs and provide guidelines for fluid replacement before and after exercise.
5. Explain the causes of cold-related disorders and how to prevent frostnip, superficial and deep frostbite and hypothermia, and how to treat a cold-related emergency when it occurs.
6. Distinguish between the signs and symptoms of diabetic coma and those of insulin shock; describe the proper treatment for each.
7. Identify common cardiovascular and pulmonary complications resulting from participation in exercise.
8. Identify the signs, symptoms, and management of common orthopedic problems; classify injuries into mild, moderate, and severe; and recommend appropriate modification of exercise programs when injury occurs.
9. Describe procedures to check vital signs.
10. Describe artificial respiration and cardiopulmonary techniques for adults.

The health fitness instructor (HFI) must be prepared to safely handle an emergency medical situation should it occur. This chapter will discuss injury prevention, injury recognition, and common treatment approaches as well as planning for and handling a medical emergency situation.

PREVENTING INJURIES

Certain inherent risks are associated with participation in physical activity. The HFI should be aware of those risks and take steps to control factors that increase the risk of injury. Advanced planning, training in injury recognition and emergency care, adequate equipment and facilities, and counseling in the selection of activities all help to reduce the possibility of injury. The following is a brief discussion of the factors contributing to injury and steps that can be taken to reduce injury risk (2-9, 11, 12, 16, 17).

Controlling Injury Risk

Injury risk in competitive athletic events is controlled by game rules. In exercise programs where games are used for aerobic activity, injury risk may be reduced by controlling the tempo of the activity or by modifying existing rules to enhance participant safety (e.g., limiting body contact, using a softer ball).

The HFI should encourage participants to seek professional advice regarding the selection and fitting of proper equipment. The equipment most commonly used, and most widely abused, is footwear. Inadequate protection of the foot is a major contributor to a variety of leg and lower-back problems. Improperly maintained exercise equipment and facilities also contribute to higher overall injury risk.

In this age of concern over bloodborne pathogens such as the **human immunodeficiency virus (HIV)** and **hepatitis B (HBV)**, precautions should be taken to protect both the participant and the HFI. Open cuts should be covered and change of clothing that is blood-saturated should be required. Provisions should be made to provide for necessary supplies to care safely for an open wound including latex gloves, biohazard containers, antiseptic solution, dressings, disinfectant, and a sharps container if applicable. Participants should be instructed to report all wounds immediately. The HFI should be instructed in **universal precaution** guidelines for management of acute blood exposure as well as appropriate cleaning and disposal policies for contaminated areas.

Factors Contributing to Injury

Activity implies movement, and with increased movement comes a corresponding increase in the risk of injury. In fitness programs, the frequency of injuries increases when the frequency of the exercise sessions increases and when the intensity of the exercise is maintained at the high end of the target heart rate (THR) zone (figure 21.1). The risk of injury is also heightened by increased speed of movement, as found in competitive activities; in activities requiring quick changes in direction (e.g., fitness games); and in activities that focus on smaller muscle groups. Environmental conditions such as extreme heat or cold also can increase the risk associated with physical activity. Lack of proper adaptation to the environment, as well as lack of education in the prevention, recognition, and methods of dealing with problems associated with these extreme environments, can lead to devastating results.

Age, gender, and body structure influence the risk of injury. In general, very young and very old people are at the greatest risk, and older individuals usually require longer periods of time for recovery. Because of body structure and strength differences, females are often more susceptible to injury in co-ed activities and games requiring quick changes of direction and/or body contact. For either gender, a lack or an imbalance of muscle strength, a lack of joint flexibility, and poor cardiorespiratory fitness (CRF) increases the chance of injury. Obese individuals not only have low CRF, but also the excess weight places additional stress on the weight-bearing joints. Individuals with specific medical problems such as asthma, diabetes, or known allergic reactions may need special attention to avoid potentially serious complications.

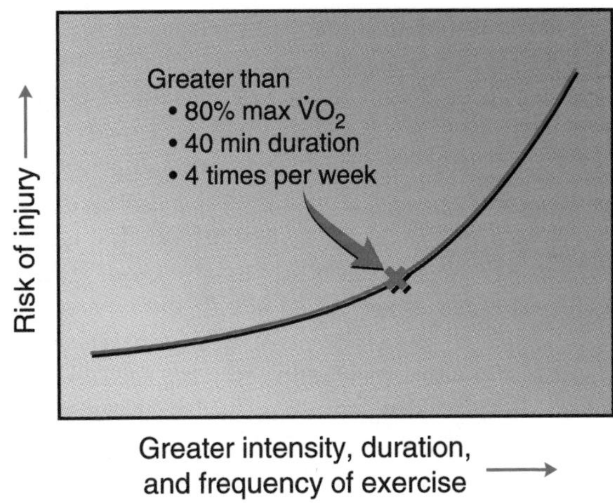

FIGURE 21.1 Increased risk of injury with too much activity.

Reducing Injury Risk

Screening participants before any physical activity program can help to reduce injury risk. The screening should highlight the major areas contributing to increased health risk. Proper screening assists the participant in recognizing problems and alerts the

human immunodeficiency virus (HIV) — A virus that destroys the body's ability to fight infection; referred to as AIDS.

hepatitis B (HBV) — A type of hepatitis (viral infection of the liver) that is transmitted by sexual or blood-to-blood contact.

universal precaution — Safety measures taken to prevent exposure to blood or other body fluids.

HFI to potential problems that could occur in an exercise session (e.g., asthma attack, diabetic shock). Proper planning for emergency situations contributes to a low overall risk. Individuals who cannot be properly supervised or given adequate care as a result of their physical problems should be referred to a program or facility that can provide the needed services. Policies to handle such referrals and all major emergency situations should be written and communicated to all HFIs involved in a fitness center.

A major factor involved in reducing the risk associated with physical activity is the design and implementation of an individual's exercise program. The program can focus attention on problems encountered in the preliminary tests, which might include

- flexibility measures;
- assessment of body-fat composition;
- evaluation of muscular strength, power, and endurance;
- posture assessment; and
- cardiovascular fitness evaluation.

The manner in which the HFI conducts the exercise program has a major bearing on the risk of injury to the participant. To highlight this point figure 21.2 contrasts the "train, don't strain" *fitness* goal with the "no pain, no gain" *performance* goal. Educating participants about the proper intensity of the exercise session (i.e., to stay in the THR zone) and how to recognize the signs and symptoms of overuse is important in reducing injury risk. The HFI should emphasize that the entire program, and each individual session, is graduated to avoid doing too much too soon. This adage is especially true for individuals who have not been involved in a regular exercise program and who have a tendency to overestimate their abilities. Overexertion can lead to chronic overuse injuries, extreme muscle soreness, and undue fatigue.

In educating participants about the signs and symptoms of overuse, the HFI should focus attention on distinguishing between simple muscle soreness and injury. Muscle soreness tends to peak 24 to 48 hr postexercise and dissipates with use and time. The signs and symptoms of injury include

- exquisite point tenderness,
- pain that persists even when the body part is at rest,
- joint pain,
- pain that does not go away after warming up,
- swelling or discoloration,
- increased pain in weight-bearing activities or with active movement, and
- changes in normal bodily functions.

1 **In Review: The HFI should be aware of inherent risks associated with activity and take steps to minimize risk by advanced planning, use of proper equipment and facilities, educating participants regarding injury recognition and**

Train,
don't strain
No pain,
no gain!
FOR FITNESS GOALS:
Exercise 40 minutes, 3 times/week
FOR PERFORMANCE GOALS:
Exercise 2 hours, 7 days/week

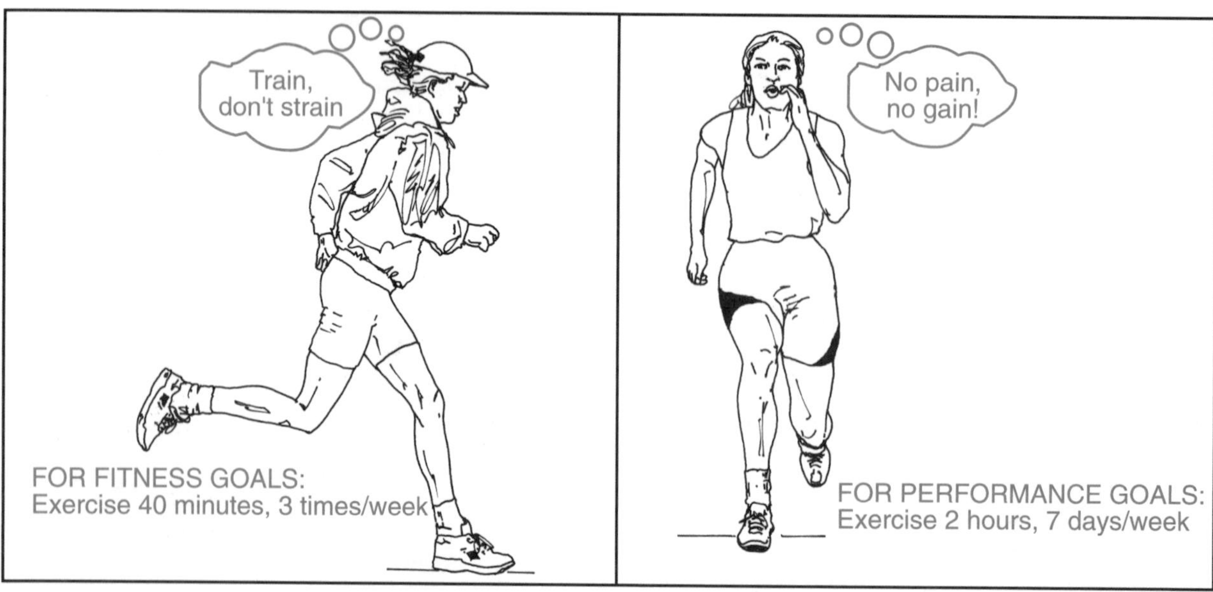

FIGURE 21.2 Fitness programs versus performance training.

care, evaluating participants to determine fitness needs and/or special health problems that may need monitoring, and giving clear guidelines for graduating activity. Follow universal precaution guidelines and use appropriate gloves, biohazard containers, sharps containers, and disinfectant to reduce the spread of bloodborne pathogens.

INJURY TREATMENT

The treatment of an injury depends on the type and severity of the injury. This section describes approaches to take with injuries that are common to fitness programs and sports (2-7, 10-15, 18, 19, 20, 21, 22).

Treating Soft-Tissue Injuries

Sprains (overstretching or tearing of ligamentous tissue) and strains (overstretching or tearing of muscle or tendon) are common injuries associated with adult fitness programs. Most significant injuries to joint structures or to soft tissue require *protection, rest,* and the immediate application of *ice, compression,* and *elevation* (**PRICE**). Figure 21.3 reinforces the PRICE concept. Usually, a wet wrap is applied first to give compression. Start distal to the injury and wrap toward the heart. Compression should be firm but not tight. If a joint structure is involved, surround the entire area with ice and secure with another elastic wrap. If the injury involves a contusion (bruise) or strain to a muscle belly, put the muscle on mild stretch before applying ice, and secure in that position if it is feasible to do so. If possible, elevate the injured part above heart level to minimize the effect of gravity and reduce bleeding into tissues. With any injury shock is a possibility, and the HFI should be prepared to handle this situation should it occur.

In most cases the participant should be informed that the application of ice should be continued anywhere from 24 to 72 hr, depending on the severity of the injury. Ice causes vasoconstriction of the blood vessels, thus helping to control bleeding into tissues. Ice also reduces the sensation of pain. Standard treatment times with ice are 15 to 20 min, with reapplication hourly or when pain is experienced. In the acute phase, when ice is not being used, the compression bandage should be in place to minimize swelling. Using ice or compression at bedtime is not necessary unless pain interferes with sleep. If this occurs, applying ice frequently (every 1 to 2 hr) may help to control the pain. Physician referral is recommended in moderate to severe cases.

An injured participant may want to apply heat sooner than is warranted. He or she needs to be informed that heat is usually applied in the later stages of an acute injury, when the risk of bleeding into tissues is minimal. In contrast, the application of heat is a common treatment for chronic inflammatory conditions as well as generalized muscle soreness. Heat causes a vasodilation of the blood vessels and reduces muscle spasm. Standard treatment time for a moist heat pack is 15 to 20 min. When in doubt about which mode of treatment to use, ice is the safer choice. Table 21.1 outlines common soft-tissue injuries, signs and symptoms, and immediate care.

2 **In Review: When injury to soft tissues does occur, proper assessment and initial treatment can reduce the possibility of further trauma and aid in the healing process (see table 21.1 for details). Protection, rest, ice, compression, and elevation (PRICE) are the important steps for immediate care of most musculoskeletal and joint injuries. Heat is often used in chronic inflammatory conditions or with general muscle soreness, and should be applied only in the later stages of an acute injury when the risk of bleeding into tissues is minimal.**

Treating Fractures

Fractures, or injury to bone, should be suspected if there is exquisite point tenderness over a bone, visual or palpable deformity, or referred pain to an area of bone with percussion or vibrational stress. X rays should be taken if a fracture is suspected. If deformity is present, do not push the bone back into place. Splint and refer to a physician. Table 21.2 gives additional procedures to follow when treating a fracture.

PRICE — The suggested treatment for minor sprains and strains: protection, rest, ice, compression, and elevation.

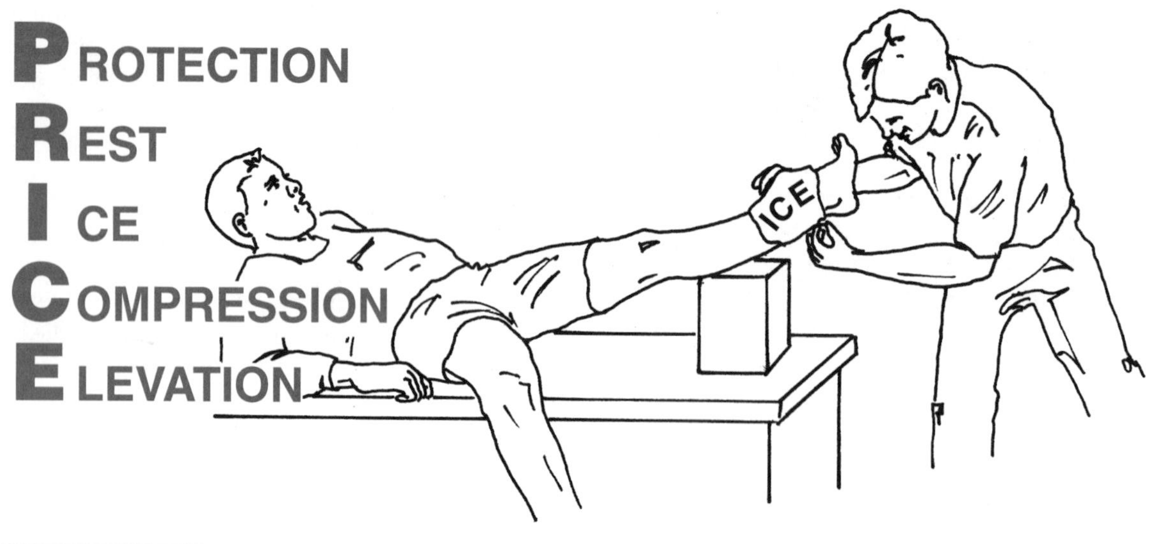

FIGURE 21.3 The PRICE method for treating sprains and strains.

Table 21.1 Soft-Tissue Injuries and Their Treatment

Injury	Signs and symptoms	Immediate care
Sprain—stretching or tearing of ligamentous tissue **Strain**—overstretching or tearing of a muscle or tendon **Contusion**—impact force that results in bleeding into the underlying tissues; a bruise	1st degree—mild injury resulting in overstretching or minor tearing of tissue. Range of motion is limited. Point tenderness is minimal. No swelling. 2nd degree—moderate injury resulting in partial tearing of tissue. Function is limited. Point tenderness and probable muscle spasm. Range of motion is painful. Swelling and/or discoloration is probable if immediate first-aid care is not given. 3rd degree—severe tearing or rupture of tissue. Exquisite point tenderness. Immediate loss of function. Swelling and muscle spasm likely to be present with discoloration appearing later. Possible palpable deformity.	Protection, rest, ice, compression, and elevation (PRICE) Usual treatment time: 15-20 min ice bag 5-7 min ice cup or ice slush How often: Moderate and severe—every hour, or when pain is experienced Less severe—as symptoms necessitate Continue with ice treatments at least 24–72 hr, depending on the severity of the injury. Refer to a physician if function is impaired. Mild to moderate strains—gradual stretching to the point of discomfort is recommended.
Heel bruise (stone bruise)—sudden abnormal force to heel area that results in trauma to underlying tissues		PRICE Pad for comfort when weight bearing is resumed

(4-7, 10, 12-19, 21, 22)

Table 21.2 Fractures and Their Treatment

Injury	Signs and symptoms	Immediate care
Fracture—disruption of bone with or without loss of continuity or external exposure, ranging from periosteal irritation to complete separation of bony parts **Simple**—bone fracture without external exposure **Compound**—bone fracture with external exposure	Acute: Direct trauma to bone resulting in disruption of continuity and immediate disability. Deformity or bony deviation. Swelling. Pain. Palpable tenderness. Referred pain or indirect point tenderness. Crepitus. False joint. Discoloration—usually becoming apparent later.	Acute: Control bleeding—elevation, pressure points, direct pressure Treat for shock. If an open fracture, control bleeding and apply a sterile dressing, prevent further disruption and infection; do not move bones back into place. Control swelling with pressure and ice, if wound is closed. Splint above and below the joint and apply traction if necessary. Protect body part from further injury. Refer to physician.
	Chronic: Low-grade inflammatory process causing proliferation of fibroblasts and generalized connective-tissue scarring. Pain progressively worsens until present all of the time. Direct point tenderness.	Chronic: Rest. Heat. Refer to physician.

(1, 3 [c, d], 13, 15, 16)

Treating Wounds and Other Skin Disorders

Another group of common injuries associated with activity programs is wounds. The major concern with an open wound is bleeding. Once bleeding is controlled, steps can be taken to give further care. This may consist of protecting from infection, covering with a bandage, treating for shock, or referring immediately to a physician for suturing. In minor cases, a thorough cleansing and application of a sterile dressing may be all that is needed. The HFI should use safety measures to prevent risk from exposure to blood. Internal bleeding is a very serious condition. The HFI should treat for shock and obtain medical assistance immediately.

Shearing and pressure forces due to poor fitting shoes and socks, poorly conditioned or sensitive skin, and uncorrected biomechanic foot disorders can lead to friction and compression injuries of the foot. Hand calluses and other skin irritations can develop from friction resulting from activities requiring frequent gripping of an object (e.g., a tennis racket or a bat) or rubbing of body parts against each other or another object (e.g., as is frequently the case in gymnastics or wrestling).

Table 21.3 outlines and provides guidelines for immediate care of wounds. Table 21.4 discusses care of common skin irritations. The HFI should use universal precautions in treating an open wound. Latex gloves should be worn when handling potentially infectious materials. Proper disposal of infectious materials and decontamination of infected areas should be routine policy.

In Review: The steps to follow in dealing with simple and compound fractures, wounds (and excessive bleeding), and other skin disorders are listed in tables 21.2, 21.3, and 21.4, respectively.

Table 21.3 Treatment of Wounds

Injury	Signs and symptoms	Immediate care
Incision—cutting of skin resulting in an open wound with cleanly cut edges and exposure of underlying tissues	Smooth edges may bleed freely. Signs of infection (see laceration)	Clean wound with soap and water, moving away from injury site. Minor cuts can be closed with a butterfly bandage or steri-strip. Apply a sterile dressing. Refer to a physician if wound needs suturing (e.g., facial cuts and large or deep wounds) or signs of infection are present.
Laceration—tearing of skin resulting in an open wound with jagged edges and exposure of underlying tissues	Jagged edges may bleed freely. Signs of infection: redness; swelling; increase in skin temperature; tender, swollen, and painful lymph glands; mild fever; and headache	Soak in antiseptic solution such as hydrogen peroxide to loosen foreign material. Clean with antiseptic soap and water using sterile technique and moving away from the injury site. Apply a sterile dressing. Instruct to seek medical attention if signs of infection are recognized. Usually refer to a physician; a tetanus shot or sutures may be needed. If injury is extensive, control bleeding, cover with thick sterile bandages, and treat for shock. Refer to a physician.
Puncture—direct penetration of tissues by a pointed object	Small opening; may bleed freely Signs of infection (see laceration)	If object is embedded deeply: Protect body part and refer to physician for removal and care. Treat for shock. Clean around wound, moving away from injury site. Allow wound to bleed freely to minimize risk of infection. Apply a sterile dressing. Puncture wounds are usually referred to a physician. A tetanus shot may be needed. Instruct individual to seek medical attention if signs of infection are present.

Table 21.3 *(continued)*

Injury	Signs and symptoms	Immediate care
Abrasion—scraping of tissues resulting in removal of the outermost layers of skin and the exposure of numerous capillaries	Superficial, reddish, irregular surface Oozing or weeping from underlying capillaries May contain dirt, debris, or bacteria embedded in tissue	Debride and flush with antiseptic solution such as hydrogen peroxide. Follow with soap-and-water cleansing. Apply a petroleum-based antiseptic agent to keep wound moist. This allows healing to take place from the deeper layers. Cover with non-adherent gauze. Instruct to seek medical help if signs of infection are recognized.
Excessive bleeding—internal or external bleeding that results in massive loss of circulating blood volumes; often results in shock and can lead to death	External hemorrhage 1. Arterial Color: bright red Flow: spurts, bleeding usually profuse 2. Venous Color: dark red Flow: steady 3. Flow: oozing	Elevate affected part above heart. Put direct pressure over the wound, using a sterile compress if possible. Apply a pressure dressing. Use pressure points. Treat for shock. Refer to a physician.
Internal bleeding—bleeding within the deep structures of the body (chest, abdominal, or pelvic cavity) and bleeding of any of the organs contained within these cavities	Internal hemorrhage—bleeding into chest, abdominal, or pelvic cavity and bleeding of any of the organs contained within these cavities. Generally, there are no external signs. However, any time an individual coughs up blood or finds blood in the urine or feces, internal hemorrhage must be suspected. The following signs are also indicative of internal bleeding: Restlessness Thirst Faintness Anxiety Cold, clammy skin Dizziness Pulse—rapid, weak, and irregular Blood pressure—significant fall	Treat for shock. Refer to hospital immediately. Don't give water or food.

(continued)

Table 21.3 (continued)

Injury	Signs and symptoms	Immediate care
Shock caused by bleeding	Restlessness Anxiety Pulse—weak, rapid Skin temperature—cold clammy, profuse sweating Skin color—pale, later cyanotic Respiration—shallow, labored Eyes—dull Pupils—dilated Thirsty Nausea and possible vomiting Blood pressure—marked fall	Maintain an open airway. Control bleeding. Elevate lower extremities approximately 12 in. (exceptions: heart problems, head injury, or breathing difficulty—place in comfortable position, usually semi-reclining, unless spinal injury is suspected, in which case do not move). Splint any fractures. Maintain normal body temperature. Avoid further trauma. Monitor vital signs and record at regular intervals—every 5 min or so. Do not feed or give any liquids.

(3 [c, d, e], 4, 5, 8, 9, 12, 13, 19, 21)

ENVIRONMENTAL CONCERNS

The environment can play an important role in the development of serious problems related to maintaining body temperature in a normal range during exercise. This section examines the factors related to an increased risk of heat- and cold-related injuries.

Heat-Related Problems

Heat illness can strike anyone. Poor physical condition, although a contributing factor, is not the primary cause. Even the most highly conditioned athlete can suffer a heat-related disorder. The exercise load and the environment can place large heat loads on an individual. Excessive heat loads stimulate a high production of sweat because evaporation of sweat is the major mechanism for cooling the body. As a result, large amounts of water may be lost during physical activity, causing an increase in the core body temperature (hyperthermia). If too much water is lost, circulatory collapse and death can occur. The following information outlines methods of recognizing dehydration (excessive loss of body fluids) and presents measures that can be used to prevent heat illness.

A water loss equal to 3% of body weight is considered safe. A 5% loss is considered borderline, and an 8% loss is considered dangerous. Water loss can be monitored by weighing participants before and after activity. Individuals who are outside the allowable 3% range from one workout to the next may have an increased risk of heat injury and should be monitored carefully if allowed to participate.

The practical experience of the military and athletic teams working in the heat and humidity has led to the development of guidelines to prevent heat injury. The HFI's application of these guidelines to adult fitness programs will enhance the enjoyment and safety of the participants. Following are the recommended guidelines for preventing heat injury:

- Acclimatize to heat and humidity by training over a period of 7 to 10 days.
- Hydrate prior to activity and frequently during activity.
- Decrease the intensity of exercise if the temperature or humidity is high; use THR as a guide.
- Monitor weight loss by weighing before and after workouts. Force the consumption of fluids if more than 3% of body weight is lost during

Table 21.4 Skin Irritations and Treatment

Skin irritation	Signs and symptoms	Immediate care
Blister—a collection of serum or blood just below the superficial layer of skin	Defined area of fluid accumulation under skin Feels hot Painful to touch	Prevent by engaging in heavy activity slowly and toughening skin by use of astringents: tannic acid or salt water soaks. Stop activity if friction area develops, apply ice, and cover irritation with a friction-proofing material or donut pad. Prevent contamination of torn blister; clean with soap and water. Refer to physician if signs of infection are present.
Callus—markedly thickened area of skin, usually over an area of pressure	Visible and excessive callus formation May be painful May have cracks or fissures May become infected May develop blisters	Prevent excessive callus formation by using an emery callus file. Take measures to reduce friction by wearing properly fitted shoes and socks, using powder or lubricant, and correcting abnormal biomechanical foot faults with orthotics. Protect susceptible areas by using special protective devices such as gloves, tape, or pad. Prevent infection by keeping callus trimmed down and using a lubricant to prevent cracks and tears in callus.
Corns		
Hard corn—thickening of skin located on toes	Local pain Inflammation and thickening of soft tissue Generally seen on top of toes and associated with hammer toe deformity	Prevent by wearing properly fitted shoes or fitting with orthotics if cause is due to abnormal foot biomechanics.
Soft corn—circular area of thickened, white macerated skin between toes and proximal head of phalanges	Pain and inflammation	Prevent with properly fitted shoes, and control moisture accumulation by keeping skin dry in between toes. Separate toes with cotton or lambs' wool.

(continued)

Table 21.4 *(continued)*

Skin irritation	Signs and symptoms	Immediate care
Ingrown toenail—leading side edge of toenail grows into soft tissue	Severe inflammation, pain, and infection	Apply hot antiseptic soaks for 20 min, 2-3 times a day, at 110-120 °F. When toenail is pliable, insert wisp of cotton under leading edge of toenail and lift from soft tissue beneath. Refer to physician or podiatrist if signs of infection are present.
Intertrigo—chafing due to excessive rubbing of body parts in combination with perspiration	Pain, inflammation, burning, itching, moistness, cracking lesion	Cleanse frequently. Use medicated drying powder.
Plantar wart—viral infection on foot, leading to a localized overgrowth of skin; can be confused with callus	Distinct edge with central core Sometimes appears to be growing inward; small black dot in center surrounded by clearer callus area Excessive thickening of skin	Donut to take pressure off of wart. Keep callus area around wart filed down (do not file down wart). See physician or podiatrist for cure and/or removal.

(4, 5, 8-12, 13, 19, 21)

activity. Minimize participation until weight is within the 3% range.

- Consume a diet high in carbohydrates; carbohydrates contain a high water content and help to maintain fluid balance.
- Wear appropriate clothing for hot or humid weather conditions. Expose as much skin surface as possible.

Further precautions include wearing light-colored clothing because it does not absorb as much heat as darker clothing. Cotton materials absorb sweat and allow evaporation to occur. Certain synthetic clothing and materials with paint screens do not absorb sweat and should be avoided.

Participants should be educated to recognize symptoms of overexertion: nausea or vomiting, extreme breathlessness, dizziness, unusual fatigue, muscle cramping, and headache. Symptoms related to heat illness include hair standing on end on chest or upper arms, body chills, headache or throbbing pressure, nausea or vomiting, labored breathing, dry lips or extreme cotton mouth, faintness (heat syncope) or muscle cramping (heat cramps), and cessation of sweating. Heat rash can also be a symptom and is due to inflammed sweat glands and usually occurs in children who have sweated profusely. If these symptoms are present, the risk for developing heat exhaustion or heat stroke rises dramatically. The participant should stop the activity and get into the shade. In addition, the participant should be instructed to ask for help if he or she is disoriented or the symptoms are severe. The HFI should provide fluids and encourage the individual to drink.

Individuals who have previously suffered from heat stroke may sustain permanent damage to the thermoregulatory system. People who do not have efficient cooling mechanisms may be highly susceptible to heat injury. Individuals who use medications such as antihistamines or diuretics, use high quantities of salt in their diet or consume **salt tablets**, or drink alcohol in large quantities (particularly prior to activity) will have a higher risk of heat injury. Furthermore, people who participate in physical activity while experiencing fever could elevate their body temperature to dangerous levels. Table 21.5

outlines the various stages of heat illness, the signs and symptoms associated with each, and guidelines for immediate care.

Be aware of environmental factors such as relative humidity and temperature. The relative humidity can be calculated by measuring dry-bulb and wet-bulb atmospheric temperatures (see chapter 14) using a sling psychrometer. As mentioned earlier, the evaporation of sweat is a primary means to lose heat during exercise. This fluid loss must be replaced to minimize health risk and maximize safe and enjoyable participation in an exercise program. For most individuals who participate in CRF programs, thirst is an adequate indicator of when to hydrate. Generally, replacing fluids as they are used is the best way to meet the demands of the body. When extreme sweating or dry atmospheric conditions are present, however, the thirst mechanism may not be able to keep up with the need for fluid intake.

Normal daily intake of fluid for the sedentary individual is between 60 and 80 oz (1.8-2.4 L). The actual fluid requirement is dependent on too many factors to establish a single recommendation for maintaining hydration. However, drinking 8 to 10 oz (240 to 300 ml) of fluid before heavy exercise, in addition to frequent hydration during activity, helps to prevent heat illness.

Loss of salt and other minerals may occur during prolonged exercise, particularly during hot and humid weather. Even so, the use of salt tablets is not recommended unless accompanied by a large intake of water. Water with 0.1% to 0.2% salt solution may be given to individuals with high water loss. Increasing the use of salt at mealtimes and consuming a high intake of water throughout the day, however, generally meets the body's need for sodium and fluid replacement.

Most **electrolyte** drinks are diluted solutions of glucose, salt, and other minerals, with added artificial flavoring. Some brands also contain as much as 200 to 300 kcal per quart of solution. Other than sodium, the minerals provided by an electrolyte solution do not provide much benefit. When sweating is profuse, large amounts of electrolyte solution may help to serve the same function as a diluted salt solution. In cases of mild to moderate sweating, the normal intake of salt in food provides adequate sodium replacement. The main advantage of using a flavored solution is that the individual might drink more than if ingesting plain water or a salt solution. However, considering the prices of commercially prepared electrolyte solutions, plain water or homemade solutions, such as the one presented next, are much more economical.

Homemade Electrolyte Solution

1 qt water
1/3 tsp salt
Some sugar for flavoring (0.5 to 1.5 Tbsp)

Fluids at a temperature of 5 to 15 °C (41 to 59 °F) are absorbed faster than fluids at other temperatures.

In Review: Inefficient body cooling mechanisms, certain medications, high intake of salt or alcohol, and exercising with a fever or in high heat and humidity may cause heat-related disorders. Heat illness is potentially deadly, and the HFI must be aware of the steps to prevent its occurrence and, simultaneously, be able to recognize the signs of heat illness and act on them (see table 21.5). Proper hydration, evaluated through a weight chart, is a good first step in prevention. Provide water before, during, and following activity to prevent dehydration.

Cold-Related Problems

Exercising in cold, windy weather can produce some potential problems if certain precautions are not taken. Considerable heat loss can occur through convective heat loss from the skin and evaporation of skin moisture. Hypothermia occurs when body heat is lost at a faster rate than it is produced and core body temperature drops below 35 °C (95 °F). Peripheral blood vessels in cold areas constrict, which conserves body heat but increases risk of frostbite. Exercising in cold, rainy weather can compound the problem by increasing the rate of evaporation. Windchill is another factor that must be taken into account. A high windchill factor can result in severe loss of body heat even when air temperature is above freezing. Additionally, exercising in cold water results

salt tablets — Generally not recommended as a means to increase salt in the diet; if used, they must be taken with large amounts of water.

electrolyte — Particles that in solution convey an electrical charge. Most electrolyte drinks are diluted solutions of glucose, salt, and other minerals, with added artificial flavoring. Other than sodium, the minerals provided by an electrolyte solution do not provide much benefit.

Table 21.5 Heat-Related Problems and Their Treatment

Heat illness	Signs and symptoms	Immediate care
Heat cramps—spasmodic muscular contraction caused by exertion in extreme heat	Muscle cramping (calf is very common) Multiple cramping (very serious)	Isolated cramps: Direct pressure to the cramp and release, stretch muscle slowly and gently, apply gentle massage, and ice. Multiple cramps: Danger of heat stroke; treat as heat exhaustion.
Heat exhaustion—collapse with or without loss of consciousness, suffered in conditions of heat and high humidity, largely resulting from the loss of fluid and salt by sweating	Profuse sweating Cold, clammy skin Normal temperature or slightly elevated Pale Dizzy Weak, rapid pulse Shallow breathing Nausea Headache Loss of consciousness	Move individual out of the sun to a well-ventilated area. Place in shock position (feet elevated 12-18 in.); prevent heat loss or gain. Gently massage the extremities. Apply gentle range-of-motion movement to the extremities. Force consumption of fluids. Reassure the individual. Monitor body temperature and other vital signs. Refer to a physician.
Heat stroke—final stage of heat exhaustion in which the thermoregulatory system shuts down to conserve depleted fluid levels	Generally no perspiration Dry skin Very hot Temperature as high as 106 °F Skin color bright red or flushed (dark-pigmented individuals will have ashen skin) Rapid, strong pulse Labored breathing	Treat as an extreme medical emergency. Transport to hospital quickly. Remove as much clothing as possible without exposing the individual. Cool quickly, starting at the head and continuing down the body; use any means possible (fan, hose down, pack in ice). Wrap in cold, wet sheets for transport. Treat for shock; if breathing is labored, place in a semi-reclining position.
Heat syncope—fainting or excessive loss of strength because of excessive heat	Headache Nausea	Normal intake of fluids

(4, 5, 19, 20, 21, 23)

in even faster loss of body temperature than if exercising in the same air temperature. Cold-related problems are preventable if the following precautions are taken:

- Avoid exercising outdoors in extreme cold and wind.
- Layer clothing and remove layers as needed to avoid sweating.
- Warm up prior to exercise and avoid periods of inactivity.
- Stay dry.
- Cover face, nose, ears, fingers, and head (a great deal of heat loss occurs when the head is exposed).
- Avoid swimming or exercising in cold water, particularly when the surrounding air temperature is low.

Table 21.6 describes how to recognize and treat cold-related problems.

In Review: Exercising in cold, rainy weather or when the windchill factor is high, as well as exercising in cold water, may lead to cold-related disorders. Precautionary measures such as avoiding exposure to extreme cold, wearing removable layers, warming up prior to activity and remaining constantly active, and understanding the effect of windchill on air temperature can go a long way toward prevention of cold-related problems. See table 21.6 for specifics on how to treat cold-related problems when they occur.

Table 21.6 Cold-Related Problems and Their Treatment

Cold-related problems	Signs and symptoms	Immediate care
Deep frostbite—freezing of deep tissue, including muscle and bone	Hard, cold, numb, pale, or white area Permanent damage to tissue may be sustained.	Refer to a physician. Rapid rewarming is necessary.
Frostnip—freezing of tips of extremities such as ears, nose, or fingers, involving only the surface of the skin	Skin firm and cold Burning, itching, local redness Skin may peel or blister in a day or two.	Rewarm by applying firm pressure over the affected area, blowing warm air over the area, submerging in warm water 100 to 105 °F, and holding frostnipped area against body.
Superficial frostbite—freezing of layers of skin and subcutaneous tissue	Pale, waxy, and cold skin Purple coloring Following rewarming there may be swelling and superficial blisters. Stinging, burning, and aching may be present for several days or weeks.	Remove from cold. Rewarm area.
Hypothermia—core body temperature drops below 95 °F	Shivering Impairment of neuromuscular function Decreased ability to make decisions Muscle rigidity Hypotension Shock Death	Treat as a medical emergency. Remove from cold. Treat for shock. Immediate transport to hospital.

(4, 5, 19, 20, 21)

MEDICAL CONCERNS

Some individuals have controlled medical conditions that might be aggravated by exercise. In addition, it is important to recognize major cardiovascular and respiratory problems should they occur. This section summarizes information on some common medical concerns.

Diabetic Reactions

The HFI should be familiar with the signs and symptoms of diabetic coma and insulin shock (see table 21.7). When an emergency situation arises with a diabetic and the individual is conscious, he or she is usually able to indicate what the problem is. If the individual cannot, then ask when food was last eaten and whether insulin was taken that day. If the person has eaten but has not taken insulin, then the individual is probably going into a diabetic coma, a condition in which there is too little insulin to fully metabolize the carbohydrates consumed (hyperglycemia). If the individual has taken insulin but has not eaten, then he or she is probably suffering from insulin shock, a condition in which there is too much insulin or not enough carbohydrate to balance the insulin intake (hypogylcemia).

If the individual lapses into unconsciousness, check for a medic-alert identification tag. This may help to identify the problem. If you are undecided as to whether the individual is suffering from diabetic coma or insulin shock, give sugar. Brain damage or death can occur quickly if insulin shock is left untreated; it is a far more critical state than diabetic coma. If the problem is insulin shock, the individual should respond quickly, within 1 to 2 min; then transport the individual to a hospital as quickly as possible. If the individual is in a diabetic coma, there is little chance of seriously worsening the condition by giving sugar. Several hours of fluid and insulin therapy will be needed, under a physician's direction. Table 21.7 outlines the diabetic reactions, signs and symptoms, and immediate care of each.

> **6** **In Review: Diabetic coma is related to hyperglycemia, and insulin shock is due to hypoglycemia. Table 21.7 describes how to deal with these conditions.**

Cardiovascular and Pulmonary Complications

Cardiovascular complications can occur with injury due to decreased circulating blood volumes as may occur with bleeding, hyperthermia or hypothermia, shock, or heart attack. The HFI should be able to recognize and deal with potential complications such as **tachycardia** (excessively rapid heart beat), **bradycardia** (abnormally slow heart beat), hypertension (high blood pressure), and **hypotension** (low blood pressure).

Pulmonary complications may be observed more readily. **Apnea**, or temporary cessation of breathing, can be caused by an obstructed airway, allergic reaction, drowning, or intrathoracic injury. **Dyspnea,** or labored breathing, can be caused by hyperventilation, asthma, and chest or lung injury. **Tachypnea,** excessively rapid breathing, may be a sign of overexertion, shock, or hyperventilation. The HFI should feel comfortable assessing circulation and respiration and have the knowledge and skills to perform appropriate emergency procedures.

Most commonly seen respiratory disorders include hyperventilation, asthma, and **airway obstruction**. Hyperventilation can occur with heavy exhalation or rapid breathing, resulting in breathing out too much carbon dioxide (CO_2) and thereby reducing CO_2 levels in the blood. Low CO_2 levels may cause a feeling of dizziness, faintness, chest pains, and tingling in the feet and hands. Reassuring the individual in a calm manner, encouraging a slower breathing rate, and assisting to breathe into a paper bag will help restore CO_2 levels.

Asthma is a condition in which the smooth muscles of the bronchial tubes go into spasm; edema and inflammation of the mucous lining is triggered by exercise, changes in barometric pressure or temperature, virus, emotional upset, and noxious odors. The affected individual may appear anxious, pale, and sweaty; may cough or wheeze; and seem to be short of breath. Hyperventilation may occur resulting in dizziness, and, due to mucous secretions, the individual may frequently try to clear the throat.

The HFI should be prepared to handle an asthma attack. Generally people with asthma know how to care for themselves and will carry medication. Individuals with exercise-induced asthma often are given medication to take before activity. Encourage individuals with asthma to drink water, and promote relaxation and breathing exercises. Remove any known irritants from the environment if possible. If bronchial spasm is excessive, seek medical attention.

Table 21.7 Diabetic Reactions and Their Treatment

Diabetes	Signs and symptoms	Immediate care
Diabetic coma/hyperglycemia— loss of consciousness caused by too little insulin	May complain of a headache Confused Disoriented Stuporous Nauseated Coma Skin color—flushed Lips—cherry red Body temperature—decreased; skin—dry Breath odor—sweet, fruity Vomiting common Abdominal pain frequently present	Call for medical assistance. Little can be done unless insulin is at hand. If medical assistance is not quickly available 1. treat as shock; 2. administer fluids in large amounts by mouth, if individual is conscious; 3. maintain an open airway; 4. if individual is nauseated, turn the head to the side to prevent aspirating vomitus; and 5. do not give sugar, carbohydrates, or fats in any form. Recovery—gradual improvement over 6-12 hr. Fluid and insulin therapy should be directed by a physician.
Insulin shock/hypoglycemia— anxiety, excitement, perspiration, delirium, or coma caused by too much insulin or not enough carbohydrates to balance insulin intake	Skin color—pale (dark-pigmented individuals will appear ashen) Skin temperature—moist and clammy; cold sweat Pulse—normal or rapid Breathing—normal or shallow and slow No odor of acetone on breath Intense hunger Possible double vision	Administer sugar as quickly as possible (e.g., orange juice, candy). If individual is unconscious, place sugar granules under the tongue. If individual is unconscious or recovery is slow, call for medical assistance. Recovery—generally quick; 1 or 2 min. Refer to a physician if still unconscious or recovery is slow.

(1, 12)

tachycardia — A heart rate greater than 100 beats · min^{-1} at rest. Tachycardia may be seen in deconditioned people or people who are apprehensive about a situation (e.g., an exercise test).

bradycardia — Slow heart rate, below 60 beats · min^{-1} at rest. Bradycardia is healthy if it is the result of physical conditioning.

hypotension — Low blood pressure.

apnea — Temporary cessation of breathing; often caused by an excess amount of oxygen or too little carbon dioxide in the brain.

dyspnea — Difficult or labored breathing beyond what is expected for the intensity of work. The exercise test or activity should be stopped.

tachypnea — Excessively rapid breathing that may be a sign of overexertion, shock, or hyperventilation.

airway obstruction — Blockage of the airway; can be caused by a foreign object. Swelling is secondary to direct trauma or allergic reaction.

Airway obstruction can occur by swallowing an object or by the tongue blocking the airway. If breathing is labored but the individual is coughing forcefully, stay with the person and encourage continued coughing. If, however, the person is unsuccessful in expelling the object or the airway becomes totally blocked, have someone call for an ambulance and begin abdominal thrusts (**Heimlich maneuver**). In an unconscious victim, visually checking the airway passage or performing a finger sweep or Heimlich maneuver may dislodge a known obstruction. Generally, moving the lower jaw forward or tilting the head and lifting the chin will open an airway blocked by the tongue. **Rescue breathing** should be performed if the person has stopped breathing and repositioning the head does not change the status.

Respiratory shock, a condition in which the lungs are unable to supply enough oxygen to the circulating blood, can result in a medical emergency. Signs and symptoms include paleness of skin or cyanosis; weak, rapid pulse; rapid, shallow breathing rate; decrease in blood pressure; changes in personality including disinterest, irritability, restlessness, and excitement; extreme thirst; and in severe cases, urinary retention and fecal incontinence.

Treatment includes maintaining body heat and elevating feet and legs 12 to 18 in. If head or neck injury, or both, is suspected, protect the involved area and raise the head and shoulders. Keep the participant warm, reassure, and seek medical attention. Employ **CPR** techniques (see later section).

In Review: Common cardiovascular complications from exercise include excessively rapid or abnormally slow heart beat and high or low blood pressure. Pulmonary complications include temporary cessation of breathing, labored breathing, or airway obstruction.

COMMON ORTHOPEDIC PROBLEMS

Many injuries that are commonly referred to an orthopedic physician for diagnosis and treatment result from overuse or irritation of a chronic musculoskeletal problem. In most instances the injuries do not incapacitate the participant immediately. It may be weeks or months after the onset of pain before the participant seeks medical consultation. By this time, the **inflammation** is severe and generally prevents normal function of the part involved. In many cases a severe injury can be avoided if proper care is initiated early. Table 21.8 outlines common orthopedic problems, their causes, signs and symptoms, and general treatment guidelines.

Shin Splints

Shin splints is a catch-all expression used to describe a variety of conditions of the lower leg. It is often used to define any pain located between the knee and the ankle (usually anterior medial and lateral). A diagnosis of shin splints should be limited to conditions involving inflammation of the musculotendinous unit caused by overexertion of muscles during weight-bearing activity. A more specific diagnosis is preferred over the general term "shin splints." In any event, the physician must rule out the following conditions: stress fracture, metabolic or vascular disorder, **compartment syndrome**, and muscular strain. The physical complaints often accompanying shin splint pain include

- a dull ache in the lower leg region following workouts,
- performance and work-output decrease because of pain,
- soft-tissue pain,
- mild swelling along the area of inflammation,
- slight temperature elevation at the site of inflammation, and
- pain on moving the foot up and down.

The individual with shin splints usually has no history of trauma. The symptoms start gradually and progress if activity is not reduced. The following is the usual symptomatic treatment:

- Rest in the acute stage; reduce weight-bearing activity.
- In mild cases brought on by overuse, decrease or modify activity for a few days (e.g., choose swimming or bicycle workouts instead of running).
- Apply heat or ice before activity; use ice after activity. Heat treatments may consist of moist heat packs for 15 to 20 min or whirlpool treatments. The temperature of the whirlpool water should be approximately 100 to 106 °F. Treatment time is usually 15 to 20 min. Ice application may consist of ice-bag treatments for 15 to 20 min or ice massage/ice slush treatments for 5 to 7 min.

Treatment should begin at the first sign of pain. If pain is extreme, medical consultation should be obtained. Determination and treatment of the cause, in addition to symptomatic treatment, is necessary to prevent a recurrence of the problem. Table 21.9 sites the major causes for shin splints as well as the signs and symptoms and steps that can be taken to help prevent the onset or recurrence of lower leg pain.

Exercise Modification

Most orthopedic-related injuries can be classified as mild, moderate, or severe. When in doubt, conservative treatment is recommended. Any injury resulting in acute pain or affecting performance, and any injury in which the individual hears or feels a pop at the time of injury, should be referred to a physician. Any time conservative measures fail to result in improvement of the condition within a reasonable period of time (2 to 4 weeks), physician consultation is again recommended.

Other conditions may call for modifiying the exercise program. The participant may be obese, arthritic, or possess a history of musculoskeletal problems. Pool work is often employed with such individuals. Warm water is very therapeutic, body weight is supported, and the water generally allows for a greater range of movement. In any case, the activity should be suited to the condition. Any individual who requires exercise modification should be monitored closely. Table 21.10 summarizes the general guidelines used to classify injuries and offers suggestions for modifying activity.

8 **In Review: Table 21.8 summarizes information on how to deal with common orthopedic injuries including inflammatory reactions, tennis elbow, stress fractures, and mechanical low-back pain. Procedures for treating shin splints are described in table 21.9. A summary of how to classify an injury as mild, moderate, or severe and how to modify an exercise program to accommodate the problem is presented in Table 21.10.**

CPR AND EMERGENCY PROCEDURES

All HFIs should be well versed in CPR techniques. (Courses are generally available through the local American Heart Association or Red Cross). In an emergency situation, there is little time to think. Most reactions occur automatically. Having a plan of action and running through practice drills on a routine basis helps to ensure that proper procedures are followed in an emergency situation (1-7).

Basic Emergency Plan

First, be prepared. Make sure a phone is available for use during the exercise class, and know where the phone is located. If a phone is not available, have an alternative emergency plan in mind. The HFI should identify the **emergency medical system (EMS)** and services that are to be used (e.g., ambulance, hospital, doctor), and have a phone list located in a convenient place. Decide who is to phone for medical help in an emergency situation, and make sure that he or she knows how to direct help to the location of the injured individual. All necessary medical information

Heimlich maneuver — Procedure used to dislodge material caught in the respiratory passage, blocking the airway.

rescue breathing — Artificial respiration; used to promote oxygenation of blood in an unconscious victim who is not breathing.

respiratory shock — A condition in which the lungs are unable to supply enough oxygen to the circulating blood.

CPR — Cardiopulmonary resuscitation; established procedures to restore breathing and blood circulation.

inflammation — A reaction to injury; signs include heat, redness, pain, and swelling.

compartment syndrome — Increased pressure within a muscular compartment that compromises blood flow and nerve supply.

emergency medical system (EMS) — A system designed to handle medical emergencies; 911 or other community emergency number.

(e.g., release forms, medical history forms) should be readily available, and all emergency equipment and supplies should be easily accessible (e.g., stretcher, emergency kit and supplies, splints, ice, inhaler, money for phone call, blanket, spine board). The equipment should be checked periodically to ensure that it is in proper working order, and the supplies should be up to date. And, of course, know where the fire alarms and fire exits are located.

Remain calm to reassure the injured person and help prevent the onset of shock. Clear thinking allows for sound judgment and proper execution of rehearsed plans. In most instances speed is not necessary. Cases of extreme breathing difficulty, stoppage of breathing or circulation, choking, severe bleeding, shock, head or neck injury, heat illness, and internal injury are exceptions to this and require urgent action. Otherwise, careful evaluation and a deliberate plan of action is desirable. The HFI should have a system for evaluating and dealing with a life-threatening situation. All procedures should be conducted in a calm, professional manner.

Determine the history of the injury from direct observation of what happened, the injured person's account of what happened, or by a witness's account of the injury. If the injured person is unconscious or semiconscious and no cause is determined, check for a medic-alert identification tag.

Check vital signs—heart rate (HR), breathing, blood pressure (BP), bleeding, and so on—to determine the seriousness of the situation. The outcome of this evaluation will identify a course of action.

Table 21.8 Common Orthopedic Problems and Their Treatment

Injury	Common causes	Signs and symptoms	Treatment
Inflammatory reactions: **Bursitis**—inflammation of bursa (sac between a muscle and bone that is filled with fluid, facilitates motion, pads and helps to prevent abnormal function) **Capsulitis**—inflammation of the joint capsule **Epicondylitis**—inflammation of muscles or tendons attaching to the epicondyles of the humerous **Myositis**—inflammation of voluntary muscle **Plantar fasciitis**—inflammation of connective tissue that spans the bottom of the foot **Tendinitis**—inflammation of a tendon (a band of tough, inelastic, fibrous tissue that connects muscle to bone) **Tenosynovitis**—inflammation of a tendonous sheath **Synovitis**—inflammation of the synovial membrane (a highly vascularized tissue that lines articular surfaces)	Overuse Improper joint mechanics Improper technique Pathology Trauma Infection	Redness Swelling Pain Increased skin temperature over the area of inflammation Tenderness Involuntary muscle guarding	Ice and rest in the acute stages. If chronic, heat is generally used before exercise or activity, followed by ice after activity. Massage. Perform muscle strengthening and stretching exercises. Correct the cause of problem. If correction of the cause and symptomatic treatment does not relieve symptoms, referral to a physician is recommended; anti-inflammatory medication is usually prescribed. If disease process or infection is suspected, refer to a physician immediately.

Table 21.8 *(continued)*

Injury	Common causes	Signs and symptoms	Treatment
Tennis elbow—inflammation of the musculotendinous unit of the elbow extensors where they attach on the outer aspect of the elbow (lateral epicondylitis)	Faulty backhand mechanics—faults may include leading with the elbow, using an improper grip, dropping the racket head, or using a topspin backhand with a whipping motion Improper grip size—usually too small Racket strung too tightly Improper hitting—hitting off center, particularly if using wet, heavy balls Overuse of forearm supinators, wrist extensors, and finger extensors	Pain directly over the outer aspect of the elbow in region of the common extensor origin Swelling Increased skin temperature over the area of inflammation Pain on extension of the middle finger against resistance with the elbow extended Pain on racket gripping and extension of the wrist	Ice and rest in the acute stages. If chronic, heat is generally used before exercise or activity, followed by ice after activity. Apply deep friction massage at the elbow. Perform strengthening and stretching exercises for the wrist extensors. Correct the cause of the problem: 1. Use proper techniques. 2. Use proper grip size (when racket is gripped, there should be room for one finger to fit in the gap between the thumb and fingers). 3. Racket should be strung at the proper tension (usually between 50 and 55 lb). 4. Avoid stiff rackets that vibrate easily. Keep elbow warm, particularly in cold weather. Use a counterforce brace, a circular band that is placed just below the elbow (serves to reduce the stress at the origin of the extensors). If correction of cause and symptomatic treatment does not relieve symptoms, referral to a physician is recommended; anti-inflammatory medication is usually prescribed.

(continued)

Table 21.8 *(continued)*

Injury	Common causes	Signs and symptoms	Treatment
Stress fracture—a bone defect that occurs because of overstress to weight-bearing bones which causes an accelerated rate of remodeling. Inability of the bone to meet the demands of the stress results in a loss of continuity in the bone and periosteal irritation. Tibial stress fractures—more common in individuals with high-arched feet Fibula stress fractures—more common in pronators	Overuse or abrupt change in training program Change in running surface Change in running gait	Referred pain to the fracture site when a percussion test is used (e.g., hitting the heel may cause pain at the site of a tibial stress fracture) Pain usually localized to one spot and exquisitely tender to palpation Pain generally present all of the time but increases with weight-bearing activity; no lessening of pain after warm-up	Refer to physician. X-ray films should be obtained. Usually no crack is detected in the bone. A cloudy area becomes visible when the callus begins to form. Often this does not show up until 2-6 weeks after onset of pain. Early detection can usually be made through a bone scan or thermogram. If a stress fracture is suspected but not diagnosed, treat as a stress fracture. Running and other high-stress, weight-bearing activities should not be allowed until the fracture has healed and the bone is no longer tender to palpation. Tibial stress fractures usually take 8-10 weeks to heal; fibula stress fractures take approximately 6 weeks. When acute symptoms have subsided, bicyling and swimming activities can usually be initiated to maintain cardiovascular levels. This should be cleared with the supervising physician. If a specific cause is attributed to the development of a stress fracture, steps should be taken to correct the cause.

Table 21.8 *(continued)*

Injury	Common causes	Signs and symptoms	Treatment
Mechanical low-back pain—low-back pain that results from poor body mechanics, inflexibility of certain muscle groups, or muscular weakness	Tight low-back musculature Tight hamstrings Poor posture or postural habits Weak trunk musculature, particularly abdominals Differences in leg length because of a structural or functional problem Structural abnormality Obesity	Generalized low-back pain, usually aggravated by activity that accentuates the curve in the low back (e.g., hill running) Muscle spasm Palpable tenderness that is limited to musculature and not located directly over the spine May see a difference in pelvic height or other signs that would indicate a possible leg-length discrepancy Muscle tightness, particularly of the hamstrings, hip flexors, and low back	Any individual with acute onset of low-back pain or any signs of nerve impingement should be referred to a physician for evaluation and X ray. It is necessary to rule out structural abnormalities such as spondylolisthesis, ruptured disc, fractures, neoplasms, or possible segmental instability prior to instituting a general exercise program. Further diagnostic procedures may be warranted. Symptomatic treatment consists of ice application and referral to physician in acute cases. Chronic cases are generally treated with moist heat to reduce muscle spasm and ice after activity. Correct the causes of low-back pain: 1. Stretch tight muscles. 2. Strengthen weak muscles. 3. Do a thorough warm-up prior to activity and proper cool-down following activity. 4. Correct leg-length differences. 5. Emphasize correct postural positions. 6. If possible, correct or compensate for structural abnormalities (e.g., orthotics for a biomechanical problem).

(2, 3 [c, d], 4-8, 10, 12-19, 20)

Table 21.9 Shin-Splint Syndrome

Injury	Common causes	Signs and symptoms	Treatment
Shin splints— inflammatory reaction of the musculotendinous unit, caused by overexertion of muscles during weight-bearing activity. The following conditions must be ruled out: stress fracture, metabolic or vascular disorder, compartment syndrome, and muscular strain.	Prominent callus in metatarsal region		Keep callus filed down.
	Fallen metatarsal arch		Wear a metatarsal arch pad.
	Weak longitudinal arch	Lower longitudinal arch on one side in comparison to the opposite side	Conduct strengthening exercises for toe flexors. Wear longitudinal arch tape for support. Wear arch supports.
		Tenderness in arch area	Conduct strengthening exercises for the dorsiflexors and inverters.
	Muscular imbalance		Exercise to increase range of motion.
	Poor leg, ankle, and foot flexibility		Avoid hard surfaces.
	Improper running surface		Avoid changing from one surface to another.
	Improper running shoes		Select a shoe with good shock-absorbency qualities; be sure that the shoe is properly fitted.
	Overuse		Be flexible about changing the training program if there are signs that a great deal of physical stress is occurring. Encourage year-round conditioning. Always warm up properly.
	Biomechanical problems or structural abnormalities	Abnormal wear pattern of shoes	Refer to podiatrist or other professional specializing in foot care; orthotics may be indicated. Design a special training program to allow for individual differences (e.g., increase intensity of workouts, reduce duration).
	Improper running or skills technique		Correct technique. Perform specific stretching or strengthening exercises as well as technique work.
	Training in poor weather		Use common sense when training in cold or foul weather. Dress properly to maintain warmth. Warm up and cool down properly.

(4-6, 14)

Table 21.10 Injury Classification Criteria and Exercise Modifications

Criteria	Modifications
Mild injury	
Performance is not affected. Pain is experienced only after athletic activity. Generally, no tenderness is felt on palpation. No or minimal swelling is present. No discoloration is apparent.	Reduce activity level, modify activity to take stress off of the injured part, treat symptomatically, and gradually, and gradually return to full activity.
Moderate injury	
Performance is mildly affected or not affected at all. Pain is experienced before and after athletic activity. Mild tenderness is felt on palpation. Mild swelling may be present. Some discoloration may be present.	Rest the injured part, modify activity to take stress off of the injured part, treat symptomatically, and gradually return to full activity.
Severe injury	
Pain is experienced before, during, and after activity. Performance is definitely affected because of pain. Normal daily function is affected because of pain. Movement is limited because of pain. Moderate-to-severe point tenderness is felt on palpation. Swelling is most likely present. Discoloration may be present.	Rest completely and see a physician.

(4)

Checking Vital Signs

The following paragraphs describe vital signs and how to monitor each. Important vital signs to check include the pulse, color, body temperature, mobility, and blood pressure of the injured person.

Check heart rate. Use light finger pressure over an artery to monitor pulse rate. The most common sites are the carotid, brachial, radial, and femoral pulses. If there is no pulse and the individual is unconscious, begin CPR.

Assess color. For light-pigmented individuals, if skin, fingernail beds, lips, sclera of eyes, and mucous membranes are red, heat stroke, high blood pressure, or carbon monoxide poisoning are possible. If pale or ashen, changes in skin color could be due to shock, fright, insufficient circulation, heat exhaustion, insulin shock, or a heart attack. If bluish, the poor oxygenation of the blood could be due to an airway obstruction, respiratory insufficiency, heart failure, or some poisonings. For dark-pigmented individuals, assess nail beds, inside of lips, mouth, and tongue. Pink is the normal color for these; a bluish cast suggests shock. A grayish cast suggests shock from **hemorrhage**. A red flush at the tips of the ears suggests fever.

Take body temperature. Normal body temperature is 98.6 °F. Record temperature with a thermometer placed under the tongue (for 3 min); axilla, or armpit (10 min); or in the rectum (1 min). Cool, clammy, damp skin suggests shock or heat exhaustion; cool, dry skin indicates exposure to cold air; and hot, dry skin suggests fever or heat stroke.

Check mobility. Inability to move (paralysis) suggests injury or illness of the spinal cord or brain.

Take blood pressure. Blood pressure (BP) is usually taken at the brachial artery with a blood pressure cuff and sphygmomanometer. The following will aid in determining the problem:

- Normal BP—in men, systolic pressure, the pressure during the contraction phase of the heart, is equal to 100 plus the age of the individual up to 140 to 150 mmHg; diastolic pressure, the pressure during the relaxation phase of the heart, is equal to 65 to 90 mmHg. In females, both readings are generally 8 to 10 mmHg lower.
- Severe hemorrhage, heart attack—marked fall (20 to 30 mmHg) in blood pressure.
- Damage or rupture of vessels in the arterial circuit—BP is abnormally high (>150/>90).

hemorrhage — The escape of a large amount of blood from a vessel.

- Brain damage—rise in systolic pressure with a stable or falling diastolic pressure.
- Heart ailment—fall in systolic pressure with a rise in diastolic pressure.

Questions to Determine Course of Action

Ask the following questions to help you determine a course of action for treating injured participants.

Is the individual conscious? If not, a head, neck, or back injury is possible. If you are unsure as to why the individual is unconscious, check for a medic-alert identification tag. Assess airway, breathing, and circulation. Do not use ammonia capsules to arouse; the individual may suddenly move the head backward in response, causing additional injury. If breathing has stopped and the individual is in a prone position, he or she should be log-rolled as carefully as possible, keeping the head, neck, and spine in the same relative position, to begin CPR techniques.

If the individual is unconscious but breathing, protect from further injury. Do not move unless the individual's life is in danger. Wait for medical assistance to arrive. Make a systematic evaluation of the entire body and perform necessary first-aid procedures.

Is the individual breathing? If not, establish an airway and administer artificial respiration. Summon medical help. The following information will aid in determining the problem:

- Normal respiration—20 breaths · min^{-1}
- Respiration in well-trained individuals—6 to 8 breaths · min^{-1}
- Shock—rapid, shallow respiration
- Airway obstruction, heart disease, pulmonary disease—deep, gasping, labored breathing
- Lung damage—frothy sputum with blood at the nose and mouth, accompanied by coughing
- Diabetic acidosis—alcoholic or sweet, fruity odor to breath
- Cessation of breathing—lack of movement of abdomen and chest as well as airflow at nose and mouth

Is the individual bleeding profusely? If so, control bleeding by elevating the body part; putting direct pressure over the wound at **pressure points**; and as a last resort, putting on a tourniquet. A tourniquet should only be used in life-threatening situations in which choosing to risk a limb is a reasonable action in order to save a life. Treat for shock.

Is there evidence of a head injury? This can be determined through a history of a blow to the head or a fall onto the head, deformity of the skull, loss of consciousness, clear or straw-colored fluid coming from the nose or ears, unequal pupil size, dizziness, loss of memory, and nausea. Prevent any unnecessary movement. If it is necessary to move the individual, use a stretcher with the individual's head elevated. If the individual is unconscious, assume there is also a neck injury. Summon medical help immediately. The following information will aid in determining the problem:

- Drug abuse or nervous system disorder—constricted pupils
- Unconscious, cardiac arrest—dilated pupils
- Head injury—pupils unequal size
- Disease, poisoning, drug overdose, injury—pupils do not react to light
- Death—pupils widely dilated and unresponsive to light

Is there evidence of a neck or back injury? The history of the injury may give a clue. Other indications of a possible neck or back injury include pain directly over the spine, burning or tingling in the extremities, and loss of muscle function or strength in the extremities. When in doubt, assume there is a neck or back injury. The following information will aid in determining the problem:

- Probable injury of spinal cord—numbness or tingling in the extremities
- Occlusion of a main artery—severe pain in the extremity, with loss of cutaneous sensation
- Hysteria, violent shock, excessive drug or alcohol use—no pain

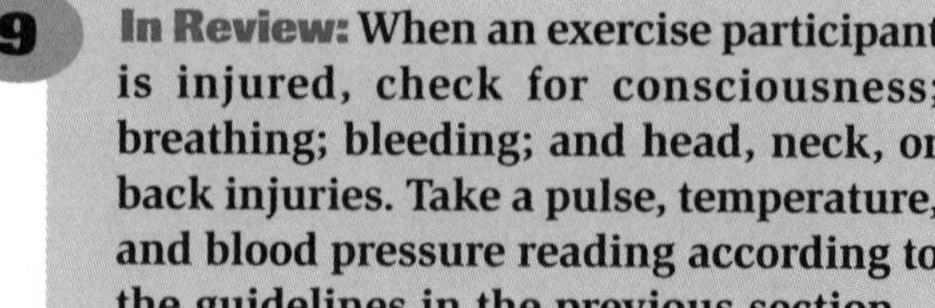
9 **In Review: When an exercise participant is injured, check for consciousness; breathing; bleeding; and head, neck, or back injuries. Take a pulse, temperature, and blood pressure reading according to the guidelines in the previous section.**

Artificial Respiration (AR) and Cardiopulmonary Resusitation (CPR)

If the HFI believes that a participant has stopped breathing, AR should be initiated. If the HFI finds that breathing has stopped and there is no pulse, he or she should initiate CPR. Although the steps presented here for AR and CPR techniques are for adults only, the HFI should review current recommended techniques for all age categories: adults, children, and infants. The following is a list of nine steps to use in mouth-to-mouth resuscitation and one-person CPR.

1. Determine responsiveness of the individual by shouting, "Are you okay?"
2. Position the victim face up and call for help (If a head or neck injury is present and the individual is breathing, do not move unless in danger).
3. Open the airway by using a jaw thrust or head tilt/chin lift.
4. Determine whether the victim is breathing. Listen and feel for air exchange. Look for chest movement.
5. If there is no breathing, pinch the nose shut and give two quick ventilations using mouth-to-mouth or mouth-to-nose technique.
6. Determine whether there is a pulse by checking the carotid artery.
7. Implement the emergency medical system—call 911 or the emergency number for your area.
8. If there is a pulse, initiate AR and ventilate once every 5 s for an adult. If there is no breathing and no pulse, initiate CPR by giving 15 compressions followed by two ventilations at a rate of 80 compressions per minute for an adult.
9. Assess the victim's condition after 1 min and approximately every 2 to 3 min thereafter.

Two-person CPR is no longer being taught in the Community CPR training. If another person who knows CPR arrives at the scene and states they know CPR, one person should go call for an ambulance, while the other rescuer gives CPR. If the initial rescuer gets tired, the second rescuer can take over at the end of a cycle of 15 compressions. The following outlines the steps in two-person CPR. Two-person CPR should be initiated only if local American Heart Association or Red Cross training teaches the procedure.

1. The second rescuer states that he or she knows CPR and asks to assist. The second rescuer then takes a position at the head when the first rescuer moves down to give chest compressions.
2. The second rescuer checks for a pulse while compressions are being given. This determines the effectiveness of the compressions. The second rescuer then tells the first rescuer to stop compressions and checks again for a pulse.
3. If a pulse is found, respiration should be checked. If there is no respiration, continue ventilation only, once every 5 s.
4. If there is no pulse, the second rescuer tells the first rescuer to continue CPR and then gives one ventilation.
5. The first rescuer follows the ventilation with five chest compressions at a rate of 60 compressions per minute for an adult.
6. The second rescuer gives one ventilation after the last compression.
7. Assess the victim's condition after 1 min and every 2 to 3 min thereafter.

10 **In Review: The procedures on how to handle a breathing emergency, assess an unconscious victim, and demonstrate proper techniques for establishing an airway and performing artificial respiration and CPR by learning the techniques were just described. HFIs must recognize their limitations and stay within the realm of their training when handling an injury or emergency situation and when giving medical advice.**

Case Studies

Refer to appendix A for suggested responses to the following case studies.

21.1

You are instructing an aerobics class when a participant collapses. On approaching the individual, you note that breathing is shallow and slow and that the skin color is pale, moist, and clammy. The individual is conscious but not alert. The individual reports double vision and an intense hunger. The individual is wearing a medical-alert tag. Answer the following questions:

a. What illness do you suspect?
b. What questions would you ask?
c. What action should you take?

pressure points — The point of application of pressure over major arteries to control bleeding.

21.2

You are leading an aerobics class and a participant collapses. You observe that the participant's skin is dry and red, breathing is labored, and pulse is rapid and strong. No trauma was experienced. Answer the following questions:

a. What heat-related illness should be suspected?
b. What is the immediate care?
c. What emergency planning should be in effect?

SOURCE LIST

1. American Academy of Orthopedic Surgeons (1977)
2. American Medical Association (1966)
3. American Red Cross (1993a, 1993b, 1993c, 1993d, 1993e)
4. Arnheim (1987)
5. Arnheim (1989)
6. Arnheim & Prentice (1993)
7. Bloomfield, Fricker, & Fitch (1992)
8. Booher & Thibadeau (1994)
9. Department of Labor, Occupational Safety & Health Administration (1991)
10. Fahey (1986)
11. Franks & Howley (1989a, 1989b)
12. Henderson (1973)
13. Klafs & Arnheim (1977)
14. Morris (1984)
15. Nieman (1990)
16. Pfeiffer & Pfeiffer (1995)
17. Rankin & Ingersoll (1995)
18. Reid (1992)
19. Ritter & Albohm (1987)
20. Scribner & Burke (1978)
21. Thygerson (1987)
22. Torg, Welsh, & Shepard (1990)
23. Williams (1988)

CHAPTER

22

Exercise Related to ECG and Medications

Daniel Martin and David R. Bassett, Jr.

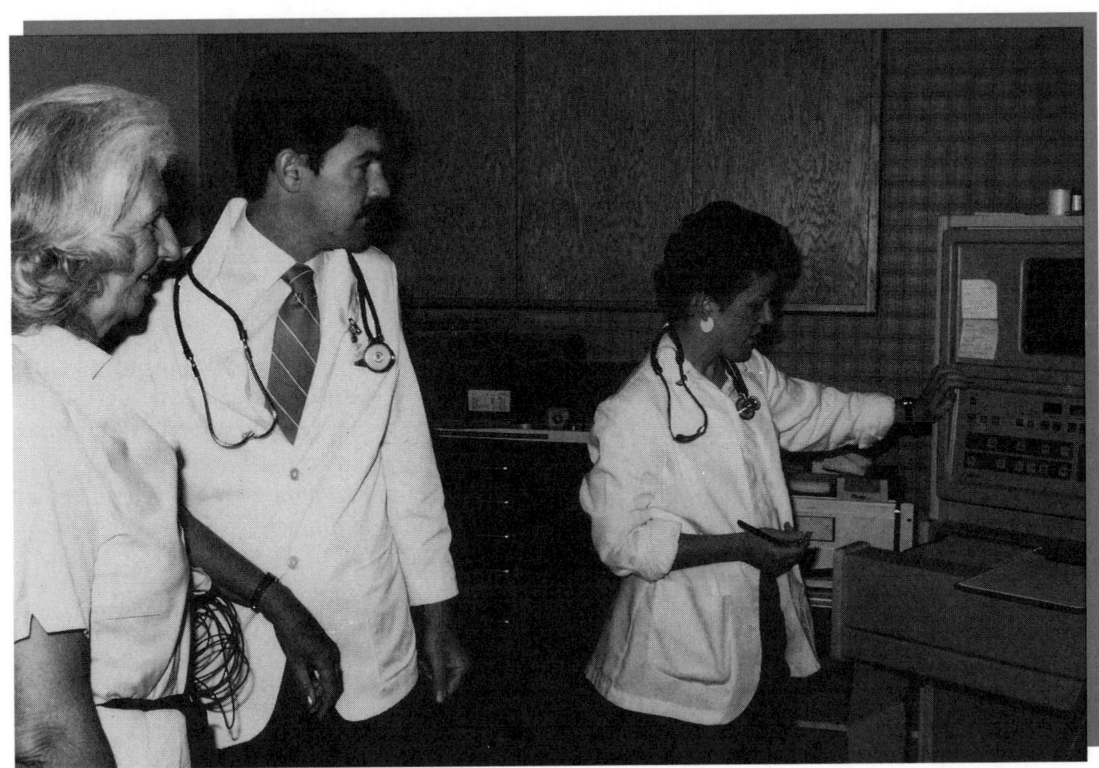

The reader will be able to: **OBJECTIVES**

1. Describe the basic anatomy of the heart.
2. Describe the basic electrophysiology of the heart.
3. Define the electrocardiogram and identify the standard settings for paper speed and amplitude.
4. Identify the basic electrocardiographic complexes and calculate heart rate from electrocardiograph rhythm strips.
5. Describe the various types of atrioventricular conduction defects and their probable impact on a subject's exercise response.
6. Identify the normal and abnormal cardiac rhythms and their significance, and predict the probable impact of the abnormal rhythms on exercise performance.
7. Describe electrocardiographic signs and biochemical markers of a heart attack.
8. List the common categories of prescription medications used to treat cardiovascular and related disease, some of the members of each category, and the probable impact of these medications on exercise performance.

The purposes of this chapter are to provide the health fitness instructor (HFI) with background information on the heart, the basics of electrocardiogram (ECG) analysis, cardiovascular medications, and how these factors affect exercise testing and prescription in the basically healthy population. This chapter is not intended to be a complete guide to ECG interpretation and cardiovascular medications; there are several excellent texts on these topics listed in the reference section (2, 6, 8-10).

UNDERSTANDING THE STRUCTURE OF THE HEART

The heart is a muscular organ, composed of four chambers: the right atrium, the right ventricle, the left atrium, and the left ventricle (see figure 22.1). The flow of blood through the heart is directed by pressure differences and valves between the chambers. Venous blood from the body enters the right atrium via the inferior and superior vena cava. From the right atrium, blood passes through the **tricuspid valve** into the right ventricle. The right ventricle pumps blood through the **pulmonary valve** into the pulmonary arteries to the lungs. In the lungs, blood gives up carbon dioxide and picks up oxygen. The oxygen-rich blood is returned to the heart via the pulmonary veins emptying into the left atrium. From the left atrium, blood passes through the **mitral valve** into the left ventricle. The left ventricle pumps oxygenated blood past the **aortic valve**, into the aorta, coronary arteries, and to the rest of the body. The left ventricle, which generates more pressure than the right ventricle, is thicker.

Coronary Arteries

The heart muscle, or **myocardium**, does not receive a significant amount of oxygen directly from blood

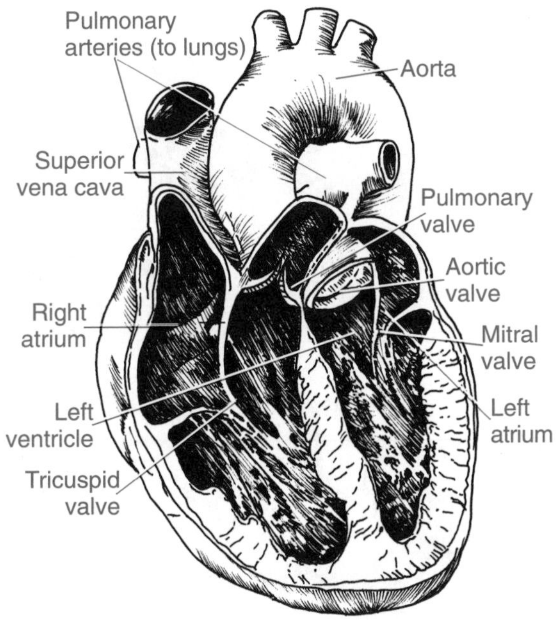

FIGURE 22.1 The chambers and valves of the heart.
Reprinted from Donnelly 1990.

in the atria or ventricles. Oxygenated blood is supplied to the myocardium via the **coronary arteries**, which lie on the surface of the heart. There are two coronary artery systems (the right and left coronary arteries), which branch off the aorta at the coronary sinus. The left main coronary artery follows a course between the left atria and pulmonary artery and branches off into the left anterior descending, or interventricular, and left circumflex arteries (figure 22.2). The left anterior descending artery follows a path along the anterior surface of the heart and lies over the interventricular septum, which separates the right and left ventricles. The left circumflex artery follows the groove between the left atrium and left ventricle on the anterior and lateral surface of the heart. The right coronary artery follows the groove separating atria and ventricles around the posterior surface of the heart and forms the posterior descending artery, or posterior interventricular artery. Numerous smaller arteries branch off each of the major arteries and form smaller and smaller arteries, finally forming the capillaries in the muscle cells where gas exchange occurs. A major obstruction in any of these coronary arteries results in a reduced blood flow to the myocardium (**myocardial ischemia**) and decreases the ability of the heart to pump blood. If the coronary arteries become blocked and the heart muscle does not receive oxygen, then a portion of the heart muscle might die, which is known as a myocardial infarction, or heart attack.

Coronary Veins

Venous drainage of the right ventricle occurs via the anterior cardiac vein, which normally has two or three major branches and eventually empties into the right atrium. The venous drainage of the left ventricle is primarily provided by the anterior interventricular vein, which roughly follows the same path as the left anterior descending artery, eventually forming the coronary sinus and emptying into the right atrium.

OXYGEN USE BY THE HEART

The myocardium is very well adapted to use oxygen to generate adenosine triphosphate (ATP). Approximately 40% of the volume of a myocardial muscle cell is composed of mitochondria, the cellular organelle responsible for producing ATP with oxygen. The oxygen consumption of the heart in a resting person is about 8 to 10 ml · min^{-1} per 100 g of myocardium;

tricuspid valve — A valve located between the right atrium and right ventricle of the heart.

pulmonary valve — A set of three crescent-shaped flaps at the opening of the pulmonary artery; also called the semilunar valves.

mitral valve — Heart valve located between the left atrium and left ventricle.

aortic valve — Heart valve located between the aorta and the left ventricle.

myocardium — The middle layer of the heart wall; involuntary, striated muscle innervated by autonomic nerves.

coronary arteries— Blood vessels that supply the heart muscle.

myocardial ischemia — A lack of oxygen for heart function caused by a reduced blood flow to the myocardium.

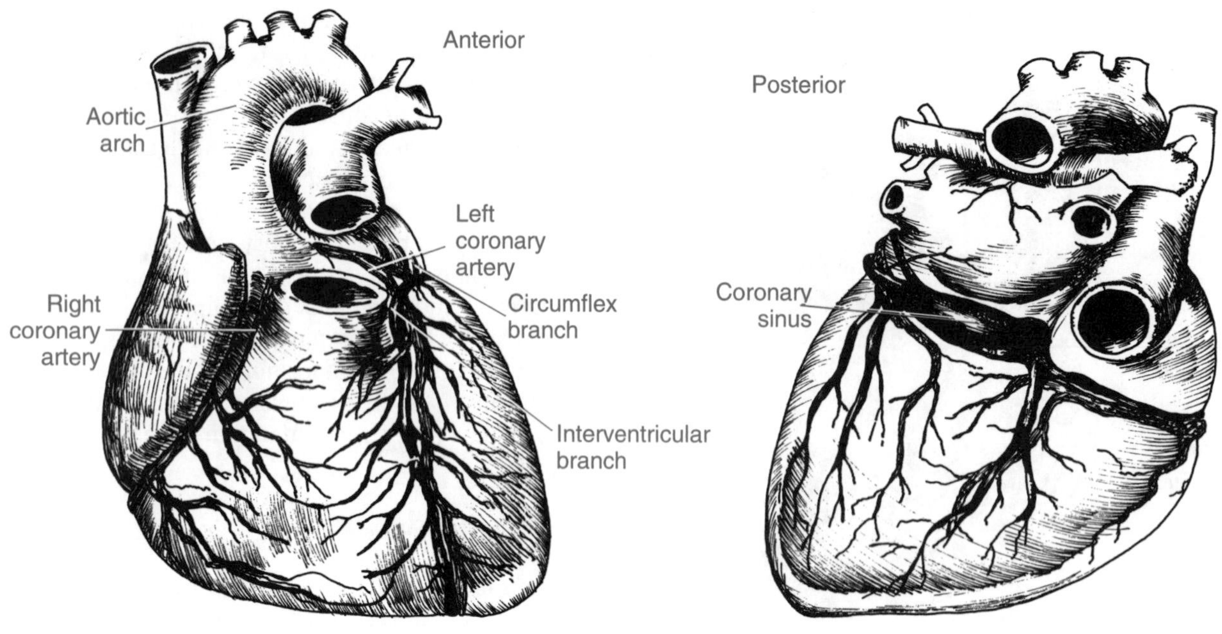

FIGURE 22.2 Coronary blood vessels.
Reprinted from Donnelly 1990.

in comparison the total resting oxygen consumption for the body is about 0.35 ml · min^{-1} per 100 g of body mass (3). Myocardial oxygen consumption can increase six to sevenfold during heavy exercise, whereas in young people the total body oxygen consumption can easily increase 12 to 15 times. Heart muscle has a limited capacity to produce energy via anaerobic pathways and depends on the delivery of oxygen to the mitochondria to produce ATP. At rest the whole body extracts only about 25% of the oxygen present in each 100 ml of arterial blood, and the body can meet its need for oxygen by simply extracting more from the blood. In contrast, the heart extracts about 75% of the oxygen available in the arterial blood. Consequently, the heart muscle's oxygen needs must be met by increasing the delivery of blood via the coronary arteries. An adequate oxygen supply to the heart is needed not only to allow the heart to pump blood but also to maintain normal electrical activity, which is covered in the next section.

1 **In Review: The heart is a muscular organ composed of four chambers: the right atrium, the right ventricle, the left atrium, and the left ventricle. The coronary arteries supply the heart muscle (myocardium) with blood, and the heart meets the increasing oxygen demands by increasing blood flow.**

ELECTROPHYSIOLOGY OF THE HEART

At rest, the insides of the myocardial cells are negatively charged and the exterior of the cells is positively charged. When the cells are depolarized (stimulated), the insides of the cells become positively charged and the exteriors of the cells become negatively charged. If a recording electrode is placed so that the wave of depolarization spreads toward the electrode, the ECG records a positive (upward) deflection. If the wave of depolarization spreads away from the recording electrode, a negative (downward) deflection will occur. When the myocardial muscle cell is completely polarized or depolarized, the ECG will not record any electrical potential but rather a flat line, known as the isoelectric line. Following depolarization, the myocardial cell undergoes repolarization to return its electrical state to what it was at rest. The steps leading from rest (complete polarization) to complete stimulation (complete depolarization) back to rest (repolarization) are shown in figure 22.3.

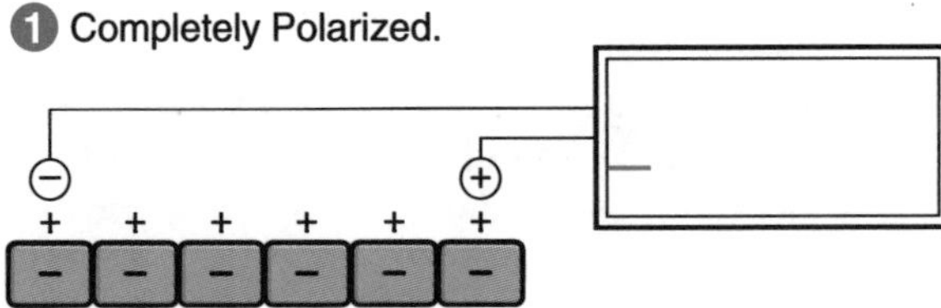

The myocardial cells shown on the left are at rest and are completely polarized. Because both of the recording electrodes are surrounded by positive charges, there is no voltage difference between them and the electrocardiogram shown on the right records the isoelectric line (0 mV).

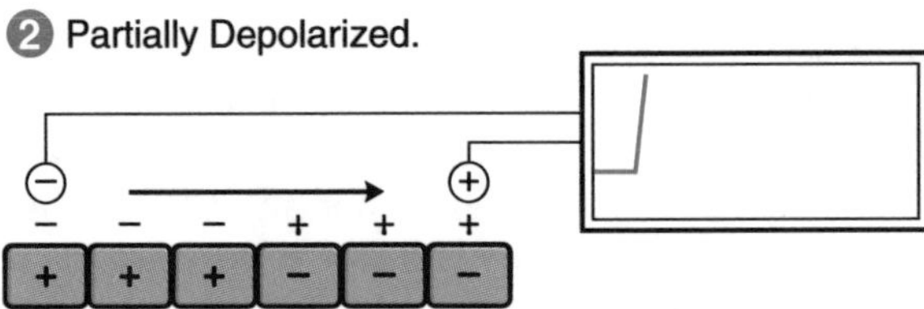

The process of depolarization (positive charges inside the cell and negative charges outside) is spreading from left to right. Because the electrode on the right is surrounded by positive charges, the ECG records a positive deflection. The amplitude of the deflection is proportional to the mass of the myocardium undergoing depolarization.

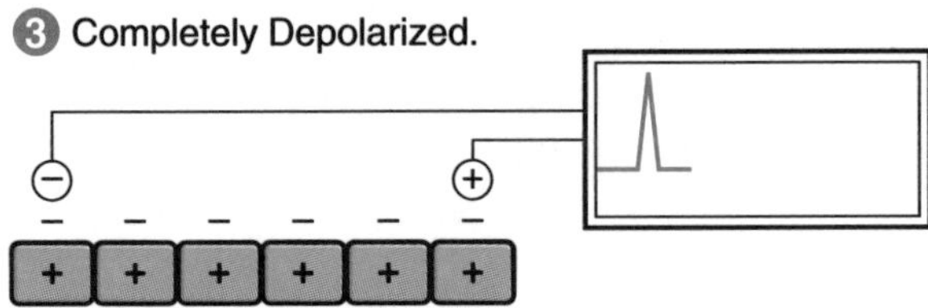

Depolarization is now complete, and both electrodes are surrounded by negative charges. Because there is no voltage difference between electrodes, the ECG is now recording 0 mV, or the isoelectric potential.

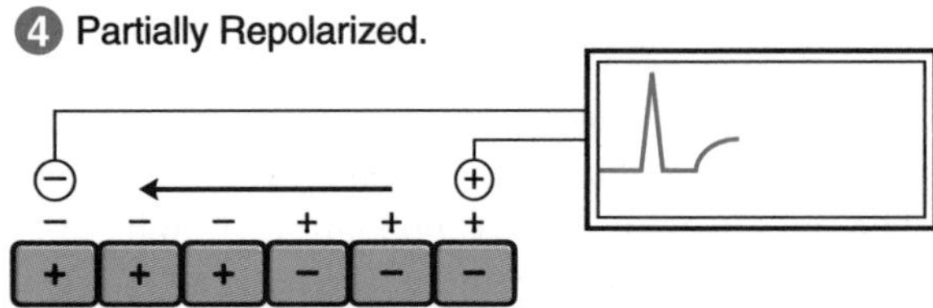

Repolarization has started from the right and is moving to the left. The ECG shows a positive (upward) deflection, because the right hand electrode is surrounded by positive charges. Note that repolarization occurs in the opposite direction from depolarization in the human heart, and this is the reason the depolarization and repolarization complexes are both normally positive. If repolarization had started on the left and moved to the right, the ECG deflection would have been negative.

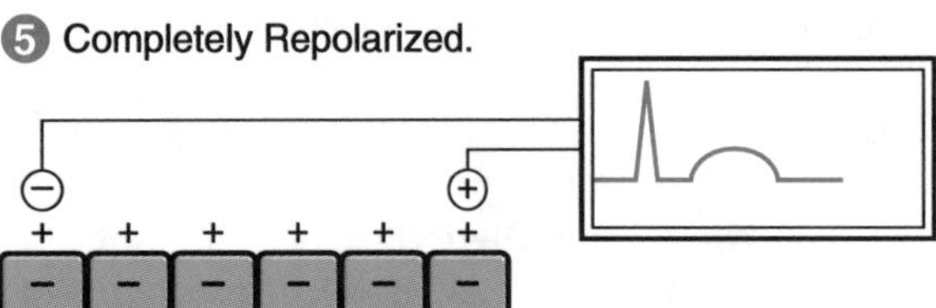

The muscle cells are now completely repolarized, or in the resting state, and the ECG records the isoelectric line. The myocardial cells are now ready to be depolarized again.

FIGURE 22.3 Steps in an electrocardiographic cycle.

CONDUCTION SYSTEM OF THE HEART

The **sinoatrial (SA) node** is the normal pacemaker of the heart and is located in the right atrium near the superior vena cava (figure 22.4). Depolarization spreads from the sinoatrial node across the atria and results in the P wave. There are three conduction tracts within the atria that conduct depolarization to the **atrioventricular (AV) node**. Impulses travel from the sinoatrial node through the atrial muscle and conduction tracts and enter the AV node, where the speed of conduction is slowed to allow the atrial

sinoatrial (SA) node — A mass of tissue in the right atrium of the heart, near the vena cava, that initiates the heartbeat.

atrioventricular (AV) node — The origin of the **bundle of His** in the right atrium of the heart. Normal electrical activity of the heart passes through the AV node prior to depolarization of the ventricles.

contraction to empty blood into the ventricles before the start of ventricular contraction. The **bundle of His** is the conduction pathway that connects the AV node with **bundle branches** in the ventricles. The right bundle branch splits off the bundle of His and forms ever-smaller branches that serve the right ventricle. The left bundle splits into two major branches that serve the thicker left ventricle. **Purkinje fibers** are the terminal branches of the bundle branches and form the link between the specialized conductive tissue and the muscle fibers. Small electrical junctions between adjacent cardiac muscle cells, known as **intercalated discs**, allow the electrical impulses to be passed from cell to cell. The intercalated discs allow for simultaneous contraction of the ventricular muscle fibers, which is needed for effective pumping action of the heart.

2 In Review: The electrical impulse originates in the SA node, located in the right atrium. From there the electrical impulse spreads to the AV node, the bundle of His, left and right bundle branches, and Purkinje fibers. Waves of depolarization then spread from cell to cell throughout the ventricular muscle. Any restriction in the blood flow to the myocardium could upset the electrical activity of the heart or cause damage to the myocardium itself.

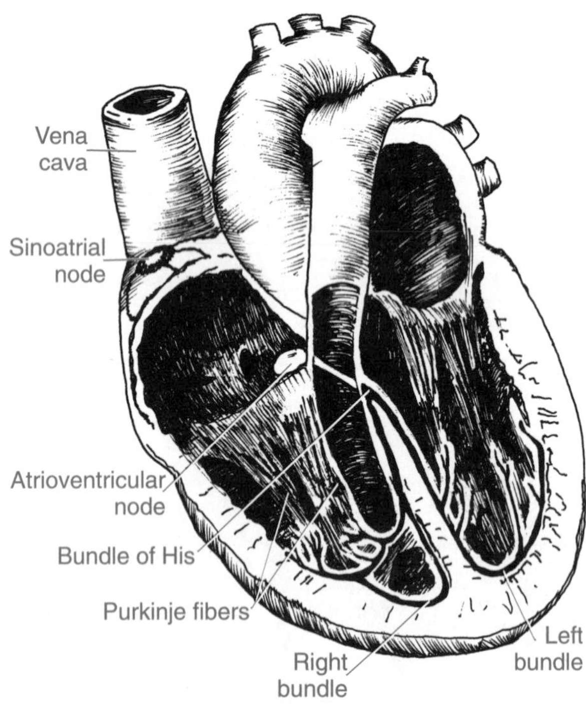

FIGURE 22.4 The electrical conduction system of the heart. These are the normal pathways used to ensure the rhythmical contraction and relaxation of the chambers of the heart.

BASIC INFORMATION FOR INTERPRETING THE ELECTROCARDIOGRAM

This section on the analysis of the ECG may appear to be beyond what an HFI should know about the topic. In fact, the physician is the person to make judgments about whether or not an ECG response is normal. However, the HFI must be aware of the basic information related to ECG interpretation to facilitate communication with the physician, program director, and exercise specialist.

A systematic approach to ECG evaluation allows the examiner to determine the heart rate, rhythm, and conduction pathways and to search for signs of ischemia or infarction. Physicians normally evaluate a 12-lead ECG, but for our purposes a single ECG lead will be adequate. The most commonly used single ECG lead for exercise testing is the CM5 (see figure 22.5), which looks very similar to lead V5 on a 12-lead ECG.

Defining the ECG

The **electrocardiogram**, or ECG, is a graphical recording of the heart's electrical activity. As waves of depolarization travel through the heart, electrical currents spread to the tissues surrounding the heart and then travel throughout the body. If recording electrodes are placed on the surface of the skin, small voltage differences can be detected between various regions of the body. Thus, the ECG is a sensitive voltmeter that records the electrical activity of the heart.

Time and Voltage

ECG paper is marked in a standard manner to allow measurement of time intervals and voltages. Time is measured on the horizontal axis, and the paper normally moves at 25 mm (millimeters) per second. Most ECG machines can be set to run at 50 or 25 mm per second, so one must know the paper speed when measuring the duration of ECG complexes. ECG

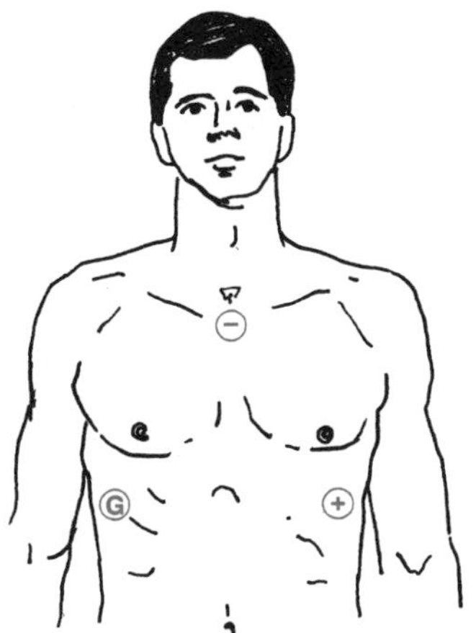

FIGURE 22.5 Lead placement for CM5: (−) negative electrode, (+) electrode, (G) ground.
Adapted from Ellestad 1994.

paper is marked with a repeating grid (see figure 22.6). Major grid lines are 5 mm apart, and at a paper speed of 25 mm per second 5 mm corresponds to 0.20 s. Minor lines are 1 mm apart, and at a paper speed of 25 mm per second, 1 mm equals 0.04 s. Voltage is measured on the vertical axis, and the calibration of the machine must be known to evaluate the ECG. The standard calibration factor is normally 0.1 mV (millivolt) per millimeter of deflection. Most ECG machines can be adjusted to reduce this factor by 50%, or double it. Like paper speed, it is very important to know the voltage calibration before evaluating an ECG. All ECG measurements in this chapter refer to a paper speed of 25 mm per s and a voltage calibration of 0.1 mV per mm.

3 In Review: The pattern of electrical activity across the heart is called the electrocardiogram (ECG). The ECG is recorded with an electrocardiograph and it provides information about the rhythm of the heart. The ECG paper speed is normally set at 25 mm per second, and at this speed each 1 mm mark represents 0.04 s. The standard calibration factor is normally 0.1 mV (millivolt) per millimeter of deflection.

Basic Electrocardiographic Complexes

The **P wave** is the graphical representation of atrial depolarization. The normal P wave is less than 0.12 s in duration and has an amplitude of 0.25 mV or less. The Ta wave is the result of atrial repolarization. It is not normally seen, as it occurs during ventricular depolarization and the larger electrical forces generated by the ventricles "hide" the Ta wave. The **Q wave** is the first downward deflection after the P wave; the Q wave signals the start of ventricular depolarization. The **R wave** is a positive deflection after the Q wave, and it is the result of ventricular depolarization. If there is more than one R wave in a single complex, the second occurrence is called R′ (R prime).

The **S wave** is a negative deflection preceded by Q or R waves, and it is also the result of ventricular depolarization. The **T wave** follows the **QRS complex**, and it represents ventricular repolarization.

bundle of His — Conduction pathway that connects the AV node with **bundle branches** in the ventricles.

bundle branch — Bundle of nerve fibers between both ventricles of the heart; conducts impulses into both ventricles (see **bundle of His**).

Purkinje fibers — The muscle-cell fibers found beneath the endocardium of the heart; the impulse-conducting network of the heart.

intercalated discs — Special junctions between adjacent cardiac muscle cells that allow electrical impulses to pass from cell to cell.

electrocardiogram — Graphical recording of the electrical activity of the heart, obtained with the electrocardiograph.

P wave — On an ECG, a small positive deflection preceding a QRS complex, indicating atrial depolarization, normally less than 0.12 s in duration with an amplitude of 0.25 mV or less.

Q wave — The initial negative deflection of the QRS complex on an ECG.

R wave — The positive deflection of the QRS complex in the ECG.

S wave — The first negative wave (preceded by Q or R waves) of the QRS complex in the ECG.

T wave — On an ECG, follows the QRS complex and represents ventricular repolarization.

QRS complex — The largest complex on an ECG, indicating a depolarization of the left ventricle, normally less than 0.1 s.

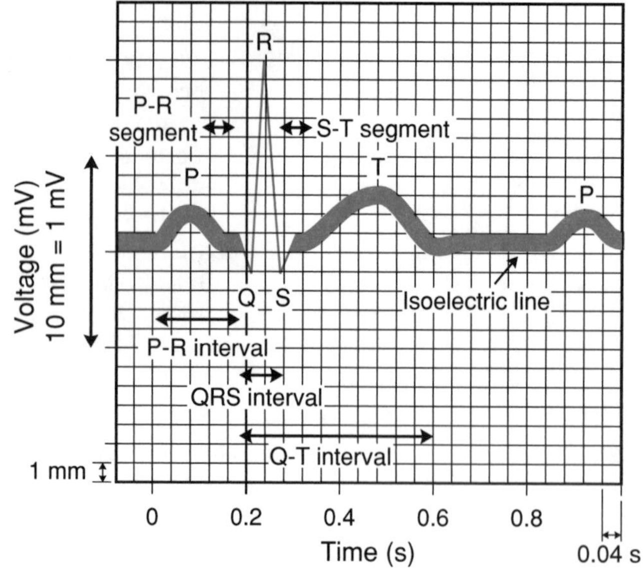

FIGURE 22.6 ECG complex with time and voltage scales.
Adapted from Goldman, *Principles of clinical electrocardiography*, 11th ed.; Appleton & Lange, 1982.

Electrocardiograph Intervals

The **R-R interval** is the time between successive R waves. An approximate heart rate (beats · min^{-1}) can be determined by dividing 1500 (60 s × 25 mm · s^{-1}) by the number of millimeters between adjacent R waves (figure 22.7a). A second method of determining heart rate is to begin with an R wave that falls on a thick black line. As you move to the right, count off the next six black lines as 300, 150, 100, 75, 60, and 50 (memorize these numbers). If the next R wave falls on one of these lines, the corresponding number indicates the heart rate. If the next R wave falls in between two thick black lines, you can estimate the heart rate by interpolation (figure 22.7b). A third method of determining heart rate is commonly used when the heart rate is irregular. With this method, you count the number of complete R-R intervals in a 6-s ECG strip and multiply by 10 (figure 22.7c).

The P-P interval represents the time between two successive atrial depolarizations. The **P-R interval** is measured from the start of the P wave to the beginning of the QRS complex. The interval is called P-R even if the first deflection following the P wave is a Q wave. The P-R interval represents the time from the start of atrial depolarization, delay through the AV node, and the start of ventricular depolarization. The upper limit for the normal P-R interval is 0.20 s or 5 small blocks.

The width of the QRS complex represents the time for depolarization of the ventricles. A normal QRS complex lasts less than 0.10 s, or 2.5 small blocks on the ECG paper. The **Q-T interval** is measured from the start of the QRS complex to the end of the T wave and corresponds to the duration of ventricular systole.

Segments and Junctions

The **P-R segment** is measured from the end of the P wave to the beginning of the QRS complex. This segment forms the isoelectric line, or baseline, from which S-T segment deviations are measured. The RS-T segment or **J point**, is the point at which the S wave ends and the S-T segment begins. The **S-T segment** is formed by the isoelectric line between the QRS complex and the T wave. This segment will be closely examined during an exercise test for depression or elevation, which may indicate the development of myocardial ischemia, or perhaps myocardial infarction. S-T segment deviation is usually measured 60 or 80 ms (milliseconds) after the J point.

4

In Review: The P wave signifies atrial depolarization, the QRS complex signifies ventricular depolarization, and the

T wave signifies ventricular repolarization. If the rhythm is regular, heart rate can be determined by dividing 1500 by the number of millimeters between successive R waves or by starting with an R wave that falls on a thick black line and counting off the next six black lines as 300, 150, 100, 75, 60, and 50 and determining at which corresponding number the next R wave occurs. If the rhythm is irregular, heart rate can be determined by counting the number of R-R intervals in a 6-s ECG strip and multiplying by 10.

Heart Rhythms

The electrocardiogram provides vital information about heart rhythms. Abnormalities in the electrical activity of the heart can be diagnosed by examining the ECG.

Sinus Rhythm

Sinus rhythm is the normal rhythm of the heart (see figure 22.8). The heart rate is 60 to 100 beats · min^{-1} and the pacemaker is the sinus node.

Sinus Bradycardia

The pacemaker is the sinus node and the rate in **sinus bradycardia** is 60 beats · min^{-1} or less (see figure 22.9). This is a normal rhythm, and it is often seen in conditioned subjects and patients taking ß-blockers.

Sinus Tachycardia

Sinus tachycardia (heart rates over 100 beats · min^{-1}) is normally seen during moderate and heavy exercise (see figure 22.10). Thus, *exercise-induced* sinus tachycardia is a perfectly normal condition. *Resting* sinus tachycardia may be seen in deconditioned people or in apprehensive patients prior to exercise testing. In these heart rhythms, the SA node is still functioning as the pacemaker.

5 **In Review: If the SA node is pacing the heart, and the heart rate is between 60 and 100 beats · min^{-1}, the heart is in normal sinus rhythm. Bradycardia is defined as a heart rate below 60 beats · min^{-1}. Tachycardia is a heart rate greater than 100 beats · min^{-1} (normally seen during moderate and heavy exercise).**

R-R interval — The time interval from the peak of the QRS of one cardiac cycle to the peak of the QRS of the next cycle.

P-R interval — The time interval between the beginning of the P wave and the QRS complex. The upper normal limit is 0.2 s. This segment is normally used as the isoelectric baseline.

Q-T interval — The time interval from the beginning of the QRS complex to the end of the T wave. The Q-T interval reflects the electrical systole of the cardiac cycle.

P-R segment — Forms the isoelectric line, or baseline, from which **S-T segment** deviations are measured.

J point — On an ECG, the point at which the S wave ends and the **S-T segment** begins.

S-T segment — The part of the ECG between the end of the QRS complex and beginning of the T wave. Depression below (or elevation above) the isoelectric line indicates ischemia.

sinus rhythm — The normal timing and sequence of the cardiac events, with the sinus node as a pacemaker; resting rate is between 60 and 100 beats · min^{-1}.

sinus bradycardia — The normal rhythm (i.e., the sinus node is the pacemaker) and sequence, with slow heart rate (below 60 beats · min^{-1} at rest). The occurrence of sinus bradycardia may be indicative of a high level of fitness, or of a mental problem such as depression.

sinus tachycardia — The normal rhythm and sequence, with a fast heart rate (above 100 beats · min^{-1} at rest). The occurrence of sinus tachycardia may be indicative of illness or stress.

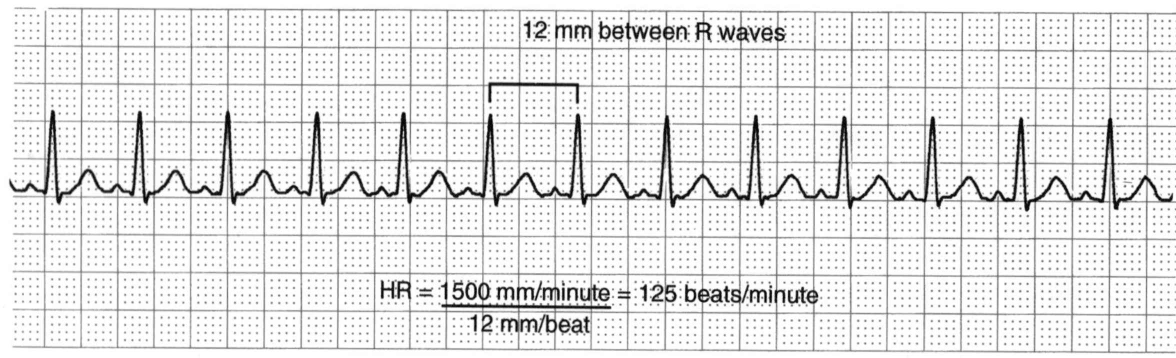

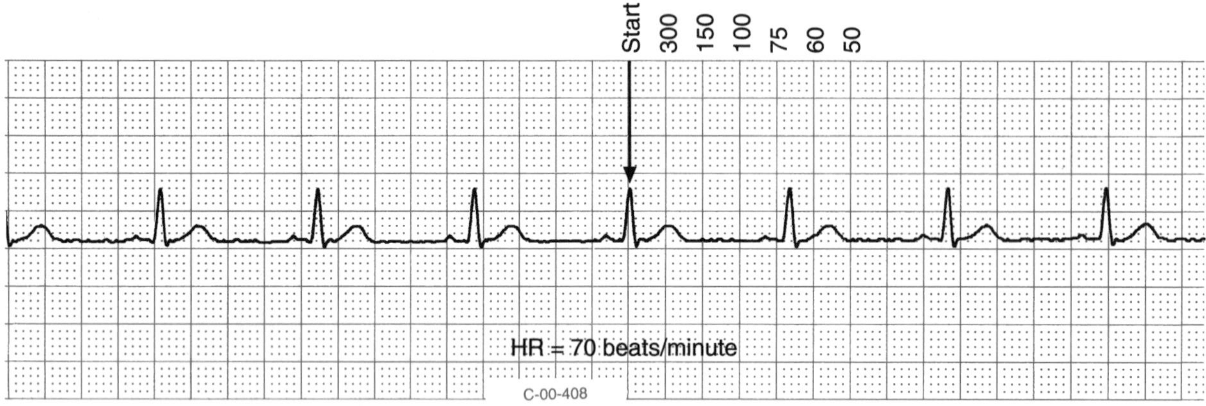

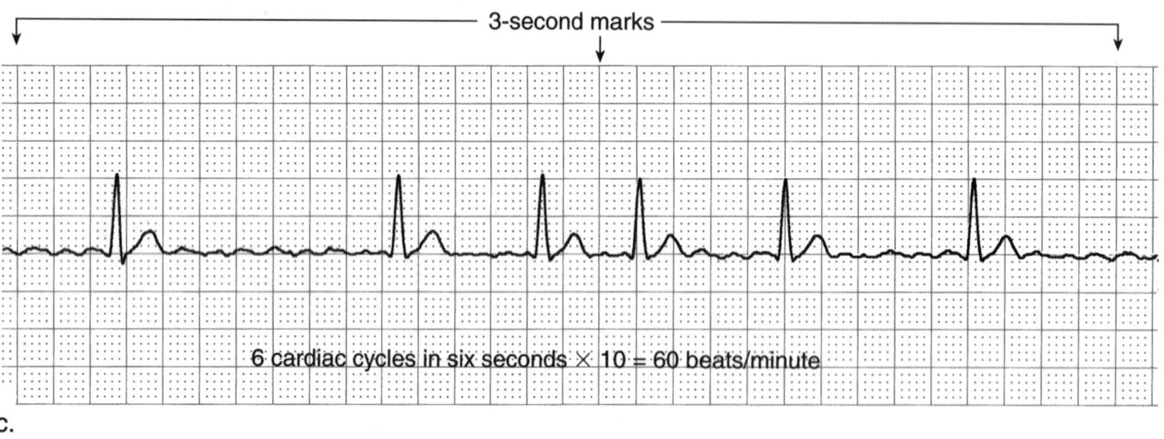

FIGURE 22.7 Three methods of determining heart rate from the electrocardiogram.

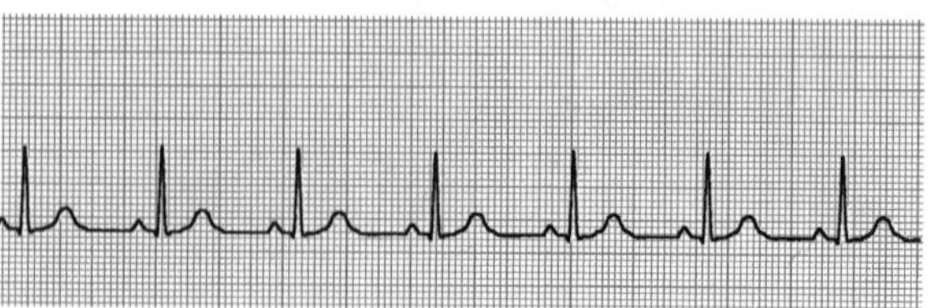

FIGURE 22.8 Normal sinus rhythm. In this example, the heart rate is 71 beats · min^{-1}.

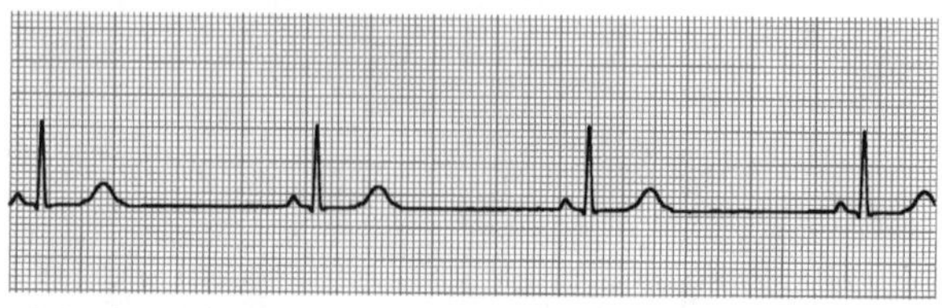

FIGURE 22.9 Sinus bradycardia. In this example, the heart rate is 35 beats · min^{-1}.

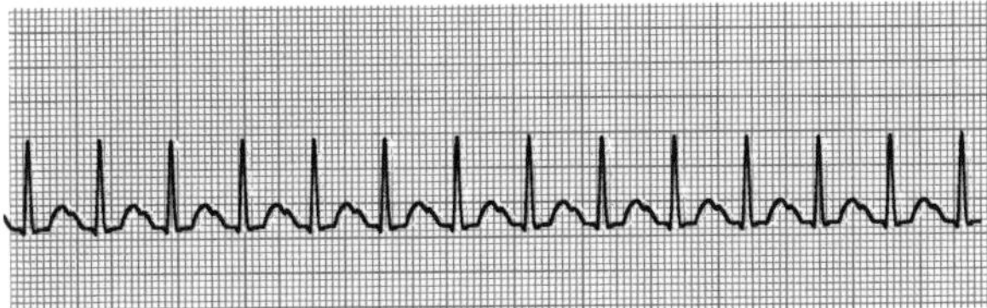

FIGURE 22.10 Sinus tachycardia. In this example, the heart rate is 143 beats · min^{-1}.

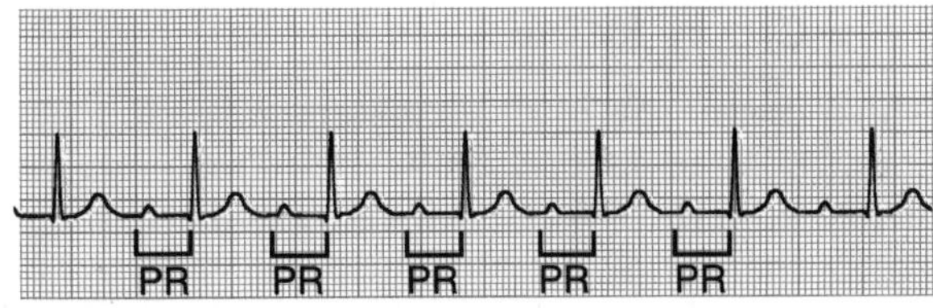

FIGURE 22.11 First degree AV block. Note the prolonged P-R interval (0.28 s in this example).

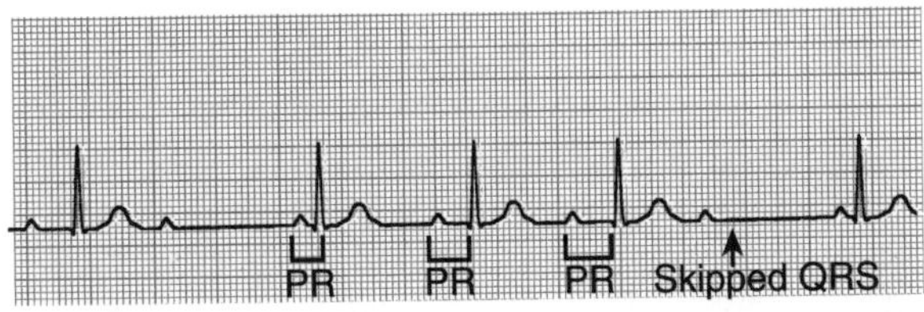

FIGURE 22.12 Mobitz Type I (Wenchebach) atrioventricular block. There is a gradually lengthening P-R interval, until finally a QRS complex is skipped.

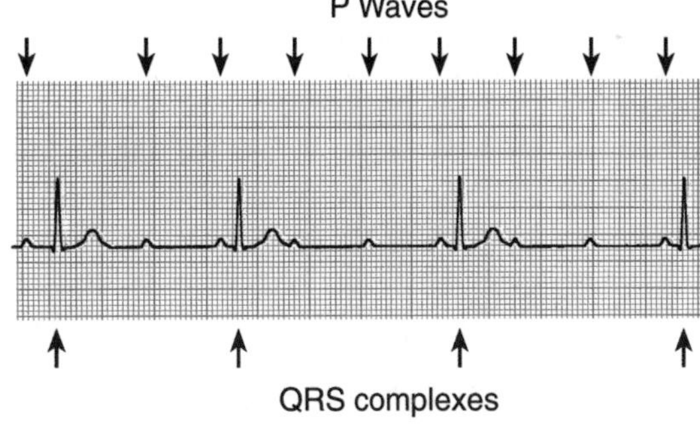

FIGURE 22.13 Mobitz Type II atrioventricular block. Occasionally, and without lengthening of the P-R interval, QRS complexes are skipped.

Atrioventricular Conduction Disturbances

Atrioventricular conduction disturbances refer to a blockage of the electrical impulse at the AV node. The blockage may be either partial or complete.

First Degree AV Block

When the P-R interval exceeds 0.20 s, and all P waves result in ventricular depolarization, a **first degree AV block** exists (see figure 22.11). Causes of a first degree AV block can include medications such as digitalis and quinidine, infections, or vagal stimulation.

Second Degree AV Block

The main distinguishing feature of **second degree AV block** is that some but not all P waves result in ventricular depolarization. There are two types of second degree AV blocks: Mobitz Type I and Mobitz Type II. **Mobitz Type I,** or Wenchebach, **AV block** is a form of second degree AV block characterized by a progressively lengthening P-R interval until an atrial depolarization fails to initiate a ventricular depolarization, and the QRS complex is skipped (see figure 22.12). This type of conduction disturbance is most commonly seen after a myocardial infarction. The site of the block is within the AV node and is probably the result of reversible ischemia.

Mobitz Type II AV block is the more serious of the second degree AV blocks, and it is characterized by atrial depolarization occasionally not resulting in ventricular depolarization with constant P-R intervals (i.e., no lengthening) (see figure 22.13). The site of the block is beyond the bundle of His, and it is usually the result of irreversible ischemia of the interventricular conduction system.

first degree AV block — The delayed transmission of impulses from atria to ventricles (in excess of 0.20 s).

second degree AV block — On an ECG, some but not all P waves precede the QRS complex and result in ventricular depolarization.

Mobitz Type I AV block — On an ECG, P-R interval progressively increases until the P wave is not followed by a QRS complex. The site of the block is within the AV node.

Mobitz Type II AV block — On an ECG, a constant P-R interval, with some but not all P waves followed by QRS. The site of the block is the bundle of His.

Third Degree AV Block

Third degree AV block is present when the ventricles contract independently of the atria (see figure 22.14). The P-R interval varies and follows no regular pattern. The ventricular pacemaker may be either the AV node, Bundle of His, Purkinje fibers, or the ventricular muscle, and it will almost always result in a slow ventricular rate of less than 50 beats · min^{-1}.

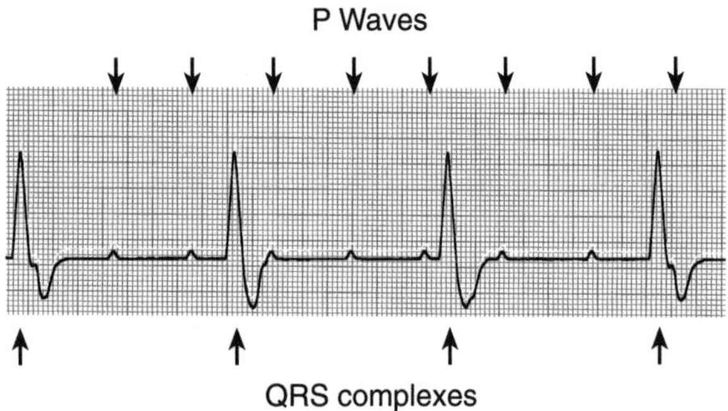

FIGURE 22.14 Third degree atrioventricular block. There is no relationship between the atrial rate (e.g., 94 beats · min^{-1}) and the ventricular rate (e.g., 36 beats · min^{-1}) indicating complete blockage of the AV node.

Arrhythmias

An arryhthmia is an irregular heart beat. Arryhthmias often arise when the myocardium becomes hyperexcitable due to a lack of blood flow or the use of stimulants.

Sinus Arrhythmia

Sinus arrhythmia is a sinus rhythm in which the R-R interval varies by more than 10% beat to beat. There is a P wave before each QRS complex, but the QRS complexes are unevenly spaced. Sinus arrhythmia is often seen in highly trained subjects and occasionally in patients taking ß-adrenergic receptor blocking medications such as Inderal®. The rhythm may be associated with respiration because HR increases with inspiration and decreases with expiration.

Premature Atrial Contraction

In **premature atrial contractions** the rhythm is irregular, and the R-R interval is short between a normal sinus beat and the premature beat (see figure 22.15). The origin of the premature beat is somewhere other than the sinus node and is known as an **ectopic focus** (an irritable spot on the myocardium that depolarizes on its own). An ectopic focus is often caused by stimulants (e.g., caffeine), antihistamines, diet pills, cold medications (e.g., ephedrine), and nicotine. Premature atrial contractions may be seen prior to exercise testing in apprehensive subjects.

Atrial Flutter

During **atrial flutter**, the atrial rate may be from 200 to 350 with a ventricular response of 60 to 160 beats · min^{-1}. The atrial rhythm is usually irregular while the ventricular rhythm is either regular or irregular. The pacemaker site during atrial flutter is not the sinoatrial node but an ectopic focus, and as a result normal P waves are not present. F waves, resembling a sawtooth pattern, may be seen (see figure 22.16). The causes of atrial flutter include increased sympathetic drive, hypoxia, and congestive heart failure.

Atrial Fibrillation

During **atrial fibrillation**, the atrial rate is 400 to 700, and the ventricular rate is usually 60 to 160 beats · min^{-1} and is irregular. Multiple pacemaker sites are present in the atria and P waves can not be discerned (see figure 22.17). The significance of atrial fibrillation in an exercise testing and training

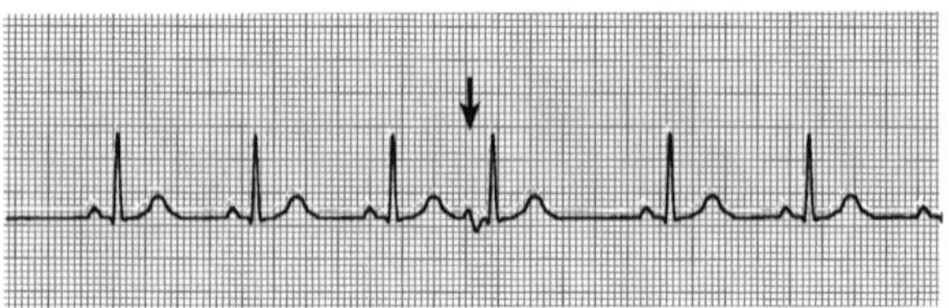

FIGURE 22.15 Premature atrial contraction. The arrow indicates a premature, disphasic P wave coming from an ectopic focus in the atria.

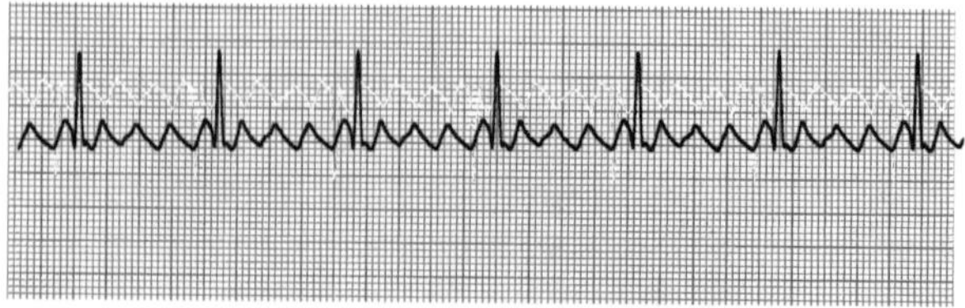

FIGURE 22.16 Atrial flutter. In atrial flutter, the atrial rate is 200-350 beats · min^{-1} (300 beats · min^{-1} in this example), but the ventricular rate is much slower.

setting lies in its effect on ventricular function. During atrial fibrillation the atria and ventricles do not work together in a coordinated fashion, and the ability of the left ventricle to maintain an adequate cardiac output may be impaired. The causes of atrial fibrillation are essentially the same as those for atrial flutter.

Premature Junctional Contraction

A **premature junctional contraction (PJC)** results when an ectopic pacemaker in the AV junctional area depolarizes the ventricles. Inverted P waves are frequently seen with PJCs as the atrial depolarization proceeds in an abnormal direction (see figure 22.18). This characteristic of PJCs may allow them to be distinguished from premature atrial contractions, which frequently have disphasic P waves. If a distinction cannot be made between these two conditions, the more general term *premature supraventricular contraction* may be used to indicate an ectopic focus above the ventricles.

If the nodal tissue is still in the refractory phase after a PJC, then normally conducted waves of depolarization initiated from the sinus node will not be conducted into the ventricles and a compensatory pause develops. Premature junctional contractions usually result in a QRS complex of normal duration, or they may slightly prolong the QRS complex. Premature junctional contractions may be caused by catecholamine-type medications, increased parasympathetic tone on the AV node, or damage to the AV node. PJCs are of little consequence, unless they occur very frequently (more than 4 to 6 PJCs per minute) or compromise ventricular function (6).

While the supraventricular arrhythmias may cause concern among exercise leaders and patients, Ellestad (8) found that the long-term prognosis of coronary artery disease patients with exercise-induced supraventricular arrhythmias does not seem to be compromised. The significance of the supraventricular arrhythmias lies in the uncoupling of coordination between the atria and ventricles and the resulting effect on the ability of the ventricles to maintain an adequate cardiac output. Recurrent atrial fibrillation may have little effect on the exercise response of an individual with good left ventricular

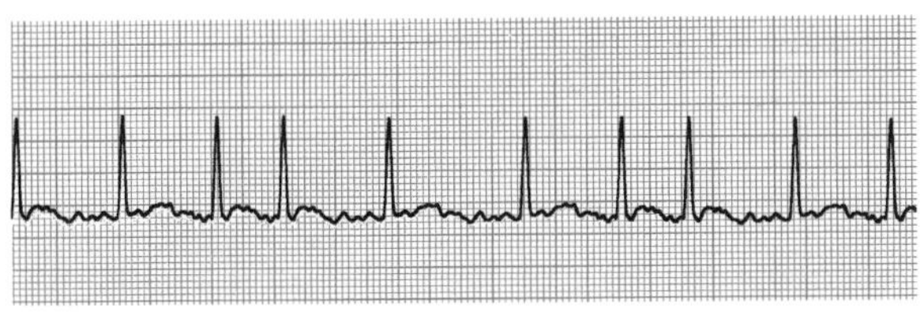

FIGURE 22.17 Atrial fibrillation. A jagged baseline and irregularly spaced QRS complexes are seen with atrial fibrillation.

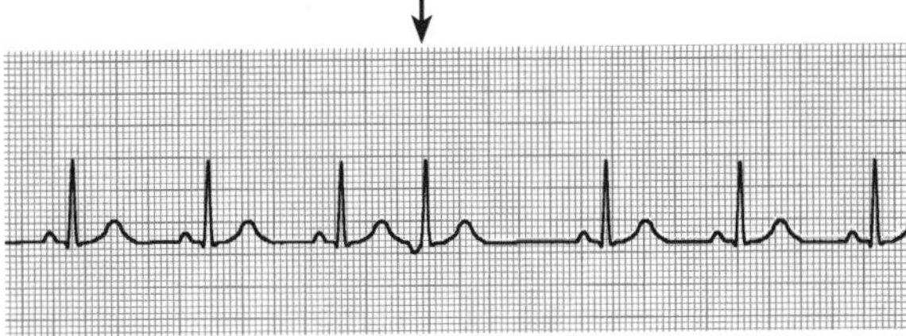

FIGURE 22.18 Premature junctional contraction. The arrow indicates a premature, inverted P wave coming from the AV node.

third degree AV block — On an ECG the QRS appears independently, P-R varies with no regular pattern, and heart rate is less than 45 beats · min^{-1}.

sinus arrhythmia — A normal variant in sinus rhythm in which the R-R interval varies by more than 10% per beat.

premature atrial contraction — On an ECG the rhythm is irregular and the R-R interval is short; the origin of the beat is somewhere other than the SA node.

ectopic focus — An irritated portion of the myocardium or electrical conducting system; gives rise to "extra beats" that do not originate from the sinoatrial node.

atrial flutter — The atrial rate is 200 to 350 while the ventricle's rate is 60 to 160 beats · min^{-1}; ECG shows a sawtooth pattern between QRS complexes.

atrial fibrillation — The atrial rate is 400 to 700 while the ventricle's rate is 60 to 160 beats · min^{-1}; P waves cannot be seen on the ECG.

premature junctional contraction (PJC) — On an ECG the ectopic pacemaker in the AV junctional area causes a QRS complex; frequently seen with inverted P waves.

function, but it may cause significant symptoms in a person with poor ventricular function.

Premature Ventricular Contractions

Premature ventricular contractions (PVCs) are the result of an ectopic focus in the His-Purkinje system, which initiates a ventricular contraction. Premature ventricular contractions have a QRS complex that is wide (>0.12 s) and bizzarely shaped (see figure 22.19). PVCs often result in the ventricles being in the refractory phase of depolarization when the normal sinus depolarization wave reaches the ventricle and a compensatory pause develops. PVCs are among the most common arrhythmias seen with exercise testing and training in coronary artery disease (CAD) patients. If PVCs have the same shape, they originate from the same site (ectopic focus) and are called *unifocal*. Multiple-shape PVCs that originate from multiple sites in the ventricles are called *multifocal* and are much more serious than unifocal PVCs. The rhythm of normal contractions alternating with PVCs is called *bigeminy*; if every third contraction is a PVC, the rhythm is called *trigeminy*. Three or more consecutive PVCs are known as **ventricular tachycardia**. If a single PVC falls on the descending portion of the T wave, the "vulnerable time," the ventricles may be thrown into fibrillation. Premature ventricular contractions have an adverse effect on the prognosis of CAD patients; generally the more complex the PVC, the more serious the problem. Ellestad (8) has shown that the combination of S-T segment depression and PVCs increases the incidence of future cardiac events.

If a PVC occurs during pulse counting, patients may report that the heart "skipped a beat" and may undercount his or her HR. They should be instructed not to increase the exercise intensity in an attempt to keep the HR in the target zone as a result of skipped beats. They should immediately reduce the exercise intensity and report the appearance or increase in number of skipped beats to the exercise leader and physician.

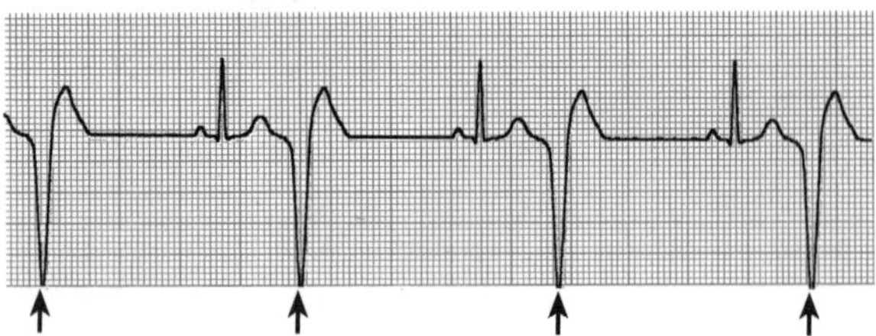

FIGURE 22.19 Premature ventricular contractions. The arrows indicate PVCs coming from a single ectopic focus in the ventricles (unifocal PVCs).

Ventricular Tachycardia

Ventricular tachycardia is present whenever three or more consecutive PVCs occur (see figure 22.20). This situation is an extremely dangerous arrhythmia that may lead to ventricular fibrillation. The rate is usually 100 to 220 beats · min^{-1}, and the heart may be unable to maintain adequate cardiac output during ventricular tachycardia. Ventricular tachycardia may be caused by the same factors that initiate PVCs; it requires immediate medical attention.

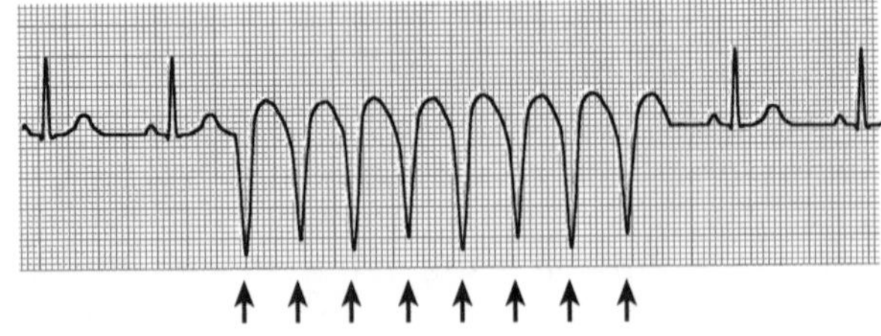

FIGURE 22.20 Ventricular tachycardia. A succession of three or more premature ventricular contractions in a row is seen in ventricular tachycardia.

Ventricular Fibrillation

Ventricular fibrillation is a life-threatening rhythm, and it requires immediate cardiopulmonary resuscitation (CPR) until a defibrillator can be used to restore a coordinated ventricular contraction; otherwise, death will result. A fibrillating heart contracts in an unorganized, quivering manner, and the heart is unable to maintain significant cardiac output. P waves and QRS complexes are not discernable; instead the electrical pattern is a fibrillatory wave (see figure 22.21).

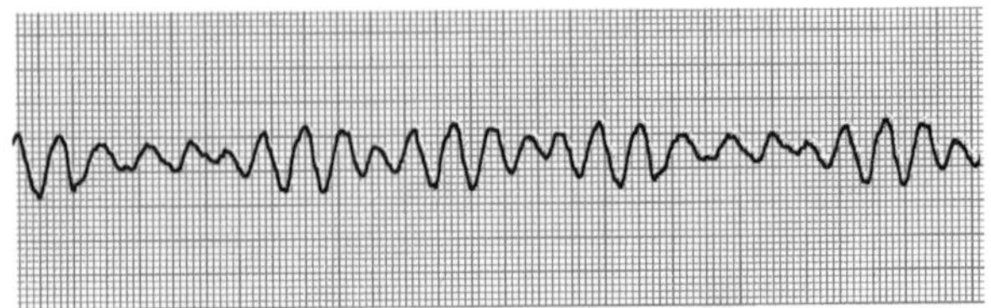

FIGURE 22.21 Ventricular fibrillation. When there are no discernable P waves or QRS complexes, the heart contracts in a disorganized, quivering manner.

6 **In Review: The ECG can be used to detect various conduction disturbances in the electrical conducting system of the heart such as first, second, or third degree AV block. The ECG can also be used to detect arrhythmias (abnormal heart rhythms) including sinus arrhythmia, premature beats, tachycardia, flutter, and fibrillation. Abnormal rhythms may limit exercise performance by decreasing cardiac output. In the case of severe arrhythmias, the HFI should terminate the exercise session and obtain immediate medical assistance.**

Myocardial Ischemia

Myocardial ischemia is a lack of oxygen in the myocardium due to inadequate blood flow. Obstruction of the coronary arteries is the most common cause of myocardial ischemia. A coronary artery is significantly obstructed if more than 50% of the diameter is occluded. A 50% reduction in diameter is equal to a loss of 75% of the arterial lumen (12). An obstructed coronary artery may be able to supply an adequate blood flow at rest, but it will probably be unable to provide enough blood and oxygen during periods of increased demand such as during exercise. Ischemia often, but not always, results in angina pectoris.

Angina pectoris is defined as pain/discomfort caused by temporary, reversible ischemia of the myocardium that does not result in death or infarction of heart muscle. The pain is often located in the center of the chest, but pain may occur in the neck, jaw, shoulders, or radiate into the arm(s) and hand(s). Angina pectoris tends to be reproducible; patients often report they get anginal symptoms at roughly the same level of exertion. During exercise, a patient experiencing anginal discomfort may deny pain, but upon further questioning, the individual will admit to the sensation of burning, tightness, pressure, or heaviness in the chest or arms. Patients frequently confuse angina pectoris with musculoskeletal pain and with the discomfort resulting from the sternal incision of coronary artery bypass surgery. Anginal pain is generally not altered by movements of the trunk or arms, while musculoskeletal pain may be decreased or increased by trunk or arm movement. Discomfort is probably not angina if the pain is changed in quality or intensity by pressing on the affected area (12).

Myocardial ischemia may cause **S-T segment depression** on the ECG during an exercise test. S-T segment depression usually occurs at a relatively constant double product. The double product equals the heart rate times systolic BP, and it is a good estimate of the amount of work the heart is doing. Three types of S-T segment depression are recognized: upsloping, horizontal, and downsloping (figure 22.22). Ellestad (8) and coworkers have shown the prognostic implications of upsloping and horizontal S-T segment depression to be roughly similar. Downsloping S-T segment depression, however, has a more adverse impact on survival.

S-T segment elevation may also occur during exercise testing. S-T segment elevation during an exercise test usually indicates the development of an **aneurysm**, or a weakened area of non-contracting myocardium and/or scar tissue.

premature ventricular contraction (PVC) — Wide, bizarrely-shaped QRS complex originating from an ectopic focus in the His-Purkinje system. The QRS interval is longer than 0.12 s in duration, and the T wave is usually in the opposite direction.

ventricular tachycardia — An extremely dangerous condition in which three or more consecutive premature ventricular contractions occur. Ventricular tachycardia may degenerate into ventricular fibrillation.

ventricular fibrillation — The heart contracts in an unorganized, quivering manner, with no discernible P waves or QRS complexes; requires immediate emergency attention.

S-T segment depression — A condition where the S-T segment of the electrocardiogram is depressed below the baseline; may signify myocardial ischemia.

S-T segment elevation — A condition where the S-T segment of the electrocardiogram is elevated above the baseline; may signify the early (acute) stages of a myocardial infarction.

aneurysm — A spindle-shaped or sac-like bulging of the wall of a blood-filled vein, artery, or ventricle.

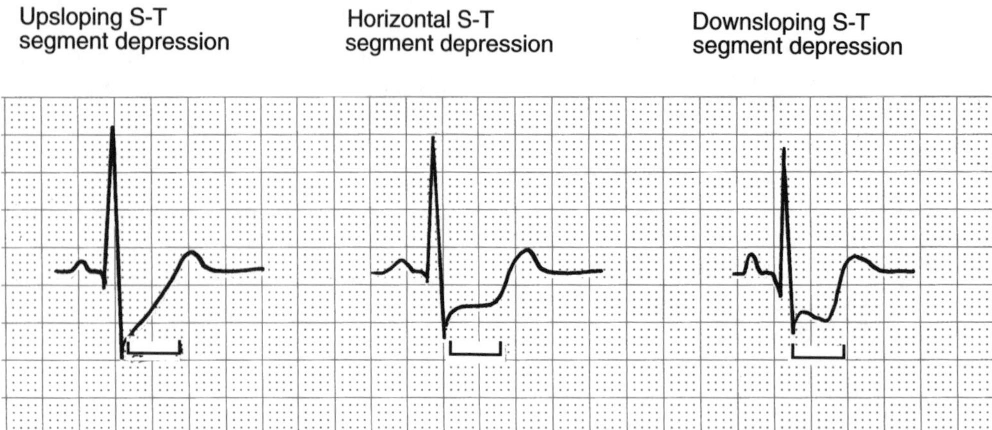

FIGURE 22.22 S-T segment depression.

Myocardial Infarction

If the myocardium is deprived of oxygen for a sufficient length of time, a portion of the myocardium dies; this is known as a myocardial infarction (MI). Pain is the hallmark symptom of a myocardial infarction. It is often very similar to anginal pain, only more severe, and may be described as a heavy feeling, squeezing in the chest, or a burning sensation. Other symptoms that may accompany a myocardial infarction are nausea, sweating, and shortness of breath.

S-T segment elevation is often the first ECG sign of an acute myocardial infarction. Later, pronounced Q waves and T wave inversion may appear in certain leads. Over time the S-T segment changes subside and the T wave returns to normal (see figure 22.23) (17). Other clinical signs of an acute myocardial infarction include elevations in cardiac muscle enzymes (serum lactate dehydrogenase [LDH] and creatine phosphokinase [CPK]), which leak into the blood after the myocardium is damaged (12).

Information from the Framingham project indicates that up to 25% of myocardial infarctions may be "silent infarctions," meaning that the infarction does not cause sufficient symptoms for the victim to seek medical attention (13). These silent infarctions may be recognized later during routine ECG examinations by the presence of significant Q waves in certain leads.

CAD patients should be instructed on a scheme of differentiating anginal attacks from possible myocardial infarctions. If an anginal attack occurs, the patient should stop the activity, if any, that precipitated the discomfort and take a nitroglycerine (NTG) tablet under the tongue. If the anginal discomfort persists after 5 min, a second sublingual NTG tablet is taken. This procedure is repeated, if needed, for a total of three NTG tablets. If the pain persists 5 min following the third NTG tablet, the patient should seek immediate medical attention (2).

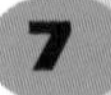

In Review: An inadequate blood flow to the myocardium often results in symptoms of chest pain (angina pectoris), but this is not always the case. The presence of S-T segment depression or elevation on the ECG can indicate the presence of inadequate blood flow (ischemia). The presence of significant Q waves on the ECG can indicate that a portion of the heart muscle has died (myocardial infarction).

CARDIOVASCULAR MEDICATIONS

A wide variety of medications are used to treat people with heart disease. Some medications control BP while others control heart rate or rhythm; still others affect the force of contraction of the ventricles. Other drugs likely to be encountered by the HFI include medications to control blood glucose concentrations, medications for patients with hyperlipidemia to control abnormal blood lipid levels, and bronchodilators for individuals with asthma. The HFI will not be prescribing medications or dealing on a day-to-day basis with patients taking these medications, but he or she will eventually encounter participants taking some of these medications. The purpose of this

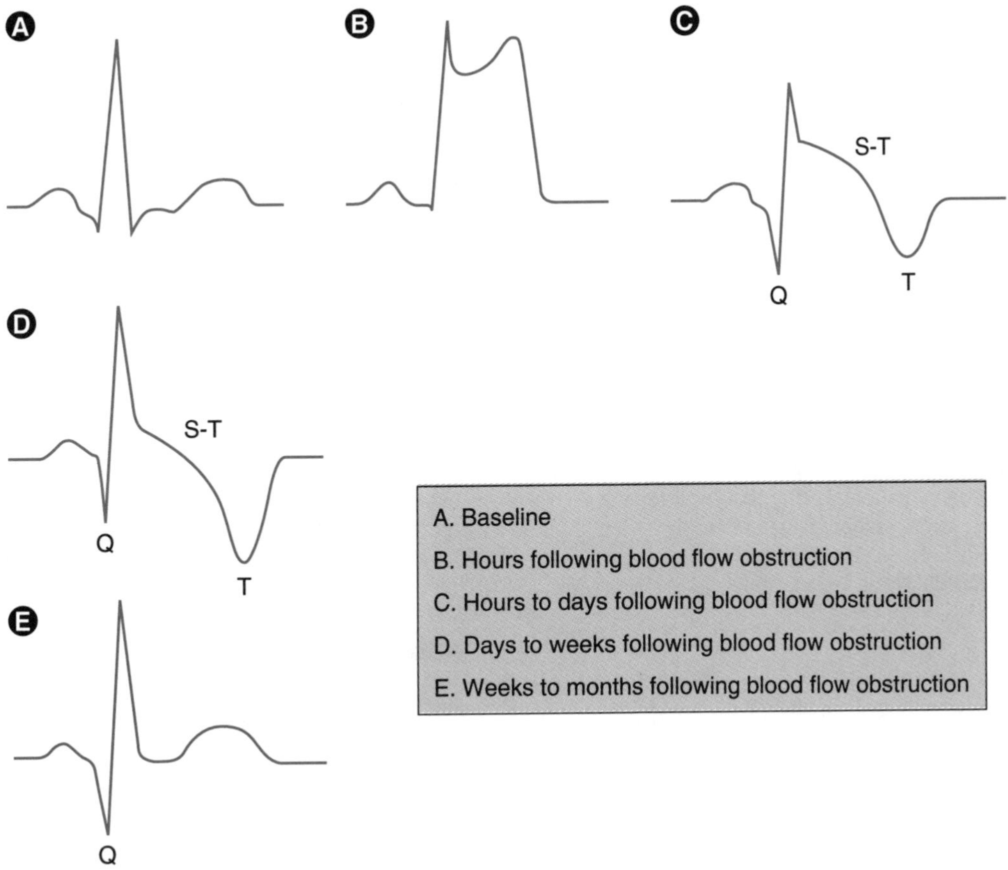

FIGURE 22.23 Evolution of ECG changes following obstruction of a coronary artery.
Reprinted from Stein, 1992, *Rapid analysis of electrocardiograms: A self-study program*, 2nd ed. By permission of Lea & Febiger.

section is to summarize the major classes of drugs, describe how they affect the exercise HR response, and indicate possible side effects.

ß-Adrenergic Blockers

ß-adrenergic blocking medications (ß-blockers) are commonly prescribed for patients with coronary artery disease, with hypertension, and occasionally for patients with migraine headaches. All of these medications compete with epinephrine and norepinephrine for the limited number of **ß-adrenergic receptors**. ß-blockers are generally used to reduce the heart rate and vigor of myocardial contraction, thus reducing the oxygen need of the heart. Because of the effect these medications have on submaximal and maximal heart rate, ß-blockers have a profound impact on the exercise prescription. Subjects should be tested on ß-blockers if they will be training on these medications. All ß-blockers lower heart rate at rest and particularly during exercise, as seen in figure 22.24.

Two types of ß-adrenergic receptors are recognized: $ß_1$ and $ß_2$. $ß_1$ receptors are found mainly in the heart, and $ß_2$ receptors are primarily located in the smooth muscle in the lungs, arterioles, intestine, uterus, and bladder. Some ß-blockers selectively block the $ß_1$ receptors in the heart. The $ß_1$-selective ("cardioselective") blockers include Sectral, Tenormin, Brevibloc, and Lopressor. Other ß-blockers are less selective and exert action on the $ß_1$ and $ß_2$ receptors. The less specific ("nonselective") ß-blockers include Inderal, Trandate, Corgard, Visken, and

beta-adrenergic blocking medications (ß-blockers) — Drugs that block receptors that respond to catecholamines (epinephrine and norepinephrine); slow heart rate.

beta-adrenergic receptors — Receptors in the heart and lungs that respond to catecholamines (epinephrine and norepinephrine).

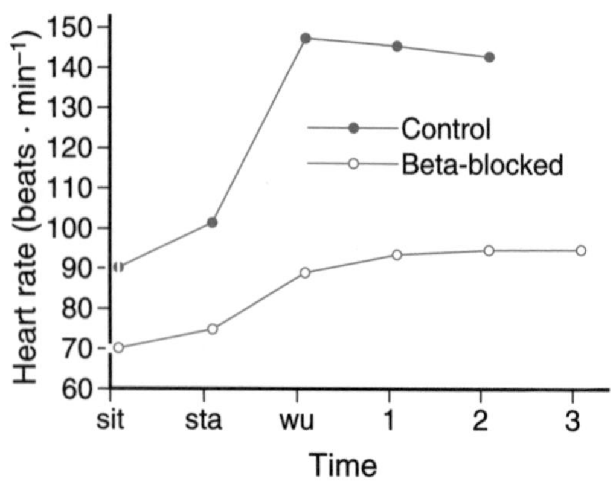

FIGURE 22.24 The heart rate before and after ß-blockade (two days of 40 mg of Inderal per day) in a very apprehensive patient during treadmill testing (sit = sitting, sta = standing, wu = warm-up at 1.0 mph, 0% grade. Minutes 1 and 2 are 2.0 mph, 0% grade. Minute 3 was at 2.0 mph, and 3.5% grade).

Blockadren. An undesirable side effect of the nonselective ß-blockers is contraction of the smooth muscle surrounding the airways in the lungs and reducing the airway lumen, which increases the work of breathing. This can result in labored breathing, shortness of breath, and other asthma-like symptoms.

Indications for the use of ß-blockers include hypertension, angina pectoris, and supraventricular arrhythmias. In addition, as previously mentioned, some ß-blockers are sometimes used to treat migraine headaches. As a general rule, nonselective ß-blocking medications are not recommended for use in patients with asthma, bronchitis, or similar lung problems. ß-blocking medications may also blunt some of the symptoms of hypoglycemia in insulin dependent diabetics, an undesirable side effect (2).

The use of Inderal and presumably other ß-blocking medications does not invalidate the THR method of prescribing exercise intensity. Hossack, Bruce, and Clark (11) have shown that the regression equations relating %HRmax to %$\dot{V}O_2$max are similar in ß-adrenergic blocked and nonblocked CAD patients. Little work has been done in this area, but it is assumed that the heart rate method of exercise prescription is valid with the other ß-blocking medications.

Because ß-blockers lower maximal HR, the use of these medications invalidates estimating THR based on taking 70% to 85% of age-adjusted, predicted HRmax (predicted HRmax = 220 − age). For example, a 40-year-old individual has a predicted HRmax of about 180, with an estimated 70% to 85% THR of 126 to 153 beats · min^{-1}. If this individual were given a ß-blocker, HRmax could easily be reduced to 150 beats · min^{-1}. If the estimated THR of 126 to 153 beats · min^{-1} were used for training, this individual would be training at maximal heart rate. Measurement of HRmax is required to calculate an appropriate THR for anyone taking ß-blockers, and testing should be repeated following any change in ß-blocking medicines.

There has been some question as to whether the use of ß-blocking medicines reduces or blocks the effectiveness of endurance training. Sable (16) reported that chronic use of Inderal diminishes the effects of endurance training in healthy, young subjects. Pratt and coworkers (15) found that chronic use of ß-adrenergic blocking medications with patients with coronary artery disease does not prevent the typical endurance training effects.

Nitrates

The **nitrates** exist in several forms including patches, ointments, long-acting tablets, and sublingual tablets, and they are used to prevent or stop attacks of angina pectoris. This class of compounds is produced from amyl nitrate (a volatile agent), which is rendered nonexplosive by adding an inert chemical such as lactose. The physiological mechanism of action is relaxation of vascular smooth muscle. Nitrate preparations relax venous smooth muscle, which reduces venous return and the quantity of blood the heart has to pump. Arterial smooth muscle is also relaxed, although to a lesser degree than venous smooth muscle, thus reducing the peripheral vascular resistance against which the heart has to pump. Both of these actions help reduce the work and oxygen requirement of the heart. Many patients use nitroglycerine (NTG) on a 24-hour basis with ointment or patches. Longer-acting tablet forms of NTG (Cardilate, Sorbitrate, and Isordil) may be taken prior to activities that are likely to provoke anginal attacks, whereas sublingual tablets (Nitrostat) are used to treat acute anginal episodes. Headaches, dizziness, and hypotension are the main side effects of NTG use (2). ß-adrenergic blocking medications may potentiate the hypotensive actions of NTG.

Calcium Channel Blockers ("Calcium Antagonists")

The **calcium channel blockers** currently include verapamil (Isoptin), nifedipine (Procardia), and diltiazem (Cardizem). These drugs interfere with the slow calcium currents during depolarization in cardiac and vascular smooth muscle. Verapamil is used primarily to treat atrial and ventricular arrhythmias, whereas nefidipine and diltiazem are used in the treatment of exertional angina and variant angina pectoris, or angina pectoris attacks that occur at rest (2).

The effects of calcium channel blockers on exercise prescription and training have received little attention. Chang and Hossack (4) showed that the regression equations relating %HRmax and %$\dot{V}O_2$max are the same in patients taking diltiazem and nonmedicated patients. Isoptin and Procardia are assumed not to alter the relationship between %HRmax and %$\dot{V}O_2$max. Calcium antagonists are not thought to affect endurance training adversely in healthy subjects or CAD patients. Duffey and coworkers (7) have shown that nifedipine does not diminish training responses in healthy, young subjects.

Antiarrhythmic Medications

Some of the more commonly used **antiarrhythmics** include Pronestyl, Norpace, Cardioquin, Quinaglute, Tambacor, Sectral, Cordarone, Tonocard, and the digitalis preparations. The ß-blocking medications are also used to treat some types of arrhythmias. With the exception of the ß-blockers, these medications will have little influence on the heart rate response to exercise; in fact, the reduction in arrhythmias may improve work capacity.

Digitalis Preparations

The **digitalis** medications are used to increase the vigor of myocardial contractions (contractility) and treat atrial flutter and fibrillation (2). In individuals with poor ventricular function, the increased contractility resulting from digitalis preparations may increase work capacity. Digitalis medications are marketed under several trade names including Lanoxin, Lanoxicaps, Purodigin, and Crystodigin. Cardiac side effects of the digitalis group include premature ventricular contractions, Wenchebach AV block, and atrial tachycardia. Digitalis drugs can cause false positive S-T segment depression during exercise testing (6). The side effects of the digitalis drugs can be potentiated by quinidine sulfate.

Antihypertensives

The **antihypertensives** can be broken down into five groups according to the mechanism of action. Drugs in the first group, *diuretics*, work by increasing the excretion of electrolytes and water. Drugs in this group include Lasix, Diamox, Diuril, Hygroton, Esidrix, Enduron, Aldactone, Hydrodiuril, and many others. This group is often used as the first treatment for hypertension. Side effects of these medications include hypokalemia, or low blood levels of potassium. Hypokalemia can induce arrhythmias and is a potentially serious problem. Diuretic-induced hypokalemia can often be prevented by increasing consumption of citrus fruits, which are high in potassium. If dietary sources of potassium prove to be ineffective, a prescription potassium supplement (K-Tab, Kay Ceil, or Slo-K) can be used (2).

The second group of antihypertensive medications is the *antiadrenergic agents*. These include drugs with the principal action at the central nervous system (CNS) level, such as clonidine (Catapres) and methyldopa (Aldomet), which reduce sympathetic outflow from the brain. This group also includes drugs that act principally on alpha-adrenergic receptors to reduce peripheral vascular resistance, such as prazosin (Minipress). In addition, this group includes those drugs that block ß-adrenergic receptors

nitrates — A class of medications used to treat angina pectoris, or chest pain.

calcium channel blockers — A class of medications that act by blocking the entry of calcium into the cell; used to treat angina, arrhythmias, and hypertension.

antiarrhythmics — Drugs that reduce the number of arrhythmias.

digitalis — A drug that augments the contraction of the heart muscle and slows the rate of conduction of cardiac impulses through the AV node.

antihypertensives — Drugs that lower blood pressure.

(see previous section) to reduce cardiac output, renin release, and sympathetic outflow from the brain.

The diuretics and the ß-blockers have the important metabolic side effect of elevating trigylceride and cholesterol levels, and impairing glucose and insulin metabolism. Thus, while they effectively lower BP and reduce the incidence of stroke and of severe kidney disease, they have a less-than-predicted effect on reducing the incidence of heart attacks.

The third group of antihypertensive medications is the *vasodilators*. These medications decrease blood pressure by relaxing vascular smooth muscle. Some of the brand names in this category are Apresoline, Apresazide, and Loniten. Side effects associated with these medications include hypotension, dizziness, and tachycardia. The active chemical in Loniten is also marketed under the name Rogaine in the form of a topical solution for use as a hair growth stimulant in male pattern baldness. Rogaine has little or no antihypertensive effect.

The fourth group of antihypertensive medications works through the renin-angiotensin system. These drugs lower blood pressure by inhibiting angiotensin-converting enzyme (ACE), which converts angiotensin I to angiotensin II. They are called *ACE inhibitors* for that reason. Some of the brand names in this category are Vasotec, Zestril, and Capoten. The ACE inhibitors are expensive, and they may produce a dry cough in 5% to 10% of patients. They have the advantages of decreasing left ventricular hypertrophy, of decreasing proteinuria in diabetic patients, and of maintaining blood lipid levels.

The fifth group of antihypertensive medications is the *calcium antagonists* (calcium channel blockers) (see page 450). As with the ACE inhibitors, this class of drugs does not have adverse effects on lipid, glucose, and insulin metabolism.

Lipid Lowering Medications

The lipid lowering medications (Questran and Colestid; Mevacor, Pravastatin, Zocor, and Lescol; Lopid and Atromid-S; nicotinic acid; and Lorelco) are used to lower cholesterol and triglycerides in individuals who are unable to adequately control lipids through diet and exercise. These lipid-lowering medications are unlikely to have any substantial effects on exercise testing or training. Patients taking these medications need to be closely followed by their physician because of potential toxic effects on the liver by some of these drugs. Some lipid lowering agents (Lopid, Atromid-S) can potentiate the effects of anticoagulants and make participants in exercise programs more susceptible to bruising.

Anticoagulants

The **anticoagulants** are used to delay the clotting process. Oral anticoagulants include Dicumarol and Coumadin. These medications are unlikely to have any direct effect on exercise testing or training, but they do increase the risk of bruising. Aspirin and some other medications (e.g., nonsteroidal anti-inflammatory drugs such as Motrin, Advil, and Nuprin) can potentiate the action of anticoagulants and increase the risk of bruising with minimal trauma.

Nicotine Gums and Patches

Nicotine gums and patches are used as smoking substitutes for individuals who are trying to stop smoking. With **nicotine gum** the nicotine is absorbed through the oral mucosa, providing sufficient plasma nicotine concentrations to curb the craving to smoke. Nicotine gums are marketed under the names Bantron and Nicorette. With transdermal nicotine patches the nicotine is absorbed through the skin. Nicotine may affect the exercise response, particularly if a person still smokes and chews nicotine gum concurrently. Nicotine may increase heart rate and blood pressure as well as the incidence of cardiac arrhythmias (1).

Bronchodilators

The **bronchodilators** are used to relax smooth muscle surrounding airways in the lungs and relieve the symptoms of asthma, bronchitis, and related lung disorders. These medications can be taken orally or from an inhaler. The inhalers are generally used for acute asthma episodes, whereas long-term bronchodilation is usually obtained with oral preparations. Most of these drugs stimulate the $ß_2$ receptors that relax bronchial smooth muscle and increase the airway lumen. Because of their ß-adrenergic stimulating effect, these medications can increase heart rate and blood pressure, although most of their effect is focused on the smooth muscle found in airways. Some of the inhaler brand names include Brethaire Inhaler, Ventolin, Alupent, Maxair, and others. The oral bronchodilators include Theobid, Aminophyllin, Theo-Dur, and many others (2).

Oral Antiglycemic Agents

A substantial number of obese participants in fitness programs have hyperglycemia, or elevated levels of blood glucose. In this condition the pancreas is able to produce insulin, but it is unable to produce sufficient quantities to maintain normal blood glucose control. This condition is called non-insulin dependent diabetes mellitus (NIDDM); often NIDDM can be controlled with **oral antiglycemic agents**. The oral antiglycemic medications work by stimulating the pancreas to secrete more insulin, which facilitates tissue uptake of glucose. The stimulating action of the oral antiglycemic medications requires a functioning pancreas. Brand names of the oral antiglycemic agents include Diabeta, Diabinese, Glucotrol, Micronase, Orinase, and Tolinase. These drugs are in the sulfonylurea class (2). Recently, a new type of oral antiglycemic drug became available (Glucophage, in the metformin class). Metformin's principal effect is to reduce insulin resistance, thereby lowering blood sugar. A serious side effect of these drugs is hypoglycemia or low blood sugar. Hypoglycemia is potentially dangerous and the HFI should be cognizant of any changes in alertness and orientation in patients taking any medication that can lower plasma glucose concentrations.

Insulin dependent diabetes mellitus (IDDM) is a more serious disorder of carbohydrate metabolism. IDDM is characterized by an absence of insulin and requires frequent insulin injections. Insulin can not be taken orally because it is a protein and would be inactivated by the digestive process. When working with an insulin dependent diabetic who is taking insulin, the HFI should be aware of the possibility of hypoglycemia. Signs of hypoglycemia include bizarre behavior and slurred speech. When individuals with IDDM are exercising, it is a good idea to have a source of sugar readily available in the event of a hypoglycemic episode. See chapter 21 for additional details on the diabetic.

Depressants

Tranquilizers are sometimes prescribed to reduce anxiety. Minor tranquilizers may lower heart rate and blood pressure by controlling anxiety, but otherwise the exercise response is not affected. With major tranquilizers, heart rate may be increased while BP is either reduced or unchanged (1). **Alcohol** is a depressant that can affect the exercise test by impairing motor coordination, balance, and reaction times. Chronic alcohol consumption tends to elevate resting and exercise BP. The acute effects of alcohol ingestion on the exercise response have been examined. During brief maximal exercise, small-to-moderate doses of alcohol exert no significant effect on oxygen uptake, stroke volume, ejection fraction, cardiac output, arteriovenous oxygen difference, and peak lactate concentration (18). However, with higher doses (blood alcohol content = 0.20 mg/dL) myocardial function may be impaired, as shown by a 6% decrease in ejection fraction (14). Alcohol intake can provoke arrhythmias at rest and during exercise.

8 **In Review: Medications are prescribed for a variety of reasons: high blood pressure, abnormal heart rhythms, elevated blood lipids, asthma, and other medical concerns. Appendix E summarizes the common categories of prescription medicines for cardiovascular and related diseases, some of the members of each category, and the impact on exercise performance.**

anticoagulant — A drug that delays blood clotting.

nicotine gum — Nicotine is absorbed through the oral mucosa, providing sufficient plasma nicotine concentrations to curb the craving to smoke.

bronchodilators — Drugs that cause a dilation of the bronchioles; provide relief from an asthma attack.

oral antiglycemic agents — A class of medications used to treat non-insulin dependent diabetes mellitus; they stimulate the pancreas to secrete more insulin.

tranquilizers — A class of medications that brings tranquillity by calming, soothing, quieting, or pacifying.

alcohol — Ethanol; a depressant that may affect the response to an exercise tolerance test.

Case Studies

Refer to appendix A for suggested responses to the following case studies.

22.1

The following ECG tracing (see Case Study figure 22.1) was obtained on a 38-year-old female prior to undergoing a graded exercise test on the treadmill.

a. Determine the heart rate (beats · min^{-1}) and the durations of the P-R interval, QRS complex, and Q-T interval (seconds).
b. What condition does she have?
c. What factors might be responsible for this condition?

22.2

A 21-year-old male college student, taking a cold medication containing ephedrine, showed the following ECG tracing at rest (see Case Study figure 22.2).

a. What type of arrhythmia does he have?
b. What is the ventricular rate?

22.3

A 57-year-old participant in your exercise program showed the following ECG tracing (see Case Study figure 22.3) while she was exercising at 3.5 mi · hr^{-1} (6% grade) on the treadmill.

a. What ECG abnormality is shown here?
b. What action should be taken?

22.4

A 55-year-old, apparently healthy male is referred to your facility for an exercise program and brings with him the results of his most recent exercise test. You notice that the participant was taking Coumadin and Inderal when he took his exercise test. Since the test, his physician has stopped the Inderal. What impact, if any would this change in medication make on the exercise prescription? (See appendix E.)

22.5

A participant in your exercise program has been taking a ß-blocking medication for several years without experiencing any significant side effects. He was recently given a prescription for Isordil and now

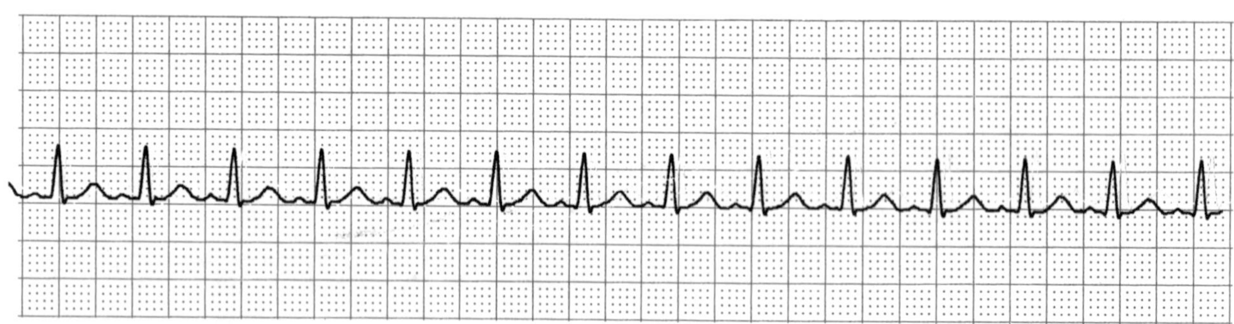

CASE STUDY FIGURE 22.1

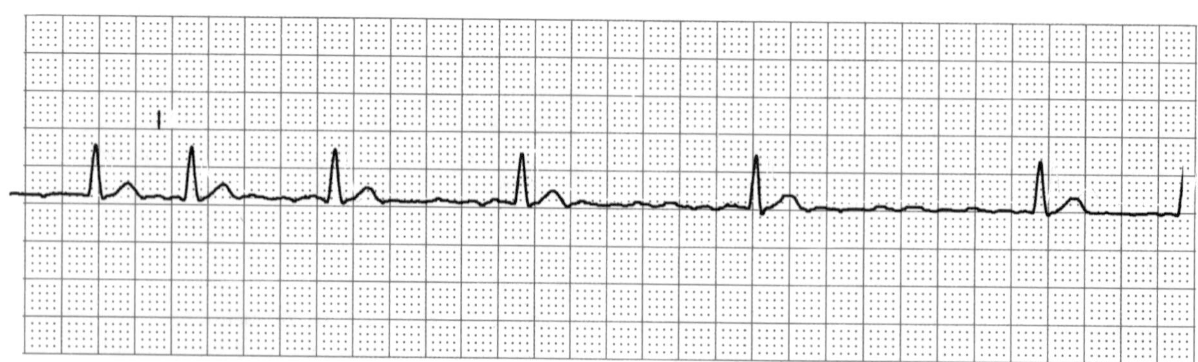

CASE STUDY FIGURE 22.2

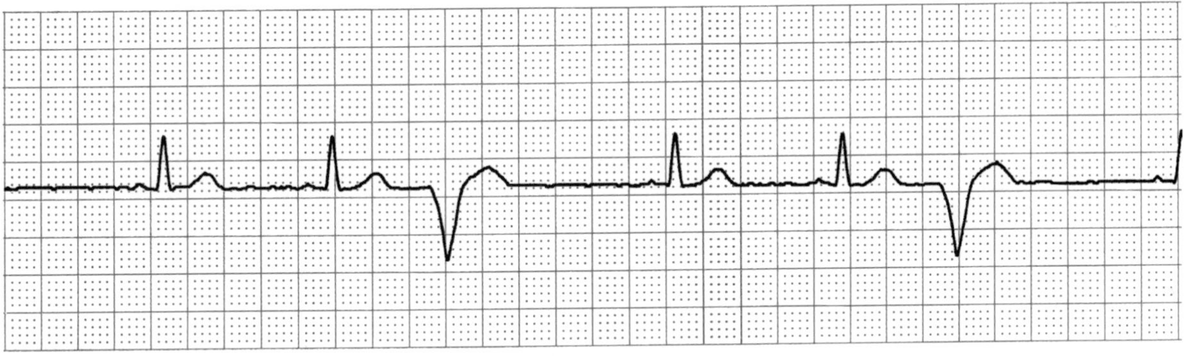

CASE STUDY FIGURE 22.3

reports that he often becomes dizzy upon standing suddenly. Could this be related to his medication? If so, why? (See appendix E .)

SOURCE LIST

1. American College of Sports Medicine (1985)
2. American Hospital Formulary Service (1993)
3. Berne & Levy (1992)
4. Chang & Hossack (1982)
5. Donnelly (1990)
6. Dubin (1989)
7. Duffey, Horwitz, & Brammell (1984)
8. Ellestad (1994)
9. Froelicher (1983)
10. Goldschlager & Goldman (1989)
11. Hossack, Bruce, & Clark (1980)
12. Hurst (1994)
13. Kannel & Abbot (1984)
14. Kelbaek et al. (1985)
15. Pratt et al. (1981)
16. Sable et al. (1982)
17. Stein (1992)
18. Williams (1991)

Chapter 23

Program Administration/ Management

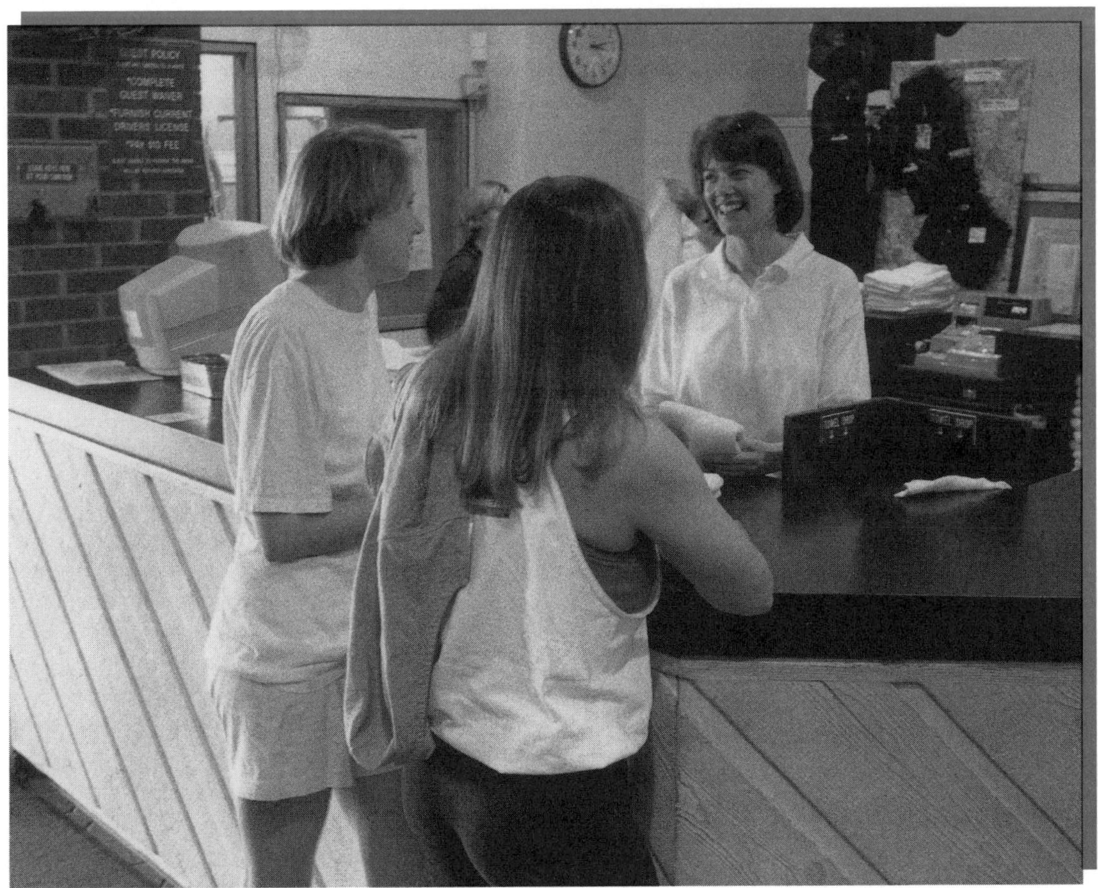

© Chris Brown

The reader will be able to: **OBJECTIVES**

1. Describe the importance of long-range planning.
2. Describe the personnel and working environment recommended for a fitness program.
3. Identify the elements of a comprehensive fitness program.
4. Explain the elements of the budget.
5. Describe the equipment recommended for a fitness program.
6. Explain the importance of communication with staff, participants, and the public.
7. Describe the importance of keeping records of all aspects of a fitness program.
8. Describe the importance of evaluation.

In small fitness programs the HFI may be in charge of administering the program, but in most cases a program director has the major administrative responsibilities. The person in charge of the program may want to consider qualifying for the ACSM Health Fitness Director certification. However, all staff personnel should have an understanding of the types of decisions that are made and the processes that are used by the program executive.

SETTING LONG-RANGE GOALS

The key concept to administration is planning. Many different programs and management styles can be successful when carefully planned; almost nothing works well over the long term without prior thought. This chapter presents the items that need to be considered in establishing a long-range plan for a fitness center and makes suggestions for dealing with responsibilities that administrators normally have in any type of program.

The program director is normally responsible for long-range planning in these areas:

- Deciding what specific classes will be offered, when, where, and for whom
- Hiring and evaluating personnel
- Preparing and executing a budget
- Maintaining communications
- Maintaining quality control

Any organization—private, public, for profit, or nonprofit—needs to clearly indicate what it wants to accomplish. The **long-range plan** includes what goals should be accomplished, what is needed to accomplish these goals, how the organization will move from where it is to where it wants to be, and what processes should be followed to implement the program. The board of directors (governing body) must approve the long-range plan. However, advisory committees (composed of key people in the community and in related groups), staff, and participants (consumers) should all have input concerning the long-range goals. The administrator facilitates the establishment of the long-range plan by working with the governing body in defining the areas that should be addressed, seeking input from appropriate individuals and groups, and providing working drafts for reactions and revisions. The program director also helps the governing body by setting realistic time lines for the draft plan, getting reactions, making modifications, and obtaining final approval. The administrator implements the plan, including periodic evaluation. The HFI's role is to provide details concerning possible fitness programs that are consistent with the aims of the fitness center and will be popular with current and potential participants. The HFI works with the fitness director in determining appropriate equipment, facilities, scheduling, personnel, and supplies.

> **1** **In Review: Long-range planning is the only way to set goals and to develop a plan for reaching them. No program can be successful without plans for program offerings, hiring and evaluating personnel, budgeting, communication, and quality control.**

MANAGING PERSONNEL

The most important aspect of any program is the quality of the staff. The recruitment, hiring, support for, and evaluation of personnel to help achieve the organization's goals is essential, time consuming, and often sensitive.

Finding Qualified Staff

The first question to consider is what types of people are needed to carry out the planned program. Fitness programs need staff personnel who can present and supervise the fitness activities. A typical fitness center needs the following personnel:

Full time

- Program director
- HFI
- Educational coordinator
- Secretary

Part time

- Medical adviser
- Fitness leaders
- Nutritionist
- Psychologist
- Physical therapist
- Equipment technician

What characteristics are desired for the staff? The qualifications include education, personal qualities, and professional competence. Gettman (2) described the many administrative responsibilities involved in a fitness program: managing, planning, supervising, educating, leading exercise, motivating, counseling, promoting, assessing, and evaluating.

During the search for specific personnel, decisions are made concerning which of these general responsibilities, and what specific tasks, will be assigned to each person. A realistic list of required and preferred qualifications is developed for each staff member. For example, an education requirement is established for each position. Requiring more education than is needed, or failing to require enough, causes problems. For fitness programs, the appropriate ACSM certification can be useful in establishing minimum qualifications. Use the certification that matches the position. See the sample job description on page 460.

Cultivating a Good Working Environment

The fitness center should provide a good working environment and accurately describe the working conditions to prospective staff members. The physical environment should be safe, clean, and cheerful, with functioning equipment, available supplies, and quick repairs when needed. The professional environment is one in which the expectations for each staff member are clearly described, and supervision is ample to assist professional growth and ensure quality performance. The psychological environment ensures that employees are valued, with their input being solicited and welcomed. They are communicated with openly and honestly, and employees feel that they have support for problems that might arise.

> **2** **In Review: Full- and part-time personnel are needed who are qualified to administer a fitness program, lead exercise, test fitness components, and deal with specific aspects of fitness including counseling participants. The working environment should be clean, safe, cheerful, well-stocked, and in good repair.**

> **long-range plan** — Includes goals to be accomplished, what is needed to accomplish the goals, how the organization will move from where it is to where it wants to be, and what processes should be followed to implement the program.

Sample Job Description
Generic Fitness Center

HEALTH FITNESS INSTRUCTOR

Qualifications

BS in physical education or related field (MS preferred)
ACSM Health Fitness Instructor Certification
Experience instructing and leading exercise in adult fitness setting
Ability to relate to people with diverse backgrounds

Responsibilities

Administer physical fitness tests
Lead physical fitness exercise sessions
Work with Program Director in
- Scheduling fitness programs and staff
- Adding variety to fitness classes
- Training new staff members

Application Process

Send a letter of application, vita, and the names, addresses, and phone numbers of three references to

Dr. Drawde Yolwob, Director
Generic Fitness Center
Yarbrogh, MI 22222

To ensure consideration for the position, applications should be received by March 1, 1997.

Title and Starting Date

The Health Fitness Instructor will begin September 1, 1997. The 12-month position includes 2 weeks of vacation and an excellent fringe-benefit package. The salary will be within the range of $32,500-$38,000, depending on qualifications.

Affirmative Action

The Generic Fitness Center encourages minority, female, and physically challenged candidates to apply for this position.

Evaluating Personnel

A clear job description that is mutually understood provides the basis for periodic evaluations. The main purpose of the evaluation is to assist the staff member in improving her- or himself. However, the evaluation is also used to determine whether or not employees are retained in the position, and if so, what merit raises should be awarded. Evaluation of the HFI includes

- the content of the fitness program;
- the manner in which the program is conducted;
- the HFI's rapport with fitness participants, other staff, and the fitness director;
- the HFI's response to emergency and unusual situations;

- the HFI's accuracy in collecting and recording test data; and
- whether the HFI has a prompt and professional manner of carrying out other assigned responsibilities.

The Sample Evaluation Checklist (form 23.1) presents questions that can be asked in an annual evaluation conference.

DEVELOPING A SUCCESSFUL PROGRAM

Painter and Haskell (7) listed four aspects of interaction between the fitness program and the participant that are necessary for developing a successful program: screening, individual program development, fitness program implementation, and maintenance.

Participant Screening

All participants should be screened before they are placed in appropriate fitness programs. Chapter 3 deals with criteria for admission to various programs. For example, people with known or suspected health problems are not allowed in fitness programs aimed to increase the positive health of apparently healthy people. The administrator ensures that the testing criteria for exclusion or referral is consistently applied and that the staff personnel leading activities are able to recognize signs and symptoms indicative of problems requiring special attention.

Fitness participants should be tested to decide whether or not they should be excluded, can enter the program only with medical clearance, or can begin immediately (see chapter 3). For people in the program, testing is important to determine the extent to which their individual objectives are being met. The test results can motivate participants to continue and can provide the basis for activity modification. Fitness testing procedures are included in chapters 3, 6, 9, and 11-13.

Part of a thorough screening process includes following the informed consent procedures established to protect participants. Informed consent has several elements, including a

- clear description of program and procedures,
- clear description of potential benefits and risks of the program,
- statement that the individual is participating voluntarily and has the right to withdraw at any time, and
- statement that each individual's data is confidential.

The first component of informed consent is to clearly describe the fitness program and all of the procedures that will be used. This description should be in writing, and each individual should read and receive a copy. In addition, each person should be given an opportunity to have any questions answered. The second element of this procedure, included in the written description of the program, is a list of the possible benefits and risks of such a program. The fitness benefits are extensive; however, the risk of certain kinds of injuries (e.g., ankle, knee) is increased, and heart attacks do occasionally happen during or after exercise. After reading the description of the program with the potential benefits and risks, the person signs the form indicating that he or she is participating voluntarily, with the provision that the individual can stop tests and all other activities at any time without penalty or coercion to continue.

Third, each individual's data is confidential unless the individual gives permission to release it. People normally agree to have their test scores used in fitness reports and research, but these reports should be presented in such a manner that an individual's test score remains confidential. An exception to this guideline is using test scores to recognize people in newsletters or news releases—in these cases, permission should be obtained (and usually is granted) from the person before publishing the individual scores. A Sample Consent Form (form 23.2) that might be used in a fitness program is shown here (see ACSM [1] for several examples of consent forms). Specific procedures should be modified to fit the particular fitness testing and program.

Programming for the Individual Participant

Although the general types of experiences offered by the organization are determined prior to staff selection, the staff can assist in fine-tuning the specific classes that will be offered to take advantage of the strengths of each staff member and provide the activities needed by each participant. Chapters 14 through 18 include suggestions and examples of activities to be included in the fitness program.

FORM 23.1

Sample Evaluation Checklist
Generic Fitness Center

Evaluation of a Health Fitness Instructor ________________________________
(Name)

Attainment of Current Goals

Did the HFI

Adhere to Center procedures? ________________________________

Make proper screening decisions? ________________________________

Administer tests efficiently, with accurate results and good records? ________________

Provide appropriate content for the exercise sessions? ________________________

Conduct the sessions with enthusiasm? ________________________________

Provide a variety of fitness activities? ________________________________

Relate well with the clients? ________________________________

Provide comprehensive training and supervision of new staff members? ______________

Understand and carry out emergency procedures? ________________________

Make suggestions for improvement in all aspects of the Center's activities and procedures? _______

____

Make efforts to improve in identified areas of weakness? ________________________

Accomplish things not listed as specific goals for this year? ______________________

Evaluation of Past Activities

What responsibilities were carried out (be specific)

Very well? ____

Adequately, but could be improved? ________________________________

Below expectations that must be corrected? ________________________________

Future Goals

What responsibilities should be

Continued? ____

Added? ____

Deleted or handled by someone else? ________________________________

What additional knowledge, skills, and so forth are needed? ________________________

____

How will they be obtained? ____

____

How can the evaluation process be improved? ________________________________

____

FORM 23.2

Sample Consent Form
Generic Fitness Center

Informed Consent for Physical Fitness Test

In order to more safely carry on an exercise program, I hereby consent, voluntarily, to exercise tests. I shall perform a graded exercise test by riding a cycle ergometer or walking/running on a treadmill. Exercise will begin at a low level and be advanced in stages. The test may be stopped at any time because of signs of fatigue. I understand that I may stop the test at any time because of my feelings of fatigue or discomfort or for any other personal reason.

I understand that the risks of this testing procedure may include disorders of heart beats, abnormal blood pressure response, and, very rarely, a heart attack. I further understand that selection and supervision of my test is a matter of professional judgment.

I also understand that skinfold measurements will be taken at (number) sites to determine percent body fat and that I will complete a sit-and-reach test and a curl-up test to evaluate factors related to low-back function.

I desire such testing so that better advice regarding my proposed exercise program may be given to me, but I understand that the testing does not entirely eliminate risk in the proposed exercise program.

I understand that information from my tests may be used for reports and research publications. I understand that my identity will not be revealed.

I understand that I can withdraw my consent or discontinue participation in any aspect of the fitness testing or program at any time without penalty or prejudice toward me.

I have read the statements above and have had all of my questions answered to my satisfaction.

____

Signed

____

Witness

____

Date

(Copy for participant and for program records.)

Implementing and Maintaining the Program

Scheduling of personnel and facilities requires attention to the types of programs being offered, the desires of consumers for specific times, and the optimal work performance from staff. Priorities are established to ensure that the more important objectives receive the needed staff and facilities. Public relations are enhanced by making the facilities available to other groups, although that is usually a lower priority. Guidelines should be established to ensure that the top-priority activities have adequate time. For example, the main exercise room might be scheduled for classes first, then other peak times could be set aside for members to use it on their own. Community groups can reserve it only during specific nonpeak times of the day. A form like the Sample Form for Use of Facility by Outside Group (form 23.3) could be used to lease the facilities to local groups.

Safety and Legal Concerns

The main concern for the fitness program is that it be conducted safely for everyone permitted to par-

FORM 23.3

Sample Form for Use of Facility by Outside Group
Generic Fitness Center

Use of facility

Name of group: ______________________________

Person responsible for the group: ______________________________

Name: ______________________________

Phone: ______________________________

Purpose for use of building: ______________________________

Estimated number of participants: ______________________________

Age range of participants: ______________________________

Room(s) desired: ______________________________

Date(s) & Time(s)	Date	Time
First choice:	________	________
Second choice:	________	________
Third choice:	________	________

On behalf of the group desiring to lease a part of the Generic Fitness Center, I have read and agree to follow the regulations for the building. Our group understands that the security deposit may be used for any damage that occurs as a result of our group's activities. In addition, we will reimburse the Generic Fitness Center for any damages that exceed the deposit.

____
Signed

____
Witness

____
Date

ticipate in the program. Fortunately, the same kinds of things done to make the program safe also help protect the program legally. Chapter 21 includes detailed procedures to prevent and deal with injuries and emergencies, including CPR procedures, that are essential for all staff members who will be in contact with fitness participants.

Liability

The program and its staff have a responsibility to perform the procedures as described in a professional manner, watch for any danger signs that might indicate a problem, and take appropriate actions to stop the activity before problems occur. Herbert and

Herbert (3) suggested common potential **liability** problems. These are failure to

- monitor and/or stop a GXT, using professional judgment;
- evaluate participants' physical capabilities or impairments that would need special attention;
- recommend a safe exercise intensity;
- instruct participants adequately on safe activities and proper use of equipment;
- supervise exercise and advise individuals regarding restrictions or modifications needed during unsupervised exercise;
- assign participants to levels of monitoring, supervision, and emergency medical support commensurate with health status;
- perform in a nonnegligent manner;
- refrain from giving advice construed to represent diagnosis of a medical condition;
- refer participants to medical or other professionals based on appropriate signs or symptoms; and
- maintain proper and confidential records.

If problems do occur, take the appropriate actions to deal with minor problems and get immediate help for major problems. Professional organizations (e.g., AAHPERD, ACSM) have arrangements with insurance carriers to provide liability insurance for individuals. Staff members should be encouraged to have this type of insurance. In addition, the organization should include liability for the program and facilities in its insurance coverage.

No amount of informed-consent procedures can justify **negligence**. Participants and facilities must be supervised. Staff personnel should be trained in appropriate emergency procedures, which need to be followed. Failure to do so, or failure to act in a manner fitting for a fitness professional, constitutes negligence. If injury or death occur as a result of the negligence, then the leader and program are legally liable.

Although getting the participant's consent does not prevent legal actions or protect against negligence, it does indicate that the program is concerned with the participant and has acted in good faith.

Concern for safety includes regular checks of the equipment and facilities and periodic reviews of the procedures used by the staff both in testing and in the classes. Records showing when the review, training, and practice were carried out should be kept in the central office. Participants should be strongly encouraged to wear helmets for cycling, skating, and other activities and eye protectors for racquetball and similar sports.

Emergency Procedures

Written **emergency procedures** should be established, and staff members should be trained to carry them out. Local emergency services to be used are contacted to help establish the procedure and comprehend the procedure to be followed. For example, in a hospital program, the fitness participants can use the emergency facilities and procedures provided for all patients. However, in a program outside a medical facility, it will be important to have separate emergency procedures and equipment to deal with minor injuries, as well as life-threatening emergencies. The Sample Emergency Procedures form (form 23.4) can be modified for a specific situation.

3 **In Review: A comprehensive fitness program includes screening, individual program development, fitness program implementation, and maintenance. Decisions need to be consistent concerning screening of potential participants. Scheduling of the facilities, activities, and appropriate testing are important aspects of the administration of a fitness program. Participants should be given good information and advice, facilities and programs must be supervised, and unusual events should be responded to professionally.**

DEVELOPING A BUDGET

The **budget** is one aspect of long-range planning. Careful inventory; assessment of needs; and a balance among personnel, equipment, facilities, and other expenses provide the maximum service for the minimum cost. A suggested budget process includes the steps outlined in form 23.5. The Sample Monthly

liability — Legal responsibility.

negligence — The failure to provide reasonable care, or the care required by the circumstances. The person and/or program is legally liable for injury that results from this failure.

emergency procedures — Plan of action to follow in emergency situations.

budget — A financial plan including estimated income and expenditure.

FORM 23.4

Sample Emergency Procedures
Generic Fitness Center

Cardiac Emergency

1. Do NOT move the victim, except to try to get him or her into a lying position.
2. Check for breathing and pulse; if absent, begin CPR immediately.
3. Call, or have someone call, the Emergency Room at ________**(name)**________

   Hospital ____**(phone number)**____, ext. ______**(number)**______.
4. Read the statement above the phone to the contact person:

(Statement to be posted by all phones:)

This is ____**(name)**____ at the ____**(name)**____ Fitness Center. We have a cardiac emergency. Please send an ambulance to the ____**(name)**____ Street entrance of the ____**(name)**____ building, at ______**(address)**______.

5. Send someone to get Dr. ____**(name)**____, whose schedule is posted by the phone [this is for centers that have medical personnel on the site].
6. Continue CPR until medical personnel arrive, then follow their instructions.

Other Serious Accidents or Injuries

For any of the following:

Airway problems of any type
Unconsciousness
Head injury
Bleeding from ear, nose, or mouth
Neck or back injuries
Limb injury with obvious deformity
Severe chest pains

1. Do NOT move the person, except to try to get her or him into a lying position, with feet elevated (unless you suspect back injuries).
2. Contact ambulance and medical personnel—same as cardiac emergencies.
3. Treat for shock.
4. Control bleeding.

Other Injuries or Accidents

1. Do not allow a sick or injured person to sit, stand, or walk until you are sure that his or her condition warrants it.
2. Do not encourage a person who is "feeling bad" to begin or continue working out.
3. Check on people who have questionable symptoms in the locker room.
4. For less serious injuries, a first-aid kit is available at______**(place)**______.

As soon as the situation is under control, inform ____**(person)**____ about the accident, complete accident report, and turn in to ____**(name or place)**____ within 24 hr.

Your suggestions for improving these instructions and the emergency procedures are welcome—talk to ______**(name)**______.

FORM 23.5

Sample Budget Process
Generic Fitness Center

1. What are the purposes of your program?
2. Describe the current program.
3. What are your current expenditures:
   A. Personnel
   B. Facilities
      (1) Loan repayment
      (2) Insurance
      (3) Maintenance and repairs
      (4) Utilities
      (5) Taxes
   C. Supplies
   D. Other
4. What is your current income:
   A Membership
   B. Insurance
   C. Gifts
   D. Investments
   E. Other
5. A. What changes should be made in your program (e.g., classes, workshops, personnel, facilities, equipment, renovation, repair) over the next 5 years?
   B. For each of these changes, indicate the change in cost and potential income.
   C. Can the changes be phased in in logical steps?
6. A. What are potential sources of increased revenue?
   B. What is needed to achieve this increased revenue?
   C. How much will it cost to secure the additional funding?
   D. What will be the net increase for each potential source of money?
7. What is a reasonable estimate for income for each year over the next 5 years?
8. What aspects of the program can be supported with this income for each year?
9. If the income exceeds expectations, what additional aspects of the program should be added?
10. If the income falls short of expectations, what aspects of the program can be reduced or eliminated?

Budget Report (form 23.6) is adapted from Musser (6). A more detailed example of a fitness budget can be found in Patton et al. (8).

Using Third-Party Payments

Insurance companies have always invested in health by providing health education, supporting research, and providing payment for treatment of health problems (e.g., postcardiac rehabilitation programs). More recently, they have offered incentives for healthy behaviors such as lower premiums for nonsmokers and cash paybacks for people who do not use their medical insurance for a set period of time. A logical extension of these policies is for the insurance companies to provide payment for preventive programs and incentives for individuals who are physically active. With increasing evidence of the health benefits of fitness programs emphasizing a variety of healthy behaviors, the program director should approach insurance companies with proposals for third-party payment for some of the services and for premium incentives for people engaging in healthy behaviors.

FORM 23.6

Sample Monthly Budget Report

Item	For June Budgeted	For June Actual	Year-to-date Budgeted	Year-to-date Actual
Revenues				
Membership				
Cardiac rehab				
Fitness tests				
Wellness programs				
Other				
Total				
Expenses				
Salaries				
Administrative				
Professional				
Clerical				
Commissions				
Materials				
GXT				
Wellness				
Office				
Towels				
Other				
Overhead				
Telephone				
Maintenance				
Heat/air cond.				
Rent				
Contracts				
Other				
Total				
Balance				
Compared with 1 year ago				

Adapted from Musser 1988.

Budgeting for Personnel and Facilities

The biggest part of the budget involves salary and benefits for the staff. Relatively high base salaries and benefits, with regular increments based on evaluations, can assist the program in employing people with better qualifications. An attractive salary and benefits package results in higher job satisfaction, higher quality performance, and a lower turnover rate. Administrators attempting to economize in terms of staff salaries, benefits, and raises often find out that it is false economy.

Other regular and ongoing expenses are for insurance, maintenance, and repair of facilities. People are often tempted to ignore regular maintenance and repair, but keeping the facilities in good shape is more efficient than incurring major expenses as a result of not having done so. New or expanded facilities are usually handled in a separate fund-raising campaign and are not part of the normal budget process.

4 **In Review: Financial management is a major part of long-range planning. The budget should be based on realistic estimates of income and expenditures, with the flexibility to adjust for unexpected developments. Salary and benefits for personnel and facility maintenance and repair are the biggest parts of the budget.**

ACQUIRING EQUIPMENT AND SUPPLIES

Equipment should be available so participants may accomplish their goals; this equipment should be kept in good condition. However, programs often go beyond what is needed in terms of equipment. For a beginning program, exercise tests can be done without the most expensive treadmill. Gas analysis equipment, necessary for many research projects, is a luxury for a beginning fitness program. Much of the muscular strength and endurance needed for fitness can be gained with strength exercises with minimal weights, thus expensive resistive exercise machines are not needed. Many program administrators use nice-looking equipment to sell their programs, when the fitness benefits might be accomplished better with activities requiring very little equipment supervised by qualified personnel. Some testing equipment is needed, but once again, inexpensive items are often satisfactory for the essential fitness tests.

Testing and exercise equipment will vary with the specific program options. The Suggestions for Testing and Exercise Equipment (4) on page 470 presents some recommendations for acquiring equipment, listing the minimum requirements and more advanced possibilities.

Ordering Supplies

The supplies for the testing equipment and for the participant's use of the facilities must be kept in stock, with a procedure for identifying what is needed. Normally, one person is designated to be in charge of checking supplies on a regular basis. Other staff members report potential shortages to this one person. Guidelines for ordering equipment and supplies include the following:

- Order early
- Order on the basis of accurate inventory and estimate of needs—including replacement of old equipment, new equipment, and supplies for all programs
- Buy from suppliers who have a good record of service
- Each year, ask all involved personnel in the process to make suggestions to improve the system

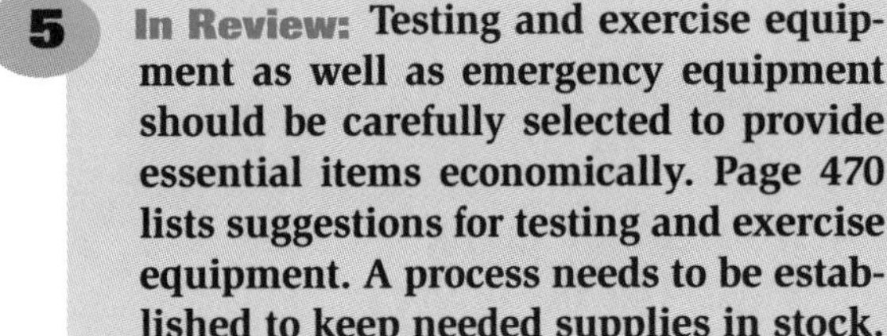

5 **In Review: Testing and exercise equipment as well as emergency equipment should be carefully selected to provide essential items economically. Page 470 lists suggestions for testing and exercise equipment. A process needs to be established to keep needed supplies in stock.**

COMMUNICATING EFFECTIVELY

One of the traits of the successful administrator is the quality of **communication** with staff, program participants, and the public. Open and honest communication is essential so that staff personnel know

communication — Interaction, often verbal, to share information and emotions.

Suggestions for Testing and Exercise Equipment

TESTING EQUIPMENT

Area	Minimum	Advanced
Health status	Forms	Microcomputer
Cardiorespiratory	Walking/running track	Cycle ergometer
	Bench	Treadmill
	RPE scale	Oxygen analysis
		ECG
		Blood pressure
		Lipid assays
Relative leanness	Scale	Underwater tank
	Tape measure	
	Skinfold calipers	
Abdominal strength/endurance	Mat	
Midtrunk flexibility	Sit-and-reach box	
Upper-body strength/endurance	Modified pull-up bar	Weights, machines

EXERCISE EQUIPMENT

Area	Minimum	Advanced
Cardiorespiratory	Walking/running track	Cycle ergometer
Relative leanness	Bench	Treadmill
		Pool
		Stair climbing
		Rowing machine
		Skiing machine
Abdominal strength/endurance	Mat	
Midtrunk flexibility	Mat	
Upper-body strength/endurance	Mat	Free weights
	Modified pull-up bar	Isokinetic machines
		Pull-up bars
		Dip bars

what is expected and how they are being evaluated. The staff personnel need to feel appreciated and encouraged to try to find better ways of accomplishing the goals. Many advances in organizations come from staff personnel who are encouraged to help find better ways to improve the content and procedures of the program.

The consumers need basic information concerning what the fitness program can (and cannot) do for them, with periodic progress reports and educational information to enhance their positive health knowledge and status. Mini-lectures during warm-up, bulletin boards, and newsletters all have been used to help educate participants. New forms of electronic communication (e.g., e-mail) can be used to communicate with current and potential participants. The information should be accurate, brief, and to the point.

Fitness programs have a responsibility to help educate the public concerning positive health—its definition and components and recommendations for its achievement. Communicate the beneficial effects of fitness programs on health, with corresponding benefits for the family, community, and work performance, via the mass media and with interested groups such as local industry.

6 **In Review: The fitness program administrator must provide clear and helpful information to staff, fitness participants, and the public. Staff need to understand what is expected of them and how they are being evaluated. Participants need to know what the program can and cannot do for them and how they are progressing in their fitness goals. The public should be educated about the benefits of positive health and how to achieve it.**

KEEPING RECORDS

Careful, systematic collection of personal and testing information, properly recorded and filed, provides the basis for much of the communication with the board, staff, and participants. This information can also be used to evaluate the effectiveness of various programs and the extent to which the long-range goals are being met. Keep records of staff training, including a demonstration of competence in emergency and safety procedures.

Forms like the Sample Accident/Injury Form (form 23.7) can be used to keep a record of all accidents and injuries. Be sure to follow up to determine the status of the individual's recovery. The completed form provides a check on whether staff personnel used appropriate emergency procedures; it is essential to have this record when questions are raised about a particular incident.

What information is needed? How is it obtained? What forms are used? Where is the information stored? How is it retrieved? When is it used? Who evaluates particular programs? Address these questions before the beginning of the program. After a reasonable amount of time working with the procedure, reevaluate it to determine whether modifications would make it better. Computers are increasingly used for these tasks. It is essential to get professional assistance in setting up the procedures for computer use, so that they can be used effectively.

In Review: The fitness program administrator should keep complete and accurate records of all aspects of the fitness program, including screening, testing, and accidents so that the effectiveness of the program can be evaluated and the handling of emergencies can be documented.

EVALUATING THE PROGRAM

Evaluation has been mentioned throughout this chapter. A value judgment should be based on the best data available concerning the extent to which the program objectives are being reached. How many people are included in the fitness program? What kind of body composition, CRF, and low-back function changes have been made? Do the participants enjoy the activities? How many dropouts were there? Why? How many injuries? Why? What can be done to help more people make better fitness gains, and decrease the number of dropouts and injuries? Are some staff members better than others in some of these areas? What can be done to help staff personnel maintain their strengths and improve in their weak areas?

In addition to this type of continuing evaluation of the program, it is helpful to have a formal evaluation of the program periodically (e.g., every 3 to 5 years). Mitchell and Blair (5) described the necessary steps and offered helpful suggestions for developing and conducting a program evaluation. They provide assistance in setting up the evaluation (questions to be asked, evaluation design), collecting, analyzing, and reporting the information.

Evaluating the Cost-Effectiveness of Fitness Programs

Good fitness programs cost a substantial amount of money for personnel, facilities, equipment, and

evaluation — The determination or judgment of the value or worth of something or someone. In a fitness setting, an evaluation determines the health or fitness status of an individual based on his or her characteristics, signs, symptoms, behaviors, and test results.

FORM 23.7

Sample Accident/Injury Form

1. ______________________________ ____________________
   Name of victim Date
2. Describe, in detail, the nature of the injury or health problem:
3. Describe, in detail, how the accident occured:
4. List, in order, the things you or other staff members did in response to the incident:
5. Describe any problems encountered in dealing with the situation:
6. List the names of people who witnessed the accident and emergency procedures performed:

Turn in this form, within 24 hr of the accident, to ______**(name or place)**______.

Your suggestions concerning safety, emergency procedures, and/or this form are welcome. Please talk to ______**(name)**______.

supplies, in addition to the cost of clothing, time, and travel for the participant. Shephard (9) reviewed the potential benefits for the individual and for businesses that sponsor a fitness program for their employees. Program directors should ask the questions in the box on page 473 to determine if their program is cost-effective. Shephard summarized **cost-effectiveness** research evidence as follows: "The currently available cost-benefit figures are encouraging in suggesting that benefits outweigh immediate program costs by a substantial margin" (p. 57).

Evaluating Cost-Effectiveness

Have the individuals in our programs achieved these benefits?

- Enhanced quality of life
  Do they feel better?
  Is their mood improved?
  Have they experienced an increased range of experiences?
- Improved personal appearance, self-image, and health
- Lower risk of major health problems
- Potential increase in the length of their life

Has the industry in which our participants work experienced these benefits?

- Improved corporate image, worker satisfaction, and productivity
- Decrease in absenteeism, employee turnover, injury rate, and medical costs

Evaluating Quality

The most important element of a program is setting up procedures to try to ensure a high standard of quality in all information, personal contact, and activities that are conducted in the name of the fitness program. One aspect of establishing high standards is to ensure the inclusiveness of the program. All people should feel welcome in the program regardless of gender, ethnic background, or social class. The administrator should ask these questions to determine if the program is achieving this atmosphere:

- Have I employed a staff with varied backgrounds?
- Is the staff trained to be sensitive to people from different backgrounds?
- Are our programs scheduled at convenient times and places?
- Do we try to contact various groups within the community?
- Have we provided ways for people with low incomes to participate?
- Do we have a policy where inappropriate (e.g., sexist or racist) comments or actions by staff members or participants will not be tolerated?

8 **In Review: Evaluation of the program is a continual process to ensure that quality information and inclusive programs are being provided in a cost-effective manner.**

cost-effectiveness — Assessment of the cost versus the benefits of a program.

Case Studies

You can check your answers by referring to appendix A.

23.1

The Fitness Director where you work asks you to evaluate four part-time fitness instructors. What steps would you take?

23.2

The fitness program Board of Directors asks for an evaluation of the fitness goals of the program. The Program Director asks you to be in charge of the evaluation. What would you do?

Source List

1. American College of Sports Medicine (1995)
2. Gettman (1988b)
3. Herbert & Herbert (1988)
4. Howley (1988)
5. Mitchell & Blair (1988)
6. Musser (1988)
7. Painter & Haskell (1988)
8. Patton, Corry, Gettman, & Graf (1986)
9. Shephard (1990)

See the Bibliography at the end of the book for a complete source listing.

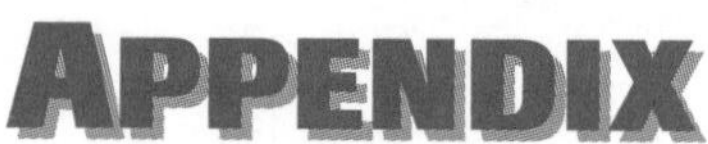

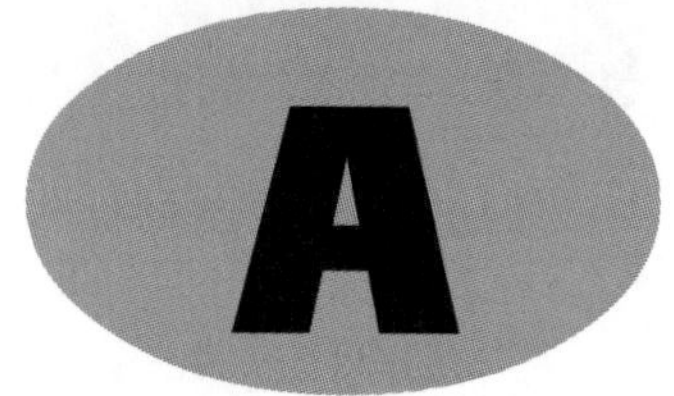

Case Study Answers

1.1

You might respond by admitting that there are risks related to exercise, with 7 deaths per year for every 100 000 exercisers. However, more people die while sleeping, or after eating and yet few people advocate the cessation of those activities. In addition, the risks of deterioration of the cardiovascular system through sedentary living causes a much higher risk of major health problems than being active. Finally, risks can be minimized by starting very slowly and gradually increasing the amount and intensity of work done during exercise.

1.2

You might begin by stating that the CDC recommendations were aimed at individuals who are currently sedentary and not individuals who are habitually active and involved in strenuous exercise. In addition, you might indicate that participation in more strenuous exercise is associated with other health-related benefits (increases in cardiorespiratory fitness [$\dot{V}O_2$max]) that cannot be realized with moderate exercise.

2.1

You would help Fred to see that his goals are primarily health-related goals at this time. After engaging in moderate-intensity exercise, he may want to add fitness goals to his list. Susan, on the other hand, has already reached her health and fitness goals—she now has performance goals. You would help her analyze the various underlying factors and skills needed to compete in soccer, and suggest some training to help her improve in these areas.

3.1

Encourage the woman to begin moderate-intensity exercise, using the walking program in chapter 17. Recommend that she get a health screening, including body composition, blood pressure, and blood profile. If the breathlessness continues or gets worse with regular exercise, she should see her personal physician. After she reaches the final stage of the walking program, recommend that she have physical fitness testing to determine appropriate vigorous-intensity exercise.

3.2

It appears that his elevated heart rate and blood pressure may be an anxious response to a new environment. Talk with him about the kinds of activities he enjoys. Explain the procedures of the GXT, indicating again that he can stop whenever he wants to and that the fitness center has never had problems on the test. Have him walk around the center to look at the various fitness stations. When he returns, have him sit, and show him how to relax when he exhales. Retake his HR and BP. If they are lower, then continue with the GXT, giving him extra attention (e.g., frequently asking how he is doing during the test). If HR and BP remain high, ask him to come back for a second visit at a time that is convenient for him when the center will not be busy. Give him a relaxation program to try at home.

3.3

a. John's major risk factors include age, hypertension, cigarette smoking, physical inactivity, and total/HDL ratio >5. Secondary risk factors include percent body fat, stress, and gender (male).

b. Nonpharmacological intervention programs might include smoking cessation classes, stress management classes, dietary counseling, and initiation of moderate physical activity.

4.1

The lactate threshold is the point during a graded exercise test when the blood lactic acid concentration suddenly increases. The lactate threshold has been used as an indicator of performance, in that the speed at which it occurs is closely related to the speed that can be maintained in distance runs (10K or marathon). As she improves her training, the lactate threshold occurs later into the GXT, indicating that she can maintain a faster pace in distance runs.

4.2

You need to confirm your client's feeling that the heart is stronger after training and, as a result, can pump more blood out per beat (increased stroke volume). As a result, the heart does not have to beat as many times to deliver the same amount of oxygen to the tissues. This is a more efficient way for the heart to pump blood, and in fact, the heart does not have to work as hard.

4.3

You might begin with a brief statement indicating that running speed in distance races is related to the amount of oxygen the runner can deliver to the muscles. The more oxygen that can be delivered, the faster the running speed. The elite female distance runner differs from the elite male distance runner in three ways that have a bearing on this issue: Heart size is smaller and she cannot pump as much oxygen-rich blood to the muscle per minute; the oxygen content of her blood is lower due to the lower hemoglobin concentration; and she is also carrying relatively more body fat that would have a negative impact on sustained running speed, even at the same level of fitness.

5.1

Explain to the exerciser that the same muscles that are used to push against the weights, the hip and knee extensor muscles, are working to control the descent. The press requires concentric contraction; the return requires eccentric contraction. Both kinds of contractions lead to increases in strength.

5.2

When she's doing the wrist curls with her palms down (radioulnar pronated position), the wrist extensors are the contracting muscles; in the palms up position (supinated position), the wrist flexors are the working muscles. The wrist flexors are usually stronger than the wrist extensors.

The explanation is different for the pull-ups. The elbow flexor muscles are working regardless of the radioulnar joint position. However, when the palms are facing away (pronation), the distal tendon of the biceps brachii muscle is wrapped around the radius bone and therefore this muscle cannot exert as much force as when the palms are facing toward the body (supinated position).

5.3

He should make a conscious effort to maintain a backward pelvic tilt. He should also keep his arms in front of his head instead of by his ears and his knees slightly flexed to help him maintain the backward tilt.

6.1

You might begin with a brief description of what cardiorespiratory fitness is, and indicate that the best measure (the "gold standard") of cardiorespiratory fitness is the direct measurement of maximal aerobic power ($\dot{V}O_2max$). You could show a picture of someone taking a graded exercise test during which $\dot{V}O_2max$ is measured, and point out the cost and complexity of the measurement. Finally, provide evidence showing that the average speed maintained during a running test (Cooper's 1.5-mi or 12-min run) is closely related to the subject's actual $\dot{V}O_2max$, providing "criterion validity" for the running test.

6.2

The reference point for the scale is the "zero" established when the free-swinging pendulum stops, with the cycle on a flat surface. All scale values are relative to this zero, and if the zero is off, all scale readings will be off. If the pendulum is not at zero when no weight is attached, the entire scale is off by the amount the zero value is off. For example, if the scale reads .25 kg when no weight is attached each value is shifted .25 kg upward when known weights are attached.

6.3

If he is really insistent about the comparisons, you might show him a table of values for elite, and "ordinary" people, to give a better sense of perspective. The primary reason for doing the fitness testing to estimate $\dot{V}O_2max$ is to provide (a) a good starting point for selecting activities for the fitness program, and (b) to have a point of reference to show improvements with training. This latter reason could be used as a starting point to discuss expected changes with training, and the fact that low cardiovascular risk does not demand "elite" values for cardiorespiratory fitness, values that few can achieve.

7.1

$$3.5\ \text{mi} \cdot \text{hr}^{-1} \cdot 26.8\ \text{m} \cdot \text{min}^{-1} = 93.8\ \text{m} \cdot \text{min}^{-1}$$

$$93.8\ \text{m} \cdot \text{min}^{-1}\left(\frac{0.1\ \text{ml} \cdot \text{kg}^{-1} \cdot \text{min}^{-1}}{\text{m} \cdot \text{min}^{-1}}\right) +$$

$$3.5\ \text{ml} \cdot \text{kg}^{-1} \cdot \text{min}^{-1} = 12.9\ \text{ml} \cdot \text{kg}^{-1} \cdot \text{min}^{-1}$$

$$12.9\ \text{ml} \cdot \text{kg}^{-1} \cdot \text{min}^{-1} \cdot 75\ \text{kg} =$$

$$968\ \text{ml} \cdot \text{min}^{-1} \text{ or } .97\ \text{L} \cdot \text{min}^{-1}$$

$$.97\ \text{L} \cdot \text{min}^{-1} \cdot 5\ \text{kcal} \cdot \text{L}^{-1} = 4.85\ \text{kcal} \cdot \text{min}^{-1}$$

$$4.85\ \text{kcal} \cdot \text{min}^{-1} \cdot 30\ \text{min} = 146\ \text{kcal}$$

7.2

$$100\ \text{W} \cdot \frac{6.1\ \text{kpm} \cdot \text{min}^{-1}}{\text{W}} = 610\ \text{kpm} \cdot \text{min}^{-1}$$

$$(610\ \text{kpm} \cdot \text{min}^{-1} \cdot 2\ \text{ml} \cdot \text{kpm}^{-1}) +$$

$$(60\ \text{kg} \cdot 3.5\ \text{ml} \cdot \text{kg}^{-1} \cdot \text{min}^{-1}) = 1430\ \text{ml} \cdot \text{min}^{-1}$$

$$\text{or } 1.43\ \text{L} \cdot \text{min}^{-1}$$

7.3

$$3\ \text{mi} \cdot 1610\ \text{m} \cdot \text{mi}^{-1} =$$

$$4830\ \text{m} \div 24\ \text{min} = 201\ \text{m} \cdot \text{m}^{-1}$$

$$201\ \text{m} \cdot \text{min}^{-1}\left(\frac{0.2\ \text{ml} \cdot \text{kg}^{-1} \cdot \text{min}^{-1}}{\text{m} \cdot \text{min}^{-1}}\right) +$$

$$3.5\ \text{ml} \cdot \text{kg}^{-1} \cdot \text{min}^{-1} = 43.7\ \text{ml} \cdot \text{kg}^{-1} \cdot \text{min}^{-1}$$

$$43.7\ \text{ml} \cdot \text{kg}^{-1} \cdot \text{min}^{-1} \cdot 70\ \text{kg} =$$

$$3059\ \text{ml} \cdot \text{min}^{-1} \text{ or } 3.06\ \text{L} \cdot \text{min}^{-1}$$

$$3.06\ \text{L} \cdot \text{min}^{-1} \cdot 5\ \text{kcal} \cdot \text{L}^{-1} =$$

$$15.3\ \text{kcal} \cdot \text{min}^{-1} \cdot 24\ \text{min} = 367\ \text{kcal}$$

7.4

12 METs = 12 kcal · kg^{-1} · hr^{-1} · 70% = 8.4 kcal · kg^{-1} · hr^{-1}

8.4 kcal · $\text{kg}^{-1} \cdot \text{hr}^{-1}$ · 85 kg = 714 kcal/hr · 0.5 hr = 357 kcal

7.5

You might indicate the cost of traveling 1 m/min jogging is about twice that (0.2 ml · kg^{-1} · min^{-1}) for walking (0.1 ml · kg^{-1} · min^{-1}) due to the extra energy needed to propel the body off the ground and absorb the force of impact on each step. You might provide a summary table he can use describing the caloric cost of walking and running 1 mi.

8.1

Carbohydrate: 2100 kcal · .58 · (1 g/4 kcal) = 304 g
Saturated fat: 2100 kcal · .10 · (1 g/9 kcal) = 23 g
Unsaturated fat: 2100 kcal · .20 · (1 g/9 kcal) = 46 g
Protein: 2100 kcal · .12 · (1 g/4 kcal) = 63 g

8.2

A possible outline follows:

A. Dietary Goals (use overhead of pie chart from text)
   1. Carbohydrates—55%-60% of total calories
   2. Fats—30% of total calories, with 10% from saturated fat
   3. Protein—about 10%-15% of total calories, but enough to meet the RDA of 0.8 g · kg^{-1} · day^{-1} for sedentary or 1-1.5 g · kg^{-1} · day^{-1} for athletes.

B. Food Guide Pyramid (use overhead of pyramid from text)
   1. Pyramid base—that on which the rest of the food selections stand—is carbohydrates.
      a. Provide real example of servings (bring to presentation)
         1. Indicate that the range of SERVINGS is such to meet the energy needs of a wide variety of people
      b. Fruits and vegetables—the next level
         1. Emphasize variety and provide examples of what a SERVING means for each
      c. Milk—emphasize meeting calcium (and protein) need, provide examples of low-fat choices to meet needs. Provide examples of what constitutes a serving.
      d. Meats—Emphasize low-fat choices to keep caloric value low while meeting protein needs. Bring examples of a SERVING to class.
      e. Fats, Oils, and Sweets—Emphasize using these sparingly to keep calorie and fat content of diet in proper range

9.1

A. WHR = 76/108 = 0.70

B. %BF (see formulas in text):
   using sum of triceps, suprailiac, and abdominal = 92 mm

   D_b = 1.089733 – 0.0009245(S3) + 0.0000025$(S3)^2$ – 0.0000979(age)

   D_b = 1.02045
   %BF = 495/D_b – 450 = 35.1%

using sum of triceps, suprailiac, and thigh = 107 mm

D_b = 1.099421 – 0.0009929(S3) + 0.0000023(S3)^2 – 0.0001392(age)

D_b = 1.01186

%BF = 495/D_b – 450 = 39.2%

C. Relative weight = 170/123 = 138.2%

D. Target weight (assume 37.2% body fat – the average of the 2 values above)

Fat free mass = total body weight – (total body weight × %BF) = 170 – (170 × .372) = 106.8 lb

$$\text{Target body weight} = \frac{\text{FFM}}{1-\left(\frac{\text{Desired \%BF}}{100}\right)} =$$

106.8/[1 – (25/100)] = 142.4 lb

10.1

A. $$\text{Target body weight} = \frac{\text{FFM}}{1-\left(\frac{\text{Desired \%BF}}{100}\right)} =$$

152.65/(1 – .2) = 190.8 lb

B. RMR = 88.362 + (4.799 × height) + (13.397 × weight) – (5.677 × age)

RMR = 88.362 + (4.799 × 182.88) + (13.397 × 97.7) – (5.677 × 50) = 1991 kcal/day

C. Daily caloric need = 1991/0.7 = 2844 kcal/day

D. Recommended daily caloric intake and exercise plan

Purpose is to create a caloric deficit of 3500 to 7000 kcal per week.

- Intake = 2400 kcal/day
- Exercise = 200 kcal/day (initially, then work up to 300 kcal/day)
- This will equal a total caloric deficit of approximately 644 kcal/day (4500 kcal/week or approximately 1.3 lb).

11.1

The requirement that sedentary middle-age participants take a maximal, unmonitored test at the beginning of their fitness program is inappropriate. You might suggest, in place of the 1.5-mi run, the use of the 1-mi-walk test, which should be used after the participants have demonstrated that they can comfortably walk 1 mi.

11.2

His estimated $\dot{V}O_2max$ = 37.8 ml · kg^{-1} · min^{-1}. His level of cardiorespiratory fitness is adequate for most activities and just short of being "good" for his age group.

11.3

The heart rate response of 100 beats · min^{-1} at the work rate of 300 kpm · min^{-1} should have been ignored. The heart rate values should have been extrapolated to 170 beats · min^{-1}, and the vertical line dropped from that point would indicate a work rate of about 1050 kpm · min^{-1}, equal to a $\dot{V}O_2$ of 2.4 L · min^{-1}. This equals 8.4 METs (2400 ml · min^{-1} ÷ 81.7 kg = 29.4 ml · kg^{-1} · min^{-1} ÷ 3.5 ml · kg^{-1} · min^{-1} = 8.4 METs).

11.4

The graph should have ignored the heart rate value of 96 beats · min^{-1}. The line was extrapolated to 190 beats · min^{-1} and the vertical line dropped from that point indicated a value of about 16.75% grade, which is equal to a $\dot{V}O_2$ of about 35.6 ml · kg^{-1} · min^{-1} (see chapter 8). This is 10.2 METs, or 1.94 L · min^{-1}.

12.1

A possible outline for the presentation follows:

A. Effects of resistance training
  1. Improvements in muscle endurance
     a. Capillary and mitochondria changes
  2. Improvements in muscle strength
     a. Neuromuscular changes
     b. Increases in muscle size
        1. Hyperplasia
        2. Hypertrophy
           a. Gender differences
              1. Hormone differences
  3. Recommendations for training
     a. RM
     b. Sets
     c. Weekly schedule

12.2

Lactic acid is not related to delayed onset muscle soreness (DOMS). The soreness could be related to a variety of factors including actual damage to skeletal muscle and connective tissue involved in the different lifts. Exercises requiring eccentric muscle contractions seem to cause more muscle soreness than exercises using primarily concentric contractions. The severity of DOMS can be reduced by using a warm-up, and progressing gradually through the weight lifting program (doing too little rather than too much).

13.1

Sacral angle should be at least 80° (a book or a board on edge placed against the sacrum would be snug if it were 90°). Next examine the curvature of the spine; it should be smooth with no evident flatness or hypermobility in any one particular area. Arm-leg length discrepancy might also be a factor (e.g., long arms in relation to legs).

13.2

Most false positives in the administration of the Thomas test result when the individual being tested brings his/her thigh too close to the chest. This can result in excessive posterior rotation of the pelvis which, in turn, can make it appear that the hip flexors are tight.

14.1

If a person has a normal response to a GXT, HR and systolic blood pressure increase with each stage of the test, whereas the diastolic pressure remains the same or decreases slightly. In addition, the ECG response shows no significant S-T segment depression or elevation, and no significant arrhythmias occur. In these cases it can be assumed that the last load achieved on the test represents the true functional capacity (max METs). The GXT presented in Case Study 14.1 is representative of such a test.

Paul has normal resting BP and a negative family history for CHD. Risk factors include a relatively high percentage of body fat (indicating obesity), sedentary lifestyle, and a poor blood lipid profile. Based on these findings, THR range of 158 to 177 beats · min^{-1} was calculated (60%-80% $\dot{V}O_2max$ as measured during the maximal GXT); this HR range corresponds to work rates equal to 6.3 to 8.4 METs. Initially, he will work at or below the lower end of the calculated THR range, with the emphasis on the duration of activity (see chapter 17). As he becomes more active he will be able to work within the THR range, depending, of course, on his interests. He was referred for nutritional counseling to improve his blood lipid profile. Paul has an estimated HRmax of 174 beats · min^{-1}; his measured HR was 24 beats · min^{-1} higher. Given the inherent biological variation in the estimated HRmax, use the measured values when they are available.

14.2

Mary's maximal aerobic power was estimated to be about 1.65 L · min^{-1} by extrapolating the HR/work rate relationship to the predicted maximal heart rate (see chapter 11). This is equivalent to a $\dot{V}O_2max$ of 27 ml · kg^{-1} · min^{-1}, or 7.7 METs.

Her blood chemistry values and BP are normal. Her family history is negative for CHD. Her HR response to the test is normal and indicates poor cardiorespiratory fitness. The low maximal aerobic power is related to the sedentary lifestyle, the cigarette smoking (carbon monoxide), and the 30% body fatness. She was encouraged to participate in a smoking-cessation program and was given the names of two local professional groups.

The recommended exercise program emphasized the low end of the THR zone (70% HRmax: 127 beats · min^{-1}) with long duration. She preferred a walking program to begin with because of the freedom it gave her schedule. She was given the walking program in chapter 17 and was asked to record her HR response to each of the exercise sessions.

A body fatness goal of 22% resulted in a target body weight of 121 lb (55 kg). She did not feel the need for dietary counseling at this time, but she agreed to record her food intake for 10 days to determine the patterns of eating behavior that would be beneficial to change (see chapters 8 and 10). She made an appointment for a meeting with the HFI in 2 weeks to discuss the progress with her program.

15.1

A. Free weights
   1. Load is constant throughout the range of motion
   2. Effort of muscle varies to adapt to load throughout the range of motion
   3. Requires the involvement of secondary muscles during the lift to stabilize a joint or maintain posture
   4. Requires a spotter for safety in some of the lifts

B. Variable resistance equipment
   1. Load varies throughout the range of motion of the joint due to cam or pulley arrangement in the machine
   2. Muscle effort is relatively constant throughout the lift
   3. Machines tend to isolate the muscle group(s) involved in a lift
   4. Weights are supported and spotting is not normally required

15.2

General guidelines for improving muscle strength include doing 3 sets with a 6- to 10-RM resistance, 3 days per week for the major muscle groups. For muscle endurance, the intensity is decreased (for example, 15- to 25-RM), with sets and days per week remaining the same.

16.1

Although it is possible that this exercise might be appropriate for some individuals with well-developed abdominal musculature, it is not an appropriate exercise to give the masses since the quality of the movement is so critical. The individual with extremely well-developed abdominal muscles may be able to perform this exercise and keep his or her low back in contact with the exercise surface throughout its execution; however, the individual with weaker abdominals and/or tight hip flexors will invariably anteriorly tilt the pelvis and the resulting lumbar lordosis places the lumbar vertebra in a potentially compromising position. Undoubtedly the physical therapists that use this activity use it only as a test on a one-to-one basis; this enables them to immediately stop the activity if they believe it is compromising to any individual.

16.2

It is good that the exercise leader emphasizes the importance of not doing ballistic stretches even from the sitting position; however, there are other factors that he/she should also consider. This maneuver is a fair exercise for use in attempting to improve hamstring extensibility. However, if the individual has extremely tight hamstrings (i.e., if the sacrum should be less than 80°-90° with the exercise surface in the sit-and-reach), the forward stretching from this position could potentially stretch the tissues of the low back instead of the hamstrings. Therefore, for the individual with fairly tight hamstrings the sit-and-reach exercise may be contraindicated; the standing toe touch could be worse because of the effect of gravity on the moment arm of force.

16.3

Although isometric exercises have become less popular as a strength development activity in most applications (joint injury would be an exception), they can be used most appropriately for strengthening trunk musculature, assuming the exerciser does not have high blood pressure. The oblique curl could be particularly advantageous since the internal and external oblique muscles would have an important role in stabilization of the spine. This factor may decrease the likelihood of having low-back problems; for the individual who is symptomatic, the development of these muscles in this way may enable the individual to better maintain his/her neutral spine and avoid postures which exacerbate his/her condition.

17.1

Topics to address include:

- attention to signs and symptoms that indicate problems and directions to act on them with a visit to their physician,
- proper shoes,
- clothing appropriate for the season,
- site (e.g., safety, surface, lighting),
- buddy system where possible to encourage participation, and
- alternate place in poor weather (shopping mall).

17.2

Before beginning an aerobic dance class, the participant should be able to walk 4 mi at a brisk pace with comfort. The appropriate transition from a walking program would be into a low-intensity, low-impact aerobics class. The participant should stay at the low end of the THR zone during this transition period and increase the intensity of the class only after these low-intensity, low-impact sessions can be comfortably completed.

18.1

Exercise increases the rate at which glucose can be removed from the blood with no change in the insulin level. The diabetic would *not* increase insulin intake since that would cause the blood glucose concentration to decrease and precipitate a hypoglycemic episode. The diabetic might increase carbohydrate intake and/or decrease the injected insulin to keep blood glucose under control.

18.2

a. It would be important to find out if she has worked with her physician and is currently not experiencing problems with her current medication. In addition, ask if she carries a bronchodilator with her to class, and determine that she knows to use it at the onset of wheezing. Lastly, pay special attention to her during the early phases of the class.

b. She should begin with a long warm-up period, and do exercises at the low end of the THR range in 5-min segments, with a recovery between segments.

19.1

You need to approach this situation from several different directions. First of all, talk with Jim privately, indicating that you are glad about his running interest but that he should not commit the center or other participants to participation in road races without checking with you and the others. Explain that some of the members might enjoy running if the emphasis is on finishing the race, not winning, and that others will not have any interest in road races. In the class, you should encourage those who have been running several miles per week at the THR to consider entering one road race just to try it. Their emphasis should be on setting their own paces, and their goal should be to finish the race. Finally, make it clear that running in road races is not for everyone—it is not necessary for fitness improvement; and in fact, it falls into the performance category, just like playing racquetball, tennis, soccer, or some other sport. Performance sports are good options for people who enjoy them; but they are not essential for fitness goals, and they involve higher risks of injury.

19.2

You might guess that Linda's days are full of interaction with people—children, employees, employers, and the public. The walking and jogging programs provided her with some time to be alone with her own thoughts without dealing with other people. You might start the conversation by telling Linda that you have missed her the past couple of weeks. Ask her what she liked about the first few months of the fitness program, what her fitness goals are, and what could be done to help her. If your guess about her wanting to be alone is correct, then emphasize that continuing in the running program is a good option for her exercise. You might suggest that she try cycling or swimming laps just for variety for some of her workouts. It is important for her to realize that it's okay for her to choose to have her individual exercise schedule and to tailor her program to her own interests.

20.1

Dana is in the preparation stage and has low exercise self-efficacy. She has had a bad experience with exercise in the past, so you want to educate her about what to expect at the beginning of an exercise program and make sure the prescription is appropriate for her fitness level. Use the evaluation to give her a realistic idea of her current fitness level and how much progress she can expect based on a sensible prescription. In setting goals with her, find out what *she* wants to achieve. Brainstorm about barriers to exercise and how to counter them. Identify supports and ways she could reward herself during the program. Target her low exercise self-efficacy with a beginner aerobic class and individual attention and encouragement, especially during the first few weeks. A behavioral contract with Mike doing something she wants him to do when she meets short-term goals could provide incentives and support she will need to keep her program going.

20.2

Jack is in the action stage, and he is especially susceptible to relapse. You could call him to find out the next time he will be walking and make plans to join him that day. On your walk, provide support for his efforts and talk about relapse prevention. Extra work at the end of the term is a high-risk situation for him, discouraging him and increasing the risk of relapse. Talk with him about readjusting his goals during this busy time, making the new short-term goals realistic and reachable. One option would be 15-min "walk breaks" during the days he can't get to the facility after work to give him more miles and help manage stress. Praise him for how far he has come and for continuing even though he is very busy. Help him see that the high-risk situation is time limited, and brainstorm about ways he can reward himself for the walking he can do. Recruit veteran walkers to provide support and encouragement.

21.1

a. Suspect insulin shock.

b. Ask the following questions: What happened? Are you a diabetic? Have you taken your insulin today? Have you eaten?

c. Check her medic-alert tag. If insulin shock is still suspected, administer sugar (orange juice, candy, sugar granules). If she is unconscious or her recovery is slow (greater than 1 to 2 min), refer to a physician.

21.2

a. Suspect heat stroke.

b. Implement EMS—call 911. This is a medical emergency. Cool quickly starting at the head and work down. Expose as much skin surface as possible. Monitor vital signs. Treat cramps by stretching and applying ice, direct pressure, and gentle massage. Treat for shock. Wrap in cold wet sheets for transport.

c. Emergency plans and materials should include
   - access to cooling agents, such as water, ice, ice towels, cool environment;
   - access to phone, with knowledge of EMS;
   - knowledge of roles in emergency: person in charge, who assists person in charge, person responsible for making emergency phone call, who is to meet and direct the emergency vehicle to the injured; and
   - knowledge of rules to move person if necessary.

22.1

a. HR = 1500/12 = 125 beats · min^{-1}

   P-R interval duration = 0.12 s
   QRS complex duration = 0.08 s
   Q-T interval duration = 0.32 s

b. Sinus tachycardia—fast heart rate over 100 beats · min^{-1}

c. Common causes of sinus tachycardia are anxiety, nervousness, caffeine, or low fitness level.

22.2

a. Atrial fibrillation—jagged baseline with irregularly spaced PVCs

b. Ventricular rate = 6 cardiac cycles in a 6-s strip × 10 = 60 beats · min^{-1}

22.3

a. Trigeminy—every third heart beat is a PVC

b. You should gradually decrease treadmill speed and grade, and notify the physician.

22.4

Because the person was on Inderal (a nonselective ß-blocker) at the time of his exercise test, his heart rate would have been suppressed. Now that he is no longer taking the medication, his previously calculated target HR will be too low. The exercise intensity should be adjusted upward.

22.5

Isordil contains nitroglycerin and is used to reduce the chance of having an angina attack. The drug relaxes vascular smooth muscle and might cause pooling of blood in the extremities. This pooling could cause a decrease in blood pressure and result in symptoms of dizziness.

23.1

You might use the following steps in your evaluation:

A. What are the expectations (based on written job descriptions, and conversations with both the Fitness Director and the Instructors)?

B. How can each expectation be evaluated?

C. Set up a procedure (including communication with both the Fitness Director and Instructors) to evaluate each component of the job.

D. Share your evaluation with the Instructors, giving them a chance to add comments, before submitting it to the Fitness Director.

23.2

You might include the following in your evaluation:

A. Clear description of the fitness goals (long-range plan, official mission statements, statement from the Program Director).

B. Identify aspects of the program that relate to each goal (e.g., exercise to music classes and improvement in cardiorespiratory fitness).

C. Set up specific tests to determine each of the fitness goals, measuring before and after various experiences.

D. Set up systematic ways to determine individual satisfaction, enjoyment, and injuries associated with various aspects of the program.

E. Analyze the positive (and negative) changes that have occurred.

F. Recommend ways to improve future fitness goals.

APPENDIX

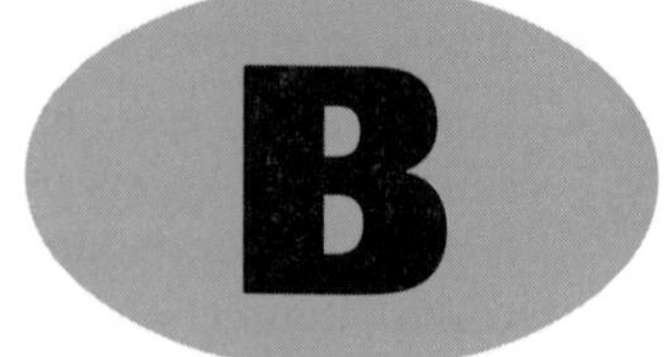

Calculation of Oxygen Uptake and Carbon Dioxide Production

CALCULATION OF OXYGEN CONSUMPTION ($\dot{V}O_2$)

The air we breathe is composed of 20.93% oxygen (O_2), 0.03% carbon dioxide (CO_2), and the balance, 79.04%, nitrogen (N_2). When we exhale, the fraction of the air represented by O_2 is decreased and the fraction represented by CO_2 is increased. To calculate the volume of O_2 used by the body ($\dot{V}O_2$), we simply subtract the number of liters of O_2 exhaled from the number of liters of O_2 inhaled. Equation 1 summarizes these words.

(1) Oxygen consumption =
[Volume of O_2 inhaled] –
[Volume of O_2 exhaled]

Now, using VO_2 to mean volume of *oxygen* used, V_I to mean volume of *air* inhaled, V_E to mean volume of *air* exhaled, F_{IO_2} to mean fraction of oxygen in inhaled air, and F_{EO_2} to mean fraction of oxygen in exhaled air, equation 1 can be written:

(2) $VO_2 = [V_I \cdot F_{IO_2}] - [V_E \cdot F_{EO_2}]$

You know that $F_{IO_2} = 0.2093$ and F_{EO_2} will be determined on an oxygen analyzer. Consequently, you are left with only two unknowns, the volume of air (liters) inhaled (V_I) and the volume of air (liters) exhaled (V_E). It appears that you must measure both volumes, but fortunately, this is not necessary. It was determined years ago that N_2 is neither used nor produced by the body. Consequently, the number of liters of N_2 inhaled must equal the number of liters of N_2 exhaled. Equation 3 states this equality using the symbols mentioned earlier.

(3) $V_I \cdot F_{IN_2} = V_E \cdot F_{EN_2}$

This is a very important relationship because it permits you to calculate V_E when V_I is known or vice versa. Using equation 3 here are two formulas, one to give V_E when V_I is known, and one to give V_I when V_E is known.

$$V_I = \frac{V_E \cdot F_{EN_2}}{F_{IN_2}} \qquad V_E = \frac{V_I \cdot F_{IN_2}}{F_{EN_2}}$$

Now that you know how to do this, there is only one other piece to the puzzle needed to permit you to calculate $\dot{V}O_2$. The value for F_{IN_2} is constant (0.7904) so we must determine F_{EN_2}. When the expired gas sample is analyzed you will obtain a value for F_{EO_2} and F_{ECO_2}, but not F_{EN_2}. However, since all the gas fractions must add up to 1.0000, you can calculate F_{EN_2}. (In the same way, we calculated F_{IN_2}: 1.0000 – .0003 (CO_2) – .2093 (O_2) = .7904.)

Problem: Calculate F_{EN_2} when F_{EO_2} = .1600 and F_{ECO_2} = .0450

Answer: F_{EN_2} = 1.0000 – .1600 – .0450 = .7950

The following problem shows how these equations are used. Given that V_I equals 100 L, F_{EO_2} = .1600, and F_{ECO_2} = .0450, calculate V_E.

$$V_E \cdot F_{EN_2} = V_I \cdot F_{IN_2}, \text{so } V_E = \frac{V_I \cdot F_{IN_2}}{F_{EN_2}}$$

$$F_{IN_2} = .7904 \text{ and}$$

$$F_{EN_2} = 1.0000 - .1600 - .0450 = .7950$$

$$V_E = 100 \text{ L} \cdot \frac{.7904}{.7950} = 99.4 \text{ L}$$

At this point, the equation for VO_2 can be rewritten, using V_I, V_E, F_{IO_2}, and F_{EO_2}.

$$VO_2 = V_I \cdot F_{IO_2} - V_E \cdot F_{EO_2}$$

Assuming that you measure only V_I this formula is rewritten:

$$VO_2 = V_I \cdot F_{IO_2} - \frac{V_I \cdot F_{IN_2}}{F_{EN_2}} \cdot F_{EO_2}$$

V_I can be factored out of this equation, so:

$$VO_2 = V_I \left[F_{IO_2} - \frac{F_{IN_2}}{F_{EN_2}} \cdot F_{EO_2} \right]$$

We will repeat the last two steps assuming that V_E is the volume that is measured and then factor out V_E.

$$\dot{V}O_2 = \frac{V_E \cdot F_{EN_2}}{F_{IN_2}} \cdot F_{IO_2} - V_E \cdot F_{EO_2} =$$

$$V_E \left[\frac{F_{EN_2}}{F_{IN_2}} \cdot F_{IO_2} - F_{EO_2} \right]$$

At this point you know how to calculate VO_2. If you ever get stuck, always go back to the formula: $VO_2 = V_I \cdot F_{IO_2} - V_E \cdot F_{EO_2}$ and simply substitute for V_E or V_I, depending on what was measured.

Some comments:

1. You must always match the volume measurement with the F_{EO_2} and F_{ECO_2} values measured in that expired volume. If you measure V_I for 2 min, you must have a single 2-min bag of expired gas to get F_{EO_2} and F_{ECO_2} values. If you measure a 30-s volume your expired bag must be collected over those 30 s.
2. VO_2 and VCO_2 are usually expressed in liters/min: the *rate* at which O_2 is used or CO_2 is produced per minute. To signify this *rate*, we write $\dot{V}O_2$ (read Vee dot). You would convert 30-s or 2-min volumes to 1-min values before making calculations of $\dot{V}O_2$.

Sample problem:

$$\dot{V}_I = 100 \text{ L/min}, \ F_{EO_2} = .1600, \ F_{ECO_2} = .0450$$

Calculate $\dot{V}O_2$:

$$\dot{V}O_2 = \dot{V}_I \cdot F_{IO_2} - \dot{V}_E \cdot F_{EO_2}$$

$$\dot{V}_E = \frac{\dot{V}_I \cdot F_{IN_2}}{F_{EN_2}}$$

$$\dot{V}O_2 = \dot{V}_I \cdot F_{IO_2} - \frac{\dot{V}_I \cdot F_{IN_2}}{F_{EN_2}} \cdot F_{EO_2}$$

$$= \dot{V}_I \left[F_{IO_2} - \frac{F_{IN_2}}{F_{EN_2}} \cdot F_{EO_2} \right]$$

$$F_{EN_2} = 1.0000 - .1600 - .0450 = .7950$$

$$\dot{V}O_2 = 100 \text{ L/min} \left[.2093 - \frac{.7904}{.7950} \cdot .1600 \right]$$

$$= 5.02 \text{ L/min}$$

The volume (let's assume that $\dot{V}_E$ was measured) used in the above equations was measured at room temperature (23 °C) and at the barometric pressure of that moment (740 mmHg). The environmental conditions under which the volume was measured are called ambient conditions. If this volume of gas were transported to 10 000 feet above sea level, where the barometric pressure is lower, the volume would increase because of the reduced pressure. The volume of a gas varies inversely with pressure (at a constant temperature). Another factor influencing the volume of a gas is the temperature. If that volume, measured at 23 °C, were placed in a refrigerator at 0 °C, the volume of gas would decrease. The volume of gas varies directly with the temperature (at constant pressure).

Since the volume ($\dot{V}_E$) is influenced by both pressure and temperature, the value measured as O_2 used ($\dot{V}O_2$) might reflect changes in pressure or temperature, rather than a change in workload, training, and so on. Consequently, it would be convenient to express $\dot{V}_E$ in such a way as to make measurements comparable when they are obtained under different environmental conditions. This is done by standardizing the temperature, barometric pressure, and water vapor pressure at which the volume is expressed. By convention, volumes are expressed at Standard Temperature and Pressure, Dry (STPD): 273 °K (equals 0 °C), 760 mmHg pressure (sea level), and with no water vapor pressure. When $\dot{V}O_2$ is expressed STPD you can calculate the number of molecules of oxygen actually used by the body because *at STPD one mole of oxygen equals 22.4 L.*

Let's make the correction to STPD one step at a time. Let's assume that a volume ($\dot{V}_E$) was measured at 740 mmHg, 23 °C and equaled 100 L/min. This *expired* volume is *always* saturated with water vapor.

To correct for temperature you use 273 °K as the standard (0 °C).

$$\text{Volume} \times \frac{273\ °\text{K}}{273\ °\text{K} + x\ °\text{C}} = \frac{273\ °\text{K}}{273 + 23}$$

$$100\ \text{L/min} \times \frac{273\ °\text{K}}{296\ °\text{K}} = 92.23\ \text{L/min}$$

When we make corrections for pressure we must remove the effect of water vapor pressure because the gas volume is adjusted on the basis of the standard pressure (760 mmHg) which is a dry pressure.

To correct the volume to the standard 760 mmHg pressure (dry) use:

$$\text{Volume} \times \frac{\text{barometric pressure} - \text{water vapor pressure}}{760\ \text{mmHg (dry)}}$$

Water vapor pressure is dependent on two things: the temperature and the relative humidity. In expired gas the gas volume is saturated (100% relative humidity). Consequently, you can obtain a value for water vapor pressure directly from the table in the next column.

Going back to our pressure correction:

$$92.23\ \text{L/min} \times \frac{740 - 21.1}{760} = 87.24\ \text{L/min (STPD)}$$

To combine the temperature and pressure correction:

Temperature (°C)	Saturation water vapor pressure (mmHg)
18	15.5
19	16.5
20	17.5
21	18.7
22	19.8
23	21.1
24	22.4
25	23.8
26	25.2
27	26.7

$$100\ \text{L/min} \times \frac{273\ °\text{K}}{273\ °\text{K} + 23} \times \frac{740 - 21.1}{760} =$$
87.24 L/min (STPD)

A special note must be made here. If you are using an inspired (inhaled) volume ($\dot{V}_I$), you are rarely dealing with a gas saturated with water vapor. Consequently, when you correct for pressure you must find what the water vapor is in the inspired air. You do this by finding the relative humidity of the air. You then multiply this value by the water vapor pressure value for saturated air at whatever the temperature is. To clarify, if your volume in the above example was $\dot{V}_I$ and had a relative humidity of 50%, the pressure correction would have been:

$$\text{Volume} \times \frac{740 - (.50 \times 21.1\ \text{mmHg})}{760\ \text{mmHg}}$$

While this may seem like a minor point, it is critical to the accurate measurement of $\dot{V}O_2$ that the proper water vapor correction be used. When you do calculations for $\dot{V}O_2$ you usually find the STPD factor first since you will be multiplying this factor by each volume measured.

Problem: Given $\dot{V}_I$ = 100 L/min, F_{EO_2} = .1700, F_{ECO_2} = .0385. The temperature = 20 °C, barometric pressure = 740 mmHg, and the relative humidity = 30%.

Answer:

$$\text{STPD factor} = \frac{740\ \text{mmHg} - (.30)17.5\ \text{mmHg}}{760} \times \frac{273\ °\text{K}}{273\ °\text{K} + 20\ °\text{C}} = .900$$

100 L/min × .900 = 90 L/min STPD

$$\dot{V}O_2 = \dot{V}_{I_{STPD}} \left[F_{IO_2} - \frac{F_{IN_2}}{F_{EN_2}} \cdot F_{EO_2} \right]$$

$$\dot{V}O_2 = 90 \text{ L/min} \left[.2093 - \frac{.7904}{.7915} \cdot .1700 \right]$$

$$\dot{V}O_2 = 3.56 \text{ L/min}$$

CARBON DIOXIDE PRODUCTION ($\dot{V}CO_2$)

When O_2 is used, CO_2 is produced. The ratio of CO_2 production ($\dot{V}CO_2$) to O_2 consumption ($\dot{V}O_2$) is an important measurement in metabolism. This ratio ($\dot{V}CO_2 \div \dot{V}O_2$) is called the respiratory exchange ratio and is abbreviated as "R."

How do we measure $\dot{V}CO_2$? We start at the same step as for $\dot{V}O_2$:

$$\dot{V}CO_2 = \text{liters of } CO_2 \text{ expired} - \text{liters of } CO_2 \text{ inspired} = \dot{V}_E \cdot F_{ECO_2} - \dot{V}_I \cdot F_{ICO_2}$$

The steps to follow are the same as for measuring $\dot{V}O_2$. Always use an STPD volume in your calculations. The following is the equation to use when $\dot{V}_I$ is measured:

$$\dot{V}CO_2 = \dot{V}_{I_{STPD}} \left[\frac{F_{IN_2}}{F_{EN_2}} \cdot F_{ECO_2} - F_{ICO_2} \right]$$

The following steps summarize the calculations for $\dot{V}CO_2$ and R for the previous problem.

$$\dot{V}CO_2 = 90 \text{ L/min} \left[\frac{.7904}{.7915} \cdot .0385 - .0003 \right] = 3.43 \text{ L/min}$$

$$R = \dot{V}CO_2 \div \dot{V}O_2 = 3.43 \text{ L/min} \div 3.56 \text{ L/min}$$

$$R = .96$$

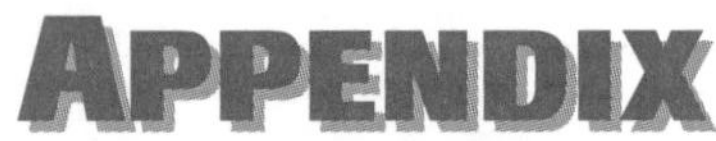

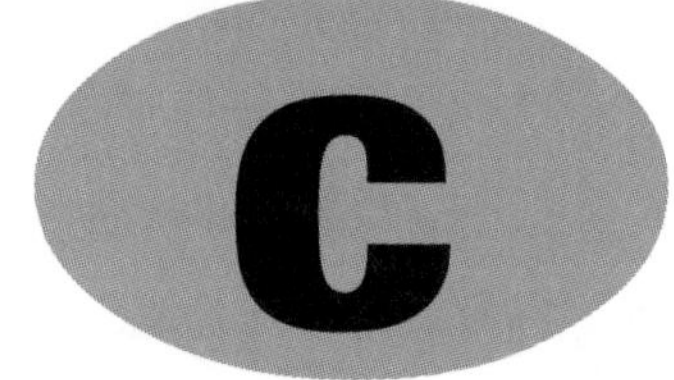

Energy Costs of Various Physical Activities

Compendium of Physical Activities

METS	Activity category	Specific activity
8.5	Bicycling	Bicycling, BMX or mountain
4.0	Bicycling	Bicycling, < 10 mph, general, leisure, to work or for pleasure
6.0	Bicycling	Bicycling, 10-11.9 mph, leisure, slow, light effort
8.0	Bicycling	Bicycling, 12-13.9 mph, leisure, moderate effort
10.0	Bicycling	Bicycling, 14-15.9 mph, racing or leisure, fast, vigorous effort
12.0	Bicycling	Bicycling, 16-19 mph, racing/not drafting or > 19 mph drafting, very fast, racing general
16.0	Bicycling	Bicycling, > 20 mph, racing, not drafting
5.0	Bicycling	Unicycling
5.0	Conditioning exercise	Bicycling, stationary, general
3.0	Conditioning exercise	Bicycling, stationary, 50 W, very light effort
5.5	Conditioning exercise	Bicycling, stationary, 100 W, light effort
7.0	Conditioning exercise	Bicycling, stationary, 150 W, moderate effort
10.5	Conditioning exercise	Bicycling, stationary, 200 W, vigorous effort
12.5	Conditioning exercise	Bicycling, stationary, 250 W, very vigorous effort
8.0	Conditioning exercise	Calisthenics (e.g., push-ups, pull-ups, sit-ups), heavy, vigorous effort
4.5	Conditioning exercise	Calisthenics, home exercise, light or moderate effort, general (example: back exercises), going up & down from floor
8.0	Conditioning exercise	Circuit training, general
6.0	Conditioning exercise	Weight lifting (free weight, nautilus or universal-type), power lifting or body building, vigorous effort
5.5	Conditioning exercise	Health club exercise, general
6.0	Conditioning exercise	Stair-treadmill ergometer, general
9.5	Conditioning exercise	Rowing, stationary ergometer, general
3.5	Conditioning exercise	Rowing, stationary, 50 W, light effort
7.0	Conditioning exercise	Rowing, stationary, 100 W, moderate effort
8.5	Conditioning exercise	Rowing, stationary, 150 W, vigorous effort
12.0	Conditioning exercise	Rowing, stationary, 200 W, very vigorous effort
9.5	Conditioning exercise	Ski machine, general

METS	Activity category	Specific activity
6.0	Conditioning exercise	Slimnastics
4.0	Conditioning exercise	Stretching, hatha yoga
6.0	Conditioning exercise	Teaching aerobic exercise class
4.0	Conditioning exercise	Water aerobics, water calisthenics
3.0	Conditioning exercise	Weight lifting (free, nautilus or universal-type), light or moderate effort, light workout, general
1.0	Conditioning exercise	Whirlpool, sitting
6.0	Dancing	Aerobic, ballet or modern, twist
6.0	Dancing	Aerobic, general
5.0	Dancing	Aerobic, low impact
7.0	Dancing	Aerobic, high impact
4.5	Dancing	General
5.5	Dancing	Ballroom, fast (disco, folk, square)
3.0	Dancing	Ballroom, slow (e.g., waltz, foxtrot, slow dancing)
4.0	Fishing and hunting	Fishing, general
4.0	Fishing and hunting	Digging worms, with shovel
5.0	Fishing and hunting	Fishing from river bank and walking
2.5	Fishing and hunting	Fishing from boat, sitting
3.5	Fishing and hunting	Fishing from river bank, standing
6.0	Fishing and hunting	Fishing in stream, in waders
2.0	Fishing and hunting	Fishing, ice, sitting
2.5	Fishing and hunting	Hunting, bow and arrow or crossbow
6.0	Fishing and hunting	Hunting, deer, elk, large game
2.5	Fishing and hunting	Hunting, duck, wading
5.0	Fishing and hunting	Hunting, general
6.0	Fishing and hunting	Hunting, pheasants or grouse
5.0	Fishing and hunting	Hunting, rabbit, squirrel, prairie chick, raccoon, small game
2.5	Fishing and hunting	Pistol shooting or trap shooting, standing
2.5	Home activities	Carpet sweeping, sweeping floors
4.5	Home activities	Cleaning, heavy or major (e.g., wash car, wash windows, mop, clean garage), vigorous effort
3.5	Home activities	Cleaning, house or cabin, general
2.5	Home activities	Cleaning, light (dusting, straightening up, vacuuming, changing linen, carrying out trash), moderate effort
2.3	Home activities	Wash dishes-standing or in general (not broken into stand/walk components)
2.3	Home activities	Wash dishes; clearing dishes from table-walking
2.5	Home activities	Cooking or food preparation-standing or sitting or in general (not broken into stand/walk components)
2.5	Home activities	Serving food, setting table-implied walking or standing

METS	Activity category	Specific activity
2.5	Home activities	Cooking or food preparation-walking
2.5	Home activities	Putting away groceries (e.g., carrying groceries, shopping without a grocery cart)
8.0	Home activities	Carrying groceries upstairs
3.5	Home activities	Food shopping, with grocery cart
2.0	Home activities	Standing-shopping (non-grocery shopping)
2.3	Home activities	Walking-shopping (non-grocery shopping)
2.3	Home activities	Ironing
1.5	Home activities	Sitting, knitting, sewing, light wrapping (presents)
2.0	Home activities	Implied standing-laundry, fold or hang clothes, put clothes in washer or dryer, packing suitcase
2.3	Home activities	Implied walking-putting away clothes, gathering clothes to pack, putting away laundry
2.0	Home activities	Making bed
5.0	Home activities	Maple syruping/sugar bushing (including carrying buckets, carrying wood)
6.0	Home activities	Moving furniture, household
5.5	Home activities	Scrubbing floors, on hands and knees
4.0	Home activities	Sweeping garage, sidewalk or outside of house
7.0	Home activities	Moving household items, carrying boxes
3.5	Home activities	Standing-packing/unpacking boxes, occasional lifting of household items, light-moderate effort
3.0	Home activities	Implied walking-putting away household items-moderate effort
9.0	Home activities	Move household items upstairs, carrying boxes or furniture
2.5	Home activities	Standing-light (pump gas, change light bulb, etc.)
3.0	Home activities	Walking-light, noncleaning (ready to leave, shut/lock doors, close windows, etc.)
2.5	Home activities	Sitting-playing with child(ren)-light
2.8	Home activities	Standing-playing with child(ren)-light
4.0	Home activities	Walk/run-playing with child(ren)-moderate
5.0	Home activities	Walk/run-playing with child(ren)-vigorous
3.0	Home activities	Child care: sitting/kneeling-dressing, bathing, grooming, feeding, occasional lifting of child-light effort

METS	Activity category	Specific activity
3.5	Home activities	Child care: standing-dressing, bathing, grooming, feeding, occasional lifting of child-light effort
3.0	Home repair	Airplane repair
4.5	Home repair	Automobile body work
3.0	Home repair	Automobile repair
3.0	Home repair	Carpentry, general, workshop
6.0	Home repair	Carpentry, outside house, installing rain gutters
4.5	Home repair	Carpentry, finishing or refinishing cabinets or furniture
7.5	Home repair	Carpentry, sawing hardwood
5.0	Home repair	Caulking, chinking log cabin
4.5	Home repair	Caulking, except log cabin
5.0	Home repair	Cleaning gutters
5.0	Home repair	Excavating garage
5.0	Home repair	Hanging storm windows
4.5	Home repair	Laying or removing carpet
4.5	Home repair	Laying tile or linoleum
5.0	Home repair	Painting, outside house
4.5	Home repair	Painting, papering, plastering, scraping, inside house, hanging sheet rock, remodeling
3.0	Home repair	Put on and removal of tarp-sailboat
6.0	Home repair	Roofing
4.5	Home repair	Sanding floors with a power sander
4.5	Home repair	Scrape and paint sailboat or powerboat
5.0	Home repair	Spreading dirt with a shovel
4.5	Home repair	Wash and wax hull of sailboat, car, powerboat, airplane
4.5	Home repair	Washing fence
3.0	Home repair	Wiring, plumbing
0.9	Inactivity, quiet	Lying quietly, reclining (watch television), lying quietly in bed-awake
1.0	Inactivity, quiet	Sitting quietly (riding in a car, listening to a lecture or music, watch television or a movie)
0.9	Inactivity, quiet	Sleeping
1.2	Inactivity, quiet	Standing quietly (standing in a line)
1.0	Inactivity, light	Recline-writing
1.0	Inactivity, light	Recline-talking or talking on phone
1.0	Inactivity, light	Recline-reading
5.0	Lawn and garden	Carrying, loading or stacking wood, loading/unloading or carrying lumber
6.0	Lawn and garden	Chopping wood, splitting logs
5.0	Lawn and garden	Clearing land, hauling branches
5.0	Lawn and garden	Digging sandbox
5.0	Lawn and garden	Digging, spading, filling garden
6.0	Lawn and garden	Gardening with heavy power tools, tilling a garden (see occupation, shoveling)
5.0	Lawn and garden	Laying crushed rock

METS	Activity category	Specific activity
5.0	Lawn and garden	Laying sod
5.5	Lawn and garden	Mowing lawn, general
2.5	Lawn and garden	Mowing lawn, riding mower
6.0	Lawn and garden	Mowing lawn, walk, hand mower
4.5	Lawn and garden	Mowing lawn, walk, power mower
4.5	Lawn and garden	Operating snow blower, walking
4.0	Lawn and garden	Planting seedlings, shrubs
4.5	Lawn and garden	Planting trees
4.0	Lawn and garden	Raking lawn
4.0	Lawn and garden	Raking roof with snow rake
3.0	Lawn and garden	Riding snow blower
4.0	Lawn and garden	Sacking grass, leaves
6.0	Lawn and garden	Shoveling, snow, by hand
4.5	Lawn and garden	Trimming shrubs or trees, manual cutter
3.5	Lawn and garden	Trimming shrubs or trees, power cutter
2.5	Lawn and garden	Walking, applying fertilizer or seeding a lawn
1.5	Lawn and garden	Watering lawn or garden, standing or walking
4.5	Lawn and garden	Weeding, cultivating garden
5.0	Lawn and garden	Gardening, general
3.0	Lawn and garden	Implied walking/standing-picking up yard, light
1.5	Miscellaneous	Sitting, card playing, playing board games
2.0	Miscellaneous	Standing-drawing (writing), casino gambling
1.3	Miscellaneous	Sitting-reading, book, newspaper, etc.
1.8	Miscellaneous	Sitting-writing, desk work
1.8	Miscellaneous	Standing-talking or talking on the phone
1.5	Miscellaneous	Sitting-talking or talking on the phone
1.8	Miscellaneous	Sitting-studying, general, including reading and/or writing
1.8	Miscellaneous	Sitting-in class, general, including note-taking or class discussion
1.8	Miscellaneous	Standing-reading
1.8	Music playing	Accordion
2.0	Music playing	Cello
2.5	Music playing	Conducting
4.0	Music playing	Drums
2.0	Music playing	Flute (sitting)
2.0	Music playing	Horn
2.5	Music playing	Piano or organ
3.5	Music playing	Trombone
2.5	Music playing	Trumpet
2.5	Music playing	Violin
2.0	Music playing	Woodwind
2.0	Music playing	Guitar, classical, folk (sitting)
3.0	Music playing	Guitar, rock and roll band (standing)

METS	Activity category	Specific activity
4.0	Music playing	Marching band, playing an instrument, baton twirling (walking)
3.5	Music playing	Marching band, drum major (walking)
4.0	Occupation	Bakery, general
2.3	Occupation	Bookbinding
6.0	Occupation	Building road (including hauling debris, driving heavy machinery)
2.0	Occupation	Building road, directing traffic (standing)
3.5	Occupation	Carpentry, general
8.0	Occupation	Carrying heavy loads, such as bricks
8.0	Occupation	Carrying moderate loads upstairs, moving boxes (16-40 lb)
2.5	Occupation	Chambermaid
6.5	Occupation	Coal mining, drilling coal, rock
6.5	Occupation	Coal mining, erecting supports
6.0	Occupation	Coal mining, general
7.0	Occupation	Coal mining, shoveling coal
5.5	Occupation	Construction, outside, remodeling
3.5	Occupation	Electrical work, plumbing
8.0	Occupation	Farming, baling hay, cleaning barn, poultry work
3.5	Occupation	Farming, chasing cattle, nonstrenuous
2.5	Occupation	Farming, driving harvester
2.5	Occupation	Farming, driving tractor
4.0	Occupation	Farming, feeding small animals
4.5	Occupation	Farming, feeding cattle
8.0	Occupation	Farming, forking straw bales
3.0	Occupation	Farming, milking by hand
1.5	Occupation	Farming, milking by machine
5.5	Occupation	Farming, shoveling grain
12.0	Occupation	Fire fighter, general
11.0	Occupation	Fire fighter, climbing ladder with full gear
8.0	Occupation	Fire fighter, hauling hoses on ground
17.0	Occupation	Forestry, ax chopping, fast
5.0	Occupation	Forestry, ax chopping, slow
7.0	Occupation	Forestry, barking trees
11.0	Occupation	Forestry, carrying logs
8.0	Occupation	Forestry, felling trees
8.0	Occupation	Forestry, general
5.0	Occupation	Forestry, hoeing
6.0	Occupation	Forestry, planting by hand
7.0	Occupation	Forestry, sawing by hand
4.5	Occupation	Forestry, sawing, power
9.0	Occupation	Forestry, trimming trees
4.0	Occupation	Forestry, weeding
4.5	Occupation	Furriery
6.0	Occupation	Horse grooming
8.0	Occupation	Horse racing, galloping
6.5	Occupation	Horse racing, trotting
2.6	Occupation	Horse racing, walking

METS	Activity category	Specific activity
3.5	Occupation	Locksmith
2.5	Occupation	Machine tooling, machining, working sheet metal
3.0	Occupation	Machine tooling, operating lathe
5.0	Occupation	Machine tooling, operating punch press
4.0	Occupation	Machine tooling, tapping and drilling
3.0	Occupation	Machine tooling, welding
7.0	Occupation	Masonry, concrete
4.0	Occupation	Masseur, masseuse (standing)
7.0	Occupation	Moving, pushing heavy objects, 75 lb or more (desks, moving van work)
2.5	Occupation	Operating heavy duty equipment/automated, not driving
4.5	Occupation	Orange grove work
2.3	Occupation	Printing (standing)
2.5	Occupation	Police, directing traffic (standing)
2.0	Occupation	Police, driving a squad car (sitting)
1.3	Occupation	Police, riding in a squad car (sitting)
8.0	Occupation	Police, making an arrest (standing)
2.5	Occupation	Shoe repair, general
8.5	Occupation	Shoveling, digging ditches
9.0	Occupation	Shoveling, heavy (more than 16 lb · min^{-1})
6.0	Occupation	Shoveling, light (less than 10 lb · min^{-1})
7.0	Occupation	Shoveling, moderate (10-15 lb · min^{-1})
1.5	Occupation	Sitting-light office work, in general (chemistry lab work, light use of handtools, watch repair or micro-assembly, light assembly/repair)
1.5	Occupation	Sitting-meetings, general, and/or with talking involved
2.5	Occupation	Sitting; moderate (heavy levers, riding mower/forklift, crane operation)
2.5	Occupation	Standing; light (bartending, store clerk, assembling, filing, xeroxing, put up Christmas tree)
3.0	Occupation	Standing; light/moderate (assemble/repair heavy parts, welding, stocking, auto repair, pack boxes for moving, etc.), patient care (as in nursing)
3.5	Occupation	Standing; moderate (assembling at fast rate, lifting 50 lb, hitch/twisting ropes)
4.0	Occupation	Standing; moderate/heavy (lifting more than 50 lb, masonry, painting, paper hanging)
5.0	Occupation	Steel mill, fettling

METS	Activity category	Specific activity
5.5	Occupation	Steel mill, forging
8.0	Occupation	Steel mill, hand rolling
8.0	Occupation	Steel mill, merchant mill rolling
11.0	Occupation	Steel mill, removing slag
7.5	Occupation	Steel mill, tending furnace
5.5	Occupation	Steel mill, tipping molds
8.0	Occupation	Steel mill, working in general
2.5	Occupation	Tailoring, cutting
2.5	Occupation	Tailoring, general
2.0	Occupation	Tailoring, hand sewing
2.5	Occupation	Tailoring, machine sewing
4.0	Occupation	Tailoring, pressing
6.5	Occupation	Truck driving, loading and unloading truck (standing)
1.5	Occupation	Typing, electric, manual or computer
6.0	Occupation	Using heavy power tools such as pneumatic tools (jackhammers, drills, etc.)
8.0	Occupation	Using heavy tools (not power) such as shovel, pick, tunnel bar, spade
2.0	Occupation	Walking on job, less than 2.0 mph (in office or lab area), very slow
3.5	Occupation	Walking on job, 3.0 mph, in office, moderate speed, not carrying anything
4.0	Occupation	Walking on job, 3.5 mph, in office, brisk speed, not carrying anything
3.0	Occupation	Walking, 2.5 mph, slowly and carrying light objects less than 25 lb
4.0	Occupation	Walking, 3.0 mph, moderately and carrying light objects less than 25 lb
4.5	Occupation	Walking, 3.5 mph, briskly and carrying objects less than 25 lb
5.0	Occupation	Walking or walk downstairs or standing, carrying objects about 25-49 lb
6.5	Occupation	Walking or walk downstairs or standing, carrying objects about 50-74 lb
7.5	Occupation	Walking or walk downstairs or standing, carrying objects about 75-99 lb
8.5	Occupation	Walking or walk downstairs or standing, carrying objects about 100 lb and over
3.0	Occupation	Working in scene shop, theater actor, backstage, employee
6.0	Running	Jog/walk combination (jogging component of less than 10 min)
7.0	Running	Jogging, general
8.0	Running	Running, 5 mph (12 min · mi^{-1})
9.0	Running	Running, 5.2 mph (11.5 min · mi^{-1})
10.0	Running	Running, 6 mph (10 min · mi^{-1})
11.0	Running	Running, 6.7 mph (9 min · mi^{-1})
11.5	Running	Running, 7 mph (8.5 min · mi^{-1})
12.5	Running	Running, 7.5 mph (8 min · mi^{-1})
13.5	Running	Running, 8 mph (7.5 min · mi^{-1})
14.0	Running	Running, 8.6 mph (7 min · mi^{-1})
15.0	Running	Running, 9 mph (6.5 min · mi^{-1})
16.0	Running	Running, 10 mph (6 min · mi^{-1})
18.0	Running	Running, 10.9 mph (5.5 min · mi^{-1})
9.0	Running	Running, cross-country
8.0	Running	Running, general
8.0	Running	Running, in place
15.0	Running	Running, stairs, up
10.0	Running	Running, on a track, team practice
8.0	Running	Running, training, pushing wheelchair, marathon wheeling
3.0	Running	Running, wheeling, general
2.5	Self-care	Standing-getting ready for bed, in general
1.0	Self-care	Sitting on toilet
2.0	Self-care	Bathing (sitting)
2.5	Self-care	Dressing, undressing (standing or sitting)
1.5	Self-care	Eating (sitting)
2.0	Self-care	Talking and eating or eating only (standing)
2.5	Self-care	Sitting or standing-grooming (washing, shaving, brushing teeth, urinating, washing hands, put on makeup)
4.0	Self-care	Showering, toweling off (standing)
1.5	Sexual activity	Active, vigorous effort
1.3	Sexual activity	General, moderate effort
1.0	Sexual activity	Passive, light effort, kissing, hugging
3.5	Sports	Archery (nonhunting)
7.0	Sports	Badminton, competitive
4.5	Sports	Badminton, social singles and doubles, general
8.0	Sports	Basketball, game
6.0	Sports	Basketball, nongame, general
7.0	Sports	Basketball, officiating
4.5	Sports	Basketball, shooting baskets
6.5	Sports	Basketball, wheelchair
2.5	Sports	Billiards
3.0	Sports	Bowling
12.0	Sports	Boxing, in ring, general
6.0	Sports	Boxing, punching bag
9.0	Sports	Boxing, sparring

METS	Activity category	Specific activity
7.0	Sports	Broomball
5.0	Sports	Children's games (hopscotch, 4-square, dodgeball, playground apparatus, T-ball, tetherball, marbles, jacks, arcade games)
4.0	Sports	Coaching: football, soccer, basketball, baseball, swimming, etc.
5.0	Sports	Cricket (batting, bowling)
2.5	Sports	Croquet
4.0	Sports	Curling
2.5	Sports	Darts, wall or lawn
6.0	Sports	Drag racing, pushing or driving a car
6.0	Sports	Fencing
9.0	Sports	Football, competitive
8.0	Sports	Football, touch, flag, general
2.5	Sports	Football or baseball, playing catch
3.0	Sports	Frisbee playing, general
3.5	Sports	Frisbee, ultimate
4.5	Sports	Golf, general
5.5	Sports	Golf, carrying clubs
3.0	Sports	Golf, miniature, driving range
5.0	Sports	Golf, pulling clubs
3.5	Sports	Golf, using power cart
4.0	Sports	Gymnastics, general
4.0	Sports	Hacky sack
12.0	Sports	Handball, general
8.0	Sports	Handball, team
3.5	Sports	Hang gliding
8.0	Sports	Hockey, field
8.0	Sports	Hockey, ice
4.0	Sports	Horseback riding, general
3.5	Sports	Horseback riding, saddling horse
6.5	Sports	Horseback riding, trotting
2.5	Sports	Horseback riding, walking
3.0	Sports	Horseshoe pitching, quoits
12.0	Sports	Jai alai
10.0	Sports	Judo, jujitsu, karate, kick boxing, tae kwan do
4.0	Sports	Juggling
7.0	Sports	Kickball
8.0	Sports	Lacrosse
4.0	Sports	Moto-cross
9.0	Sports	Orienteering
10.0	Sports	Paddleball, competitive
6.0	Sports	Paddleball, casual, general
8.0	Sports	Polo
10.0	Sports	Racquetball, competitive
7.0	Sports	Racquetball, casual, general
11.0	Sports	Rock climbing, ascending rock
8.0	Sports	Rock climbing, rapelling
12.0	Sports	Rope jumping, fast
10.0	Sports	Rope jumping, moderate, general
8.0	Sports	Rope jumping, slow
10.0	Sports	Rugby
3.0	Sports	Shuffleboard, lawn bowling

METS	Activity category	Specific activity
5.0	Sports	Skateboarding
7.0	Sports	Skating, roller
3.5	Sports	Sky diving
10.0	Sports	Soccer, competitive
7.0	Sports	Soccer, casual, general
5.0	Sports	Softball or baseball, fast or slow pitch, general
4.0	Sports	Softball, officiating
6.0	Sports	Softball, pitching
12.0	Sports	Squash
4.0	Sports	Table tennis, ping pong
4.0	Sports	Tai chi
7.0	Sports	Tennis, general
6.0	Sports	Tennis, doubles
8.0	Sports	Tennis, singles
3.5	Sports	Trampoline
4.0	Sports	Volleyball, competitive, in gymnasium
3.0	Sports	Volleyball, noncompetitive; 6-9 member team, general
8.0	Sports	Volleyball, beach
6.0	Sports	Wrestling (one match = 5 min)
7.0	Sports	Wallyball, general
2.0	Transportation	Automobile or light truck (not a semi) driving
2.0	Transportation	Flying airplane
2.5	Transportation	Motor scooter, motor cycle
6.0	Transportation	Pushing plane in and out of hangar
3.0	Transportation	Driving heavy truck, tractor, bus
7.0	Walking	Backpacking, general
3.5	Walking	Carrying infant or 15-lb load (e.g., suitcase), level ground or downstairs
9.0	Walking	Carrying load upstairs, general
5.0	Walking	Carrying 1- to 15-lb load, upstairs
6.0	Walking	16- to 24-lb load, upstairs
8.0	Walking	Carrying 25- to 49-lb load, upstairs
10.0	Walking	Carrying 50- to 74-lb load, upstairs
12.0	Walking	Carrying 74 + -lb load, upstairs
7.0	Walking	Climbing hills with 0- to 9-lb load
7.5	Walking	Climbing hills with 10- to 20-lb load
8.0	Walking	Climbing hills with 21- to 42-lb load
9.0	Walking	Climbing hills with 42 + -lb load
3.0	Walking	Downstairs
6.0	Walking	Hiking, cross-country
6.5	Walking	Marching, rapidly, military
2.5	Walking	Pushing or pulling stroller with child
6.5	Walking	Race walking
8.0	Walking	Rock or mountain climbing
8.0	Walking	Up stairs, using or climbing up ladder
4.0	Walking	Using crutches

METS	Activity category	Specific activity
2.0	Walking	Walking, less than 2.0 mph, level ground, strolling, household walking, very slow
2.5	Walking	Walking, 2.0 mph, level, slow pace, firm surface
3.0	Walking	Walking, 2.5 mph, firm surface
3.0	Walking	Walking, 2.5 mph, downhill
3.5	Walking	Walking, 3.0 mph, level, moderate pace, firm surface
4.0	Walking	Walking, 3.5 mph, level, brisk, firm surface
6.0	Walking	Walking, 3.5 mph, uphill
4.0	Walking	Walking, 4.0 mph, level, firm surface, very brisk pace
4.5	Walking	Walking, 4.5 mph, level, firm surface, very, very brisk
3.5	Walking	Walking, for pleasure, work break, walking the dog
5.0	Walking	Walking, grass track
4.0	Walking	Walking, to work or class
2.5	Water activities	Boating, power
4.0	Water activities	Canoeing, on camping trip
7.0	Water activities	Canoeing, portaging
3.0	Water activities	Canoeing, rowing, 2.0-3.9 mph, light effort
7.0	Water activities	Canoeing, rowing, 4.0-5.9 mph, moderate effort
12.0	Water activities	Canoeing, rowing, >6 mph, vigorous effort
3.5	Water activities	Canoeing, rowing, for pleasure, general
12.0	Water activities	Canoeing, rowing, in competition, or crew or sculling
3.0	Water activities	Diving, springboard or platform
5.0	Water activities	Kayaking
4.0	Water activities	Paddleboat
3.0	Water activities	Sailing, boat and board sailing, windsurfing, ice sailing, general
5.0	Water activities	Sailing, in competition
3.0	Water activities	Sailing, Sunfish/Laser/Hobby Cat, keel boats, ocean sailing, yachting
6.0	Water activities	Skiing, water
7.0	Water activities	Skimobiling
12.0	Water activities	Skin diving or scuba diving as frogman
16.0	Water activities	Skin diving, fast
12.5	Water activities	Skin diving, moderate
7.0	Water activities	Skin diving, scuba diving, general
5.0	Water activities	Snorkeling
3.0	Water activities	Surfing, body or board
10.0	Water activities	Swimming laps, freestyle, fast, vigorous effort
8.0	Water activities	Swimming laps, freestyle, slow, moderate or light effort
8.0	Water activities	Swimming, backstroke, general
10.0	Water activities	Swimming, breaststroke, general
11.0	Water activities	Swimming, butterfly, general
11.0	Water activities	Swimming, crawl, fast (75 yd · min^{-1}), vigorous effort
8.0	Water activities	Swimming, crawl, slow (50 yd · min^{-1}), moderate or light effort
6.0	Water activities	Swimming, lake, ocean, river
6.0	Water activities	Swimming, leisurely, not lap swimming, general
8.0	Water activities	Swimming, sidestroke, general
8.0	Water activities	Swimming, synchronized
10.0	Water activities	Swimming, treading water, fast, vigorous effort
4.0	Water activities	Swimming, treading water, moderate effort, general
10.0	Water activities	Water polo
3.0	Water activities	Water volleyball
5.0	Water activities	Whitewater rafting, kayaking, or canoeing
6.0	Winter activities	Moving ice house (set up/drill holes, etc.)
5.5	Winter activities	Skating, ice, 9 mph or less
7.0	Winter activities	Skating, ice, general
9.0	Winter activities	Skating, ice, rapidly, more than 9 mph
15.0	Winter activities	Skating, speed, competitive
7.0	Winter activities	Ski jumping (climb up carrying skis)
7.0	Winter activities	Skiing, general
7.0	Winter activities	Skiing, cross-country, 2.5 mph, slow or light effort, ski walking
8.0	Winter activities	Skiing, cross-country, 4.0-4.9 mph, moderate speed and effort, general
9.0	Winter activities	Skiing, cross-country, 5.0-7.9 mph, brisk speed, vigorous effort
14.0	Winter activities	Skiing, cross-country, >8.0 mph, racing
16.5	Winter activities	Skiing, cross-country, hard snow, uphill, maximum
5.0	Winter activities	Skiing, downhill, light effort
6.0	Winter activities	Skiing, downhill, moderate effort, general
8.0	Winter activities	Skiing, downhill, vigorous effort, racing
7.0	Winter activities	Sledding, tobogganing, bobsledding, luge
8.0	Winter activities	Snow shoeing
3.5	Winter activities	Snowmobiling

Additional values

2.0	Home activities (weaving at loom, sitting)
1.8	Music playing (accordion)
6.0	Occupation: lifting 22 lb 1 m
8.0	Occupation: lifting 45 lb 1 m
11.0	Occupation: lifting 65 lb 1 m
8.0	Walking, ice climbing
8.0	Sports: rollerskiing, 10 mph, no grade

METS	Activity category	Specific activity
10.0	Sports: rollerskiing, 11 mph, no grade	
11.0	Sports: rollerskiing, 12 mph, no grade	
12.0	Sports: rollerskiing, 9 mph, 6% grade	
7.5	Sports: in-line skating, 10 mph	
8.5	Sports: in-line skating, 11 mph	
10.0	Sports: in-line skating, 12 mph	
7.0	Water activities: underwater swimming, 1 mph	
9.0	Winter activities: figure skating	
14.0	Winter activities: skiing, competitive, short periods	

From Ainsworth, B.E., Haskell, W.L., Leon, A.S., Jacobs, D.R., Jr., Montoye, H.J., Sallis, J.F., and Paffenbarger, R.S. (1993). Compendium of physical activities: Classification of energy costs of human physical activities. *Medicine and Science in Sports and Exercise*, **25**, 71-80. Additional values from Montoye, H.J., Kemper, H.C.G., Saris, W.H.M., and Washburn, R.A. (1996). *Measuring physical activity and energy expenditure*. Champaign, IL: Human Kinetics.

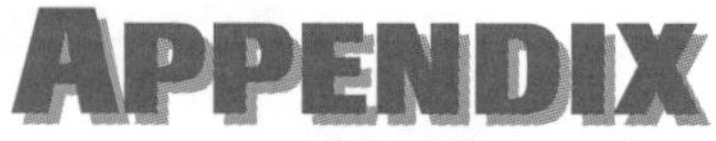

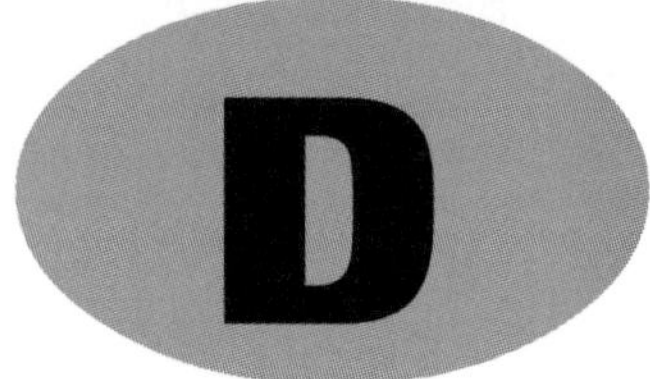

Recommended Dietary Allowances and Intakes

Estimated Safe and Adequate Daily Dietary Intakes of Selected Vitamins and Minerals[a]

		Vitamins		Trace elements[b]				
Category	Age (years)	Biotin (μg)	Pantothenic acid (mg)	Copper (mg)	Manganese (mg)	Fluoride (mg)	Chromium (μg)	Molybdenum (μg)
Infants	0-0.5	10	2	0.4-0.6	0.3-0.6	0.1-0.5	10-40	15-30
	0.5-1	15	3	0.6-0.7	0.6-1.0	0.2-1.0	20-60	20-40
Children	1-3	20	3	0.7-1.0	1.0-1.5	0.5-1.5	20-80	25-50
and	4-6	25	3-4	1.0-1.5	1.5-2.0	1.0-2.5	30-120	30-75
adolescents	7-10	30	4-5	1.0-2.0	2.0-3.0	1.5-2.5	50-200	50-150
	11 +	30-100	4-7	1.5-2.5	2.0-5.0	1.5-2.5	50-200	75-250
Adults		30-100	4-7	1.5-3.0	2.0-5.0	1.5-4.0	50-200	75-250

[a]Because there is less information on which to base allowances, these figures are not given in the main table of RDA and are provided here in the form of ranges of recommended intakes.

[b]Because the toxic levels for many trace elements may be only several times usual intakes, the upper levels for the trace elements given in this table should not be habitually exceeded.

Food and Nutrition Board, National Academy of Sciences—National Research Council Recommended Dietary Allowances[a], Revised 1989* (Designed for the maintenance of good nutrition of practically all healthy people in the United States)

							Fat-soluble vitamins				Water-soluble vitamins							Minerals						
	Age (years) or condition	Weight[b] (kg)	Weight[b] (lb)	Height[b] (cm)	Height[b] (in.)	Protein (g)	Vitamin A (μg R.E.)[c]	Vitamin D (μg)[d]	Vitamin E (mg α-T.E.)[e]	Vitamin K (μg)	Vitamin C (mg)	Thiamin (mg)	Riboflavin (mg)	Niacin (mg N.E.)[f]	Vitamin B_6 (mg)	Folate (μg)	Vitamin B_{12} (μg)	Calcium (mg)	Phosphorus (mg)	Magnesium (mg)	Iron (mg)	Zinc (mg)	Iodine (μg)	Selenium (μg)
Infants	0.0-0.5	6	13	60	24	13	375	7.5	3	5	30	0.3	0.4	5	0.3	25	0.3	400	300	40	6	5	40	10
	0.5-1.0	9	20	71	28	14	375	10	4	10	35	0.4	0.5	6	0.6	35	0.5	600	500	60	10	5	50	15
Children	1-3	13	29	90	35	16	400	10	6	15	40	0.7	0.8	9	1.0	50	0.7	800	800	80	10	10	70	20
	4-6	20	44	112	44	24	500	10	7	20	45	0.9	1.1	12	1.1	75	1.0	800	800	120	10	10	90	20
	7-10	28	62	132	52	28	700	10	7	30	45	1.0	1.2	13	1.4	100	1.4	800	800	170	10	10	120	30
Males	11-14	45	90	157	62	45	1000	10	10	45	50	1.3	1.5	17	1.7	150	2.0	1200	1200	270	12	15	150	40
	15-18	66	145	176	69	59	1000	10	10	65	60	1.5	1.8	20	2.0	200	2.0	1200	1200	400	12	15	150	50
	19-24	72	160	177	70	58	1000	10	10	70	60	1.5	1.7	19	2.0	200	2.0	1200	1200	350	10	15	150	70
	25-50	79	174	176	70	63	1000	5	10	80	60	1.5	1.7	19	2.0	200	2.0	800	800	350	10	15	150	70
	51 +	77	170	173	68	63	1000	5	10	80	60	1.2	1.4	15	2.0	200	2.0	800	800	350	10	15	150	70
Females	11-14	46	101	157	62	46	800	10	8	45	50	1.1	1.3	15	1.4	150	2.0	1200	1200	280	15	12	150	45
	15-18	55	120	163	64	44	800	10	8	55	60	1.1	1.3	15	1.5	180	2.0	1200	1200	300	15	12	150	50
	19-24	58	128	164	65	46	800	10	8	60	60	1.1	1.3	15	1.6	180	2.0	1200	1200	280	15	12	150	55
	25-50	63	138	163	64	50	800	5	8	65	60	1.1	1.3	15	1.6	180	2.0	800	800	280	15	12	150	55
	51 +	65	143	160	63	50	800	5	8	65	60	1.0	1.2	13	1.6	180	2.0	800	800	280	10	12	150	55
Pregnant						60	800	10	10	65	70	1.5	1.6	17	2.2	400	2.2	1200	1200	320	30	15	175	65
Lactating	1st 6 months					65	1300	10	12	65	95	1.6	1.8	20	2.1	280	2.6	1200	1200	355	15	19	200	75
	2nd 6 months					62	1200	10	11	65	90	1.6	1.7	20	2.1	260	2.6	1200	1200	340	15	16	200	75

[a]The allowances, expressed as average daily intakes over time, are intended to provide for individual variations among most normal people as they live in the United States under usual environmental stresses. Diets should be based on a variety of common foods in order to provide other nutrients for which human requirements have been less well defined.

[b]Weights and heights of reference adults are actual medians for the U.S. population of the designated age, as reported by NHANES II. The median weights and heights of those under 19 years of age were taken from Hamill et al. (1979). The use of these figures does not imply that the height to weight ratios are ideal.

[c]Retinol equivalents. 1 retinol equivalent = 1 μg retinol or 6 μg ß-carotene.

[d]As cholecalciferol, 10 μg cholecalciferol = 400 I.U. of vitamin D.

[e]α-Tocopherol equivalents. 1 mg d-α tocopherol = 1 α-T.E.

[f]1 N.E. (niacin equivalent) is equal to 1 mg of niacin or 60 mg of dietary tryptophan.

*Reprinted with permission from *Recommended Dietary Allowances, 10th Edition.* © 1989 by the National Academy of Sciences. Published by National Academy Press.

Estimated Sodium, Chloride, and Potassium Minimum Requirements of Healthy People[a]

Age	Weight (kg)[a]	Sodium (mg)[ab]	Chloride (mg)[ab]	Potassium (mg)[c]
Months				
0-5	4.5	120	180	500
6-11	8.9	200	300	700
Years				
1	11.0	225	350	1000
2-5	16.0	300	500	1400
6-9	25.0	400	600	1600
10-18	50.0	500	750	2000
> 18[d]	70.0	500	750	2000

[a]No allowance has been included for large, prolonged losses from the skin through sweat.

[b]There is no evidence that higher intakes confer any health benefit.

[c]Desirable intakes of potassium may considerably exceed these values (~3500 mg for adults).

[d]No allowance included for growth. Values for those below 18 years assume a growth rate at the 50th percentile reported by the National Center for Health Statistics (Hamill et al., 1979) and averaged for males and females.

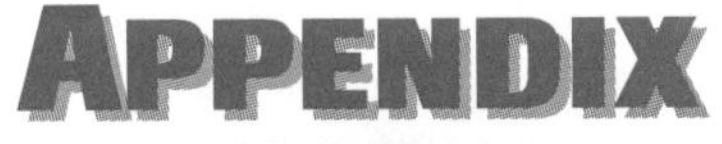

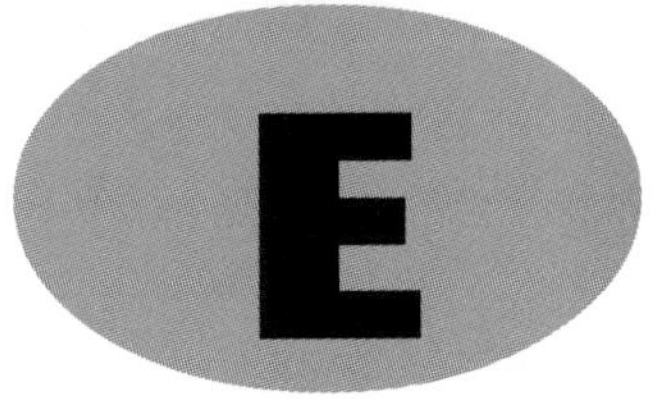

Medications and Their Effects

Generic and Brand Names of Common Drugs by Class

Generic name	Brand name
Beta blockers	
Acebutolol	Sectral
Atenolol	Tenormin
Metoprolol	Lopressor, Toprol
Nadolol	Corgard
Pindolol	Visken
Propranolol	Inderal
Timolol	Blocadren
Carteolol	Cartrol
Betaxolal	Kerlone
Bisoprolol	Zebeta
Penbutolol	Levatol
Alpha$_1$ blockers	
Prazosin	Minipress
Terazosin	Hytrin
Doxazosin	Cardura
Alpha and beta blocker	
Labetalol	Trandate, Normodyne
Antiadrenergic agents without selective receptor blockade	
Clonidine	Catapres
Guanabenz	Wyntensin
Guanethidine	Ismelin
Guanfacine	Tenex
Methyldopa	Aldomet
Reserpine	Serapasil
Guanadrel	Hylorel

Generic name	Brand name
Nitrates and nitroglycerin	
Isosorbide dinitrate	Isordil, Diltrate
Nitroglycerin	Nitrostat, Nitrolingual spray
Nitroglycerin ointment	Nitrol ointment
Nitroglycerin patches	Transderm Nitro, Nitro-Dur II, Nitrodisc
Isosorbide mononitrate	Ismo, Monoket
Pentaerythritol tetranitrate	Cardilate
Calcium channel blockers	
Diltiazem	Cardizem
Nifedipine	Procardia, Adalat
Verapamil	Calan, Isoptin
Nicardipine	Cardene
Amlodipine	Norvasc
Felodipine	Plendil
Isradipine	DynaCirc
Nimodipine	Nimotop
Bepridil	Vascor
Digitalis	
Digoxin	Lanoxin
Diuretics	
Thiazides	
Hydrochlorothiazide (HCTZ)	Esidrix

Generic and Brand Names of Common Drugs by Class *(continued)*

Generic name	Brand name
Diuretics *(continued)*	
"Loop"	
Furosemide	Lasix
Bumetanide	Bumex
Ethacrynic acid	Edecrin
Potassium-sparing	
Spironolactone	Aldactone
Triamterene	Dyrenium
Amiloride	Midamor
Combinations	
Triamterene and hydrochlorothiazide	Dyazide, Maxzide
Amiloride and hydrochlorothiazide	Moduretic
Others	
Metolazone	Zaroxolyn
Peripheral vasodilators (nonadrenergic)	
Hydralazine	Apresoline
Minoxidil	Loniten
Angiotensin-converting enzyme (ACE) inhibitors	
Catopril	Capoten
Enalapril	Vasotec
Lisinopril	Prinivil, Zestril
Ramipril	Altace
Benazepril	Lotensin
Fosinopril	Monopril
Quinapril	Accupril
Antiarrhythmic agents	
Class I	
IA	
Quinidine	Quinidex, Quinaglute
Procainamide	Pronestyl, Procan SR
Disopyramide	Norpace
IB	
Tocainide	Tonocard
Mexiletine	Mexitil
Lidocaine	Xylocaine, Xylocard

Reprinted from American College of Sports Medicine 1995.

Generic name	Brand name
Antiarrhythmic agents *(continued)*	
Class I *(continued)*	
IC	
Encainide	Enkaid
Flecainide	Tambocor
Multiclass	
Ethmozine	Moricizine
Class II	
ß-Blockers	
Class III	
Amiodarone	Cordarone
Bretylium	Bretylol
Sotalol	Betapace
Class IV	
Calcium channel blockers	
Sympathomimetic agents	
Ephedrine	Adrenalin
Epinephrine	Alupent
Metaproterenol	Proventil, Ventolin
Albuterol	Bronkosol
Isoetharine	Brethine
Cromolyn sodium	Intal
Antihyperlipidemic agents	
Cholestyramine	Questran
Colestipol	Colestid
Gemfibrozil	Lopid
Lovastatin	Mevacor
Nicotinic acid (niacin)	Nicobid, Nicolar, Slo-Niacin
Probucol	Lorelco
Pravastatin	Pravachol
Simvastatin	Zocor
Fluvastatin	Lescol
Other	
Dipyridamole	Persantine
Warfarin	Coumadin
Pentoxifylline	Trental

Effects of Medications on Heart Rate, Blood Pressure, the Electrocardiogram (ECG), and Exercise Capacity

Medications	Heart rate	Blood pressure	ECG	Exercise capacity
I. Beta blockers (including labetalol)	↓* (R and E)	↓ (R and E)	↓ HR* (R) ↓ ischemia‡ (E)	↑ in patients with angina; ↓ or ↔ in patients without angina
II. Nitrates	↑ (R) ↑ or ↔ (E)	↓ (R) ↓ or ↔ (E)	↑ HR (R) ↑ or ↔ HR (E) ↓ ischemia‡ (E)	↑ in patients with angina; ↔ in patients without angina; ↑ or ↔ in patients with congestive heart failure (CHF)
III. Calcium channel blockers				
Felodipine Isradipine Nicardipine Nifedipine	↑ or ↔ (R and E)	↓ (R and E)	↑ or ↔ HR (R and E) ↓ ischemia‡ (E)	↑ in patients with angina; ↔ in patients without angina
Bepridil Diltiazem Verapamil	↓ (R and E)		↓ HR (R and E) ↓ ischemia‡ (E)	
IV. Digitalis	↓ in patients with atrial fibrillation and possibly CHF Not significantly altered in patients with sinus rhythm	↔	May produce non-specific S-T/T wave changes (R) May produce S-T segment depression (E)	Improved only in patients with atrial fibrillation or in patients with CHF
V. Diuretics	↔	↔ or ↓ (R and E)	↔ (R) May cause PVCs and "false positive" test results if hypokalemia occurs May cause PVCs if hypomagnesemia occurs (E)	↔, except possibly in patients with CHF
VI. Vasodilators, nonadrenergic	↑ or ↔ (R and E)	↓ (R and E)	↑ or ↔ (R and E)	↔, except ↑ or ↔ in patients with CHF
ACE inhibitors	↔	↓ (R and E)	↔	↔, except ↑ or ↔ in patients with CHF
Alpha-adrenergic blockers	↔	↓ (R and E)	↔	↔
Anti-adrenergic agents without selective blockade of peripheral receptors	↓ or ↔ (R and E)	↓ (R and E)	↓ or ↔ HR (R and E)	↔

Medications	Heart rate	Blood pressure	ECG	Exercise capacity
VII. Antiarrhythmic agents		All antiarrhythmic agents may cause new or worsened arrhythmias (proarrhythmic effect)		
Class I				
Quinidine Disopyramide	↑ or ↔ (R and E)	↓ or ↔ (R) ↔ (E)	↑ or ↔ HR (R) May prolong QRS and Q-T intervals (R) Quinidine may result in "false negative" test results (E)	↔
Procainamide	↔	↔	May prolong QRS and Q-T intervals (R) May result in "false positive" test results (E)	↔
Phenytoin Tocainide Mexiletine	↔	↔	↔	↔
Flecainide Moricizine	↔	↔	May prolong QRS and Q-T intervals (R) ↔ (E)	↔
Propafenone	↓ (R) ↓ or ↔ (E)	↔	↓ HR (R) ↓ or ↔ HR (E)	↔
Class II Beta blockers (see I.)				
Class III Amiodarone	↓ (R and E)	↔	↓ HR (R) ↔ (E)	↔
Class IV Calcium channel blockers (see III.)				
VIII. Bronchodilators	↔	↔	↔	Bronchodilators ↑ exercise capacity in patients limited by bronchospasm
Anticholinergic agents Methylxanthines	↑ or ↔ (R and E)	↔	↑ or ↔ HR May produce PVCs (R and E)	
Sympathomimetic agents	↑ or ↔ (R and E)	↑, ↔, or ↓ (R and E)	↑ or ↔ HR (R and E)	↔
Cromolyn sodium	↔	↔	↔	↔
Corticosteroids	↔	↔	↔	↔
IX. Hyperlipidemic agents	Clofibrate may provoke arrhythmias, angina in patients with prior myocardial infarction Dextrothyroxine may ↑ HR and BP at rest and during exercise, provoke arrhythmias, and worsen myocardial ischemia and angina Nicotinic acid may ↓ BP Probucol may cause Q-T interval prolongation All other hyperlipidemic agents have no effect on HR, BP, and ECG			↔

Medications	Heart rate	Blood pressure	ECG	Exercise capacity
X. Psychotropic medications				
Minor tranquilizers	May ↓ HR and BP by controlling anxiety. No other effects.			
Antidepressants	↑ or ↔ (R and E)	↓ or ↔	Variable (R) May result in "false positive" test results (E)	
Major tranquilizers	↑ or ↔ (R and E)	↓ or ↔	Variable (R) May result in "false positive" or "false negative" test results (E)	
Lithium	↔	↔	May result in T wave changes and arrhythmias (R and E)	
XI. Nicotine	↑ or ↔ (R and E)	↑ (R and E)	↑ or ↔ HR May provoke ischemia, arrhythmias (R and E)	↔, except ↓ or ↔ in patients with angina
XII. Antihistamines	↔	↔	↔	↔
XIII. Cold medications with sympathomimetic agents	Effects similar to those described in sympathomimetic agents, although magnitude of effects is usually smaller			↔
XIV. Thyroid medications Only levothyroxine	↑ (R and E)	↑ (R and E)	↑ HR. May provoke arrhythmias ↑ ischemia (R and E)	↔, unless angina worsened
XV. Alcohol	↔	Chronic use may have role in ↑ BP (R and E)	May provoke arrhythmias (R and E)	↔
XVI. Hypoglycemic agents Insulin and oral agents	↔	↔	↔	↔
XVII. Dipyridamole	↔	↔	↔	↔
XVIII. Anticoagulants	↔	↔	↔	↔
XIX. Anti-gout medications	↔	↔	↔	↔
XX. Antiplatelet medications	↔	↔	↔	↔
XXI. Pentoxifylline	↔	↔	↔	↑ or ↔ in patients limited by intermittent claudication
XXII. Caffeine	Variable effects depending upon previous use Variable effects on exercise capacity May provoke arrhythmias			
XXIII. Diet pills	↑ or ↔	↑ or ↔	↑ or ↔ HR	

Key: ↑ = increase, ↔ = no effect, ↓ = decrease.
*Beta-blockers with ISA lower resting HR only slightly.
‡May prevent or delay myocardial ischemia (see text).
R = rest; E = exercise.

Bibliography

Abraham, W.M. (1977). Factors in delayed muscle soreness. *Medicine and Science in Sports,* **9**, 11-20.

Ainsworth, B.E., Haskell, W.L., Leon, A.S., Jacobs, D.R., Jr., Montoye, H.J., Sallis, J.F., & Paffenbarger, R.S. (1993). Compendium of physical activities: Classification of energy costs of human physical activities. *Medicine and Science in Sports and Exercise,* **25**, 71-80.

Allerheiligen, W.B. (1994). Speed development and plyometric training. In T.R. Baechle (Ed.), *Essentials of strength training and conditioning* (pp. 314-344). Champaign, IL: Human Kinetics.

American Academy of Orthopedic Surgeons. (1977). *Emergency care and transportation of the sick and injured* (2nd ed.). Menasha, WI: George Banta.

American Alliance for Health, Physical Education, Recreation and Dance. (1984). *Technical manual: Health-related physical fitness*. Reston, VA: Author.

American Alliance for Health, Physical Education, Recreation and Dance. (1988). *Physical best*. Reston, VA: Author.

American Association for Active Lifestyles (1995). *Physical best and individuals with disabilities*. Reston, VA: AAHPERD.

American College of Obstetricians and Gynecologists (ACOG). (1994). Exercise during pregnancy and the postpartum period. *ACOG Technical Bulletin #189.*

American College of Sports Medicine. (1975). Prevention of heat injuries during distance running. *Medicine and Science in Sports,* **7**, vii-viii.

American College of Sports Medicine. (1978). The recommended quality and quantity of exercise for developing and maintaining fitness in healthy adults. *Medicine and Science in Sports and Exercise,* **10**, vii-x.

American College of Sports Medicine. (1980). *Guidelines for graded exercise testing and exercise prescription* (2nd ed.). Philadelphia: Lea & Febiger.

American College of Sports Medicine. (1985). The prevention of thermal injuries during distance running. *Medicine and Science in Sports and Exercise,* **19**, 529-533.

American College of Sports Medicine. (1987). Position stand on the use of anabolic-androgenic steroids in sports. *Medicine and Science in Sports and Exercise,* **19**, 534-539.

American College of Sports Medicine. (1990). The recommended quantity and quality of exercise for developing and maintaining cardiorespiratory and muscular fitness in healthy adults. *Medicine and Science in Sports and Exercise,* **22**, 265-274.

American College of Sports Medicine. (1991). *Guidelines for exercise testing and prescription* (4th ed.). Philadelphia: Lea & Febiger.

American College of Sports Medicine. (1993a). Position stand: Physical activity, physical fitness, and hypertension. *Medicine and Science in Sports and Exercise,* **25**, i-x.

American College of Sports Medicine. (1993b) Summary statement: Workshop on physical activity and public health. *Sports Medicine Bulletin,* **28**, 7.

American College of Sports Medicine. (1995). *ACSM's guidelines for exercise testing and prescription* (5th ed.). Baltimore: Williams & Wilkins.

American College of Sports Medicine. (1996). Position stand on exercise and fluid replacement. *Medicine and Science in Sports and Exercise*, **28**, i-vii.

American Diabetes Association. (1985). *Fact sheet on diabetes*. Alexandria, VA: Author.

American Diabetes Association. (1990). Diabetes and exercise: Position statement. *Diabetes Care*, **13**, 804-805.

American Diabetes Association. (1994). Position statement: Nutritional recommendations and principles for people with diabetes mellitus. *Diabetes Care*, **17**, 519-522.

American Dietetic Association. (1987). Nutrition for physical fitness and athletic performance for adults. *ADA Reports*, **87**, 933-939.

American Dietetic Association & Canadian Dietetic Association. (1993). Position of the American Dietetic Association and the Canadian Dietetic Association: Nutrition for physical fitness and athletic performance for adults. *Journal of the American Dietetic Association*, **93**, 691-696.

American Heart Association. (1987a). *Diet and coronary heart disease*. Dallas: Author.

American Heart Association. (1987b). *Heartsaver manual: A student handbook for cardiopulmonary resuscitation*. Dallas: Author.

American Heart Association. (1992). Statement on exercise. *Circulation*, **86**, 340-344.

American Heart Association Committee Report. (1982). Rationale of the diet-heart statement of the American Heart Association. *Nutrition Today*, Sept./Oct., 16-20; Nov./Dec., 15-19.

American Heart Association Committee on Stress, Strain, and Heart Disease. (1977). Report. *Circulation*, **55**, 1-11.

American Hospital Formulary Service. (1993). *Drug information '93*. Bethesda, MD: American Society of Hospital Pharmacists.

American Medical Association. (1966). *Standard nomenclature of athletic injuries*. Chicago: Author.

American Psychiatric Association. (1994). *Diagnostic and statistical manual of mental disorders* (4th ed.). Washington, DC: American Psychiatric Press.

American Red Cross (1993a). *Adult CPR*. St. Louis: C.V. Mosby.

American Red Cross (1993b). *Community CPR*. St. Louis: C.V. Mosby.

American Red Cross (1993c). *Community first aid and safety*. St. Louis: C.V. Mosby.

American Red Cross (1993d). *Emergency response*. St. Louis: C.V. Mosby.

American Red Cross (1993e). *Preventing disease transmission*. St. Louis: C.V. Mosby.

Andersen, P. (1975). Capillary density in skeletal muscle of man. *Acta Physiological Scandinavian*, **95**, 203-205.

Appell, H.J. (1990). Muscular atrophy following immobilization. *Sports Medicine*, **10**, 42-58.

Arnheim, D.D. (1987). *Essentials of athletic training*. St.Louis: Times Mirror/Mosby.

Arnheim, D.D. (1989). *Modern principles of athletic training*. St. Louis: Times Mirror/Mosby.

Arnheim, D.D., & Prentice, W.E. (1993). *Principles of athletic training*. St. Louis: C.V. Mosby.

Asmussen, E., & Bonde-Peterson, F. (1974). Storage of elastic energy in skeletal muscles in man. *Acta Physiological Scandinavian*, **91**, 385-392.

Åstrand, I. (1960). Aerobic work capacity in men and women with special reference to age. *Acta Physiologica Scandinavica*, **49**(Suppl. 169), 1-92.

Åstrand, P.-O. (1952). *Experimental studies of physical working capacity in relation to sex and age*. Copenhagen: Ejnar Munksgaard.

Åstrand, P.-O. (1979). *Work tests with the bicycle ergometer*. Varberg, Sweden: Monark-Crescent AB.

Åstrand, P.-O. (1984). Principles of ergometry and their implications in sport practice. *International Journal of Sports Medicine*, **5**, 102-105.

Åstrand, P.-O., & Rhyming, I. (1954). A nomogram for calculation of aerobic capacity (physical fitness) from pulse rate during submaximal work. *Journal of Applied Physiology*, **7**, 218-221.

Åstrand, P.-O., & Rodahl, K. (1977, 1986). *Textbook of work physiology* (1st, 2nd, and 3rd eds.). New York: McGraw-Hill.

Åstrand, P.-O., & Saltin, B. (1961). Maximal oxygen uptake and heart rate in various types of muscular activity. *Journal of Applied Physiology*, **16**, 977-981.

Atha, J. (1981). Strengthening muscle. *Exercise and Science Reviews*, **9**, 1-73.

Babcock, M., Paterson, D.H., & Cunningham, D.A. (1994). Effects of aerobic endurance training on gas exchange kinetics of older men. *Medicine and Science in Sports and Exercise*, **26**, 447-452.

Baechle, T.R. (1994). *Essentials of strength training and conditioning*. Champaign, IL: Human Kinetics.

Balke, B. (1963). A simple field test for assessment of physical fitness. *Civil Aeromedical Research Institute Report*, 63-66. Oklahoma City: Civil Aeromedical Research Institute.

Balke, B. (1970). *Advanced exercise procedures for evaluation of the cardiovascular system* (Monograph). Milton, WI: Burdick.

Balke, B., & Ware, R.W. (1959). An experimental study of "physical fitness" of Air Force personnel. *Armed Forces Medical Journal*, **10**, 675-688.

Barnard, R.J., Gardner, G.W., Diaco, N.V., MaCalpin, R.N., & Kattus, A.A. (1973). Cardiovascular responses to sudden strenuous exercise—heart rate, blood pressure and ECG. *Journal of Applied Physiology*, **34**, 833-837.

Barnham, J.N. (1960). *A comparison of the effectiveness of isometric and isotonic exercise when performed at different frequencies per week*. Unpublished doctoral dissertation, Louisiana State University.

Barrow, M. (1992). *Understanding cardiovascular diseases*. Gainesville, FL: Cor-Ed.

Bassett, D.R., Jr. (1994). Skeletal muscle characteristics: Relationships to cardiovascular risk factors. *Medicine and Science in Sports and Exercise*, **26**, 957-966.

Bassett, D.R., Jr., Giese, M.D., Nagle, F.J., Ward, A., Raab, D.M., & Balke, B. (1985). Aerobic requirements of overground versus treadmill running. *Medicine and Science in Sports and Exercise*, **17**, 477-481.

Bassett, D.R., Sr., & Zweifler, A.J. (1990). Risk factors and risk factor management. In G.B. Zelenock, L.G. D'Alecy, J.C. Fantone, III, M. Shlafer, & J.C. Stanley (Eds.), *Clinical ischemic syndromes* (pp. 15-46). St. Louis: C.V. Mosby.

Battie, M.C., Videman, T., Gill, K., Moneta, G.B., Nyman, R., Kaprio, J., & Koskenvuo, M. (1991). Smoking and lumbar intervertebral disc degeneration: An MRI study of identical twins. *Spine*, **16**(9), 1015-1021.

Baum. (1961). *Sphygmomanometers, principles and precepts*. (1961). New York: Author.

Benson, H. (1975). *The relaxation response*. New York: Morrow.

Berg, K.E. (1986). *Diabetic's guide to health and fitness*. Champaign, IL: Life Enhancement (Human Kinetics).

Berger, M., & Kemmer, F.W. (1990). Discussion: Exercise, fitness, and diabetes. In C. Bouchard, R.J. Shephard, T. Stephens, J.R. Sutton, & B.D. McPherson (Eds.), *Exercise, fitness, and health* (pp. 491-495). Champaign, IL: Human Kinetics.

Berger, R.A., & Hardage, B. (1967). Effect of maximum loads for each of ten repetitions on strength improvement. *Research Quarterly*, **38**, 715-718.

Berman, L.B., & Sutton, J.R. (1986). Exercise and the pulmonary patient. *Journal of Cardiopulmonary Rehabilitation*, **6**, 52-61.

Berne, R.M, & Levy, M.N. (1992). *Cardiovascular physiology* (6th ed.). St. Louis: C.V. Mosby.

Berning, J.R. (1995). Nutritional concerns of recreational endurance athletes with an emphasis on swimming. In C.G.R. Jackson (Ed.), *Nutrition for the recreational athlete* (pp. 55-68). Boca Raton: CRC Press.

Biering-Sorensen, F. (1984). Physical measurements as risk indicators for low back trouble over a one-year period, *Spine*, **9**, 106.

Bjorntrop, P. (1985). Regional patterns of fat distribution. *Annals of Internal Medicine*, **103**, 994-995.

Blair, S.N., Kohl, H.W., III, Barlow, C.E., Paffenbarger, R.S., Jr., Gibbons, L.W., & Marcera, C.A. (1995). Changes in physical fitness and all-cause mortality. *Journal of the American Medical Association*, **273**, 1093-1098.

Blair, S.N., Kohl, H.W., III, Paffenbarger, R.S., Jr., Clark, D.G., Cooper, K.H., & Gibbons, L.W. (1989). Physical fitness and all-cause mortality. *Journal of the American Medical Association*, **262**, 2395-2401.

Blair, S.N., Painter, P., Pate, R.R., Smith, L.K., & Taylor, C.B. (Eds.) (1988). *Resource manual for guidelines for exercise testing and prescription*. Philadelphia: Lea & Febiger.

Bloomfield, J., Fricker, P.A., & Fitch, K.P. (Eds.). (1992). *Textbook of science and medicine in sport*. Champaign, IL: Human Kinetics.

Booher, J.M., & Thibadeau, G.A. (1994). *Athletic injury assessment* (3rd ed.). St. Louis: C.V. Mosby.

Borenstein, D., & Wiesel, S. (1989). *Low back pain: Medical diagnosis and comprehensive management*. Philadelphia: W.B. Saunders.

Borg, G.A.V. (1982). Psychological bases of physical exertion. *Medicine and Science in Sports and Exercise*, **14**(5), 377-381.

Bouchard, C., Lesage, R., Lortie, G., Simoneau, J., Hamel, P., Boulay, M., Perusse, L., Theriault, G., & Leblank, C. (1986). Aerobic performance in brothers, dizygotic and monozygotic twins. *Medicine and Science in Sports and Exercise*, **18**, 639-646.

Bouchard, C., & Perusse, L. (1994). Heredity, activity level, fitness, and health. In C. Bouchard, R.J. Shephard, & T. Stephens (Eds.), *Physical activity, fitness, and health* (pp. 106-118). Champaign, IL: Human Kinetics.

Bouchard, C., Perusse, L., Leblanc, C., Tremblay, A., & Theriault, G. (1988). Inheritance of the amount and distribution of human body fat. *International Journal of Obesity*, **12**, 205-215.

Bouchard, C., Shephard, R.J., & Stephens, T. (Eds.). (1994). *Physical activity, fitness, and health*. Champaign, IL: Human Kinetics.

Bouchard, C., Shephard, R.J., Stephens, T., Sutton, J.R., & McPherson, B.D. (Eds.). (1990a). *Exercise, fitness, and health: A consensus of current knowledge*. Champaign, IL: Human Kinetics.

Bouchard, C., Shephard, R.J., Stephens, T., Sutton, J.R., & McPherson, B.D. (1990b). Exercise, fitness, and health: The consensus statement. In C. Bouchard, R.J. Shephard, T. Stephens, J.R. Sutton, & B.D. McPherson (Eds.), *Exercise, fitness, and health: A consensus of current knowledge* (pp. 3-28). Champaign, IL: Human Kinetics.

Bransford, D.R., & Howley, E.T. (1977). The oxygen cost of running in trained and untrained men and women. *Medicine and Science in Sports*, **9**, 41-44.

Braun, B., Zimmermann, M.B., & Kretchmer, N. (1995). Effects of exercise intensity on insulin sensitivity in women with non-insulin-dependent diabetes mellitus. *Journal of Applied Physiology*, **78**, 300-306.

Breslow, L. (1990). Lifestyle, fitness, and health. In C. Bouchard, R.J. Shephard, T. Stephens, J.R. Sutton, & B.D. McPherson (Eds.), *Exercise, fitness, and health: A consensus of current knowledge* (pp. 155-163). Champaign, IL: Human Kinetics.

Brooks, G.A. (1985). Anaerobic threshold: Review of the concept, and directions for future research. *Medicine and Science in Sports and Exercise*, **17**, 22-31.

Brooks, G.A., Fahey, T.D., & White, T.P. (1996). *Exercise physiology: Human bioenergetics and its application* (2nd ed.). Mountain View, CA: Mayfield.

Brotherhood, J.R. (1984). Nutrition and sports performance. *Sports Medicine*, **1**, 350-389.

Brown, D.R. (1990). Exercise, fitness, and mental health. In C. Bouchard, R.J. Shephard, T. Stephens, J.R. Sutton, & B.D. McPherson (Eds.), *Exercise, fitness, and health: A consensus of current knowledge* (pp. 607-626). Champaign, IL: Human Kinetics.

Brownell, K.D. (1994). *The LEARN program for weight control*. Dallas: American Health.

Brownell, K.D., & Kramer, F.M. (1989). Behavioral management of obesity. *Medical Clinics of North America*, **73**, 185-201.

Bruce, R.A. (1972). Multistage treadmill test of submaximal and maximal exercise. In American Heart Association (Ed.), *Exercise testing and training of apparently healthy individuals: A handbook for physicians* (pp. 32-34). New York: American Heart Association.

Brysasco, V., & Crimi, E. (1994). Allergy and sports: Exercise-induced asthma. *International Journal of Sportsmedicine*, **15**, S184-S186.

Bubb, W.J., Martin, A.D., & Howley, E.T. (1985). Predicting oxygen uptake during level walking at speeds of 80 to 130 meters per minute. *Journal of Cardiac Rehabilitation*, **5**(10), 462-465.

Burton, A.C., & Edholm, O.G. (1955). *Man in a cold environment*. London, England: Edward Arnold.

Buskirk, E.R., & Bass, D.E. (1974). Climate and exercise. In W.R. Johnson & E.R. Buskirk (Eds.), *Science and medicine of exercise and sport* (pp. 190-205). New York: Harper & Row.

Buskirk, E.R., & Hodgson, J.L. (1987). Age and aerobic power: The rate of change in men and women. *Federation Proceedings*, **46**, 1824-1829.

Byrnes, W.C., Clarkson, P.M., & Katch, F.I. (1985). Muscle soreness following resistive exercise with and without eccentric contraction. *Research Quarterly for Exercise and Sport*, **56**, 283-285.

Cady, L.D., Bischoff, D.P., & O'Connell, E.R., et al. (1979). Strength and fitness and subsequent back injuries in firefighters. *Journal of Occupational Medicine*, **21**, 269.

Cailliet, R. (1988). *Low back pain syndrome* (4th ed.). Philadelphia: F.A. Davis.

Caiozzo, V.J., Perrine, J.J., & Edgerton, V.R. (1981). Training induced alterations of the in vivo force velocity relationship of human muscle. *Journal of Applied Physiology: Respiratory, Environmental, and Exercise Physiology*, **51**, 750-754.

Campaigne, B.N., & Lampman, R.M. (1994). *Exercise in the clinical management of diabetes*. Champaign, IL: Human Kinetics.

Canadian Association for Health, Physical Education, Recreation and Dance. (1994). *The Canadian active living challenge*. Gloucester, Ontario: Author

Cantu, D.C. (1982). *Diabetes and exercise*. Ithaca, NY: Mouvement.

Carpenter, M.W. (1994). Physical activity, fitness, and health of the pregnant mother and fetus. In C. Bouchard, R.J. Shephard, & T. Stephens (Eds.), *Physical activity, fitness, and health* (pp. 967-979). Champaign, IL: Human Kinetics.

Caspersen, C.J., Powell, K.E., & Christensen, G.M. (1985). Physical activity, exercise, and physical fitness: Definition and distinctions for health-related research. *Public Health Reports*, **100**, 126-131.

Centers for Disease Control and Prevention. (1996a). *Guidelines for nutrition for adolescents*. Atlanta: Author.

Centers for Disease Control and Prevention. (1996b). *Guidelines for physical activity for adolescents.* Atlanta: Author.

Centers for Disease Control and Prevention, Division of Adolescent School Health. (1995). *Coordinated school health.* Atlanta: Author.

Chang, K., & Hossack, K.F. (1982). Effect of diltiazem on heart rate responses and respiratory variables during exercise: Implications for exercise prescription and cardiac rehabilitation. *Journal of Cardiac Rehabilitation,* **2**, 326-332.

Chilibeck, P.D., Sale, D.C., & Webber, C.E. (1995). Exercise and bone mineral density. *Sports Medicine,* **19**, 103-122.

Chodzko-Zajko, W. (1996). Physical capabilities, psychological responses, and the aging process. *Quest,* **48**(3), 311-329.

Chrischilles, E., Sherman, T., & Wallace, R. (1994). Cost and health effects of osteoporosis fractures. *Bone,* **15**, 377-386.

Christian, J.L. & Greger, J.L. (1985). *Nutrition for Living.* Redwood City, CA: Benjamin/Cummings.

Clarke, D.H. (1973). Adaptations in strength and muscular endurance resulting from exercise. In J. H. Wilmore (Ed.), *Exercise and Sports Science Reviews* (Vol. 1, pp. 73-102). New York: Academic Press.

Clarke, D.H., & Clarke, H.H. (1984). *Research processes in physical education, recreation, and health.* Englewood Cliffs, NJ: Prentice Hall.

Clarke, H.H. (1966). *Muscular strength and endurance in man.* Englewood Cliff, NJ: Prentice Hall.

Clarke, H.H. (1974). *Development of muscular strength and endurance.* Washington, DC: President's Council on Physical Fitness and Sports.

Clarke, H.H., Bailey, T.L., & Shay, C.L. (1952). New objective strength test of muscle groups by cable tension methods. *Research Quarterly,* **23**, 136.

Clarkson, P.M., Byrnes, W.C., McCormick, K.M., Turcotte, L.P., & White, J.S. (1986). Muscle soreness and serum creatine kinase activity following isometric, eccentric and concentric exercise. *International Journal of Sports Medicine,* **7**, 152-155.

Claytor, R.P. (1985). *Selected cardiovascular, sympathoadrenal, and metabolic responses to one-leg exercise training.* Unpublished doctoral dissertation, University of Tennessee, Knoxville.

Coggan, A.R., & Coyle, E.F. (1991). Carbohydrate ingestion during prolonged exercise: Effects on metabolism and performance. In J.O. Holloszy (Ed.), *Exercise and Sport Sciences Reviews* (Vol. 19, pp. 1-40). Baltimore: Williams & Wilkins.

Conroy, B.P., & Earle, R.W. (1994). Bone, muscle, and connective tissue adaptations to physical activity. In T.R. Baechle (Ed.), *Essentials of strength training and conditioning.* Champaign, IL: Human Kinetics.

Cooper Institute for Aerobics Research. (1992). *The Prudential FITNESSGRAM Test Administration Manual.* Dallas: Author.

Cooper, K.H. (1977). *The aerobics way.* New York: Bantam Books.

Corbin, C.B., Dowell, L.J., Lindsey, R., & Tolson, H. (1978). *Concepts in physical education.* Dubuque, IA: Brown.

Corbin, C.B., & Lindsey, R. (1991). *Concepts of physical fitness* (7th ed.). Dubuque, IA: Brown.

Costill, D.L. (1988). Carbohydrates for exercise: Dietary demands of optimal performance. *International Journal of Sports Medicine,* **9**, 1-18.

Costill, D.L., Daniels, J., Evans, W., Fink, W., Krahenbuhl, G., & Saltin, B. (1976). Skeletal muscle enzymes and fiber composition in male and female track athletes. *Journal of Applied Physiology,* **40**, 149-154.

Cottrell, R.R. (1992). *Weight control.* Guilford, CT: Dushkin.

Courneya, K.S., & McAuley, E. (1996). Cognitive mediators of the social influence-exercise adherence relationship: A test of the theory of planned behavior. *Journal of Behavioral Medicine,* **18**, 499-515.

Coyle, E.F. (1988). Detraining and retention of training-induced adaptations. In S.N. Blair, P. Painter, R.R. Pate, L.K. Smith, & C.B. Taylor (Eds.), *Resource manual for guidelines for exercise testing and prescription.* Philadelphia: Lea & Febiger.

Coyle, E.F., Hemmert, M.K., & Coggan, A.R. (1986). Effects of detraining on cardiovascular responses to exercise: Role of blood volume. *Journal of Applied Physiology,* **60**, 95-99.

Coyle, E.F., Martin, W.H., III, Bloomfield, S.A., Lowry, O.H., & Holloszy, J.O. (1985). Effects of detraining on responses to submaximal exercise. *Journal of Applied Physiology,* **59**, 853-859.

Coyle, E.F., Martin, W.H., III, Sinacore, D.R., Joyner, M.J., Hagberg, J.M., & Holloszy, J.O. (1984). Time course of loss of adaptation after stopping prolonged intense endurance training. *Journal of Applied Physiology,* **57**, 1857-1864.

Cunningham, J.J. (1991). Body composition as a determinant of energy expenditure: A synthetic review and a proposed general prediction equation. *American Journal of Clinical Nutrition,* **54**, 963-969.

Cureton, K.J., Sparling, P.B., Evans, B.W., Johnson, S.M., Kong, U.D., & Purvis, J.W. (1978). Effect of experimental alterations in excess weight on aerobic capacity and distance-running performance. *Medicine and Science in Sports*, **10**, 194-199.

Cureton, K.J., & Warren, G.L. (1990). Criterion-referenced standards for youth health-related fitness tests: A tutorial. *Research Quarterly for Exercise and Sports*, **61**, 7-19.

Dalsky, G.P., Stocke, K.S., Ehsani, A.A., Slatoplsky, E., Lee, W.C., & Birge, S.J. (1988). Weight-bearing exercise training and lumbar bone mineral content in post menopausal women. *Annals of Internal Medicine*, **108**, 824-828.

Daniels, J., Oldridge, N., Nagle, F., & White, B. (1978). Differences and changes in VO_2 among young runners 10-18 years of age. *Medicine and Science in Sports*, **10**, 200-203.

Daniels, J.T. (1985). A physiologist's view of running economy. *Medicine and Science in Sports and Exercise*, **17**, 332-338.

Davis, J.H. (1985). Anaerobic threshold: Review of the concept and directions for future research. *Medicine and Science in Sports and Exercise*, **17**, 6-18.

Dehn, M.M., & Mullins, C.B. (1977). Physiologic effects and importance of exercise in patients with coronary artery disease. *Cardiovascular Medicine*, **2**, 365.

DeLorme, T.L., & Watkins, A.L. (1948). Techniques of progressive resistance exercise. *Archives of Physical Medicine*, **29**, 263-271.

Dempster, P., & Aitkens, S. (1995). A new air displacement method for the determination of human body composition. *Medicine and Science in Sports and Exercise*, **27**, 1692-1697.

Department of Labor. Occupational Safety and Health Administration (1991). *Occupational exposure to bloodborne pathogens: Final rule*. Atlanta: Federal Register. Vol. 56., No. 235. Rules and Regulations.

Deprés, J-P., Bouchard, C., & Malina, R.M. (1990). Physical activity and coronary heart disease risk factors during childhood and adolescence. In K.B. Pandolf (Ed.), *Exercise and Sports Sciences Reviews*, **18**, 243-261.

Desmedt, J.E., & Godaux, E. (1977). Ballistic contractions in man: Characteristics recruitment pattern of single motor units of the tibialis muscle. *Journal of Physiology*, **264**, 673-694.

deVries, H.A. (1980). *Physiology of exercise for physical education and athletics* (3rd ed.). Dubuque, IA: Brown.

Dill, D.B. (1965). Oxygen cost of horizontal and grade walking and running on the treadmill. *Journal of Applied Physiology*, **20**, 19-22.

Dionne, F.T., Turcotte, L., Thibault, M-C., Boulay, M.R., Skinner, J.S., & Bouchard, C. (1991). Mitochondrial DNA sequence polymorphism, $\dot{V}O_2$max, and response to endurance training. *Medicine and Science in Sports and Exercise*, **23**, 177-185.

Dishman, R.K. (1990). Determinants of participation in physical activity. In C. Bouchard, R.J. Shephard, T. Stephens, J.R. Sutton, & B.D. McPherson (Eds.), *Exercise, fitness, and health* (pp. 75-101). Champaign, IL: Human Kinetics.

Dishman, R.K., & Buckworth, J. (1996). Adherence to physical activity. In W.P. Morgan (Ed.), *Physical activity and mental health* (pp. 63-80). Washington: Taylor & Francis.

Dishman, R.K., & Gettman, L.R. (1980). Psychobiologic influences in exercise adherence. *Journal of Sport Psychology*, **2**, 295-310.

Dodd, S., Powers, S.K., Callender, T., & Brooks, E. (1984). Blood lactate disappearance at various intensities of recovery exercise. *Journal of Applied Physiology*, **57**, 1462-1465.

Donnelly, J.E. (1990) *Living anatomy* (2nd ed.) Champaign, IL: Human Kinetics.

Doxey, G.E., Fairbanks, B., Housh, T.H., Johnson, G.O., Datch, F., and Lohman, T. (1987). Body composition round table: Part I. Scientific considerations. *National Strength and Conditioning Association Journal*, **9**, 14-15.

Drewnowski, A. (1994). Mechanisms of appetite and body weight regulation. In G.L. Blackburn & B.S. Kanders (Eds.), *Obesity: Pathophysiology, psychology, and treatment*. New York: Chapman & Hall.

Drinkwater, B.L. (1994). Physical activity, fitness, and osteoporosis. In C. Bouchard, R.J. Shephard, & T. Stephens (Eds.), *Physical activity, fitness, and health* (pp. 724-736). Champaign, IL: Human Kinetics.

Drinkwater, B.L., Denton, J.E., Kupprat, I.C., Talag, T.S., & Horvath, S.M. (1976). Aerobic power as a factor in women's response to work within hot environments. *Journal of Applied Physiology*, **41**, 815-821.

Dubin, D. (1989). *Rapid interpretation of EKGs* (4th ed.). Tampa, FL: Cover.

Duda, J. (1996). Goals: Process vs. outcome. *Quest*, **48**(3), 290-302.

Duffey, D.J., Horwitz, L.D., & Brammell, H.L. (1984). Nifedipine and the conditioning response. *American Journal of Cardiology*, **53**, 908-911.

Durstine, J.L., & Haskell, W.L. (1994). Effects of exercise training on plasma lipids and lipoproteins. In J.O. Holloszy (Ed.), *Exercise and Sport Sciences Reviews* (Vol. 22, pp. 477-521). Baltimore: Williams & Wilkins.

Durstine, J.L., King, A.C., Painter, P.L., Roitman, J.L., Zwiren, L.D., & Kenney, W.L. (1993). *ACSM's resource manual for guidelines for exercise testing and prescription* (2nd ed.). Philadelphia: Lea & Febiger.

Edington, D.W., & Edgerton, V.R. (1976). *The biology of physical activity*. Boston: Houghton Mifflin.

Eggleston, P.A. (1986). Pathophysiology of exercise-induced asthma. *Medicine and Science in Sports and Exercise*, **18**, 318-321.

Ekblom, B., Åstrand, P.O., Saltin, B., Stenberg, J., & Wallstrom, B. (1968). Effect of training on circulatory response to exercise. *Journal of Applied Physiology*, **24**, 518-528.

Ekelund, L.G., Haskell, W.L., Johnson, J.L., Wholey, F.S., Criqui, M.H., & Sheps, D.S. (1988). Physical fitness as a prevention of cardiovascular mortality in asymptomatic North American men. *New England Journal of Medicine*, **319**, 1379-1384.

Ellestad, M. (1994). *Stress testing: Principles and practice*. Philadelphia: F.A. Davis.

Erling, J., & Oldridge, N.B. (1985). Effects of a spousal-support program on exercise compliance with cardiac rehabilitation. *Medicine and Science in Sports and Exercise*, **17**, 284.

Ewy, G.A., & Bressler, R. (1982). *Current cardiovascular therapy*. New York: Raven Press.

Expert Panel on Detection, Evaluation, and Treatment of High Blood Cholesterol in Adults. (1993). Summary of the Second Report of the National Cholesterol Education Program (NCEP) Expert Panel on Detection, Evaluation, and Treatment of High Blood Cholesterol in Adults (Adult Treatment Panel II). *Journal of the American Medical Association*, **269**, 3015-3023.

Fagard, R.H. & Tipton, C.M. (1994). Physical activity, fitness, and hypertension. In C. Bouchard, R.J. Shephard, & T. Stephens (Eds.), *Physical activity, fitness, and health* (pp. 633-655). Champaign, IL: Human Kinetics.

Fahey, T.D. (1986). *Athletic training*. Mountain View, CA: Mayfield.

Faulkner, J.A., Roberts, D.E., Elk, R.L., & Conway, J. (1971). Cardiovascular responses to submaximum and maximum effort cycling and running. *Journal of Applied Physiology*, **30**, 457-461.

Faulkner, R.A., Sprigings, E.S., McQuarrie, A., & Bell, R.D. (1988). *Partial curl-up research project final report*. Report submitted to the Canadian Fitness and Lifestyle Research Institute.

Fleck, S.J., & Dean, L.S. (1987). Resistance-training experience and the pressor response during resistance exercise. *Journal of Applied Physiology*, **63**, 116-120.

Fleck, S.J., & Kraemer, W.J. (1987). *Designing resistance training programs*. Champaign, IL: Human Kinetics.

Fleck, S.J., & Schutt, R.C. (1985). Types of strength training. *Clinics in Sports Medicine*, **4**, 159-168.

Folinsbee, L.J. (1990). Discussion: Exercise and the environment. In C. Bouchard, R.J. Shephard, T. Stephens, J.R. Sutton, & B.D. McPherson (Eds.), *Exercise, fitness, and health* (pp. 179-183). Champaign, IL: Human Kinetics.

Food and Nutrition Board, National Research Council. (1989). *Recommended Dietary Allowances* (10th ed.). Washington, DC: National Academy Press.

Foster, C., Hare, J., Taylor, M., Goldstein, T., Anholm, J., & Pollock, M.L. (1984). Prediction of oxygen uptake during exercise testing in cardiac patients and healthy volunteers. *Journal of Cardiac Rehabilitation*, **4**, 537-542.

Foster G.D., & Wadden T.A. (1994). The psychology of obesity, weight loss, and weight regain: Research and clinical findings. In G.L. Blackburn & B.S. Kanders (Eds.), *Obesity: Pathophysiology, psychology, and treatment* (pp. 140-166). New York: Chapman & Hall.

Fox, E.L., Bowers, R.W., & Foss, M.L. (1993). *The physiological basis for exercise and sport* (5th ed.). Madison, WI: Brown and Benchmark.

Franklin, B.A. (1985). Exercise testing, training, and arm ergometry. *Sports Medicine*, **2**, 100-119.

Franklin, B.A. (1988). Program factors that influence exercise adherence: Practical adherence skills for the clinical staff. In R.K. Dishman (Ed.), *Exercise adherence* (pp. 237-258). Champaign, IL: Human Kinetics.

Franklin, B.A., Hellerstein, H.K., Gordon, S., & Timmis, G.C. (1986). Exercise prescription of the myocardial infarction patient. *Journal of Cardiopulmonary Rehabilitation*, **6**, 62-79.

Franklin, B.A., Oldridge, N.B., Stoedefalke, K.G., & Loechel, W.E. (1990). *On the ball*. Carmel, IN: Benchmark Press.

Franks, B.D. (1979). Methodology of the exercise ECG test. In E. K. Chung (Ed.), *Exercise electrocardiography: Practical approach* (pp. 46-61). Baltimore: Williams & Wilkins.

Franks, B.D. (1983). Physical warm-up. In M.H. Williams (Ed.), *Ergogenic aids in sports* (pp. 340-375). Champaign, IL: Human Kinetics.

Franks, B.D. (1989). *YMCA youth fitness test*. Champaign, IL: Human Kinetics.

Franks, B.D. (1995). What is stress? *Quest*, **46**(1), 1-7.

Franks, B.D., & Howley, E.T. (1989a). *Fitness facts: The healthy living handbook*. Champaign, IL: Human Kinetics.

Franks, B.D., & Howley, E.T. (1989b). *Fitness leaders' handbook*. Champaign, IL: Human Kinetics.

Franz, M.J. (1987). Exercise and the management of diabetes mellitus. *Journal of the American Dietetic Association*, **87**, 872-880.

Friden, J., Sjostrom, M., & Ekblom, B. (1983). Myofibrillar damage following intense eccentric exercise in man. *International Journal of Sports Medicine*, **4**, 170-176.

Froelicher, V.F. (1983). *Exercise testing and training*. Chicago: Year Book Medical.

Frohlich, E.D., Grim, C., Labarthe, D.R., Maxwell, M.H., Perloff, D., & Weidman, W.H. (1988). Recommendations for human blood-pressure determination by sphygmomanometers. *Circulation*, **77**, 501A-514A.

Frontera, W.R., Meredith, C.N., O'Reilly, K.P., Knuttgen, W.G., & Evans, W.J. (1988). Strength conditioning in older men: Skeletal muscle hypertrophy and improved function. *Journal of Applied Physiology*, **64**, 1038-1044.

Garrick, J.G., & Requa, R.K. (1988). Aerobic dance—A review. *Sports Medicine*, **6**, 169-179.

Gerhard, H., & Schachter, E.N. (1980). Exercise-induced asthma. *Postgraduate Medicine*, **67**, 91-102.

Gettman, L.R. (1988a). Fitness testing. In S.N. Blair, P. Painter, R. Pate, L.K. Smith, & C.B. Taylor (Eds.), *Resource manual guidelines for exercise testing and prescription* (pp. 161-170). Philadelphia: Lea & Febiger.

Gettman, L.R. (1988b). Management skills required for exercise programs. In S.N. Blair, P. Painter, R. Pate, L.K. Smith, & C.B. Taylor (Eds.), *Resource manual guidelines for exercise testing and prescription* (pp. 377-389). Philadelphia: Lea & Febiger.

Gettman, L.R. (1993). Fitness testing. In L.L. Durstine, A.C. King, P.L. Painter, J.L. Roitman, L.D. Zwiren, & P.A. Malvern (Eds.), *ACSM's resource manual for guidelines for exercise testing and prescription* (2nd ed.). Philadelphia: Lea & Febiger.

Gettman, L.R., Ayres, J.J., Pollock, M.L., & Jackson, A. (1978). The effect of circuit weight training on strength, cardiorespiratory function and body composition of adult men. *Medicine and Science in Sports*, **10**, 171-176.

Gettman, L.R., & Pollock, M.L. (1981). Circuit weight training: A critical review of its physiological benefits. *The Physician and Sportsmedicine*, **9**, 44-66.

Giacca, A., Shi, Z.Q., Marliss, E.B., Zinman, B., & Vranic, M. (1994). Physical activity, fitness, and Type I diabetes. In C. Bouchard, R. J. Shephard, & T. Stephens (Eds.), *Physical activity, fitness, and health* (pp. 656-668). Champaign, IL: Human Kinetics.

Gibson, R.S. (1993). *Nutritional assessment: A laboratory manual*. New York: Oxford University Press.

Giese, M.D. (1988). Organization of an exercise session. In S.N. Blair, P. Painter, R. Pate, L.K. Smith, & C.B. Taylor (Eds.), *Resource manual guidelines for exercise testing and prescription* (pp. 244-247). Philadelphia: Lea & Febiger.

Gisolfi, C., & Wenger, C.B. (1984). Temperature regulation during exercise: Old concepts, new ideas. In R. Terjung (Ed.), *Exercise and Sports Science Reviews* (Vol. 12, pp. 339-372). Lexington, MA: Collamore Press.

Gisolfi, G.V., & Cohen, J. (1979). Relationships among training, heat acclimation, and heat tolerance in men and women: The controversy revisited. *Medicine and Science in Sports*, **11**, 56-59.

Gleeson, P.B., Protas, E.J., LeBlanc, A.D., Schneider, V.S., & Evans, H.J. (1990). Effects of weight lifting on bone mineral density in premenopausal women. *Journal of Bone Mineral Research*, **5**, 153-158.

Golding, L.A., Myers, C.R., & Sinning, W.E. (1989). *The Y's way to physical fitness*. Champaign, IL: Human Kinetics.

Goldman, H.I., & Becklake, M.R. (1959). Respiratory function tests. *American Review of Tuberculosis and Pulmonary Disease*, **79**, 457-467.

Goldschlager, N., & Goldman, M.J. (1989). *Principles of clinical electrocardiography*. San Mateo, CA: Appleton & Lange.

Goodman, L.S., & Gilman, A. (Eds.). (1975). *The pharmacological basis of therapeutics*. New York: Macmillan.

Gorely, T., & Gordon, S. (1995). An examination of the transtheoretical model and exercise behavior in older adults. *Journal of Sport and Exercise Psychology*, **17**, 312-324.

Gowitzke, B.A., & Milner, M. (1988). *Scientific bases of human movement* (3rd ed.). Baltimore: Williams & Wilkins.

Gracovetsky, S. (1988). *The spinal engine*. New York: Springer-Verlag.

Gracovetsky, S., & Farfan, H. (1986). The optimum spine. *Spine*, **11**, 543-572.

Gray, H. (1994). *Anatomy of the human body*. Philadelphia: Lea & Febiger.

Grilo, C.M., Brownell, K.D., & Stunkard, A.J. (1993). The metabolic and psychological importance of exercise in weight control. In A.J. Stunkard & T.A. Wadden (Eds.), *Obesity: Theory and therapy* (2nd ed.). New York: Raven Press.

Grover, R., Reeves, J., Grover, E., & Leathers, J. (1967). Muscular exercise in young men native to 3,100 m altitude. *Journal of Applied Physiology*, **22**, 555-564.

Gudat, U., Berger, M., & Lefèbvre, P.J. (1994). Physical activity, fitness, and non-insulin-dependent diabetes mellitus. In C. Bouchard, R.J. Shephard, & T. Stephens (Eds.), *Physical activity, fitness, and health* (pp. 669-683). Champaign, IL: Human Kinetics.

Hagberg, J.M. (1990). Exercise, fitness, and hypertension. In C. Bouchard, R.J. Shephard, T. Stephens, J.R. Sutton, & B.D. McPherson (Eds.), *Exercise, fitness, and health* (pp. 455-466). Champaign, IL: Human Kinetics.

Hagberg, J.M. (1994). Physical activity, fitness, health, and aging. In C. Bouchard, R.J. Shephard, & T. Stephens (Eds.), *Physical activity, fitness, and health* (pp. 993-1005). Champaign, IL: Human Kinetics.

Hagberg, J.M., Mullin, J.P., Giese, M.D., & Spitznagel, E. (1981). Effect of pedaling rate on submaximal exercise responses of competitive cyclists. *Journal of Applied Physiology*, **51**, 447-451.

Hall, S.J. (1995). *Basic biomechanics* (2nd ed.). St. Louis: C.V. Mosby.

Hamill, J., & Knutzen, K. (1995). *Biomechanical basis of human movement*. Baltimore: Williams & Wilkins.

Hanson, P. (1988). Clinical exercise testing. In S.N. Blair, P. Painter, R. Pate, L.K. Smith, & C.B. Taylor (Eds.), *Resource manual for guidelines for exercise testing and prescription* (pp. 205-222). Philadelphia: Lea & Febiger.

Hanson, P.G., & Zimmerman, S.W. (1979). Exertional heatstroke in novice runners. *Journal of the American Medical Association*, **242**, 154-157.

Hardy, J.D., & Bard, P. (1974). Body temperature regulation. In V.B. Mountcastle (Ed.), *Medical physiology: Vol 2.* (13th ed., pp. 1305-1342). St. Louis: C.V. Mosby.

Hart, L.E., & Sutton, J.R. (1987). Environmental considerations for exercise. *Cardiology Clinics*, **5**, 245-258.

Haskell, W.L. (1978). Design and implementation of cardiac conditioning programs. In N.K. Wenger & H.K. Hellerstein (Eds.), *Rehabilitation of the coronary patient* (pp. 203-241). New York: John Wiley & Sons.

Haskell, W.L. (1984). The influence of exercise on the concentrations of triglyceride and cholesterol in human plasma. In R.L. Terjung (Ed.), *Exercise and Sports Sciences Reviews* (Vol. 12, pp. 205-244). Lexington, MA: Collamore.

Haskell, W.L. (1985). Physical activity and health: Need to define the required stimulus. *American Journal of Cardiology*, **55**, 4D-9D.

Haskell, W.L. (1994). Dose-response issues from a biological perspective. In C. Bouchard, R.J. Shephard, & T. Stevens (Eds.), *Physical activity, fitness, and health* (pp. 1030-1039). Champaign, IL: Human Kinetics.

Haskell, W.L. (1995). Physical activity in the prevention and management of coronary heart disease. *PCPFS Physical Activity and Fitness Research Digest*, **2**(1).

Haskell, W.L. (1996a). Background and definitions. In S. Blair (Ed.), *Surgeon General's Report: Physical Activity and Health.* Washington, DC: Health and Human Services.

Haskell, W.L. (1996b). Personal communication.

Haskell, W.L., Savin, W., Oldridge, N., & DeBusk, R. (1982). Factors influencing estimated oxygen uptake during exercise testing soon after myocardial infarction. *American Journal of Cardiology*, **50**, 299-304.

Hay, J.G., & Reid, J.G. (1988). *The anatomical and mechanical bases of human motion.* Englewood Cliffs, NJ: Prentice Hall.

Hayward, M.G., & Keatinge, W.R. (1981). Roles of subcutaneous fat and thermoregulatory reflexes in determining ability to stabilize body temperature in water. *Journal of Physiology* (London), **320**, 229-251.

Heaney, R.P. (1987). The role of calcium in prevention and treatment of osteoporosis. *The Physician and Sportsmedicine*, **15**(11), 83-88.

Heinzelmann, F., & Bagley, R.W. (1970). Response to physical activity programs and their effects on health behavior. *Public Health Reports*, **86**, 905-911.

Hellerstein, H.K., & Franklin, B.A. (1984). Exercise testing and prescription. In N.K. Wenger & H.K. Hellerstein (Eds.), *Rehabilitation of the coronary patient* (2nd ed., pp. 197-284). New York: John Wiley & Sons.

Henderson, J. (1973). *Emergency medical guide* (3rd ed.). St. Louis: C.V. Mosby.

Herbert, W.G., & Herbert, D.L. (1988). Legal considerations. In S.N. Blair, P. Painter, R. Pate, L.K. Smith, & C.B. Taylor (Eds.), *Resource manual for guidelines for exercise testing and prescription* (pp. 395-399). Philadelphia: Lea & Febiger.

Hermansen, L., & Watchtlova, M. (1971). Capillary density of skeletal muscle in well-trained and untrained men. *Journal of Applied Physiology*, **30**, 860-863.

Hettinger, R., & Muller, E. (1953). Muskelleistung and muskeltraining. *Arbeits Physiology*, **15**, 111-126.

Heymsfield, S.B., Lichtman, S., Baumgartner, R.N., Wang, J., Kamen, Y., Aliprantis, A., & Pierson, R.N. (1990). Body composition of humans: Comparison of two improved four-compartment models that differ in expense, technical complexity, and radiation exposure. *American Journal of Clinical Nutrition*, **52**, 52-58.

Heyward, V.H. (1991). *Advanced fitness assessment and exercise prescription* (2nd ed.). Champaign, IL: Human Kinetics.

Hickson, R.C., Bomze, H.A., & Holloszy, J.O. (1977). Linear increase in aerobic power induced by a strenuous program of endurance exercise. *Journal of Applied Physiology: Respiratory, Environmental, and Exercise Physiology*, **42**, 372-376.

Hickson, R.C., Bomze, H.A., & Holloszy, J.O. (1978). Faster adjustment of O_2 uptake to the energy requirement of exercise in the trained state. *Journal of Applied Physiology: Respiratory, Environmental, and Exercise Physiology*, **44**, 877-881.

Hickson, R.C., Foster, C., Pollock, M.L., Galassi, T.M., & Rich, S. (1985). Reduced training intensities and loss of aerobic power, endurance, and cardiac growth. *Journal of Applied Physiology*, **58**, 492-499.

Hickson, R.C., Kanakis, C., Jr., Davis, J.R., Moore, A.M., & Rich, S. (1982). Reduced training duration effects on aerobic power, endurance, and cardiac growth. *Journal of Applied Physiology*, **53**, 225-229.

Hickson, R.C., & Rosenkoetter, M.A. (1981). Reduced training frequencies and maintenance of increased aerobic power. *Medicine and Science in Sports and Exercise*, **13**, 13-16.

Hill, J.O., Drougas, H.J., & Peters, J.C. (1994). Physical activity, fitness, and moderate obesity. In C. Bouchard, R.J. Shephard, & T. Stephens (Eds.), *Physical activity, fitness, and health* (pp. 684-695). Champaign, IL: Human Kinetics.

Hoffman, R.M., & Garewal, H.S. (1995). Antioxidants and the prevention of coronary heart disease. *Archives of Internal Medicine*, **155**, 241-246.

Holden, J.H., Darga, L.L., Olson, S.M., Stettner, D.C., Ardito, E.A., & Lucas, C.P. (1992). Long-term follow-up of patients attending a combination very-low calorie diet and behaviour therapy weight loss programme. *International Journal of Obesity*, **16**, 605-613.

Holloszy, J.O., & Coyle, E.F. (1984). Adaptations of skeletal muscle to endurance exercise and their metabolic consequences. *Journal of Applied Physiology: Respiratory, Environmental, and Exercise Physiology*, **56**, 831-838.

Holmer, I. (1979). Physiology of swimming man. In R.S. Hutton & D.I. Miller (Eds.), *Exercise and Sport Sciences Reviews* (Vol. 7, pp. 87-123). Salt Lake City: Franklin Institute.

Hopkins, D.R., & Hoeger, W.W.K. (1992). A comparison of the sit-and-reach test and the modified sit-and-reach test in the measurement of flexibility in males. *Journal of Applied Sport Science*, **6**, 7-10.

Horvath, S.M. (1981). Exercise in a cold environment. In D.I. Miller (Ed.), *Exercise and Sport Sciences Reviews* (Vol. 9, pp. 221-263). Salt Lake City: Franklin Institute.

Horvath, S.M., Raven, P.R., Dahms, T.E., & Gray, D.J. (1975). Maximal aerobic capacity of different levels of carboxyhemoglobin. *Journal of Applied Physiology*, **38**, 300-303.

Hossack, K.F., Bruce, R.A., & Clark, L.J. (1980). Influence of propranolol on exercise prescription of training heart rates. *Cardiology*, **65**, 47-58.

Howley, E.T. (1980). Effect of altitude on physical performance. In G.A. Stull & T.K. Cureton (Eds.), *Encyclopedia of physical education, fitness, and sports: Training, environment, nutrition, and fitness* (pp. 177-187). Salt Lake City: Brighton.

Howley, E.T. (1988). The exercise testing laboratory. In S.N. Blair, P. Painter, R.R. Pate, L.K. Smith, & C.B. Taylor (Eds.), *Resource manual for guidelines for exercise testing and prescription* (pp. 406-413). Philadelphia: Lea & Febiger.

Howley, E.T., Bassett, D.R., Jr., & Welch, H.G. (1995). Criteria for maximal oxygen uptake—review and commentary. *Medicine and Science in Sports and Exercise*, **24**, 1055-1058.

Howley, E.T. & Franks, B.D. (1986). *Health/fitness instructor's handbook*. Champaign, IL.: Human Kinetics.

Howley, E.T., & Glover, M.E. (1974). The caloric costs of running and walking 1 mile for men and women. *Medicine and Science in Sports*, **6**, 235-237.

Howley, E.T., & Martin, D. (1978). Oxygen uptake and heart-rate responses measured during rope skipping. *Tennessee Journal of Health, Physical Education and Recreation*, **16**, 7-8.

Hughson, R.L., Green, H.J., Houston, M.E., Thompson, J.A., MacLean, D.R., & Sutton, J.R. (1980). Heat injuries in Canadian mass-participation runs. *Canadian Medicine Medical Association Journal*, **122**, 1141-1144.

Hultman, E. (1967). Physiological role of muscle glycogen in man, with special reference to exercise. *Circulation Research*, **20-21** (Suppl. 1), 99-114.

Hurst, J.W. (1994). *Diagnostic atlas of the heart.* Philadelphia, PA: Lippincott-Raven.

Imrie, D., & Barbuto, L. (1988). *The back power program.* Toronto: Stoddart.

Inger, F. (1979). Effects of endurance training on muscle fiber ATP-ase activity, capillary supply, and mitochondrial content of man. *Journal of Physiology*, **294**, 419-432.

Issekutz, B., Birkhead, N.C., & Rodahl, K. (1962). The use of respiratory quotients in assessment of aerobic power capacity. *Journal of Applied Physiology*, **17**, 47-50.

Jackson, A.S., & Pollock, M.L. (1978). Generalized equations for predicting body density of men. *British Journal of Nutrition*, **40**, 497-504.

Jackson, A.S., & Pollock, M.L. (1985). Practical assessment of body composition. *The Physician and Sportsmedicine*, **13**, 76-90.

Jackson, A.S., Pollock, M.L., & Ward, A. (1980). Generalized equations for predicting body density of women. *Medicine and Science in Sports and Exercise*, **12**, 175-182.

Jacobsen, E. (1938). *Progressive relaxation.* Chicago: University of Chicago Press.

Jennings, G. L., Deakin, G., Korner, P., Meredith, I., Kingwell, B., & Nelson, L. (1991). What is the dose-response relationship between exercise training and blood pressure? *Annals of Medicine*, **23**, 313-318.

Johnson, C.C., & Slemenda, C. (1987). Osteoporosis: An overview. *The Physician and Sportsmedicine*, **15**(11), 65-68.

Johnson, M.D. (1994). Disordered eating. In R. Agostini (Ed.), *Medical and orthopedic issues of active and athletic women* (pp. 141-151). Philadelphia: Hanley & Belfus.

Joint Committee on Detection, Evaluation, and Treatment of High Blood Pressure. (1993). Fifth Report of the Joint Committee on Detection, Evaluation, and Treatment of High Blood Pressure (JNCV). *Archives of Internal Medicine*, **153**, 154-183.

Jones, N.L., Berman, L.B., Bartkiewig, P.D., & Oldridge, N.B. (1987). Chronic obstructive respiratory disorders. In J.S. Skinner (Ed.), *Exercise testing and exercise prescription for special cases* (pp. 175-187). Philadelphia: Lea & Febiger.

Jones, W.H.S. (Trans.). (1953). *Regimen (Hippocrates)*. Cambridge, MA: Harvard University Press.

Kannel, W.B. (1990). Contribution of the Framingham study to preventive cardiology. *Journal of the American College of Cardiology*, **15**, 206-211.

Kannel, W.B., & Abbot, R.D. (1984). Incidence and prognosis of unrecognized myocardial infarction. *New England Journal of Medicine*, **311**, 1144-1147.

Kaplan, N.M. (1994). *Clinical hypertension* (6th ed.). Baltimore: Williams & Wilkins.

Karvonen, M.J., Kentala, E., & Mustala, O. (1957). The effects of training heart rate: A longitudinal study. *Annales Medicinae Experimentalis et Biologiae Fenniae*, **35**, 307-315.

Kasch, F.W., Boyer, J.L., Van Camp, S.P., Verity, L.S., & Wallace, J.P. (1990). The effects of physical activity and inactivity on aerobic power in older men (a longitudinal study). *The Physician and Sportsmedicine*, **18**(4), 73-83.

Kasch, F.W., Wallace, J.P., & Van Camp, S.P. (1985). Effects of 18 years of endurance exercise on the physical work capacity of older men. *Journal of Cardiopulmonary Rehabilitation*, **5**, 308-312.

Kasch, F.W., Wallace, J.P., Van Camp, S.P., & Verity, L.S (1988). A longitudinal study of cardiovascular stability in active men aged 45 to 65 yrs. *The Physician and Sportsmedicine*, **16**(1), 117-126.

Kasser, S.L. (1995). *Inclusive games: Movement fun for everyone.* Champaign, IL: Human Kinetics.

Katch, F.I., & McArdle, W.D. (1977). *Nutrition and weight control.* Boston: Houghton Mifflin.

Katch, F.I., Pechar, G.S., Pardew, D., & Smith, L.E. (1975). Neuro-motor specificity of isokinetic bench training in women. *Medicine and Science in Sports*, **7**, 77.

Katz, R.M. (1986). Prevention with and without the use of medications for exercise-induced asthma. *Medicine and Science in Sports and Exercise*, **18**, 331-333.

Katz, R.M. (1987, July). Coping with exercise-induced asthma in sports. *The Physician and Sportsmedicine*, **15**, 100-112.

Keeley, J., Mayer, T.G., Cox, R., Gatchel, R.J., Smith, J., & Mooney, V. (1986). Quantification of lumbar function. Part 5: Reliability of range-of-motion measures in the sagittal plane and an in vivo torso rotation measurement technique. *Spine*, **11**, 31-37.

Kelbaek, H., Gjorup, T., Floistrup, S., Hartling, O., Christensen, N., & Godtfredsen, J. (1985). Acute effects of alcohol on left ventricular function in healthy subjects at rest and during upright exercise. *American Journal of Cardiology*, **55**, 164-167.

Kibler, W.B., Chandler, T.J., & Stracener, E.S. (1992). Musculoskeletal adaptations and injuries due to overtraining. In J.O. Holloszy (Ed.), *Exercise and Sport Science Reviews* (vol. 20, pp. 99-126). Baltimore: Williams & Wilkins.

King, A.C. (1994). Clinical and community interventions to promote and support physical activity participation. In R.K. Dishman (Ed.), *Advances in exercise adherence* (pp. 183-212). Champaign, IL: Human Kinetics.

King, A.C., & Martin, J.E. (1993). Exercise adherence and maintenance. In J.L. Durstine, A.C. King, P.L. Painter, J.L. Roitman, & L.D. Zwiren (Eds.), *Resource manual for guidelines for exercise testing and prescription* (pp. 443-454). Philadelphia: Lea & Febiger.

Kirkendall, W.M., Feinlieb, M., Freis, E.D., & Mark, A.L. (1980). Recommendations for human blood-pressure determination by sphygmomanometers. *Circulation*, **62**, 1146A-1155A.

Kisselle, J., & Mazzeo, K. (1983). *Aerobic dance*. Englewood, CO: Morton.

Klafs, C.E., & Arnheim, D.D. (1977). *Modern principles of athletic training*. St. Louis: C.V. Mosby.

Kline, G.M., Porcari, J.P., Hintermeister, R., Freedson, P.S., Ward, A., McCarron, R.F., Ross, J., & Rippe, J.M. (1987). Estimation of VO_2max from a 1-mile track walk, gender, age, and body weight. *Medicine and Science in Sports and Exercise*, **19**, 253-259.

Knapik, J.J., Mawdsley, R.H., & Ramos, M.U. (1983). Angular specificity and test mode specificity of isometric and isokinetic strength training. *Journal of Orthopedic Sports Physical Therapy*, **5**, 58-65.

Knapp, D.N. (1988). Behavior management techniques and exercise promotion. In R.K. Dishman (Ed.), *Exercise adherence* (pp. 203-235). Champaign, IL: Human Kinetics.

Knoebel, L.K. (1984). Energy metabolism. In E. Selkurt (Ed.), *Physiology* (5th ed.). Boston: Little, Brown.

Kohl, H.W., & McKenzie, J.D. (1994). Physical activity, fitness, and stroke. In C. Bouchard, R.J. Shephard, & T. Stephens (Eds.), *Physical activity, fitness, and health* (pp. 609-621). Champaign, IL: Human Kinetics.

Kohrt, W.M. (1995). Body composition by DXA: Tried and true? *Medicine and Science in Sports and Exercise*, **27**, 1349-1353.

Kramer, J.W. (1994). General adaptations to resistance and endurance training programs. In T.R. Baechle (Ed.), *Essentials of strength training and conditioning* (pp. 127-150). Champaign, IL: Human Kinetics.

Kreighbaum, E., & Barthels, K.M. (1996). *Biomechanics* (4th ed.). Minneapolis: Burgess.

Kriska, A.M., Blair, S.N., & Pereira, M.A. (1994). The potential role of physical activity in the prevention of non-insulin-dependent diabetes mellitus: The epidemiological evidence. In J.O. Holloszy (Ed.), *Exercise and Sports Sciences Reviews* (Vol. 22, pp. 121-143). Baltimore: Williams & Wilkins.

Kuczmarski, R.J., Flegal, K.M., Campbell, S.M., & Johnson, C.L. (1994). Increasing prevalence of overweight among U.S. adults: The National Health and Nutrition Examination Surveys, 1960 to 1991. *Journal of the American Medical Association*, **272**, 205-211.

Kyllo, L.B., & Landers, D.M. (1995). Goal setting in sport and exercise: A research synthesis to resolve the controversy. *Journal of Sport and Exercise Psychology*, **17**, 117-137.

Lakka, T.A., Venalainen, J.M., Rauramaa, R., et al. (1994). Relation of leisure-time activity and cardiorespiratory fitness to the risk of acute myocardial infarction in men. *New England Journal of Medicine*, **330**, 1549-1554.

Lamb, D.R. (1984). *Physiology of exercise* (2nd ed.). New York: Macmillan.

Landers, D.M. (1995). Performance, stress, and health: Overall reaction. *Quest*, **46**(1), 123-135.

Landers, D.M., & Petruzzello, S.J. (1994). Physical activity, fitness, and anxiety. In C. Bouchard, R.J. Shephard, & T. Stephens (Eds.), *Physical activity, fitness, and health* (pp. 868-882). Champaign, IL: Human Kinetics.

Larsson, L. (1982). Physical training effects on muscle morphology in sedentary males at different ages. *Medicine and Science in Sports and Exercise*, **14**, 203-206.

Laubach, L.L. (1976). Comparative muscular strength of men and women: A review of the literature. *Aviation, Space and Environmental Medicine*, **47**, 534-542.

Lavery, M.A., & Loewy, J.W. (1993). Identifying predictive variables for long-term weight change after participation in a weight loss program. *Journal of the American Dietetic Association*, **93**, 1017-1024.

Lee, I.M. (1994). Physical activity, fitness, and cancer. In C. Bouchard, R.J. Shephard, & T. Stephens (Eds.), *Physical activity, fitness, and health* (pp. 814-831). Champaign, IL: Human Kinetics.

Lee, I.M., Hsieh, C., & Paffenbarger, R.S. (1995). Exercise intensity and longevity in men. *Journal of the American Medical Association*, **273**, 1179-1184.

Leon, A.S., Cormett, J., Jacobs, D.R., & Rauramaa, R. (1987). Leisure-time physical activity levels and risk of coronary heart disease and death: The multiple risk factor intervention trial. *Journal of the American Medical Association*, **258**, 2388-2395.

Lichtman, S.W., Pisarska, K., Berman, E.R., Pestone, M., Dowling, H., Offenbacher, E., Weisel, H., Heshka, S., Matthews, D.E., & Heymsfield, S.B. (1992). Discrepancy between self-reported and actual caloric intake and exercise in obese subjects. *New England Journal of Medicine*, **327**, 1893-1898.

Liemohn, W., Martin, S., Sharpe, G., & Thompson, J. (1996). The effect of ankle posture on sit-and-reach test performance. *Medicine and Science in Sport and Exercise*, **28**(5), 57.

Liemohn, W., & Sharpe, G. (1992). Muscular strength and endurance, flexibility, and low-back function. In E.T. Howley & B.D. Franks (Eds.), *Health fitness instructor's handbook* (pp. 179-196). Champaign, IL: Human Kinetics.

Liemohn, W.P., Sharpe, G.L., & Wasserman, J. (1994). Lumbosacral movement in the sit-and-reach and in Cailliet's protective-hamstring stretch. *Spine*, **19**, 2127–2130.

Lind, A.R., & McNicol, G.W. (1967). Muscular factors which determine the cardiovascular responses to sustained and rhythmic exercise. *Canadian Medical Association Journal*, **96**, 706-713.

Lindsay, R. (1987). Estrogen and osteoporosis. *The Physician and Sportsmedicine*, **15**(11), 105-108.

Lohman, T.G. (1986). Applicability of body composition techniques and constants for children and youth. In K.B. Pandolf (Ed.), *Exercise and Sports Sciences Reviews* (Vol. 14, pp. 325-356). New York: MacMillan.

Lohman, T.G. (1992). *Advances in body composition assessment*. Champaign, IL: Human Kinetics.

Lohman, T.G., Roche, A.F., & Martorell, R. (1988). *Anthropometric standardization reference manual*. Champaign, IL: Human Kinetics.

Londeree, B.R., & Ames, S.A. (1976). Trend analysis of the %VO_2max-HR regression. *Medicine and Science in Sports*, **8**, 122-125.

Londeree, B.R., & Moeschberger, M.L. (1982). Effect of age and other factors on maximal heart rate. *Research Quarterly for Exercise and Sport*, **53**, 297-304.

Lotgering, F.K., Gilbert, R.D., & Longo, L.D. (1984). The interactions of exercise and pregnancy: A review. *American Journal of Obstetrics and Gynecology*, **149**, 560-568.

Lotgering, F.K., Gilbert, R.D., & Longo, L.D. (1985). Maternal and fetal responses to exercise during pregnancy. *Physiological Reviews*, **65**, 1-36.

Luciano, D.S., Vander, A.J., & Sherman, J.H. (1978). *Human function and structure*. New York: McGraw-Hill.

Luttgens, K. Deutsch, H., & Hamilton, N. (1992). *Kinesiology* (8th ed.). Madison, WI: Brown and Benchmark.

MacDougall, J.D., Ray, S., McCartney, N., Sale, D., Lee, P., & Gardner, S. (1988). Substrate utilization during weight lifting. *Medicine and Science in Sports and Exercise*, **20**, S66.

MacDougall, J.D., Tuxen, D., Sale, D.G., Moroz, J.R., & Sutton, J.R. (1985). Arterial blood-pressure response to heavy resistance exercise. *Journal of Applied Physiology*, **58**, 785-790.

Mahler, D. A. (1993). Exercise-induced asthma. *Medicine and Science in Sports and Exercise*, **25**, 554-561.

Makker, H.K., & Holgate, S.T. (1994). Mechanisms of exercise-induced asthma. *European Journal of Clinical Investigation*, **24**, 571-585.

Marcus, B.H., Rossi, J.S., Selby, V.C., Niaura, R.S., & Abrams, D.B. (1992). The stages and processes of exercise adoption and maintenance in a worksite setting. *Health Psychology*, **11**, 386–395.

Marcus, B.H., & Simkin, L.R. (1994). The transtheoretical model: Applications to exercise behavior. *Medicine and Science in Sports and Exercise*, **26**, 1400-1404.

Margaria, R., Cerretelli, P., Aghemo, P., & Sassi, J. (1963). Energy cost of running. *Journal of Applied Physiology*, **18**, 367-370.

Maritz, J.S., Morrison, J.F., Peter, J., Strydom, N.B., & Wyndham, C.H. (1961). A practical method of estimating an individual's maximal oxygen uptake. *Ergonomics*, **4**, 97-122.

Marlatt, G.A., & Gordon, J.R. (1985). *Relapse prevention: Maintenance strategies in addictive behavior change.* New York: Guilford Press.

Marlatt, G.A., & Parks, G.A. (1982). Self-management of addictive behavior. In P. Karoly & F.H. Kanfer (Eds.), *Self-management and behavior change: From theory to practice* (pp. 443-488). New York: Pergamon Press.

Mathews, D.K., & Fox, E.L. (1976). *The physiological basis of physical education and athletics* (2nd ed.). Philadelphia: W. B. Saunders.

Mazzeo, J.W. (1984). *Shape-up*. Englewood, CO: Morton.

McArdle, W.D., Katch, F.I., & Katch, V.L. (1981). *Exercise physiology*. Philadelphia: Lea & Febiger.

McArdle, W.D., Katch, F.I., & Katch, V.L. (1991). *Exercise physiology, energy, nutrition, and human performance* (3rd ed.). Philadelphia: Lea & Febiger.

McArdle, W.D., Katch, F.I., & Katch, V.L. (1996). *Exercise physiology, energy, nutrition, and human performance* (4th ed.). Baltimore: Williams & Wilkins.

McArdle, W.D., Katch, F.I., & Pechar, G.S. (1973). Comparison of continuous and discontinuous treadmill and bicycle tests for max VO_2. *Medicine and Science in Sports,* **5**(3), 156-160.

McArdle, W.D., & Magel, J.R. (1970). Physical work capacity and maximum oxygen uptake in treadmill and bicycle exercise. *Medicine and Science in Sports,* **2**(3), 118-123.

McArdle, W.D., Magel, J.R., Gergley, T.J., Spina, R.J., & Toner, M.M. (1984). Thermal adjustment to cold-water exposure in resting men and women. *Journal of Physiology: Respiratory Environment Exercise Physiology*, **56**, 1565-1571.

McArdle, W.D., Magel, J.R., Spina, R.J., Gergley, T.J., & Toner, M.M. (1984). Thermal adjustments to cold-water exposure in exercising men and women. *Journal of Applied Physiology,* **56**, 1572-1577.

McCartney, N. (1994). Physical activity, fitness, and the physically disabled (Neuromuscular disorders). In C. Bouchard, R.J. Shephard, & T. Stephens (Eds.), *Physical activity, fitness, and health* (pp. 840-850). Champaign, IL: Human Kinetics.

McCrory, M.A, Gomez, T.D., Bernauer, E.M., & Molé, P.A. (1995). Evaluation of a new air displacement plethysmograph for measuring human body composition. *Medicine and Science in Sports and Exercise,* **27**, 1686-1691.

McKenzie, D.C., McLuckie, S.L., & Stirling, D.R. (1994). The protective effects of continuous and interval exercise in athletes with exercise-induced asthma. *Medicine and Science in Sports and Exercise*, **26**, 951-956.

McKenzie, R. (1981). Exercises. In R. McKenzie (Ed.), *The lumbar spine—mechanical diagnosis and therapy* (p. 49). Upper Hutt, New Zealand: Spinal.

McSwegin, P.J., & Pemberton, C.L. (1993). Exercise leadership: Key skills and characteristics. In J.L. Durstine, A.C. King, P.L. Painter, J.L. Roitman, L.D. Zwiren, & W.L. Kenney (Eds.), *ACSM's resource manual for guidelines for exercise testing and prescription* (2nd ed., pp. 319-326). Philadelphia: Lea & Febiger.

Micheli, L.J. (1983). Overuse injuries in children's sports: The growth factor. *The Orthopedic Clinics of North America,* **14**, 337-360.

Middleton, E. (1980). A rational approach to asthma therapy. *Postgraduate Medicine*, **67**, 107-123.

Miracle, V.A. (1986). Pulmonary exercise program: A model for pulmonary rehabilitation. *Journal of Cardiopulmonary Rehabilitation*, **6**, 368-371.

Mitchell, B.S., & Blair, S.N. (1988). Evaluation of preventive and rehabilitation exercise programs. In S.N. Blair, P. Painter, R. Pate, L.K. Smith, & C.B. Taylor (Eds.), *Resource manual for guidelines for exercise testing and prescription* (pp. 414-420). Philadelphia: Lea & Febiger.

Moffroid, M.T., & Whipple, R.H. (1970). Specificity of speed of exercise. *Physical Therapy,* **50**, 1699-1704.

Molé, P.A. (1990). Impact of energy intake and exercise on resting metabolic rate. *Sports Medicine,* **10**, 72-87.

Montoye, H.J., & Ayen, T. (1986). Body-size adjustment for oxygen requirement in treadmill walking. *Research Quarterly for Exercise and Sport,* **57**, 82-84.

Montoye, H.J., Ayen, T., Nagle, F., & Howley, E.T. (1986). The oxygen requirement for horizontal and grade walking on a motor-driven treadmill. *Medicine and Science in Sports and Exercise*, **17**, 640-645.

Montoye, H.J., Kemper, H.C.G., Saris, W.H.M., & Washburn, R.A. (1996). *Measuring physical activity and energy expenditure.* Champaign, IL: Human Kinetics.

Moore, S. (1994). Physical activity, fitness, and atherosclerosis. In C. Bouchard, R.J. Shephard, & T. Stephens (Eds.), *Physical activity, fitness, and health* (pp. 570-578). Champaign, IL: Human Kinetics.

Morgan, D.W., Bransford, D.R., Costill, D.L., Daniels, J.T., Howley, E.T., & Krahenbuhl, G.S. (1995). Variation in the aerobic demand of running among trained and untrained subjects. *Medicine and Science in Sports and Exercise*, **27**, 404-409.

Morgan, W.P. (1994). Physical activity, fitness, and depression. In C. Bouchard, R.J. Shephard, & T. Stephens (Eds.), *Physical activity, fitness, and health* (pp. 851-867). Champaign, IL: Human Kinetics.

Morris, A.F. (1984). *Sports medicine: Prevention of athletic injuries*. Dubuque, IA: Brown.

Morris, J.N., Clayton, D.G., Everitt, N.G., Semmence, A.M., & Burgess, E.H. (1990). Exercise in leisure time: Coronary attack and death rates. *British Heart Journal*, **63**, 325-334.

Musser, J.W. (1988). Budget considerations. In S.N. Blair, P. Painter, R. Pate, L.K. Smith, & C.B. Taylor (Eds.), *Resource manual for guidelines for exercise testing and prescription* (pp. 390-394). Philadelphia: Lea & Febiger.

Nachemson, A. (1975). Towards a better understanding of low-back pain: A review of the mechanics of the lumbar disc. *Rheumatology and Rehabilitation*, **14**, 129-143.

Nachemson, A.L., Andersson, G.B.J., & Schultz, A.B. (1986). Valsalva maneuver biomechanics: Effects on lumbar trunk loads of elevated intraabdominal pressures. *Spine*, **11**, 476-479.

Nagle, F.J., Balke, B., Baptista, G., Alleyia, J., & Howley, E. (1971). Compatibility of progressive treadmill, bicycle, and step tests based on oxygen-uptake responses. *Medicine and Science in Sport*, **3**, 149-154.

Nagle, F.J., Balke, B., & Naughton, J.P. (1965). Gradational step tests for assessing work capacity. *Journal of Applied Physiology*, **20**, 745-748.

National Institutes of Health. (1985). *Health implications of obesity: NIH Consensus Development Conference Statement*. Bethesda, MD: Author.

National Institutes of Health. (1994a). *Bioelectrical impedance analysis in body composition measurement: NIH Technology Assessment Conference Statement*. Bethesda, MD: Author.

National Institutes of Health. (1994b). *Optimal calcium intake: NIH Consensus Development Conference Statement*. Bethesda, MD: Author.

National Institutes of Health. (1996). Consensus Development Conference. *Physical Activity and Cardiovascular Health*. Rockville, VA: Author.

National Institutes of Health Technology Assessment Conference Panel. (1993). Methods for voluntary weight loss and control: Technology Assessment Conference Statement. *Annals of Internal Medicine*, **119**(7 pt 2), 764-770.

National Research Council, Committee on Diet and Health. (1989). *Diet and health: Implications for reducing chronic disease risk*. Washington, DC: National Academy Press.

National Research Council, Food and Nutrition Board. (1989). *Recommended Dietary Allowances* (10th ed.). Washington, DC: National Academy Press.

Nattiv, A., Yeager, K., Drinkwater, B., & Agostini, R. (1994). The female athlete triad. In R. Agostini (Ed.), *Medical and orthopedic issues of active and athletic women* (pp. 169-174). Philadelphia: Hanley & Belfus.

Naughton, J.P., & Haider, R. (1973). Methods of exercise testing. In J.P. Naughton, H.R. Hellerstein, & L.C. Mohler (Eds.), *Exercise testing and exercise training in coronary heart disease* (pp. 79-91). New York: Academic Press.

New Games Foundation. (1976). *The new games book*. Garden City, NY: Dolphin Books.

Nieman, D.C. (1990). *Fitness and sports medicine: An introduction*. Palo Alto, CA: Bull.

Nilsson, B.E., & Westlin, N.E. (1977). Bone density in athletes. *Clinical Orthopedics and Related Research*, **7**, 179-182.

Noble, B.J., Borg, G.A.V., Cafarelli, E., Robertson, R.J., & Pandolf, K.B. (1982). Symposium on recent advances in the study and clinical use of perceived exertion. *Medicine and Science in Sports and Exercise*, **14**, 376-411.

O'Connor, B., Simmons, J., & O'Shea, P. (1989). *Weight training today*. St. Paul: West.

Oldridge, N.B. (1988). Qualities of an exercise leader. In S.N. Blair, P. Painter, R.R. Pate, L.K. Smith, & C.B. Taylor (Eds.), *Resource manual for guidelines for exercise testing and prescription* (pp. 239-243). Philadelphia: Lea & Febiger.

Oldridge, N.B., Haskell, W.L., & Single, P. (1981). Carotid palpation, coronary heart disease, and exercise rehabilitation. *Medicine and Science in Sports and Exercise*, **13**, 6-8.

Oteghen, S.L. (1975). Two speeds of isokinetic exercise as related to the vertical jump performance of women. *Research Quarterly*, **46**, 78-84.

Paffenbarger, R.S., & Hale, W.E. (1975, March 13). Work activity and coronary heart mortality. *New England Journal of Medicine*, **292**, 545-550.

Paffenbarger, R.S., Hyde, R.T., & Wing, A.L. (1986, March 6). Physical activity, all-cause mortality, and longevity of college alumni. *New England Journal of Medicine*, **314**, 605-613.

Paffenbarger, R.S., Hyde, R.T., & Wing, A.L. (1990). Physical activity and physical fitness as determinants of health and longevity. In C. Bouchard, R.J. Shephard, T. Stephens, J.R. Sutton, & B.D. McPherson (Eds.), *Exercise, fitness, and health* (pp. 33-48). Champaign, IL: Human Kinetics.

Paffenbarger, R.S., Jr., Hyde, R.T., Wing, A.L., Lee, I.M., Jung, D.L., & Kampert, J.B. (1993). The association of changes in physical-activity level and other lifestyle characteristics with mortality among men. *New England Journal of Medicine*, **328**, 538-545.

Painter, P., & Haskell, W.L. (1988). Decision making in programming exercise. In S.N. Blair, P. Painter,

R.R. Pate, L.K. Smith, C.B. Taylor (Eds.), *Resource manual for guidelines for exercise testing and prescription* (pp. 256-262). Philadelphia: Lea & Febiger.

Park Nicollet Medical Foundation (1995). *The activity pyramid.* Minneapolis: Author.

Park, R.S. (1989). *Measurement of physical fitness: A historical perspective.* Washington, DC: ODPHP National Health Information Center.

Pate, R.R., Pratt, M., Blair, S.N., Haskell, W.L., Marcera, C.A., & Bouchard, C. (1995). Physical activity and public health: A recommendation from the Centers for Disease Control and Prevention and the American College of Sports Medicine. *Journal of the American Medical Association,* **273**, 402-407.

Patton, R.W., Corry, J.M., Gettman, L.R., & Graf, J. (1986). *Implementing health/fitness programs.* Champaign, IL: Human Kinetics.

Peters, T.J., & Waterman, R.H. (1982). *In search of excellence.* New York: Warner Books.

Pfeiffer, R.P. & Pfeiffer, B.C. (1995). *Concepts of athletic training.* Boston: Jones and Bartlett.

Pierson, W.E., Covert, D.S., Koenig, J.Q., Namekta, T., & Shin Kim, Y. (1986). Implications of air pollution effects on athletic performance. *Medicine and Science in Sports and Exercise,* **18**, 322-327.

Plowman, S.A. (1993). Physical fitness and healthy low back function. *PCPFS Physical Activity and Fitness Research Digest,* **1**(3).

Plowman, S.A. (1994). Stress, hyperreactivity, and health. *Quest,* **46**(1), 78-99.

Pollock, M.L., Gettman, L.R., Mileses, C.A., Bah, M.D., Durstine, J.L., & Johnson, R.B. (1977). Effects of frequency and duration of training on attrition and incidence of injury. *Medicine and Science in Sports,* **9**, 31-36.

Pollock, M.L., & Wilmore, J.H. (1990). *Exercise in health and disease* (2nd ed.). Philadelphia: W.B. Saunders.

Pollock, M.L., Wilmore, J.H., & Fox, S.M. (1978). *Health and fitness through physical activity.* New York: John Wiley & Sons.

Pope, M.H., Bevins, T., & Wilder, D., et al. (1985). The relationship between anthropometric, postural, muscular, and mobility characteristics of males ages 18-55. *Spine,* **10**, 644.

Pothier, B., & Allen, M.W.E. (1991). Kinesiology and the degenerative joint. *Rheumatology Disease Clinics of North America,* **16**, 989-1002.

Powell, K.E., Thompson, P.D., & Caspersen, C.J. (1987). Physical activity and the incidence of coronary heart disease. *Annual Review of Public Health,* **8**, 253-287.

Powers, S., Dodd, S., Deason, R., Byrd, R., & McKnight, T. (1983). Ventilatory threshold, running economy, and distance-running performance of trained athletes. *Research Quarterly for Exercise and Sport,* **54**, 179-182.

Powers, S., Riley, W., & Howley, E. (1980). A comparison of fat metabolism in trained men and women during prolonged aerobic work. *Research Quarterly for Exercise and Sport,* **52**, 427-431.

Powers, S.K., Dodd, S., & Beadle, R.E. (1985). Oxygen-uptake kinetics in trained athletes differing in VO_2max. *European Journal of Applied Physiology,* **54**, 306-308.

Powers, S.K., & Dodd, S.L. (1996). *Total fitness exercise, nutrition, and wellness.* Needham Heights, MA: Allyn & Bacon.

Powers, S.K., & Howley, E.T. (1990, 1994, 1997). *Exercise physiology.* Madison, WI: Brown & Benchmark.

Pratt, C.M., Welton, D.E., Squires, W.G., Kirby, T.E., Hartung, G.H., & Miller, R.R. (1981). Demonstration of training effect during chronic ß-adrenergic blockade in patients with coronary artery disease. *Circulation,* **64**, 1125-1129.

President's Council on Physical Fitness and Sports. (1995a). Ad Council. *Newsletter,* **95**(2), 1.

President's Council on Physical Fitness and Sports. (1995b). *The PCPFS strategic plan: Meeting the Healthy People 2000 Objectives for Physical Activity and Fitness.* Washington, DC: Author.

President's Council on Physical Fitness and Sports. (1996). *Presidential Sports Award.* Washington, DC: Author.

Prochaska, J.O., & Marcus, B.H. (1994). The transtheoretical model: Applications to exercise. In R.K. Dishman (Ed.), *Advances in exercise adherence* (pp. 161-180). Champaign, IL: Human Kinetics.

Pugh, L.G.C. (1964). Deaths from exposure in Four Inns Walking Competition, March 14-15, 1964. *Lancet,* **1**, 1210-1212.

Pugh, L.G.C., & Edholm, O.G. (1955). The physiology of Channel swimmers. *Lancet,* **2**, 761-768.

Ragg, K.E., Murray, T.F., Karbonit, L.M., & Jump, D.A. (1980). Errors in predicting functional capacity from a treadmill exercise stress test. *American Heart Journal,* **100**, 581-583.

Rankin, J.M. & Ingersoll, C.H. (1995). *Athletic training management: Concepts and applications.* St. Louis: C.V. Mosby.

Rasch, P.J. (1989). *Kinesiology and applied anatomy* (7th ed.). Philadelphia: Lea & Febiger.

Raven, P.B. (1980). Effects of air pollution on physical performance. In G.A. Stull & T.K. Cureton

(Ed.), *Encyclopedia of physical education: Physical fitness, training, environment and nutrition related to performance* (Vol. 2, pp. 201-216). Salt Lake City: Brighton.

Raven, P.B., Drinkwater, B.L., Ruhling, R.O., Bolduan, N., Taguchi, S., Gliner, J., & Horvath, S.M. (1974). Effect of carbon monoxide and peroxyacetyl nitrate on man's maximal aerobic capacity. *Journal of Applied Physiology*, **36**, 288-293.

Reid, D. (1992). *Sports injury assessment and rehabilitation*. New York: Churchill Livingston.

Richter, E.R., & Galbo, H. (1986). Diabetes, insulin, and exercise. *Sports Medicine*, **3**, 275-288.

Ritter, M.A., & Albohm, M.J. (1987). *Your inquiry: A commonsense guide to sports injuries*. Indianapolis: Benchmark Press.

Robergs, R.A., Pearson, D.R., Costill, D.L., Fink, W.J., Pascoe, D.D., Benedict, M.A., Lambert, C.P., & Zachweija, J.J. (1991). Muscle glycogenolysis during differing intensities of weight-resistance exercise. *Journal of Applied Physiology*, **70**, 1700-1706.

Robinson, D. (1990, July 22). Stressbusters. *Parade Magazine*, p. 12.

Robinson, S. (1938). Experimental studies of physical fitness in relation to age. *Arbeitsphysiologie*, **10**, 251-323.

Ross, C.E., & Morowsky, J. (1983). Social epidemiology of overweight: A substantive and methodological investigation. *Journal of Health and Social Behavior*, **24**, 288-298.

Rothenberg, R.E. (1987). *Medical dictionary and health manual*. New York: Times Mirror.

Rowell, L.B. (1969). Circulation. *Medicine and Science in Sports*, **1**, 15-22.

Rowell, L.B. (1986). *Human circulation-regulation during physical stress*. New York: Oxford University Press.

Rowland, T. W. (1990). *Exercise and children's health*. Champaign, IL: Human Kinetics.

Roza, A.M., & Shizgal, H.M. (1984). The Harris-Benedict Equation reevaluated: Resting energy requirements and the body cell mass. *American Journal of Clinical Nutrition*, **40**, 168-182.

Ruud, J.S., & Wolinsky, I. (1995). Nutritional concerns of recreational strength athletes. In C.G.R. Jackson (Ed.), *Nutrition for the recreational athlete* (pp. 55-68). Boca Raton, FL: CRC Press.

Ryan, A.S., Treuth, M.S., Rubin, M.A., Miller, J.P., Nicklas, B.J., Landis, D.M., Pratlet, R.E., Libanati, C.R., Gundberg, C.M., & Hurley, B.F. (1994). Effects of strength training in bone mineral density: Hormonal and bone turnover relationships. *Journal of Applied Physiology*, **77**, 1678-1684.

Saal, J.S., & Saal, J.A. (1991). Strength training and flexibility. In A.H. White & R. Anderson (Eds.), *Conservative care of low back pain*. Baltimore: Williams & Wilkins.

Sable, D.L., Brammell, H.L., Sheehan, M.W., Nies, A.S., Gerber, J., & Horwitz, L.D. (1982). Attenuation of exercise conditioning by ß-adrenergic blockade. *Circulation*, **65**, 679-684.

Safrit, J. (1995). *Complete guide to youth fitness testing*. Champaign, IL: Human Kinetics.

Sale, D.G. (1987). Influence of exercise and training on motor unit activation. In K.B. Pandolf (Ed.), *Exercise and Sport Sciences Reviews* (Vol. 15, pp. 95-151). New York: MacMillan.

Sale, D.G. (1988). Neural adaptations to resistance training. *Medicine and Science in Sports and Exercise*, **20**, S135-S145.

Saltin, B. (1969). Physiological effects of physical conditioning. *Medicine and Science in Sports*, **1**, 50-56.

Saltin, B., & Gollnick, P.D. (1983). Skeletal muscle adaptability: Significance for metabolism and performance. In L.D. Peachey, R.H. Adrian, & S.R. Geiger (Eds.), *Handbook of physiology* (pp. 555-631). Baltimore: Williams & Wilkins.

Saltin, B., Henriksson, J., Nygaard, E., Anderson, P., & Jansson, E. (1977). Fiber types and metabolic potentials of skeletal muscles in sedentary man and endurance runners. *Annals of the New York Academy of Science*, **301**, 3-29.

Saltin, B., & Hermansen, L. (1966). Esophageal, rectal, and muscle temperature during exercise. *Journal of Applied Physiology*, **21**, 1757-1762.

Sandvick, L., Erikssen, J., Thaulow, E., et al. (1993). Physical fitness as a predictor of mortality among healthy middle-aged Norwegian men. *New England Journal of Medicine*, **328**, 533-537.

Saris, W.H.M. (1993). The role of exercise in the dietary treatment of obesity. *International Journal of Obesity*, **17**(Suppl. 1), S17-S21.

Sawka, M.N., Francesconi, R.P., Young, A.J., & Pandolf, K.B. (1984). Influence of hydration level and body fluids on exercise performance in the heat. *Journal of the American Medical Association*, **252**(9), 1165-1169.

Sawka, M.N., Young, A.J., Francesconi, R.P., Muza, S.R., & Pandolf, K.B. (1985). Thermoregulatory and blood responses during exercise at graded hypohydration levels. *Journal of Applied Physiology*, **59**, 1394-1401.

Schutte, J.E., Townsend, E., Hugg, J., Shoup, R., Malina, R., & Blomqvist, C. (1984). Density of lean body mass is greater in Blacks than in Whites. *Journal of Applied Physiology: Respira-*

tory, Environmental, and Exercise Physiology, **56**, 1647-1649.

Schwade, J., Blomqvist, C.G., & Shapiro, W. (1977). A comparison of the response to arm and leg work in patients with ischemic heart disease. *American Heart Journal*, **94**, 203-208.

Scribner, K., & Burke, E. (Eds.). (1978). *Relevant topics in athletic training*. New York: Mouvement.

Sedlock, D.A., Knowlton, R.G., Fitzgerald, P.I., Tahamont, M.V., & Schneider, D.A. (1983). Accuracy of subject-palpated carotid pulse after exercise. *The Physician and Sportsmedicine*, **11**(4), 106-116.

Servedio, F.J., Bartels, R.L., Hamlin, R.L., Teske, D., Shaffer, T., & Servedio, A. (1985). The effects of weight training using Olympic style lifts on various physiological variables in pre-pubescent boys. *Medicine and Science in Sports and Exercise*, **17**, 158.

Sewall, L., & Micheli, L. J. (1984). Strength development in children. *Medicine and Science in Sports and Exercise*, **16**, 158.

Shaper, A.G. & Wannamethee, G. (1991). Physical activity and ischemic heart disease in middle-aged British men. *British Heart Journal*, **66**, 384-394.

Sharkey, B.J. (1990). *Physiology of fitness* (3rd ed.). Champaign, IL: Human Kinetics.

Sharp, R.L., Costill, D.L., Fink, W.J., & King, D.S. (1986). Effects of eight weeks of bicycle ergometer sprint training on human muscle buffer capacity. *International Journal of Sports Medicine*, **7**, 13-17.

Shephard, R. (1996). Exercise, independence, and quality of life in the elderly. *Quest*, **48**(3), 354-365.

Shephard, R.J. (1970). Computer programs for solution of the Åstrand nomogram and the calculation of body surface area. *Journal of Sports Medicine and Physical Fitness*. **10**, 206-210.

Shephard, R.J. (1976). Exercise and chronic obstructive lung disease. In J. Keogle & R.S. Hutton (Eds.), *Exercise and Sport Sciences Reviews* (Vol. 4, pp. 263-296). Santa Barbara, CA: Journal Publishing Affiliates.

Shephard, R.J. (1984). Tests of maximal oxygen uptake: A critical review. *Sports Medicine*, **1**, 99-124.

Shephard, R.J. (1988). PAR-Q, Canadian home fitness test, and exercise screening alternatives. *Sports Medicine*, **5**, 185-195.

Shephard, R.J. (1990). Costs and benefits of an exercising versus a nonexercising society. In C. Bouchard, R.J. Shephard, T. Stephens, J.R. Sutton, & B.D. McPherson (Eds.), *Exercise, fitness, and health* (pp. 49-60). Champaign, IL: Human Kinetics.

Sherman, W.M. (1983). Carbohydrates, muscle glycogen, and muscle glycogen super compensation. In M.H. Williams (Ed.), *Ergogenic aids in sports* (pp. 3-26). Champaign, IL: Human Kinetics.

Sherman, W.M., & Wimer, G.S. (1991). Insufficient carbohydrate during training: Does it impair performance? *Sports Nutrition*, **1**, 28-44.

Sime, W.E. (1990). Discussion: Exercise, fitness, and mental health. In C. Bouchard, R.J. Shephard, T. Stephens, J.R. Sutton, & B.D. McPherson (Eds.), *Exercise, fitness, and health* (pp. 627-633). Champaign, IL: Human Kinetics.

Sime, W.E., & McKinney, M.E. (1988). Stress management applications in the prevention and rehabilitation of coronary heart disease. In S.N. Blair, P. Painter, R.R. Pate, L.K. Smith, & C.B. Taylor (Eds.), *Resource manual for guidelines for exercise testing and prescription* (pp. 367-374). Philadelphia: Lea & Febiger.

Sinaki, M., Lutness, M.P., & Ilstrup, D.M., et al. (1989). Lumbar spondylolisthesis: Retrospective comparison and three-year follow-up of two conservative treatment programs. *Archives of Physical Medicine & Rehabilitation*, 594.

Siri, W.E. (1961). Body composition from fluid space and density: Analysis of methods. In J. Brozek & A. Henschel (Eds.), *Techniques for measuring body composition* (pp. 223-244). Washington, DC: National Academy of Sciences.

Siscovick, D.S., Weiss, N.S., Fletcher, R.H., & Lasky, T. (1984). Habitual vigorous exercise and primary cardiac arrest: Effect of other risk factors on the relationship. *Journal of Chronic Disease*, **37**, 625-631.

Sizer, F., & Whitney, E. (1994). *Hamilton and Whitney's nutrition: Concepts and controversies*. St Paul: West.

Sly, R.M. (1986). History of exercise-induced asthma. *Medicine and Science in Sports and Exercise*, **18**, 314-317.

Smith, E.L. (1984). Special considerations in developing exercise programs for the older adult. In J.D. Matarazzo, N.E. Miller, S.M. Weiss, J.A. Herd, & S.M. Weiss (Eds.), *Behavioral health: A handbook of health enhancement and disease prevention* (pp. 525-546). New York: John Wiley & Sons.

Smith, E.L., & Gilligan, C. (1987). Effects of inactivity and exercise on bone. *The Physician and Sportsmedicine*, **15**(11), 91-102.

Smith, E.L., Smith, K.A., & Gilligan, C. (1990). Exercise, fitness, osteoarthritis, and osteoporosis. In C. Bouchard, R.J. Shephard, T. Stephens, J.R. Sutton, & B.D. McPherson (Eds.), *Exercise, fitness, and health* (pp. 517-528). Champaign, IL: Human Kinetics.

Smith, E.L., & Stoedefalke, K.G. (1978). *Aging and exercise*. Unpublished manuscript.

Smith, N.J. (1976). *Food for sport*. Palo Alto, CA: Bull.

Snow-Harter, C., Bousxein, M.S., & Lewis, B.T., Carter, D.R., & Marcus, R. (1992). Effects of resistance and endurance exercise on bone mineral status of young women: A randomized exercise intervention trial. *Journal of Bone Mineral Research*, **7**, 761-769.

Snow-Harter, C., & Marcus, R. (1991). Exercise, bone mineral density, and osteoporosis. In J.O. Holloszy (Ed.), *Exercise and Sports Science Reviews*. (vol. 19, pp. 351-388). Baltimore: Williams & Wilkins.

Sonstroem, R.J. (1988). Psychological models. In R.K. Dishman (Ed.), *Exercise adherence* (pp. 125-153). Champaign, IL: Human Kinetics.

Soukup, J.T., & Kovaleski, J.E. (1993). A review of the effects of resistance training for individuals with diabetes mellitus. *Diabetes Education*, **19**, 307-312.

Sova, R. (1995). *Water fitness after 40*. Champaign, IL: Human Kinetics.

Staron, R.S., Leonardi, M.J., Karapondo, D.L., Malicky, E.S., Falkel, J.E., Hagerman, F.C., & Hikida, R.S. (1991). Strength and skeletal muscle adaptations in heavy-resistance-trained women after detraining and retraining. *Journal of Applied Physiology*, **70**, 631-640.

Stein, E. (1992). *Rapid analysis of electrocardiograms: A self-study program* (2nd ed.). Philadelphia: Lea & Febiger.

Stephens, T. (1987). Secular trends in adult physical activity: Exercise boom or busy? *Research Quarterly for Exercise and Sport*, **58**, 94-105.

Stockdale-Woolley, R., Haggerty, M.C., & McMahon, P.M. (1986). The pulmonary rehabilitation program at Norwalk Hospital. *Journal of Cardiopulmonary Rehabilitation*, **6**, 505-518.

Stone, M.H. (1990). Muscle conditioning and muscle injuries. *Medicine and Science in Sports and Exercise*, **22**, 457-462.

Stone, M. H., & O'Bryant, H. S. (1987). *Weight training: A scientific approach*. Minneapolis: Burgess International.

Stunkard, A.J., Sørensen, T.I.A., Hanis, C., Teasdale, T.W., Chakraborty, R., Schull, W.J., & Schulsinger, F. (1986). An adoption study of human obesity. *New England Journal of Medicine*, **314**, 193-198.

Sullivan, M.K., Dejulia, J.J., & Worrell, T.W. (1992). Effect of pelvic position and stretching method on hamstring muscle flexibility. *Medicine and Science in Sports and Exercise*, **24**, 1383-1389.

Sutton, J.R. (1990). Exercise and the environment. In C. Bouchard, R.J. Shephard, T. Stephens, J.R. Sutton, & B.D. McPherson (Eds.), *Exercise, fitness, and health* (pp. 165-178). Champaign, IL: Human Kinetics.

Tanaka, K., & Matsuura, Y. (1984). Marathon performance, anaerobic threshold, and onset of blood lactate accumulation. *Journal of Applied Physiology*, **57**, 640-643.

Tate, C.A., Hyek, J.E., & Taffet, G.E. (1994). Mechanism for the responses of cardiac muscle to physical activity in old age. *Medicine and Science in Sports and Exercise*, **26**, 561-567.

Taylor, C.B., & Miller, N.H. (1988). Basic psychologic principles related to group exercise programs. In S.N. Blair, P. Painter, R.R. Pate, L.K. Smith, & C.B. Taylor (Eds.), *Resource manual for guidelines for exercise testing and prescription* (pp. 329-334). Philadelphia: Lea & Febiger.

Taylor, H.L., Buskirk, E.R., & Henschel, A. (1955). Maximal oxygen intake as an objective measure of cardiorespiratory performance. *Journal of Applied Physiology*, **8**, 73-80.

Tesch, P.A. (1988). Skeletal muscle adaptations consequent to long-term heavy-resistance exercise. *Medicine and Science in Sports and Exercise*, **20**, S124-S132.

Thistle, H.G., Hislop, H.J., & Moffroid, M. (1967). Isokinetic contraction: A new concept of resistance exercise. *Archives of Physical Medicine and Rehabilitation*, **48**, 279-282.

Thompson, C.E., & Wankel, L.M. (1980). The effects of perceived activity choice upon frequency of exercise behavior. *Journal of Applied Social Psychology*, **10**, 436-443.

Thompson, C.W. (1994). *Manual of structural kinesiology*. St. Louis: C.V. Mosby.

Thompson, P.D. (1988). The safety of exercise testing and participation. In S.N. Blair, P. Painter, R.R. Pate, L.K. Smith, & C.B. Taylor (Eds.), *Resource manual for guidelines for exercise testing and prescription* (pp. 273-277). Philadelphia: Lea & Febiger.

Thompson, P.D. & Fahrenbach, M.C. (1994). Risks of exercising: Cardiovascular including sudden cardiac death. In C. Bouchard, R.J. Shephard, & T. Stephens (Eds.), *Physical activity, fitness, and health* (pp. 1019-1028). Champaign, IL: Human Kinetics.

Thygerson, A.L. (1987). *First aid and emergency care workbook.* Boston: Jones & Bartlett.

Tommaso, C.L., Lesch, M., & Sonnenblick, E.H. (1984). Alterations in cardiac function in coronary heart disease, myocardial infarction, and coronary bypass surgery. In N.K. Wenger & H.K. Hellerstein (Eds.), *Rehabilitation of the coronary patient* (pp. 41-66). New York: John Wiley & Sons.

Torg, J.S., Welsh, P.R., & Shepard, R.J. (1990). *Current therapy in sports medicine.* St. Louis: C.V. Mosby.

United States Department of Agriculture. (1992). The Food Guide Pyramid. *Home and Garden Bulletin Number 252.*

United States Department of Agriculture. (1996). *Dietary guidelines for American adults.* Washington, DC: U.S. Government Printing Office.

United States Department of Health and Human Services. (1991). *Healthy People 2000: National Health Promotion and Disease Prevention Objectives* (publication no. PHS 91-50212). Washington, DC: Author.

United States Department of Health and Human Services. (1994). *Healthy People 2000: Review, 1994.* Washington, DC: Author.

United States Department of Health and Human Services. (1996). *Surgeon General's Report on Physical Activity and Health.* Washington, DC: Author.

Vander, A.J., Sherman, J.H., & Luciano, D.S. (1985). *Human physiology.* (4th ed.). New York: McGraw-Hill.

Voy, R.O. (1986). The U.S. Olympic Committee experience with exercise-induced bronchospasm—1984. *Medicine and Science in Sports and Exercise,* **18**, 328-330.

Vranic, M., & Wasserman, D. (1990). Exercise, fitness, and diabetes. In C. Bouchard, R.J. Shephard, T. Stephens, J.R. Sutton, & B.D. McPherson (Eds.), *Exercise, fitness, and health* (pp. 467-490). Champaign, IL: Human Kinetics.

Wadden, T.A., & Stunkard, A.J. (1993). Psychosocial consequences of obesity and dieting: Research and clinical findings. In A.J. Stunkard & T.A. Wadden (Eds.), *Obesity: Theory and therapy* (2nd ed.). New York: Raven Press.

Wathen, D., & Roll, F. (1994). Training methods and modes. In T.R. Baechle (Ed.), *Essentials of strength training and conditioning.* Champaign, IL: Human Kinetics.

Welle, S., Forbes, G.B., Statt, M., Barnard, R.R., & Amatruda J.M. (1992). Energy expenditure under free-living conditions in normal-weight and overweight women. *American Journal of Clinical Nutrition,* **55**, 14-21.

Weltman, A., Levine, S., Seip, R.L., & Tran, Z.V. (1988). Accurate assessment of body composition in obese females. *American Journal of Clinical Nutrition,* **48**, 1179-1183.

Weltman, A., Seip, R.L., & Tran Z.V. (1987). Practical assessment of body composition in obese males. *Human Biology,* **59**, 523-536.

Wenger, N.K., & Hellerstein, H.K. (1984). *Rehabilitation of the coronary patient* (2nd ed.). New York: John Wiley & Sons.

Wenger, N.K., & Hurst, J.W. (1984). Coronary bypass surgery as a rehabilitative procedure. In N.K. Wenger & H.K. Hellerstein (Eds.), *Rehabilitation of the coronary patient* (pp. 115-132). New York: John Wiley & Sons.

Westcott, W.L. (1991). Muscular strength and endurance. In M. Sudy (Ed.), *Personal training manual.* San Diego: American Council on Exercise.

Whatley J.E., & Poehlman E.T. (1994). Obesity and exercise. In G.L. Blackburn & B.S. Kanders (Eds.), *Obesity: Pathophysiology, psychology, and treatment* (pp. 123-139). New York: Chapman & Hall.

Whipp, B.J., & Casaburi, R. (1994). Physical activity, fitness, and chronic lung disease. In C. Bouchard, R.J. Shephard, & T. Stephens (Eds.), *Physical activity, fitness, and health* (pp. 749-761). Champaign, IL: Human Kinetics.

White, M. (1995). *Water exercise.* Champaign, IL: Human Kinetics.

Whitney, E.N., & Hamilton, E.M.N. (1987). *Understanding nutrition* (4th ed.). St. Paul: West.

Williams, M.H. (1988). *Nutrition for fitness and sport.* Dubuque, IA: Brown.

Williams, M.H. (1991). Alcohol, marijuana and beta blockers. In D.R. Lamb & M.H. Williams (Eds.), *Perspectives in exercise science and sports medicine. Vol. 4. Ergogenics: Enhancement of performance in exercise and sport.* (pp. 331-372). Dubuque, IA: Brown.

Williams, R., Binkley, J., Bloch, R., Goldsmith, C.H., & Minuk, T. (1993). Reliability of the modified-modified Schober and double inclinometer methods for measuring lumbar flexion and extension. *Physical Therapy,* **73**(1), 26–37.

Williamson, D.F., Madans, J., Anda, R.F., Kleinman, J.C., Kahn, H.S., & Byers, T. (1993). Recreational physical activity and ten-year weight change in a US national cohort. *International Journal of Obesity,* **17**, 279-286.

Williford, H.N., Scharff-Olson, M., & Blessing, D.L. (1989). The physiological effects of aerobic dance—A review. *Sports Medicine,* **8**, 335-345.

Willis, J.D., & Campbell, L.F. (1992). *Exercise psychology.* Champaign, IL: Human Kinetics.

Wilmore, J.H. (1969). A simplified method for determination of residual volume. *Journal of Applied Physiology*, **27**, 96-100.

Wilmore, J.H. (1974). Alterations in strength, body composition, and anthropometric measurements consequent to a 10-week weight training program. *Medicine and Science in Sports,* **6**, 133-138.

Wilmore, J.H., & Costill, D.L. (1994). *Physiology of sport and exercise.* Champaign, IL: Human Kinetics.

Wilmore, J.H., Parr, R.B., Girandola, R.N., Ward, P., Vodak, P.A., Barstow, T.J., Pipes, T.V., Romero, G.T., & Leslie, P. (1978). Physiological alterations consequent to circuit weight training. *Medicine and Science in Sports,* **10**, 79-84.

Wolfe, L.A., Brenner, I.K.M., & Mottola, M.F. (1994). Maternal exercise, fetal well-being and pregnancy outcome. In J.O. Holloszy (Ed.), *Exercise and Sport Sciences Reviews* (Vol. 22., pp. 145-194). Baltimore: Williams & Wilkins.

Wolfe, L.A., Hall, P., Webb, K.A., Goodman, L., Monga, M., & McGrath, M.J. (1989). Prescription of aerobic exercise during pregnancy. *Sports Medicine,* **8**, 273-301.

World Health Organization. (1986). Guidelines for the treatment of mild hypertension. *Hypertension*, **8**, 957-961.

Young, J.C. (1995). Exercise prescription for individuals with metabolic disorders. *Sports Medicine*, **19**, 44-53.

Zwiren, L.D. (1993). Exercise prescription for children. In J.L. Durstine, A.C. King, P.L. Painter, J.L. Roitman, L.D. Zwiren, & W.L. Kenney (Eds.), *ACSM's resource manual for guidelines for exercise testing and prescription* (2nd ed., pp. 409-417). Philadelphia: Lea & Febiger.

Credits

Figures

Figure 4.2 Reprinted, by permission, from A.J. Vander, J.H. Sherman, and D.S. Luciano, 1980, *Human physiology,* 3rd edition (New York: McGraw-Hill, Inc.), 212, and 216.

Figure 4.3 Reprinted, by permission, from A.J. Vander, J.H. Sherman, and D.S. Luciano, 1985, *Human physiology,* 4th edition (New York: McGraw-Hill, Inc.), 263.

Figure 4.4 Reprinted, by permission, from A.J. Vander, J.H. Sherman, and D.S. Luciano, 1985, *Human physiology,* 4th edition (New York: McGraw-Hill, Inc.), 268.

Figure 4.5 Reprinted, by permission, from D.G. Sale, 1987, Influence of exercise and training on motor unit activation. In *Exercise and sport sciences reviews*, vol. 15, edited by K.B. Pandolf (New York: McGraw-Hill, Inc.), 99.

Figure 4.19 Adapted, by permission, from J. Schwade, C.G. Blomqvist, and W. Shapiro, 1977, "A comparison of the response to arm and leg work in patients with ischemic heart disease," *American Heart Journal* 94: 206.

Figure 4.21 Adapted, by permission, from E.F. Coyle et al., 1984, "Time course of loss of adaptations after stopping prolonged intense endurance training," *Journal of Applied Physiology* 57: 1861.

Figure 4.23 Reprinted, by permission, from P.-O. Åstrand and K. Rodahl, 1986, *Textbook of work physiology*, 3rd edition (New York: McGraw-Hill), 200.

Figure 4.24 Adapted, by permission, from A.R. Lind and G.W. McNichol, 1967, "Muscular factors which determine the cardiovascular responses to sustained and rhythmic exercise," *Canadian Medical Association Journal* 96: 712.

Figure 6.1 Reprinted, by permission, from E.T. Howley, 1988, The exercise testing laboratory. In *Resource manual for guidelines for exercise testing and prescription*, American College of Sports Medicine, edited by S.N. Blair et al. (Philadelphia: Lea & Febiger), 409.

Figure 6.2 Adapted, by permission, from *Instruction manual, Monark model 818E* (Varberg, Sweden: Monark Exercise AB), 18.

Figure 6.3 Reproduced with permission. Human Blood Pressure Determination by Sphygmomanometers, 1994. Copyright American Heart Association.

Figure 11.2 Reprinted, by permission, from B. Balke, 1963, "A simple field test for the assessment of physical fitness," *Federal Aviation Agency Report* 63: 7.

Figure 11.4 Reprinted from *Y's Way to Physical Fitness*, 3rd edition, with permission of the YMCA of the USA, 101 N. Wacker Drive, Chicago, IL 60606.

Figure 11.5 Reprinted from *Y's Way to Physical Fitness*, 3rd edition, with permission of the YMCA of the USA, 101 N. Wacker Drive, Chicago, IL 60606.

Figure 12.1 Reprinted, by permission, from D.S. Luciano, A.J. Vander, and J.H. Sherman, 1978, *Human function and structure* (New York: McGraw-Hill, Inc.) 127.

Figure 12.2 Adapted, by permission, from D.G. Sale, 1988, "Neural adaptation to resistance training," *Medicine and Science in Sports and Exercise,* 20: S142.

Figure 12.3 Reproduced, by permission, from R.S. Staron et al., 1991, "Strength and skeletal muscle adaptations in heavy resistance-trained women after detraining and retraining," *Journal of Applied Physiology* 70: 631-640.

Figure A12.1 Reprinted, by permission, from W.D. McArdle, F.I. Katch, and V.I. Katch, 1991, *Exercise physiology*, 3rd edition (Philadelphia: Lea & Febiger), 453.

Figure 14.1 Reprinted, by permission, from Goodman and Gilman, 1975, *The pharmacological basis of therapeutics* (New York: Macmillan), 25.

Figure 14.2 Reprinted, by permission, from G.L. Jennings et al., 1991, "What is the dose-response relationship?" *Annals of Medicine* 23: 317.

Figure 14.3 From R. Pate et al., 1995, "Physical activity and public health," *Journal of the American Medical Association* 273(5): 404.

Figure 14.9 Reprinted, by permission, from B.A. Franklin, N.B. Oldridge, K.G. Stoedefalke, and W.F. Loechel, 1990, *On the ball* (Madison, WI: Brown & Benchmark), 15, 49.

Figure 14.10 Reprinted, by permission, from B.J. Sharkey, 1974, *Physiology of fitness and weight control* (Missoula, MT: Mountain Press Publishing Company).

Figure 15.1 From S.K. Powers and S.L. Dodd, *Total fitness, exercise, nutrition, and wellness*. Copyright © 1996 by Allyn and Bacon. Reprinted by permission.

Figure 15.2 Reprinted, by permission, from J.H. Wilmore and D.L. Costill, 1994, *Physiology of sport and exercise* (Champaign, IL: Human Kinetics), 81.

Figure 15.3 Reprinted, by permission, from J.H. Wilmore and D.L. Costill, 1994, *Physiology of sport and exercise* (Champaign, IL: Human Kinetics), 81.

Figure 15.4 Reprinted, by permission, from D. Wathen and F. Roll, 1994, Training methods and modes. In *Essentials of strength training and conditioning*, edited by T.R. Baechle (Champaign, IL: Human Kinetics), 408.

Figure 15.5 Adapted, by permission, from V.H. Heyward, 1991, *Advanced fitness assessment and exercise prescription* (Champaign, IL: Human Kinetics), 124.

Figure 15.6 Reprinted, by permission, from S.J. Fleck and W.J. Kraemer, 1987, *Designing resistance training programs* (Champaign, IL: Human Kinetics), 90.

Figure 22.1 Reprinted, by permission, from J.E. Donnelly, 1990, *Living anatomy*, 2nd edition (Champaign, IL: Human Kinetics), 199.

Figure 22.2 Reprinted, by permission, from J.E. Donnelly, 1990, *Living anatomy*, 2nd edition (Champaign, IL: Human Kinetics), 202.

Figure 22.6 Adapted, by permission, from M.J. Goldman, 1982, *Principles of clinical electrocardiography*, 11th edition (Los Altos, CA: Appleton & Lange).

Figure 22.23 Reprinted, by permission, from E. Stein, 1992, *Rapid analysis of electrocardiograms: A self-study program*, 2nd edition (Philadelphia: Lea & Febiger), 150.

Tables

Table 3.2 Reprinted, by permission, from American College of Sports Medicine, 1995, *ACSM's guidelines for exercise testing and prescription* (Baltimore: Williams & Wilkins), 25.

Table 6.2 Reprinted, by permission, from E.T. Howley, 1988, The exercise testing laboratory. In *Resource manual for guidelines for exercise testing and prescription*, American College of Sports Medicine, edited by S.N. Blair et al. (Philadelphia: Lea & Febiger), 410.

Table 7.8 Reprinted, by permission, from American College of Sports Medicine, 1980, *Guidelines for graded exercise testing and prescription*, 2nd edition (Philadelphia: Lea & Febiger), 20.

Table 8.1 Reprinted, by permission, from B.D. Franks and E.T. Howley, 1989, *Fitness facts: The healthy living handbook* (Champaign, IL: Human Kinetics), 39.

Table 8.2 Reprinted, by permission, from B.D. Franks and E.T. Howley, 1989, *Fitness facts: The healthy living handbook* (Champaign, IL: Human Kinetics), 40.

Table 9.3 Adapted, by permission, from M.L. Pollock, D.H. Schmidt, and A.S. Jackson, 1980, "Measurement of cardiorespiratory fitness and body composition in a clinical setting," *Comprehensive Therapy* 6(9): 12-27. © American Society of Contemporary Medicine and Surgery. 4711 Golf Road, Suite 408, Skokie, IL 60076.

Table 9.4 Adapted, by permission, from M.L. Pollock, D.H. Schmidt, and A.S. Jackson, 1980, "Measurement of cardiorespiratory fitness and body composition in a clinical setting," *Comprehensive Therapy* 6(9): 12-27. © American Society of Contemporary Medicine and Surgery. 4711 Golf Road, Suite 408, Skokie, IL 60076.

Table 11.2 Reprinted, by permission, from E.T. Howley and B.D. Franks, 1986, *Health/fitness instructor's handbook* (Champaign, IL: Human Kinetics).

Table 11.5 Reprinted, by permission, from G. Borg, 1985, *An introduction to Borg's RPE scale* (Ithaca, NY: Mouvement Publications), 7.

Table 11.6 Reprinted, by permission, from B.D. Franks, 1979, Methodology of the exercise ECG test. In *Exercise electrocardiography: Practical approach*, edited by E.K. Chung (Baltimore: Williams & Wilkins), 46-61.

Table 11.8 Reprinted, by permission, from P.-O. Åstrand, 1979, *Work tests with the bicycle ergometer* (Varberg, Sweden: Monark Exercise AB), 24.

Table A12.2 (p. 243) Adapted, by permission, from *The physical fitness specialist certification manual.* The Cooper Institute for Aerobics Research, Dallas, TX, revised 1997.

Table A12.3 (p. 244) Adapted, by permission, from *The physical fitness specialist certification manual.* The Cooper Institute for Aerobics Research, Dallas, TX, revised 1997.

Table A12.4 (p. 245) Adapted, by permission, from W. Liemohn and G. Sharpe, 1992, Muscular strength and endurance, flexibility and low back function. In *Health fitness instructor's handbook*, 2nd edition, edited by E.T. Howley and B.D. Franks (Champaign, IL: Human Kinetics), 193.

Table A12.5 (p. 246) Reprinted, by permission, from M.L. Pollock, J.H. Wilmore, and S.M. Fox, 1978, *Health and fitness through physical activity* (New York: John Wiley & Sons, Inc.) 109.

Table 14.3 Reprinted, by permission, from L.E. Hart and J.R. Sutton, 1987, "Environmental considerations for exercise," *Cardiology Clinics* 5: 246.

Table 15.2 Adapted, by permission, from V.H. Heyward, 1991, *Advanced fitness assessment and exercise prescription* (Champaign, IL: Human Kinetics), 122.

Table 15.3 Adapted, by permission, from V.H. Heyward, 1991, *Advanced fitness assessment and exercise prescription* (Champaign, IL: Human Kinetics), 123.

Table 15.4 Adapted, by permission, from V.H. Heyward, 1991, *Advanced fitness assessment and exercise prescription* (Champaign, IL: Human Kinetics), 125.

Table 15.6 Reprinted, by permission, from B.P. Conroy and R.W. Earle, 1994, Bone, muscle, and connective tissue adaptations to physical activity. In *Essentials of strength training and conditioning*, edited by T.R. Baechle (Champaign, IL: Human Kinetics), 55.

Table 18.1 Reprinted, by permission, from American College of Sports Medicine, 1995, *ACSM's guidelines for exercise testing and prescription* (Baltimore: Williams & Wilkins), 223.

Table 18.3 Reprinted, by permission, from N.L. Jones et al., 1987, Chronic obstructive respiratory disorders. In *Exercise testing and exercise prescription for special cases*, edited by J.S. Skinner (Philadelphia: Lea & Febiger).

Boxes

Box 10.4 (p. 196) Adapted, by permission, from M.D. Johnson, 1994, Disordered eating. In *Medical and orthopedic issues of active and athletic women*, edited by R. Agostini (Philadelphia: Hanley & Belfus, Inc.), 150.

Box 11.2 (p. 205) Reprinted, by permission, from American College of Sports Medicine, 1995, *ACSM's guidelines for exercise testing and prescription* (Baltimore: Williams & Wilkins), 42.

Box 11.5 (p. 219) Adapted, by permission, from E.T. Howley, 1988, The exercise testing laboratory. In *Resource manual for guidelines for exercise testing and prescription*, edited by S.N. Blair et al. (Philadelphia: Lea & Febiger), 406-413.

Box 11.6 (p. 220) Reprinted, by permission, from American College of Sports Medicine, 1995, *ACSM's guidelines for exercise testing and prescription* (Baltimore: Williams & Wilkins), 78.

Box 11.7 (p. 223) Reprinted, by permission, from B.D. Franks and E.T. Howley, 1989, *Fitness leader's handbook* (Champaign, IL: Human Kinetics), 87.

Box 11.8 (p. 227) Adapted, by permission, from E.T. Howley, 1988, The exercise testing laboratory. In *Resource manual for guidelines for exercise testing*, edited by S.N. Blair et al. (Philadelphia: Lea & Febiger), 413.

Box 17.1 (p. 334) Reprinted, by permission, from N. Oldridge, 1988, Qualities of an exercise leader. In *Resource manual for guidelines for exercise testing and prescription*, American College of Sports Medicine, edited by S.N. Blair et al. (Philadelphia: Lea & Febiger), 240.

Box 17.2 (p. 338) Reprinted, by permission, from B.A. Franklin et al., 1990, *On the ball* (Carmel, IN: Benchmark Press).

Sports Medicine, edited by S.N. Blair et al. (Philadelphia: Lea & Febiger), 246.

Box 17.7 (p. 348) Reprinted, by permission, from B.D. Franks and E.T. Howley, 1989, *Fitness leader's handbook* (Champaign, IL: Human Kinetics), 143.

Box 18.1 (p. 359) American College of Obstetricians and Gynecologists. Exercise During Pregnancy and the Postpartum Period. Technical Bulletin No. 189. Washington, D.C., ACOG, ©1994.

Forms

Form 6.1 Reprinted, by permission, from B.D. Franks and E.T. Howley, 1989, *Fitness leader's handbook* (Champaign, IL: Human Kinetics), 194-195.

Index

About the Authors

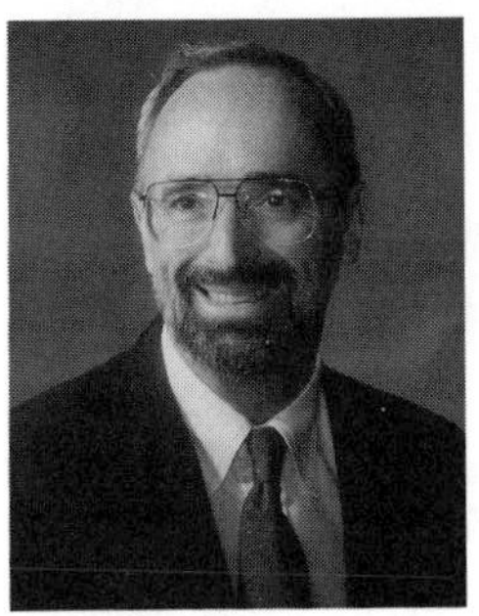

Edward T. Howley is a professor of exercise science at the University of Tennessee. He has received several honors, including the College of Education John Tunstall Outstanding Professor Award in 1995 and 1987, the University of Tennessee Alumni Association Outstanding Teacher Award in 1987, and the George F. Brady Teaching Award in 1979 and 1986. Dr. Howley holds a PhD in physical education from the University of Wisconsin at Madison and certification as a Program Director from the American College of Sports Medicine. He has also been active in the ACSM as a Fellow, as president of their southeast chapter, as a chair of their certification committee, as a faculty member in their Health/Fitness certification workshops, and as a member of the ACSM Preventive and Rehabilitative Committee, which developed the college's various certification programs.

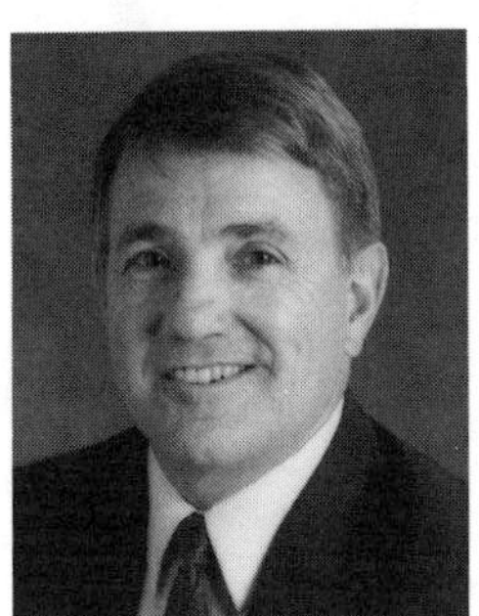

B. Don Franks received his PhD in exercise science from the University of Illinois at Urbana-Champaign in 1967. He served on the UIUC faculty until 1970 and later taught at Temple University and at the University of Tennessee at Knoxville. He was Senior Program Advisor for the President's Council on Physical Fitness and Sports in 1995. Currently he is a professor in and chair of the Department of Kinesiology at Louisiana State University. Dr. Franks is a Fellow of the ACSM, the American Academy of Kinesiology and Physical Education, and the Research Consortium of the American Alliance for Health, Physical Education, Recreation and Dance. He is also a former president of AAKPE and the Research Consortium of AAHPERD. He has received many honors, including the AAHPERD Physical Fitness Council Honor Award and the President's Council on Physical Fitness and Sports' Distinguished Service Award.

About the Contributing Authors

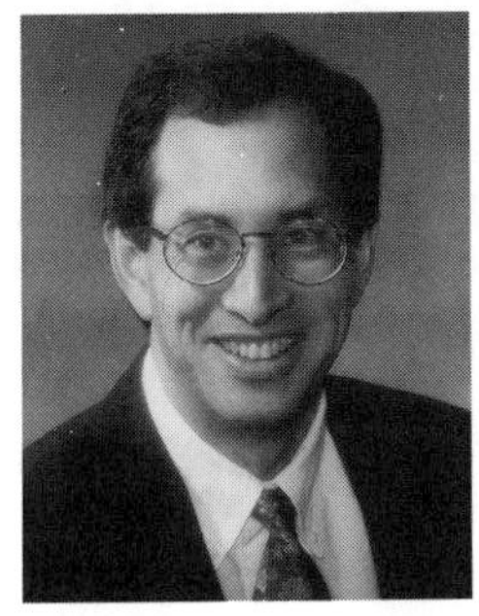

David R. Bassett, Jr., received his BS degree in biology from Oberlin College, his MS degree in biology from Ball State University, and his PhD in physical education from the University of Wisconsin at Madison. His research interests include the cardiovascular responses to assessment, and the role of exercise in the prevention of hypertension. He is currently an associate professor in the Exercise Science Unit at the University of Tennessee at Knoxville. He is a fellow of the ACSM and serves on the Executive Board of its Southeast Chapter. For recreation, he runs, swims, and rides a mountain bike.

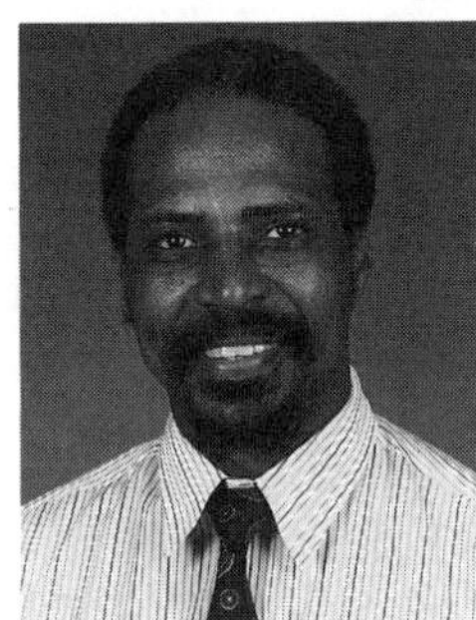

Vernon Bond, Jr., earned his BS degree in physical education from Saint Augustine's College, his MS in exercise physiology from North Carolina Central University, and his EdD in exercise physiology from the University of Tennessee. Dr. Bond is an associate professor in the Department of Kinesiology at the University of Maryland. His research interest is in the adaptive cardiovascular responses to exercise and how it influences blood pressure reactivity to physical and mental stress. He is a fellow in the ACSM.

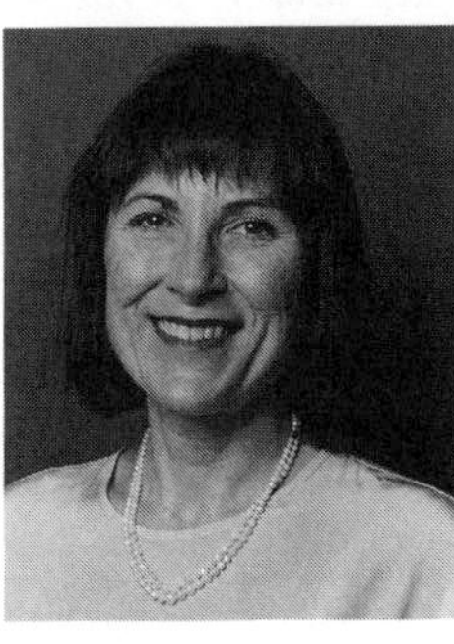

Janet Buckworth is an assistant professor in sport and exercise sciences at Ohio State University. She specialized in exercise behavior change and women's health issues. Prior to joining the Ohio State faculty in 1996, Dr. Buckworth was an assistant professor of education at Georgia College in Milledgeville, Georgia, where she also served as assistant director of the Center for Health and Lifestyle. Named a certified Health/Fitness Instructor by the ACSM in 1995, she maintains an active role in many organizations, including AAHPERD and the American Heart Association. In addition, she holds two Master's degrees, one in clinical social work, and a doctoral degree from the University of Georgia.

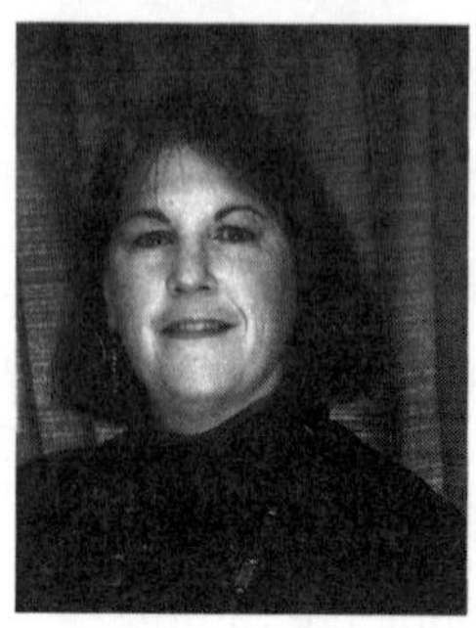

Sue Carver is presently the director of an outpatient physical therapy clinic in Little Rock, Arkansas, with Physical Therapy Clinics, Co. She graduated from Emory University with an MPT degree. She earned an MS degree in physical education with a specialization in athletic training from IU, and a BS degree in HPER from West Chester State College. She served as the Women's Athletic Trainer at the University of Tennessee from 1978 to 1982. Volunteer experiences include athletic trainer for track and field at the 1996 Summer Olympic Games in Atlanta, the 1988 U.S. Olympic Track and Field Trials (Indianapolis), the 1985 National Sports Festival (Baton Rouge) and the Olympic Training Center (Colorado Springs) in 1984.

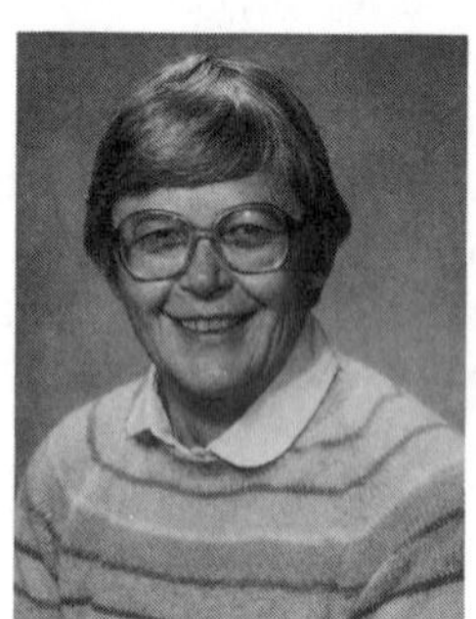

Jean Lewis received her doctorate in education (physical education with an emphasis in exercise physiology) from the University of Tennessee, Knoxville, where she is now a professor emeritus. She was involved in the establishment of undergraduate major concentrations in physical fitness and exercise physiology and has also developed courses in applied anatomy, applied kinesiology, and weight control, fitness, and exercise. Dr. Lewis was known for innovative teaching methods, which helped physical education majors understand how to apply kinesiological concepts. Recently retired, she misses the students and teaching but is enjoying working in her garden and workshop.

Wendell Liemohn received his BA from Wartburg College and his MA from the University of Iowa. After coaching and teaching on the collegiate level, he returned to the University of Iowa and completed

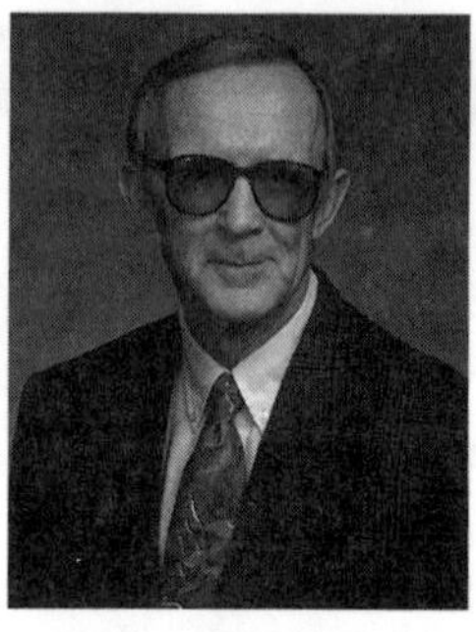

his PhD. He was on the faculty at Indiana University for 7 years and has been a professor at the University of Tennessee for the past 18 years. Most of his research at IU and his first few years at UT was related to studying psychomotor functioning in special populations. As his research interest shifted to the study of flexibility and low-back function, he started a graduate specialization in kinesiology/sports medicine at UT. While professionally active in AAHPERD, including being president of the Research Consortium, in recent years he has become active in ACSM.

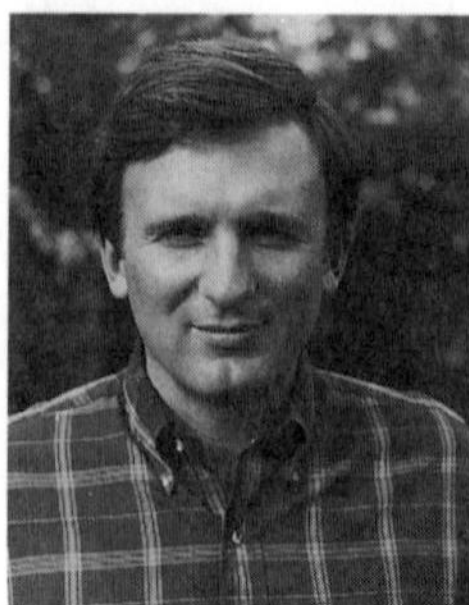

Daniel Martin earned his BS degree in physical therapy and his PhD in education from the University of Tennessee. Dr. Martin is currently an associate professor of physical therapy at the University of Florida. His research interests include exercise training and rehabilitation of lung transplant patients. His clinical activities include the rehabilitation of lung transplant patients before and after transplant and the weaning of ventilator dependent patients. He is a Fellow in the ACSM and a member of the American Physical Therapy Association. A former All-American javelin thrower at Tennessee, he now enjoys fishing in the Gulf of Mexico.

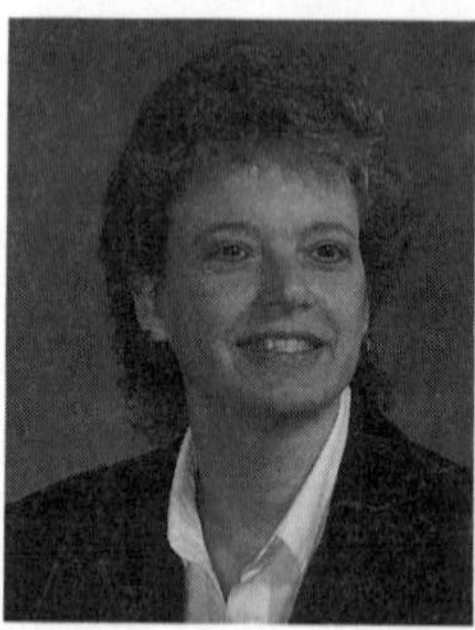

Dixie L. Thompson received BA and MA degrees from the University of North Carolina at Chapel Hill and a PhD with a specialization in exercise physiology from the University of Virginia. Dr. Thompson is currently an assistant professor in the Exercise Science Unit at the University of Tennessee, Knoxville. Her current research interests include body composition assessment, physiological performance in female athletes, substrate utilization during exercise, and the use of exercise to modify cardiovascular risk factors. When not working or walking for exercise, she can usually be found gardening, searching through antique shops, or taking in the beauty of the Smoky Mountains.